# WHO Classification of Tumours

# Breast Tumours

WHO Classification of Tumours Editorial Board

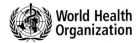

World Health Organization

**Suggested citation**

WHO Classification of Tumours Editorial Board. Breast tumours.
Lyon (France): International Agency for Research on Cancer; 2019.
(WHO classification of tumours series, 5th ed.; vol. 2).
https://publications.iarc.fr/581.

**Sales, rights, and permissions**

Print copies are distributed by WHO Press, World Health Organization, 20 Avenue Appia, 1211 Geneva 27, Switzerland
Tel.: +41 22 791 3264; Fax: +41 22 791 4857; email: bookorders@who.int; website: https://whobluebooks.iarc.fr

To purchase IARC publications in electronic format, see the IARC Publications website (https://publications.iarc.fr).

Requests for permission to reproduce or translate IARC publications – whether for sale or for non-commercial distribution – should be submitted
through the IARC Publications website (https://publications.iarc.fr/Rights-And-Permissions).

**Third-party materials**

If you wish to reuse material from this work that is attributed to a third party, such as figures, tables, or boxes, it is your responsibility to determine
whether permission is needed for that reuse and to obtain permission from the copyright holder. See *Sources*, pages 307–310. The risk of claims
resulting from infringement of any third-party-owned component in the work rests solely with the user.

**General disclaimers**

The designations employed and the presentation of the material in this publication do not imply the expression of any opinion whatsoever on the
part of WHO or contributing agencies concerning the legal status of any country, territory, city, or area, or of its authorities, or concerning the
delimitation of its frontiers or boundaries. Dotted and dashed lines on maps represent approximate border lines for which there may not yet be full
agreement.

The mention of specific companies or of certain manufacturers' products does not imply that they are endorsed or recommended by WHO or
contributing agencies in preference to others of a similar nature that are not mentioned. Errors and omissions excepted, the names of proprietary
products are distinguished by initial capital letters.

All reasonable precautions have been taken by WHO to verify the information contained in this publication. However, the published material is
being distributed without warranty of any kind, either expressed or implied. The responsibility for the interpretation and use of the material lies with
the reader. In no event shall WHO or contributing agencies be liable for damages arising from its use.

Third print run (5000 copies)

Updated corrigenda can be found at https://publications.iarc.fr

**IARC Library Cataloguing-in-Publication Data**

Names: WHO Classification of Tumours Editorial Board.
Title: Breast tumours / edited by WHO Classification of Tumours Editorial Board.
Description: Fifth edition. | Lyon: International Agency for Research on Cancer, 2019. | Series: World Health Organization classification of tumours.
| Includes bibliographical references and index.
Identifiers: ISBN 9789283245001 (pbk.) | ISBN 9789283245018 (ebook)
Subjects: MESH: Breast neoplasms.
Classification: NLM WP 15

The WHO classification of breast tumours presented in this book reflects
the views of the WHO Classification of Tumours Editorial Board that convened at
MD Anderson Cancer Center, Houston, USA, 9–11 December 2018.

For the complete list of all contributors and their affiliations, see pages 299–304.

# WHO Classification of Tumours
## Breast Tumours

| | |
|---|---|
| Edited by | The WHO Classification of Tumours Editorial Board |
| IARC Editors | Dilani Lokuhetty |
| | Valerie A. White |
| | Reiko Watanabe |
| | Ian A. Cree |
| Epidemiology | Ariana Znaor |
| Project Assistant | Asiedua Asante |
| Assistants | Anne-Sophie Hameau |
| | Laura Brispot |
| Technical Editor | Jessica Cox |
| Database | Alberto Machado |
| | Katherine Lloyd |
| Layout | Meaghan Fortune |
| Printed by | Naturaprint |
| | 74370 Argonay, France |
| Publisher | International Agency for Research on Cancer (IARC) |
| | 150 Cours Albert Thomas |
| | 69372 Lyon Cedex 08, France |

# Contents

List of abbreviations     ix

Foreword     x

TNM staging of carcinomas of the breast     1

**1   Introduction to tumours of the breast**     5

**2   Epithelial tumours of the breast**     9
    WHO classification of epithelial tumours of the breast     10
    Benign epithelial proliferations and precursors
       Introduction     11
       Usual ductal hyperplasia     13
       Columnar cell lesions, including flat epithelial atypia     15
       Atypical ductal hyperplasia     18
    Adenosis and benign sclerosing lesions
       Introduction     22
       Sclerosing adenosis     22
       Apocrine adenosis and adenoma     25
       Microglandular adenosis     28
       Radial scar / complex sclerosing lesion     30
    Adenomas
       Introduction     32
       Tubular adenoma     32
       Lactating adenoma     35
       Ductal adenoma     37
    Epithelial-myoepithelial tumours
       Introduction     39
       Pleomorphic adenoma     40
       Adenomyoepithelioma     43
       Malignant adenomyoepithelioma     46
    Papillary neoplasms
       Introduction     49
       Intraductal papilloma     52
       Papillary ductal carcinoma in situ     57
       Encapsulated papillary carcinoma     60
       Solid papillary carcinoma (in situ and invasive)     63
       Invasive papillary carcinoma     66
    Non-invasive lobular neoplasia
       Introduction     68
       Atypical lobular hyperplasia     68
       Lobular carcinoma in situ     71
    Ductal carcinoma in situ
       Introduction     75
       Ductal carcinoma in situ     76
    Invasive breast carcinoma
       General overview     82
       Invasive breast carcinoma of no special type     102
       Microinvasive carcinoma     110
       Invasive lobular carcinoma     114
       Tubular carcinoma     119
       Cribriform carcinoma     121
       Mucinous carcinoma     123
       Mucinous cystadenocarcinoma     126
       Invasive micropapillary carcinoma     128
       Carcinoma with apocrine differentiation     131
       Metaplastic carcinoma     134

    Rare and salivary gland–type tumours
       Introduction     139
       Acinic cell carcinoma     139
       Adenoid cystic carcinoma     142
       Secretory carcinoma     146
       Mucoepidermoid carcinoma     149
       Polymorphous adenocarcinoma     151
       Tall cell carcinoma with reversed polarity     153
    Neuroendocrine neoplasms
       Introduction     155
       Neuroendocrine tumour     156
       Neuroendocrine carcinoma     159

**3   Fibroepithelial tumours and hamartomas of the breast**     163
    WHO classification of fibroepithelial tumours and
       hamartomas of the breast     164
    Introduction     165
    Hamartoma     166
    Fibroadenoma     168
    Phyllodes tumour     172

**4   Tumours of the nipple**     177
    WHO classification of tumours of the nipple     178
    Introduction     179
    Epithelial tumours
       Syringomatous tumour     180
       Nipple adenoma     182
       Paget disease of the breast     184

**5   Mesenchymal tumours of the breast**     187
    WHO classification of mesenchymal tumours of the breast     188
    Introduction     189
    Vascular tumours
       Haemangioma     191
       Angiomatosis     193
       Atypical vascular lesions     195
       Postradiation angiosarcoma of the breast     197
       Primary angiosarcoma of the breast     200
    Fibroblastic and myofibroblastic tumours
       Nodular fasciitis     202
       Myofibroblastoma     204
       Desmoid fibromatosis     206
       Inflammatory myofibroblastic tumour     209
    Peripheral nerve sheath tumours
       Schwannoma     211
       Neurofibroma     213
       Granular cell tumour     215
    Smooth muscle tumours
       Leiomyoma     217
       Leiomyosarcoma     219
    Adipocytic tumours
       Lipoma     221
       Angiolipoma     223
       Liposarcoma     225
    Other mesenchymal tumours and tumour-like conditions
       Pseudoangiomatous stromal hyperplasia     228

6   Haematolymphoid tumours of the breast                    231
    WHO classification of haematolymphoid tumours
        of the breast                                        232
    Introduction                                             233
    Lymphoma
        Extranodal marginal zone lymphoma of mucosa-
            associated lymphoid tissue (MALT lymphoma)       235
        Follicular lymphoma                                  238
        Diffuse large B-cell lymphoma                        240
        Burkitt lymphoma                                     242
        Breast implant–associated anaplastic large cell
            lymphoma                                         245

7   Tumours of the male breast                               249
    WHO classification of tumours of the male breast         250
    Introduction                                             251
    Epithelial tumours
        Gynaecomastia                                        252
        Carcinoma in situ                                    255
        Invasive carcinoma                                   257

8   Metastases to the breast                                 261

9   Genetic tumour syndromes of the breast                   267
    Introduction                                             268
    BRCA1/2-associated hereditary breast and ovarian cancer
        syndrome                                             270
    Cowden syndrome                                          275
    Ataxia–telangiectasia                                    277
    Li–Fraumeni syndrome, TP53-associated                    279
    Li–Fraumeni syndrome, CHEK2-associated                   282
    CDH1-associated breast cancer                            284
    PALB2-associated cancers                                 286
    Peutz–Jeghers syndrome                                   288
    Neurofibromatosis type 1                                 290
    The polygenic component of breast cancer susceptibility  292

Contributors                                                 299

Declaration of interests                                     305

IARC/WHO Committee for ICD-O                                 306

Sources                                                      307

References                                                   311

Subject index                                                349

Previous volumes in the series                               356

# List of abbreviations

| | | | | |
|---|---|---|---|---|
| 3D | three-dimensional | | kDa | kilodalton |
| ABC | activated B cell | | M:F ratio | male-to-female ratio |
| ADP | adenosine diphosphate | | MALT | mucosa-associated lymphoid tissue |
| AJCC | American Joint Committee on Cancer | | MRI | magnetic resonance imaging |
| AR | androgen receptor | | mRNA | messenger ribonucleic acid |
| ASCO | American Society of Clinical Oncology | | N:C ratio | nuclear-to-cytoplasmic ratio |
| cAMP | cyclic adenosine monophosphate | | NAC | nipple–areola complex |
| CAP | College of American Pathologists | | NCCN | National Comprehensive Cancer Network |
| CI | confidence interval | | NOS | not otherwise specified |
| CNB | core needle biopsy | | NSE | neuron-specific enolase |
| CNS | central nervous system | | NST | of no special type |
| CT | computed tomography | | PAS | periodic acid–Schiff |
| EBV | Epstein–Barr virus | | PASD | periodic acid Schiff with diastase |
| EGTM | European Group on Tumor Markers | | PCR | polymerase chain reaction |
| ER | estrogen receptor | | PET | positron emission tomography |
| ESMO | European Society for Medical Oncology | | PR | progesterone receptor |
| FISH | fluorescence in situ hybridization | | PRS | polygenic risk score |
| FNA | fine-needle aspiration | | RNA | ribonucleic acid |
| GCB | germinal-centre B cell | | RS | recurrence score |
| H&E | haematoxylin and eosin | | RT-PCR | reverse transcriptase polymerase chain reaction |
| HIV | human immunodeficiency virus | | SEER Program | Surveillance, Epidemiology, and End Results Program |
| IARC | International Agency for Research on Cancer | | SNP | single nucleotide polymorphism |
| ICD-11 | International Classification of Diseases, 11th Revision | | TDLU | terminal duct lobular unit |
| ICD-O | International Classification of Diseases for Oncology | | Th1 cell | T helper 1 cell |
| Ig | immunoglobulin | | Th17 cell | T helper 17 cell |
| IQ | intelligence quotient | | TIL | tumour-infiltrating lymphocyte |
| kb | kilo base pair | | TNM | tumour, node, metastasis |

# Foreword

The WHO Classification of Tumours, published as a series of books (also known as the WHO Blue Books) and now as a website (https://tumourclassification.iarc.who.int), is an essential tool for standardizing diagnostic practice worldwide. The WHO classification also serves as a vehicle for the translation of cancer research into practice. The diagnostic criteria and standards that make up the classification are underpinned by evidence evaluated and debated by experts in the field. About 200 authors and editors participate in the production of each book, and they give their time freely to this task. I am very grateful for their help; it is a remarkable team effort.

This second volume of the fifth edition of the WHO Blue Books has, like the first, been led by the WHO Classification of Tumours Editorial Board, which is composed of standing members nominated by pathology organizations and expert members selected on the basis of informed bibliometric analysis. The diagnostic process is increasingly multidisciplinary, and we are delighted that several radiology and clinical experts have joined us to address specific needs.

The most conspicuous change to the format of the books in the fifth edition is that tumour types common to multiple systems are dealt with together – so there are separate chapters on haematolymphoid tumours and mesenchymal tumours. There is also a chapter on genetic tumour syndromes. Genetic disorders are of increasing importance to diagnosis in individual patients, and the study of these disorders has undoubtedly informed our understanding of tumour biology and behaviour over the past decade. The inclusion of a chapter dedicated to genetic tumour syndromes reflects this importance.

We have attempted to take a more systematic approach to the multifaceted nature of tumour classification; each tumour type is described on the basis of its localization, clinical features, epidemiology, etiology, pathogenesis, histopathology, diagnostic molecular pathology, staging, and prognosis and prediction. We have also included information on macroscopic appearance and cytology, as well as essential and desirable diagnostic criteria. This standardized, modular approach makes it easier for the books to be accessible online, but it also enables us to call attention to areas in which there is little information, and where serious gaps in our knowledge remain to be addressed.

The organization of the WHO Blue Books content now follows the normal progression from benign to malignant – a break with the fourth edition, but one we hope will be welcome.

The volumes are still organized by anatomical site (digestive system, breast, soft tissue and bone, etc.), and each tumour type is listed within a taxonomic classification that follows the format below, which helps to structure the books in a systematic manner:

- Site; e.g. breast
- Category; e.g. epithelial tumours
- Family (class); e.g. papillary neoplasms
- Type; e.g. solid papillary carcinoma
- Subtype; e.g. solid papillary carcinoma in situ

The issue of whether a given tumour type represents a distinct entity rather than a subtype continues to exercise pathologists, and it is the topic of many publications in the scientific literature. We continue to deal with this issue on a case-by-case basis, but we believe there are inherent rules that can be applied. For example, tumours in which multiple histological patterns contain shared truncal mutations are clearly of the same type, despite the differences in their appearance. Equally, genetic heterogeneity within the same tumour type may have implications for treatment. A small shift in terminology in the fifth edition is that the term "variant" in reference to a specific kind of tumour has been wholly superseded by "subtype", in an effort to more clearly differentiate this meaning from that of "variant" in reference to a genetic alteration.

The WHO Blue Books are much appreciated by pathologists and of increasing importance to practitioners of other clinical disciplines involved in cancer management, as well as to researchers. The new editorial board and I certainly hope that the series will continue to meet the need for standards in diagnosis and to facilitate the translation of diagnostic research into practice worldwide. It is particularly important that cancers continue to be classified and diagnosed according to the same standards internationally so that patients can benefit from multicentre clinical trials, as well as from the results of local trials conducted on different continents.

Dr Ian A. Cree

Head, WHO Classification of Tumours Group
International Agency for Research on Cancer
August 2019

# TNM staging of carcinomas of the breast

## Breast Tumours
(ICD-O-3 C50)

### Introductory Notes
The site is described under the following headings:
- Rules for classification with the procedures for assessing T, N, and M categories; additional methods may be used when they enhance the accuracy of appraisal before treatment
- Anatomical subsites
- Definition of the regional lymph nodes
- TNM clinical classification
- pTNM pathological classification
- G histopathological grading
- Stage

### Rules for Classification
The classification applies only to carcinomas and concerns the male as well as the female breast. There should be histological confirmation of the disease. The anatomical subsite of origin should be recorded but is not considered in classification.

In the case of multiple simultaneous primary tumours in one breast, the tumour with the highest T category should be used for classification. Simultaneous *bilateral* breast cancers should be classified independently to permit division of cases by histological type.

The following are the procedures for assessing T, N, and M categories:

| | |
|---|---|
| T categories | Physical examination and imaging, e.g., mammography |
| N categories | Physical examination and imaging |
| M categories | Physical examination and imaging |

### Anatomical Subsites
1. Nipple (C50.0)
2. Central portion (C50.1)
3. Upper-inner quadrant (C50.2)
4. Lower-inner quadrant (C50.3)
5. Upper-outer quadrant (C50.4)
6. Lower-outer quadrant (C50.5)
7. Axillary tail (C50.6)

### Regional Lymph Nodes
The regional lymph nodes are:
1. *Axillary* (ipsilateral): interpectoral (Rotter) nodes and lymph nodes along the axillary vein and its tributaries, which may be divided into the following levels:
   a) *Level I* (low-axilla): lymph nodes lateral to the lateral border of pectoralis minor muscle
   b) *Level II* (mid-axilla): lymph nodes between the medial and lateral borders of the pectoralis minor muscle and the interpectoral (Rotter) lymph nodes
   c) *Level III* (apical axilla): apical lymph nodes and those medial to the medial margin of the pectoralis minor muscle, excluding those designated as subclavicular or infraclavicular

2. *Infraclavicular (subclavicular)* (ipsilateral)
3. *Internal mammary* (ipsilateral): lymph nodes in the intercostal spaces along the edge of the sternum in the endothoracic fascia
4. *Supraclavicular* (ipsilateral)

Note
Intramammary lymph nodes are coded as axillary lymph nodes level I. Any other lymph node metastasis is coded as a distant metastasis (M1), including cervical or contralateral internal mammary lymph nodes.

### TNM Clinical Classification
**T – Primary Tumour**

| | |
|---|---|
| TX | Primary tumour cannot be assessed |
| T0 | No evidence of primary tumour |
| Tis | Carcinoma in situ |
| Tis (DCIS) | Ductal carcinoma in situ |
| Tis (LCIS) | Lobular carcinoma in situ[a] |
| Tis (Paget) | Paget disease of the nipple not associated with invasive carcinoma and/or carcinoma in situ (DCIS and/or LCIS) in the underlying breast parenchyma. Carcinomas in the breast parenchyma associated with Paget disease are categorized based on the size and characteristics of the parenchymal disease, although the presence of Paget disease should still be noted. |
| T1 | Tumour 2 cm or less in greatest dimension |
| | T1mi Microinvasion 0.1 cm or less in greatest dimension[b] |
| | T1a More than 0.1 cm but not more than 0.5 cm in greatest dimension |
| | T1b More than 0.5 cm but not more than 1 cm in greatest dimension |
| | T1c More than 1 cm but not more than 2 cm in greatest dimension |
| T2 | Tumour more than 2 cm but not more than 5 cm in greatest dimension |
| T3 | Tumour more than 5 cm in greatest dimension |
| T4 | Tumour of any size with direct extension to chest wall and/or to skin (ulceration or skin nodules)[c] |
| | T4a Extension to chest wall (does not include pectoralis muscle invasion only) |
| | T4b Ulceration, ipsilateral satellite skin nodules, or skin oedema (including peau d'orange) |
| | T4c Both 4a and 4b |
| | T4d Inflammatory carcinoma[d] |

Notes
[a] The AJCC exclude Tis (LCIS).
[b] Microinvasion is the extension of cancer cells beyond the basement membrane into the adjacent tissues with no focus more than 0.1 cm in greatest dimension. When there are multiple foci of microinvasion, the size of only the largest focus is used to classify the microinvasion. (Do not use the sum of all individual foci.) The

presence of multiple foci of microinvasion should be noted, as it is with multiple larger invasive carcinomas.

c Invasion of the dermis alone does not qualify as T4. Chest wall includes ribs, intercostal muscles, and serratus anterior muscle but not pectoral muscle.

d Inflammatory carcinoma of the breast is characterized by diffuse, brawny induration of the skin with an erysipeloid edge, usually with no underlying mass. If the skin biopsy is negative and there is no localized measurable primary cancer, the T category is pTX when pathologically staging a clinical inflammatory carcinoma (T4d). Dimpling of the skin, nipple retraction, or other skin changes, except those in T4b and T4d, may occur in T1, T2, or T3 without affecting the classification.

## N – Regional Lymph Nodes

NX   Regional lymph nodes cannot be assessed (e.g., previously removed)

N0   No regional lymph node metastasis

N1   Metastasis in movable ipsilateral level I, II axillary lymph node(s)

N2   Metastasis in ipsilateral level I, II axillary lymph node(s) that are clinically fixed or matted; or in clinically detected* ipsilateral internal mammary lymph node(s) in the *absence* of clinically evident axillary lymph node metastasis

    N2a   Metastasis in axillary lymph node(s) fixed to one another (matted) or to other structures

    N2b   Metastasis only in clinically detected* internal mammary lymph node(s) and in the *absence* of clinically detected axillary lymph node metastasis

N3   Metastasis in ipsilateral infraclavicular (level III axillary) lymph node(s) with or without level I, II axillary lymph node involvement; or in clinically detected* ipsilateral internal mammary lymph node(s) with clinically evident level I, II axillary lymph node metastasis; or metastasis in ipsilateral supraclavicular lymph node(s) with or without axillary or internal mammary lymph node involvement

    N3a   Metastasis in infraclavicular lymph node(s)

    N3b   Metastasis in internal mammary and axillary lymph nodes

    N3c   Metastasis in supraclavicular lymph node(s)

Notes

* Clinically detected is defined as detected by clinical examination or by imaging studies (excluding lymphoscintigraphy) and having characteristics highly suspicious for malignancy or a presumed pathological macrometastasis based on fine needle aspiration biopsy with cytological examination. Confirmation of clinically detected metastatic disease by fine needle aspiration without excision biopsy is designated with a (f) suffix, e.g. cN3a(f).

Excisional biopsy of a lymph node or biopsy of a sentinel node, in the absence of assignment of a pT, is classified as a clinical N, e.g., cN1. Pathological classification (pN) is used for excision or sentinel lymph node biopsy only in conjunction with a pathological T assignment.

## M – Distant Metastasis

M0   No distant metastasis

M1   Distant metastasis

## pTNM Pathological Classification

### pT – Primary Tumour

The pathological classification requires the examination of the primary carcinoma with no gross tumour at the margins of resection. A case can be classified pT if there is only microscopic tumour in a margin.

The pT categories correspond to the T categories.

Note

When classifying pT the tumour size is a measurement of the invasive component. If there is a large in situ component (e.g., 4 cm) and a small invasive component (e.g., 0.5 cm), the tumour is coded pT1a.

### pN – Regional Lymph Nodes

The pathological classification requires the resection and examination of at least the low axillary lymph nodes (level I) (see above). Such a resection will ordinarily include 6 or more lymph nodes. If the lymph nodes are negative, but the number ordinarily examined is not met, classify as pN0.

pNX   Regional lymph nodes cannot be assessed (e.g., previously removed, or not removed for pathological study)

pN0   No regional lymph node metastasis*

Note

* Isolated tumour cell clusters (ITC) are single tumour cells or small clusters of cells not more than 0.2 mm in greatest extent that can be detected by routine H and E stains or immunohistochemistry. An additional criterion has been proposed to include a cluster of fewer than 200 cells in a single histological cross section. Nodes containing only ITCs are excluded from the total positive node count for purposes of N classification and should be included in the total number of nodes evaluated. (See {229}, page 7.)

pN1   Micrometastases; or metastases in 1 to 3 axillary ipsilateral lymph nodes; and/or in internal mammary nodes with metastases detected by sentinel lymph node biopsy but not clinically detected*

    pN1mi   Micrometastases (larger than 0.2 mm and/or more than 200 cells, but none larger than 2.0 mm)

    pN1a   Metastasis in 1–3 axillary lymph node(s), including at least one larger than 2 mm in greatest dimension

    pN1b   Internal mammary lymph nodes not clinically detected

    pN1c   Metastasis in 1–3 axillary lymph nodes and internal mammary lymph nodes not clinically detected

pN2   Metastasis in 4–9 ipsilateral axillary lymph nodes, or in clinically detected* ipsilateral internal mammary lymph node(s) in the absence of axillary lymph node metastasis

    pN2a   Metastasis in 4–9 axillary lymph nodes, including at least one that is larger than 2 mm

    pN2b   Metastasis in clinically detected internal mammary lymph node(s), in the *absence* of axillary lymph node metastasis

pN3

    pN3a   Metastasis in 10 or more ipsilateral axillary lymph nodes (at least one larger than 2 mm) *or* metastasis in infraclavicular lymph nodes/ level III lymph nodes

pN3b    Metastasis in clinically detected* internal ipsilateral mammary lymph node(s) in the *presence* of positive axillary lymph node(s); or metastasis in more than 3 axillary lymph nodes *and* in internal mammary lymph nodes with microscopic or macroscopic metastasis detected by sentinel lymph node biopsy but not clinically detected

pN3c    Metastasis in ipsilateral supraclavicular lymph node(s)

## Post-treatment ypN:

- Post-treatment yp 'N' should be evaluated as for clinical (pretreatment) 'N' methods (see Section N – Regional Lymph Nodes). The modifier 'sn' is used only if a sentinel node evaluation was performed after treatment. If no subscript is attached, it is assumed the axillary nodal evaluation was by axillary node dissection.
- The X classification will be used (ypNX) if no yp post-treatment SN or axillary dissection was performed
- N categories are the same as those used for pN.

Notes

\* *Clinically detected* is defined as detected by imaging studies (excluding lymphoscintigraphy) or by clinical examination and having characteristics highly suspicious for malignancy or a presumed pathological macrometastasis based on fine needle aspiration biopsy with cytological examination.

*Not clinically detected* is defined as not detected by imaging studies (excluding lymphoscintigraphy) or not detected by clinical examination.

## pM – Distant Metastasis*

pM1    Distant metastasis microscopically confirmed

Note

\* pM0 and pMX are not valid categories.

## G Histopathological Grading

For histopathological grading of invasive carcinoma the Nottingham Histological Score is recommended.[1]

### Stage[a]

| Stage | T | N | M |
|---|---|---|---|
| Stage 0 | Tis | N0 | M0 |
| Stage IA | T1[b] | N0 | M0 |
| Stage IB | T0,T1 | N1mi | M0 |
| Stage IIA | T0,T1 | N1 | M0 |
| | T2 | N0 | M0 |
| Stage IIB | T2 | N0 | M0 |
| | T3 | N0 | M0 |
| Stage IIIA | T0,T1,T2 | N2 | M0 |
| | T3 | N1,N2 | M0 |
| Stage IIIB | T4 | N0,N1,N2 | M0 |
| Stage IIIC | Any T | N3 | M0 |
| Stage IV | Any T | Any N | M1 |

Notes

[a] The AJCC also publish a prognostic group for breast tumours.

[b] T1 includes T1mi.

Reference

1    Elston CW, Ellis IO. Pathological prognostic factors in breast cancer. I. The value of histological grade in breast cancer: experience from a large study with long-term follow-up. Histopathology 1991; 19: 403-410.

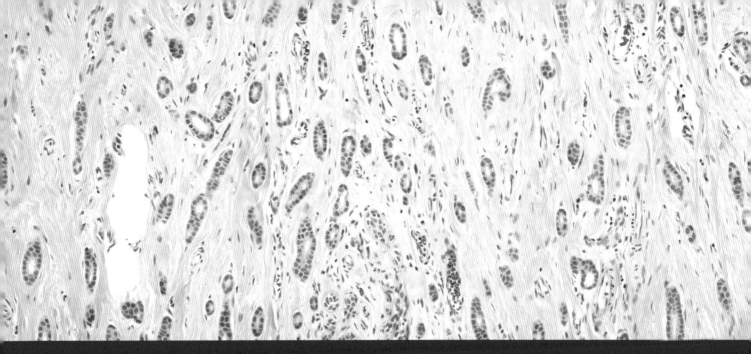

# 1

# Introduction to tumours of the breast

Edited by: Cree IA, Lokuhetty D

# Introduction to tumours of the breast

Tan PH
Ellis IO

The classification of breast tumours continues to evolve, with the integration of new knowledge from research being translated into practice. In this volume of the WHO Classification of Tumours series' fifth edition, which is an update of the fourth-edition breast tumours volume published in 2012 {1098}, the descriptions of breast tumours follow the familiar systematic approach of previous volumes, with the content now organized in sequence from benign epithelial proliferations and precursors, through benign neoplasms, to in situ and invasive breast carcinoma, followed by fibroepithelial and nipple tumours, mesenchymal and haematolymphoid neoplasms, tumours of the male breast, and genetic tumour syndromes. The ICD-O topographical coding for the anatomical sites covered in this volume is presented in Box 1.01.

A brief introduction prefaces the content pertaining to each major tumour group, to provide a general perspective and highlight key modifications. In the previous edition, the introductory first chapter focused on epidemiology, imaging, clinical features, grading, staging, molecular testing for hormone receptors and ERBB2 (HER2), posttherapy effects, core needle biopsy and FNA considerations, molecular pathology, and genomics. In the current volume, this information is now presented in the general overview that introduces the sections on invasive breast carcinoma. Core biopsy diagnosis, an important preoperative tool, is addressed in many sections. The importance of molecular pathology in aiding diagnosis is recognized, with a specific subsection for each tumour type. Essential and desirable diagnostic criteria are also included, to provide key histological clues.

Within the invasive carcinoma overview, the emerging roles of stromal response and the tumour microenvironment are discussed, with specific attention to tumour-infiltrating lymphocytes and their impact on prognosis and response to chemotherapy. Ki-67 proliferation index is not a parameter that is routinely evaluated in invasive breast carcinoma, but its role in determining molecular subtypes is acknowledged.

An important change in this edition is the conversion of mitotic count from the traditional denominator of 10 high-power fields to a defined area expressed in mm². This serves to standardize the true area over which mitoses are enumerated, because

**Box 1.01** ICD-O topographical coding for the anatomical sites covered in this volume

**C50 Breast (excluding C44.5 Skin of breast)**
C50.0 Nipple
C50.1 Central portion of breast
C50.2 Upper-inner quadrant of breast
C50.3 Lower-inner quadrant of breast
C50.4 Upper-outer quadrant of breast
C50.5 Lower-outer quadrant of breast
C50.6 Axillary tail of breast
C50.8 Overlapping lesion of breast
C50.9 Breast NOS

**Table 1.01** Score thresholds for mitotic counts based on the diameter of the high-power field and its corresponding area

| Field diameter (mm) | Field area (mm²) | Mitotic count (score) | | |
|---|---|---|---|---|
| | | 1 | 2 | 3 |
| 0.40 | 0.126 | ≤ 4 | 5–9 | ≥ 10 |
| 0.41 | 0.132 | ≤ 4 | 5–9 | ≥ 10 |
| 0.42 | 0.138 | ≤ 5 | 6–10 | ≥ 11 |
| 0.43 | 0.145 | ≤ 5 | 6–10 | ≥ 11 |
| 0.44 | 0.152 | ≤ 5 | 6–11 | ≥ 12 |
| 0.45 | 0.159 | ≤ 5 | 6–11 | ≥ 12 |
| 0.46 | 0.166 | ≤ 6 | 7–12 | ≥ 13 |
| 0.47 | 0.173 | ≤ 6 | 7–12 | ≥ 13 |
| 0.48 | 0.181 | ≤ 6 | 7–13 | ≥ 14 |
| 0.49 | 0.188 | ≤ 6 | 7–13 | ≥ 14 |
| 0.50 | 0.196 | ≤ 7 | 8–14 | ≥ 15 |
| 0.51 | 0.204 | ≤ 7 | 8–14 | ≥ 15 |
| 0.52 | 0.212 | ≤ 7 | 8–15 | ≥ 16 |
| 0.53 | 0.221 | ≤ 8 | 9–16 | ≥ 17 |
| 0.54 | 0.229 | ≤ 8 | 9–16 | ≥ 17 |
| 0.55 | 0.237 | ≤ 8 | 9–17 | ≥ 18 |
| 0.56 | 0.246 | ≤ 8 | 9–17 | ≥ 18 |
| 0.57 | 0.255 | ≤ 9 | 10–18 | ≥ 19 |
| 0.58 | 0.264 | ≤ 9 | 10–19 | ≥ 20 |
| 0.59 | 0.273 | ≤ 9 | 10–19 | ≥ 20 |
| 0.60 | 0.283 | ≤ 10 | 11–20 | ≥ 21 |
| 0.61 | 0.292 | ≤ 10 | 11–21 | ≥ 22 |
| 0.62 | 0.302 | ≤ 11 | 12–22 | ≥ 23 |
| 0.63 | 0.312 | ≤ 11 | 12–22 | ≥ 23 |
| 0.64 | 0.322 | ≤ 11 | 12–23 | ≥ 24 |
| 0.65 | 0.332 | ≤ 12 | 13–24 | ≥ 25 |
| 0.66 | 0.342 | ≤ 12 | 13–24 | ≥ 25 |
| 0.67 | 0.352 | ≤ 12 | 13–25 | ≥ 26 |
| 0.68 | 0.363 | ≤ 13 | 14–26 | ≥ 27 |
| 0.69 | 0.374 | ≤ 13 | 14–27 | ≥ 28 |

different microscopes have high-power fields of different sizes. This change will also be helpful for anyone reporting using digital systems. The score thresholds for mitotic counts based on the diameter of the high-power field and its corresponding area are presented in Table 1.01.

In the fourth edition, it was agreed that diagnosing classic medullary breast carcinoma was a challenge. It was decided then that these tumours with prominent lymphoplasmacytic infiltrates – medullary carcinoma, atypical medullary carcinoma, and invasive carcinoma of no special type (NST) with medullary features – would be grouped together under the category of carcinomas with medullary features, in recognition of their common characteristics of an immune-enriched microenvironment, basal-like expression, and occasional association with *BRCA1* mutations. In the current volume, a further step is taken: these tumours have been subsumed into a combined morphological subset under the category of invasive carcinoma NST with basal-like and medullary pattern, regarding them as part of a spectrum of tumour-infiltrating lymphocyte–rich breast cancers.

Although neuroendocrine neoplasms (NENs) are allocated their own sections, harmonized with those of other organ systems on the basis of a recent WHO workshop report {1764}, it must be emphasized that true primary neuroendocrine tumours (NETs) of the breast remain uncommon. Many breast tumours that display neuroendocrine differentiation belong to recognized entities such as hypercellular invasive mucinous carcinoma and solid papillary carcinoma of both in situ and invasive forms. Small cell neuroendocrine carcinoma (SCNEC) does arise in the breast, often admixed with invasive carcinoma NST. For well-differentiated NETs resembling carcinoid tumour, it is prudent to exclude metastasis from another site. It is recommended that the classification of breast tumours displaying neuroendocrine expression be based on the recognizable morphological tumour type, be it invasive carcinoma NST, invasive mucinous carcinoma, or solid papillary carcinoma {2040}.

One important change in the classification of fibroepithelial tumours is the removal of well-differentiated liposarcoma as a histological criterion of malignancy in breast phyllodes tumours in the absence of additional supporting microscopic alterations.

Evidence has emerged that these abnormal adipocyte populations residing within phyllodes tumours do not harbour the *MDM2* aberrations that characterize well-differentiated liposarcomas elsewhere. In light of the consensus opinion that this heterologous element does not have metastatic potential, it was agreed that its presence alone should not warrant a malignant grade in phyllodes tumours unless there are other histological changes of malignancy.

A new entity included in this volume is mucinous cystadenocarcinoma, and it is now recognized that some invasive lobular carcinomas may be associated with extracellular mucin production. The entity "tall cell carcinoma with reversed polarity" is introduced in the section about rare and salivary gland–type tumours, as there have been multiple reports of this entity, previously termed "breast tumour resembling the tall cell variant of papillary thyroid carcinoma" as well as "solid papillary carcinoma with reverse polarity", with these descriptions united by the consistent finding of *IDH2* and *PIK3CA* mutations {1243}.

In addition to new tumours now being recognized, rare tumours that were previously addressed in their own sections are now grouped together under the category of invasive carcinoma NST. These are the oncocytic, lipid-rich, glycogen-rich clear cell, and sebaceous carcinomas.

Mesenchymal tumours, haematolymphoid tumours, and genetic tumour syndromes are covered in dedicated chapters in alignment with the approach being taken throughout this fifth edition of the series.

Tumour classification is a dynamic process, integrating multiple sources of information that have emerged since the previous WHO update. Digital pathology, which is becoming widely available, can enable the application of artificial intelligence and computer learning to refine breast and other tumour classifications that ultimately facilitate appropriate therapy and accurate prognostication.

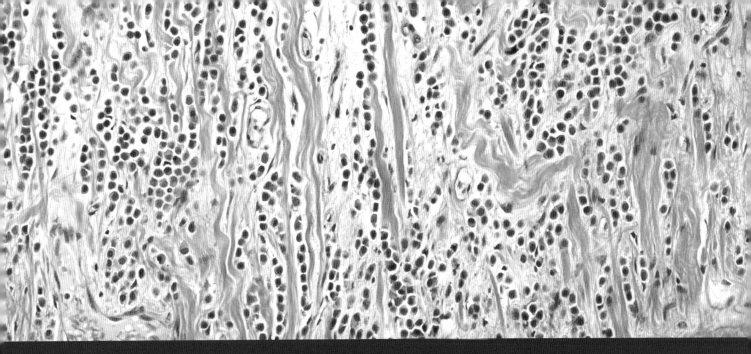

# 2

# Epithelial tumours of the breast

Edited by: Allison KH, Brogi E, Ellis IO, Fox SB, Lakhani SR, Lax SF, Sahin A, Salgado R, Sapino A, Sasano H, Schnitt SJ, Tan PH, Thompson LDR, van Diest PJ

Benign epithelial proliferations and precursors
   Usual ductal hyperplasia
   Columnar cell lesions, including flat epithelial atypia
   Atypical ductal hyperplasia
Adenosis and benign sclerosing lesions
   Sclerosing adenosis
   Apocrine adenosis and adenoma
   Microglandular adenosis
   Radial scar / complex sclerosing lesion
Adenomas
   Tubular adenoma
   Lactating adenoma
   Ductal adenoma
Epithelial-myoepithelial tumours
   Pleomorphic adenoma
   Adenomyoepithelioma
   Malignant adenomyoepithelioma
Papillary neoplasms
   Intraductal papilloma
   Papillary ductal carcinoma in situ
   Encapsulated papillary carcinoma
   Solid papillary carcinoma (in situ and invasive)
   Invasive papillary carcinoma

Non-invasive lobular neoplasia
   Atypical lobular hyperplasia
   Lobular carcinoma in situ
Ductal carcinoma in situ
Invasive breast carcinoma
   Invasive breast carcinoma of no special type
   Microinvasive carcinoma
   Invasive lobular carcinoma
   Tubular carcinoma
   Cribriform carcinoma
   Mucinous carcinoma
   Mucinous cystadenocarcinoma
   Invasive micropapillary carcinoma
   Carcinoma with apocrine differentiation
   Metaplastic carcinoma
Rare and salivary gland–type tumours
   Acinic cell carcinoma
   Adenoid cystic carcinoma
   Secretory carcinoma
   Mucoepidermoid carcinoma
   Polymorphous adenocarcinoma
   Tall cell carcinoma with reversed polarity
Neuroendocrine neoplasms
   Neuroendocrine tumour
   Neuroendocrine carcinoma

# WHO classification of epithelial tumours of the breast

**Benign epithelial proliferations and precursors**
    Usual ductal hyperplasia
    Columnar cell lesions, including flat epithelial atypia
    Atypical ductal hyperplasia

**Adenosis and benign sclerosing lesions**
    Sclerosing adenosis
8401/0  Apocrine adenoma
    Microglandular adenosis
    Radial scar / complex sclerosing lesion

**Adenomas**
8211/0  Tubular adenoma NOS
8204/0  Lactating adenoma
8503/0  Duct adenoma NOS

**Epithelial-myoepithelial tumours**
8940/0  Pleomorphic adenoma
8983/0  Adenomyoepithelioma NOS
8983/3  Adenomyoepithelioma with carcinoma
8562/3  Epithelial-myoepithelial carcinoma

**Papillary neoplasms**
8503/0  Intraductal papilloma
8503/2  Ductal carcinoma in situ, papillary
8504/2  Encapsulated papillary carcinoma
8504/3  Encapsulated papillary carcinoma with invasion
8509/2  Solid papillary carcinoma in situ
8509/3  Solid papillary carcinoma with invasion
8503/3  Intraductal papillary adenocarcinoma with invasion

**Non-invasive lobular neoplasia**
    Atypical lobular hyperplasia
8520/2  Lobular carcinoma in situ NOS
      Classic lobular carcinoma in situ
      Florid lobular carcinoma in situ
8519/2  Lobular carcinoma in situ, pleomorphic

**Ductal carcinoma in situ (DCIS)**
8500/2  Intraductal carcinoma, non-infiltrating, NOS
      DCIS of low nuclear grade
      DCIS of intermediate nuclear grade
      DCIS of high nuclear grade

**Invasive breast carcinoma**
8500/3  Infiltrating duct carcinoma NOS
8290/3  Oncocytic carcinoma
8314/3  Lipid-rich carcinoma
8315/3  Glycogen-rich carcinoma
8410/3  Sebaceous carcinoma
8520/3  Lobular carcinoma NOS
8211/3  Tubular carcinoma
8201/3  Cribriform carcinoma NOS
8480/3  Mucinous adenocarcinoma
8470/3  Mucinous cystadenocarcinoma NOS
8507/3  Invasive micropapillary carcinoma of breast
8401/3  Apocrine adenocarcinoma
8575/3  Metaplastic carcinoma NOS

**Rare and salivary gland–type tumours**
8550/3  Acinar cell carcinoma
8200/3  Adenoid cystic carcinoma
      Classic adenoid cystic carcinoma
      Solid-basaloid adenoid cystic carcinoma
      Adenoid cystic carcinoma with high-grade
        transformation
8502/3  Secretory carcinoma
8430/3  Mucoepidermoid carcinoma
8525/3  Polymorphous adenocarcinoma
8509/3  Tall cell carcinoma with reversed polarity

**Neuroendocrine neoplasms**
8240/3  Neuroendocrine tumour NOS
8240/3  Neuroendocrine tumour, grade 1
8249/3  Neuroendocrine tumour, grade 2
8246/3  Neuroendocrine carcinoma NOS
8041/3  Neuroendocrine carcinoma, small cell
8013/3  Neuroendocrine carcinoma, large cell

---

These morphology codes are from the International Classification of Diseases for Oncology, third edition, second revision (ICD-O-3.2) {921}. Behaviour is coded /0 for benign tumours; /1 for unspecified, borderline, or uncertain behaviour; /2 for carcinoma in situ and grade III intraepithelial neoplasia; /3 for malignant tumours, primary site; and /6 for malignant tumours, metastatic site. Behaviour code /6 is not generally used by cancer registries.

This classification is modified from the previous WHO classification, taking into account changes in our understanding of these lesions.

Subtype labels are indented.

# Benign epithelial proliferations and precursors: Introduction

Schnitt SJ

## Definition

Intraductal proliferative lesions are a group of cytologically and architecturally diverse proliferations, most often originating in the terminal duct lobular unit (TDLU) and confined to the mammary ductal-lobular system. They are associated with an increased risk of subsequent breast cancer, albeit of different magnitudes {558}. Some of these lesions are best considered risk indicators, whereas others are recognized as true precursors of invasive breast carcinoma (IBC). Columnar cell lesions (CCLs; columnar cell change and columnar cell hyperplasia) and flat epithelial atypia (FEA) are lesions of the TDLU that are often seen in biopsies performed because of mammographic microcalcifications. Although molecular evidence suggests that these are early precursor lesions in the low-grade breast neoplasia pathway {1950,3,192,1237,382}, limited data from epidemiological studies suggest that they are associated with a very low risk of progression to IBC {213,80,1820}.

## Site of origin and route of lesion progression

The vast majority of intraductal proliferative lesions originate in the TDLU. A substantially smaller proportion originate in larger and lactiferous ducts. CCLs and FEA arise in the TDLU and do not typically involve extralobular ducts.

## Terminology

Intraductal proliferative lesions of the breast have traditionally been divided into three categories: usual ductal hyperplasia (UDH), atypical ductal hyperplasia (ADH), and ductal carcinoma in situ (DCIS). In most cases, the histopathological distinction between different types of intraductal proliferation can be made on morphological grounds alone, particularly with standardization of histopathological criteria. However, the distinction between some of the lesions (particularly between ADH and some small, low-grade forms of DCIS) remains problematic. In addition, population-based mammography screening has resulted in increased detection of lesions that show cytological atypia with or without intraluminal proliferation that do not fulfil the combined cytological and architectural criteria for the diagnosis of ADH or DCIS. Lesions lacking appreciable proliferation have been described in the past as clinging carcinoma (monomorphic type), atypical cystic lobules, and atypical columnar cell change (among other terms), and they are currently categorized as FEA.

## Progression to IBC

Clinical follow-up studies have indicated that intraductal proliferative lesions are associated with different levels of risk for the subsequent development of IBC, ranging from approximately 1.5 times that of the reference population for UDH, to 4- to 5-fold for ADH, to 8- to 10-fold for DCIS {650}. Recent immunophenotypic and molecular genetic studies have provided new insights into these lesions and have indicated that the long-held notion of a linear progression from normal epithelium through usual hyperplasia, atypical hyperplasia, and carcinoma in situ to invasive cancer is overly simplistic; the interrelationship between these various intraductal proliferative lesions and IBC is far more complex. In brief, these data have shown that: (1) UDH shares few similarities with most ADH, DCIS, or invasive cancer; (2) ADH shares many similarities with low-grade DCIS; (3) low-grade DCIS and high-grade DCIS appear in most cases to represent genetically distinct disorders leading to distinct forms of IBC; and (4) FEA represents a clonal, neoplastic lesion that shares morphological, immunohistochemical, and molecular features with ADH and low-grade DCIS. These data support the notion that FEA, ADH, and all forms of DCIS represent intraepithelial neoplasia. The WHO Classification of Tumours Editorial Board feels that UDH is not a substantial risk factor and in most cases is unlikely to represent a precursor lesion. However, there are some genomic data to suggest that a small proportion of UDH can harbour clonal populations of cells, which indicates that clonal lesions such as ADH may occasionally arise in this setting {750,1101}. Limited data from epidemiological studies suggest that CCLs and FEA are associated with a very low risk of progression to IBC {213,80,1820}.

## Classification and grading

Emerging genetic data and the increasingly frequent detection of ADH and low-grade DCIS by mammography have raised important questions about the manner in which intraductal proliferative lesions are currently classified. Although used by pathology laboratories worldwide, the traditional classification system suffers from interobserver variability, in particular in distinguishing between ADH and some small, low-grade DCIS. Over the past decade, it has been proposed that the traditional terminology be replaced by the ductal intraepithelial neoplasia system, reserving the term "carcinoma" for invasive tumours. The ductal intraepithelial neoplasia terminology has not gained widespread acceptance in part because no new diagnostic criteria are used, and the change in terminology would therefore not help with improving interobserver variability. Molecular analysis is being refined and should help to improve the traditional classification {44,2177}. The classification of intraductal proliferative lesions should be viewed as an evolving concept that may be modified as additional molecular and genetic data become available.

## Diagnostic reproducibility

Multiple studies have assessed reproducibility in diagnosing the range of intraductal proliferative lesions, some with emphasis on borderline lesions {181,1584,1587,1784,1868,1961,1960,577}. These studies have clearly indicated that interobserver agreement is poor when no standardized criteria are used {1784}. Diagnostic reproducibility is improved with the use of standardized criteria {1868}. However, discrepancies in diagnosis persist in some cases, particularly in the distinction between ADH and limited forms of low-grade DCIS, because much of this distinction is based on quantitative rather than qualitative features {577}. In one study, consistency in diagnosis and classification did not change significantly when interpretation was confined to specific images as compared with assessment of the entire tissue section on a slide, reflecting inconsistencies secondary to differences in morphological interpretation {586}. Clinical follow-up studies have generally demonstrated increasing levels of breast cancer risk associated with UDH, ADH, and DCIS, but concerns about diagnostic reproducibility have led some to question the practice of using these risk estimates at the individual patient level {181}.

## Etiology

In general, the factors associated with the development of IBC are also associated with increased risk for the development of intraductal proliferative lesions {993,1083}.

## Genetics

The morphological similarities between invasive and in situ carcinomas of similar grade and their intimate association within the breast suggest that these proliferations are biologically related. The relationships between in situ and invasive lesions have been investigated using a variety of methods, including immunohistochemistry, loss-of-heterozygosity analysis, comparative genomic hybridization, and gene expression profiling. These data reveal close relationships between DCIS and invasive ductal carcinoma {247,248,1530,1260,1097,1246}. The distinct molecular features found in different grades of invasive carcinomas are also mirrored in preinvasive lesions of comparable morphology {1260}. Other preinvasive lesions are more difficult to position along the multistep pathways. UDH has traditionally been postulated as a precursor of ADH and DCIS. However, at the molecular level, relatively few and random chromosomal changes have been detected in UDH {1101, 92,957}. There is evidence that a minority of UDH cases may harbour genomic alterations also observed in ADH and therefore could be precursors of ADH; however, the vast majority of these lesions are not thought to progress and are more likely to be dead-end proliferations {185}. Recent data suggest that more-likely precursors of ADH and low-grade DCIS are CCLs/FEA {1950}. The hallmark genetic feature of low-grade lesions, loss of 16q, is the most frequently detected recurrent change in CCLs/FEA, and there is a degree of overlap in the molecular profile of CCLs/FEA and associated more advanced lesions {1950,1397}. Promoter methylation and copy-number alterations in breast cancer–related genes including *CCND1*, *ESR1*, and *CDH1* have been identified in CCLs, providing further evidence for their potential role in breast carcinogenesis {1950, 2173,2171,431}. Genetic alterations have also been identified in normal breast tissues, both near and away from invasive carcinoma {480,1096}. Genetic alterations have been seen independently in luminal and myoepithelial cell compartments {1096}, suggesting that the changes may have occurred very early during breast carcinoma development. Genetic alterations in the mammary stroma of patients with malignancy have also been described, and there is currently considerable interest in understanding the relationship of the stroma and epithelial cells in breast tumorigenesis and progression {1396,1259}. The significance of alterations in normal breast tissues in individual patients is unclear at present, but further investigation is likely to shed light on cancer development and potential preventive strategies in the future.

## Clinical features

The age range of women with intraductal proliferative lesions is wide, spanning 7–8 decades after adolescence. All these lesions are extremely rare before puberty; when they do occur among infants and children, they are generally a reflection of exogenous or abnormal endogenous hormonal stimulation.

## Macroscopy

The vast majority of intraductal proliferative lesions, in particular those detected mammographically, are not evident on macroscopic inspection of the specimen. CCLs and FEA are not macroscopically detectable.

# Usual ductal hyperplasia

Schnitt SJ
Purdie CA
Weaver DL

## Definition

Usual ductal hyperplasia (UDH) is an architecturally, cytologically, and molecularly heterogeneous benign epithelial proliferation primarily involving terminal duct lobular units.

## ICD-O coding

None

## ICD-11 coding

GB20.Y Other specified benign breast disease

## Related terminology

*Acceptable:* intraductal hyperplasia; hyperplasia of the usual type; hyperplasia without atypia; epitheliosis; ordinary intraductal hyperplasia.
*Not recommended:* hyperplasia (without further designation).

## Subtype(s)

None

## Localization

UDH typically involves terminal duct lobular units but may occur in extralobular ducts. UDH may also occur in association with other lesions, such as intraductal papillomas, fibroadenomas, radial scars / complex sclerosing lesions, and nipple adenomas.

## Clinical features

UDH does not present as a mass or a mammographic lesion, except in occasional instances when it may present with associated microcalcifications.

## Epidemiology

Incidence cannot easily be determined, because UDH is rarely the targeted lesion in breast biopsies. In cohorts of women who have had biopsies for lesions that proved to be benign proliferative lesions without atypia (which include UDH and other non-atypical proliferations such as sclerosing adenosis and papillomas, often admixed), UDH represents approximately 30% of diagnoses rendered, but it is the highest-risk lesion in approximately 12% of benign breast biopsies {2237}. The average patient age at the time of diagnosis is 54 years, which is about 4 years younger than in women presenting with atypical ductal hyperplasia (ADH) {830}.

## Etiology

No specific factors have been identified that are etiologically linked to UDH.

## Pathogenesis

Most studies have found no consistent genetic alterations associated with UDH {1743,183}. There is emerging evidence to suggest that activation of the PI3K/AKT/mTOR pathway is an important factor in the pathogenesis of UDH {930}. Clonal abnormalities are present at low frequencies (≤ 15%) in UDH, but the characteristic alterations seen in ADH and low-grade ductal carcinoma in situ are not found in UDH, suggesting that these lesions are markers of risk for breast cancer development, but not direct precursors in most cases {1237,192}.

## Macroscopic appearance

UDH is a microscopic finding, with no specific macroscopic appearance.

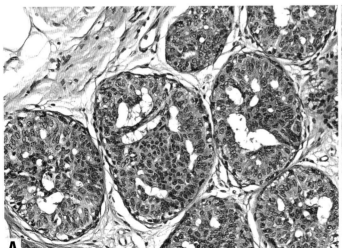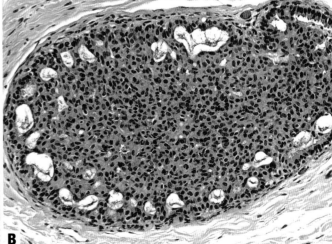

**Fig. 2.01** Usual ductal hyperplasia. **A** There is heterogeneity of epithelial cell size and shape, as well as variability of nuclear size, shape, and location. The lumina are irregular in shape. **B** In this example, the lumina are present at the periphery of the intraductal epithelial proliferation.

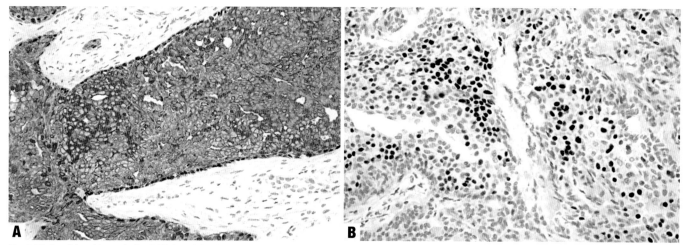

**Fig. 2.02** Usual ductal hyperplasia. **A** Triple staining demonstrates the heterogeneity of the cell population. Some cells express low-molecular-weight cytokeratins (red cytoplasmic staining) and others express high-molecular-weight cytokeratins (brown cytoplasmic staining). Myoepithelial cells at the periphery of the lesion show nuclear staining for p63 (brown nuclear staining). **B** ER immunohistochemistry shows nuclear staining of variable intensity.

## Histopathology

UDH is characterized by a cohesive proliferation of benign epithelial cells that display a haphazard orientation with respect to one another. The presence of secondary lumina or fenestrations is characteristic of this lesion. The lumina are often peripherally located and tend to be slit-like, in contrast to the very rounded, punched-out lumina seen in ADH and low-grade ductal carcinoma in situ. In some cases, the proliferation has a solid pattern and no secondary lumina are present. Occasionally, a micropapillary architecture similar to that seen in gynaecomastia may be present.

The cells of UDH are irregularly arranged, with indistinct borders. The nuclei are variably sized, often with grooves and intranuclear cytoplasmic pseudoinclusions. The cells often have a streaming or syncytial pattern, which is particularly evident in the centre of the proliferation. In contrast to the rigid bridges seen in low-grade atypical proliferations, the epithelial bridges in UDH are thin and stretched, with unevenly distributed nuclei frequently parallel to the bridge. Micropapillations, when present, have a broad base and a narrow or pinched tip, with hyperchromatic, almost pyknotic-looking nuclei. The nuclei of the cells surrounding the secondary lumina tend to run parallel to the lumina, in contrast to the formation of the new "ducts within ducts" of neoplastic intraductal proliferations, where the cells are oriented perpendicular to the spaces. An admixture of epithelial, myoepithelial, and even apocrine metaplastic epithelial cells can be seen within a proliferation of UDH. Foamy histiocytes, calcifications, and (rarely) foci of necrosis may also be seen. The presence of mitotic figures does not preclude the diagnosis of UDH. The cellular population exhibits a mixed phenotype, staining for both low-molecular-weight cytokeratins (luminal type: CK7, CK8, and CK18) and high-molecular-weight cytokeratins (basal type: CK5/6, CK14, and 34βE12 [CK903]), the latter in a heterogeneous or mosaic pattern {4}. ER staining is also heterogeneous in UDH, in contrast to the strong, diffuse staining seen in ADH and low-grade ductal carcinoma in situ {1150}.

## Cytology

FNA specimens from UDH may be highly cellular, leading to suspicion of malignancy. However, they are composed of flat, cohesive sheets of rather bland epithelial cells showing no substantial nuclear atypia. Naked bipolar nuclei are present in the background, and these are a reassuring feature. Other features may also be present (depending on any associated pathology), such as papillary structures, fibroadenoma-type stroma, calcifications, and metaplastic apocrine cells.

## Diagnostic molecular pathology

Not clinically relevant

## Essential and desirable diagnostic criteria

*Architectural features:* fenestrated, solid, or micropapillary patterns; irregular lumina of variable size and shape, often slit-like and present at the periphery of involved spaces without polarization of surrounding cells; bridges stretched and often centrally attenuated.

*Cytological features:* a heterogeneous cell population with poorly defined cell borders and variation in cell size, shape, and orientation; variation in the size, shape, and location of the nuclei, with areas of nuclear overlapping, nuclear grooves, and intranuclear cytoplasmic pseudoinclusions.

## Staging

Not clinically relevant

## Prognosis and prediction

Long-term follow-up of women with UDH indicates a slight increase in subsequent breast cancer risk, on the order of 1.5- to 2-fold. This risk is conferred on either breast and appears to be slightly higher among patients with a strong family history of breast cancer {830,650,553,386,1864}. At present, there are no prognostic factors that can predict with any reliability which patients may develop invasive breast carcinoma after a diagnosis of UDH. The magnitude of breast cancer risk associated with UDH is similar to that associated with certain reproductive factors (e.g. early menarche and late menopause) and should not alter the frequency of mammographic screening.

# Columnar cell lesions, including flat epithelial atypia

Schnitt SJ
Morris EA
Vincent-Salomon A

## Definition
Columnar cell lesions (CCLs) are clonal alterations of the terminal duct lobular unit (TDLU) characterized by enlarged, variably dilated acini lined by columnar epithelial cells. Flat epithelial atypia (FEA) is characterized by low-grade (monomorphic) cytological atypia.

## ICD-O coding
None

## ICD-11 coding
GB20.Y Other specified benign breast disease

## Related terminology
*Columnar cell lesions*
*Acceptable:* columnar cell change; columnar cell hyperplasia.
*Not recommended:* blunt duct adenosis; columnar alteration of lobules; columnar metaplasia; hyperplastic unfolded lobules; hyperplastic enlarged lobular units; enlarged lobular units with columnar alteration.

*Flat epithelial atypia*
*Acceptable:* columnar cell change with atypia; columnar cell hyperplasia with atypia.
*Not recommended:* clinging carcinoma (monomorphic type); atypical cystic lobules; atypical lobules type A.

## Subtype(s)
None

## Localization
CCLs and FEA are lesions of the TDLU of the breast.

## Clinical features
These lesions are most often detected because of the presence of grouped, amorphous calcifications on mammography. Less frequently they are an incidental microscopic finding.

## Epidemiology
Unknown

## Etiology
There are no data directly addressing the etiology of these lesions. However, given that they share immunophenotypic and molecular alterations with other lesions in the low-grade breast neoplasia pathway {382}, it is reasonable to speculate that their etiology is similar.

## Pathogenesis
The available evidence suggests that CCLs are the earliest stage in the low-grade breast neoplasia pathway and represent non-obligate precursors to atypical ductal hyperplasia (ADH), low-grade ductal carcinoma in situ (DCIS), and low-grade invasive breast carcinomas (including tubular carcinomas). Some examples of columnar cell change and columnar cell hyperplasia show genomic abnormalities as determined by assays for loss of heterozygosity (particularly losses of 16q) and comparative genomic hybridization {431,1950,4}. Although usual ductal hyperplasia has traditionally been considered the precursor to ADH, current evidence suggests that CCLs and FEA are in fact more likely precursors {1865,1950,4}. CCLs and FEA show an immunoprofile similar to that of ADH / low-grade DCIS {1865, 4}. The degree of proliferation, architectural atypia, and cytological atypia in these lesions is mirrored at the genetic level, with a stepwise increase in the number and complexity of

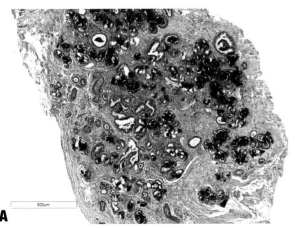

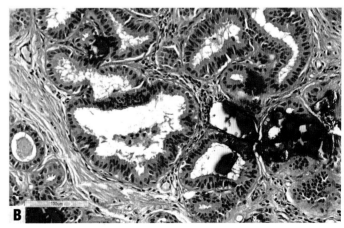

**Fig. 2.03** Columnar cell lesion. **A** Core biopsy of screen-detected calcifications reveals breast tissue with numerous calcifications within an enlarged lobule with columnar cell change. **B** Higher magnification shows ductules lined by columnar epithelial cells with vertically oriented nuclei. Focal columnar cell hyperplasia with nuclear stratification is present.

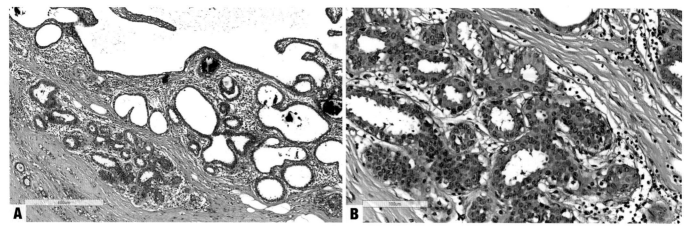

**Fig. 2.04** Flat epithelial atypia. **A** Breast tissue shows cystic changes of ductules, with luminal calcifications. **B** Higher magnification shows cuboidal epithelial cells with apical snouts, displaying mild nuclear atypia with rounded, slightly enlarged vesicular nuclei and discernible nucleoli.

chromosomal copy-number changes as defined by comparative genomic hybridization {1950,3}. Furthermore, the characteristic genetic alteration of low-grade lesions, loss of 16q, is the most frequently detected recurrent change in CCLs and FEA. It has also been demonstrated that there is a degree of overlap in the molecular genetic profile of CCL/FEA and that of associated more-advanced lesions, implying a precursor–product relationship {1950,1397}.

## Macroscopic appearance
CCLs and FEA are of microscopic size and cannot be identified on macroscopic examination.

## Histopathology
Columnar cell change and hyperplasia are characterized by TDLUs with variably enlarged and dilated acini lined by columnar epithelial cells that frequently have apical cytoplasmic snouts. The involved acini usually have irregular contours. The nuclei are typically ovoid, are regularly oriented perpendicular to the basement membrane, and have evenly dispersed chromatin and inconspicuous nucleoli. Luminal secretions and/or microcalcifications are commonly present. Lesions in which the epithelial cell lining is only 1–2 cell layers thick are categorized as columnar cell change; those with cellular stratification or tufting > 2 cell layers thick are designated columnar cell hyperplasia {1870,1652,382}. Cytological atypia is not a feature of these lesions; CCLs with cytological atypia are included within the category of FEA. Columnar cell change/hyperplasia can be reliably distinguished from FEA using established criteria {1551}.

FEA is characterized by replacement of the native epithelial cells of the TDLUs by one to several layers of mildly atypical cuboidal to columnar cells, often with apical snouts. Occasional cellular tufts or mounds may be seen, but well-developed arcades, bridges, and micropapillary formations are absent. The acini of involved TDLUs are variably distended, usually have smooth contours, and may contain secretory or floccular material that often contains microcalcifications. The nuclei of the neoplastic cells tend to be round and uniform in appearance and have inconspicuous nucleoli, similar in appearance to the nuclei that characterize low-grade DCIS {1865,1395}. Lymphoid infiltrates may be present in the intralobular stroma of involved

TDLUs. The cells of CCLs and FEA consistently demonstrate strong and diffusely nuclear staining for ER and lack staining for high-molecular-weight cytokeratins such as CK5/6 {382}.

CCLs and FEA are often seen in association with other benign changes, such as cysts and epithelial proliferative lesions. There is a strong association between these lesions and the presence of lobular neoplasia (lobular carcinoma in situ and atypical lobular hyperplasia), and FEA is frequently associated with ADH, low-grade DCIS, and low-grade invasive cancers, in particular tubular carcinoma and invasive lobular carcinoma {236,1143,288}. These observations, in conjunction with the shared molecular alterations of these lesions, support the existence of a low-grade breast neoplasia pathway.

## Cytology
A report of 10 cases of CCLs sampled by FNA described flat sheets of cells with enlarged nuclei, distinct cell borders, and finely granular cytoplasm, with atypia ranging from minimal to severe. There was substantial overlap with the cytological features of papillary neoplasms and well-differentiated adenocarcinoma. Therefore, CCLs cannot be reliably diagnosed by FNA {940}.

## Diagnostic molecular pathology
Not clinically relevant

## Essential and desirable diagnostic criteria
*Columnar cell change and columnar cell hyperplasia*
*Essential:* TDLUs with enlarged dilated acini, often with irregular contours; columnar lining epithelial cells have uniform, elongated nuclei with evenly dispersed chromatin and inconspicuous nucleoli, oriented perpendicular to the basement membrane of the involved spaces; cellular stratification or tufting > 2 cell layers thick in columnar cell hyperplasia.

*Flat epithelial atypia*
*Essential:* TDLUs with enlarged dilated acini with more-rounded contours; lined by one to several layers of mildly atypical cuboidal to columnar cells resembling the monomorphic nuclei of low-grade DCIS.

## Staging
Not clinically relevant

## Prognosis and prediction
A few follow-up studies have shown that columnar cell change and hyperplasia are associated with a slightly increased risk for the subsequent development of breast cancer (relative risk: ~1.5) {213,80}. However, the risk associated with these lesions is not clearly independent of the risk associated with concomitant proliferative lesions.

Data from a few small retrospective studies and one larger epidemiological study suggest that some cases of FEA may progress to invasive breast carcinoma, although the risk of progression appears to be very low and this lesion is not associated with the same level of breast cancer risk associated with atypical lobular hyperplasia and ADH {600,170,1820}. Therefore, FEA should not be managed in the same manner as ADH or atypical lobular hyperplasia.

Small retrospective studies have shown that as many as 30% of patients with FEA on core needle biopsy have a worse lesion at surgical excision. However, given the limitations of study design and wide variation in reported upgrade rates, the need for routine surgical excision after a diagnosis of FEA on core needle biopsy is uncertain. Surgical excision may not be necessary if a postbiopsy mammogram shows that all of the radiographical microcalcifications have been removed {502}. Radiological–pathological correlation is recommended for guiding the further management of these cases.

# Atypical ductal hyperplasia

Allison KH
Collins LC
Moriya T
Sanders ME
Visscher DW

## Definition

Atypical ductal hyperplasia (ADH) is an epithelial proliferative lesion with cytological and architectural features similar to those of low-grade ductal carcinoma in situ (DCIS) but less developed in architecture, degree of terminal duct lobular unit involvement, and contiguous extent.

## ICD-O coding

None

## ICD-11 coding

GB20.Y Other specified benign breast disease

## Related terminology

*Acceptable:* atypical intraductal hyperplasia.
*Not recommended:* atypical hyperplasia (to be used only if ductal vs lobular cannot be determined).

## Subtype(s)

None

## Localization

ADH typically occurs in the terminal duct lobular units. It can also occur within lesions such as papilloma and fibroadenoma or rarely within major lactiferous ducts.

## Clinical features

ADH is most frequently diagnosed in women undergoing screening mammography in whom microcalcifications are identified, or less commonly as an incidental finding in tissue sampled for other reasons. There are no radiological features that

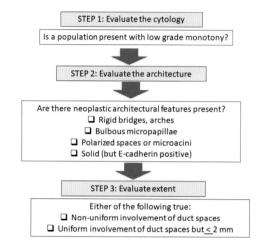

**Fig. 2.06** Process of evaluation for the diagnosis of atypical ductal hyperplasia in intraductal proliferations.

help distinguish the calcifications associated with ADH from those present in other lesions, such as columnar cell change/hyperplasia or low-grade DCIS. Proliferative lesions in general, including ADH, may also account for non-mass enhancement on breast MRI. ADH does not typically present as a mass, unless it involves a mass-forming lesion such as a papillary lesion or fibroadenoma.

## Epidemiology

The frequency of ADH diagnoses increased with the introduction of mammographic screening but has remained steady in

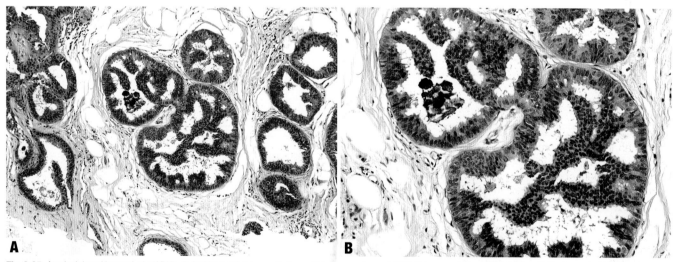

**Fig. 2.05** Atypical ductal hyperplasia (ADH). **A** Architectural changes that are within the spectrum of ADH. This example has rigid bridges of cells traversing the duct space, as well as smaller arches. **B** At higher power, early bulbous micropapillae, as well as rigid bridges and arches, are seen. The cells are monotonous and low-grade. These findings are consistent with ADH.

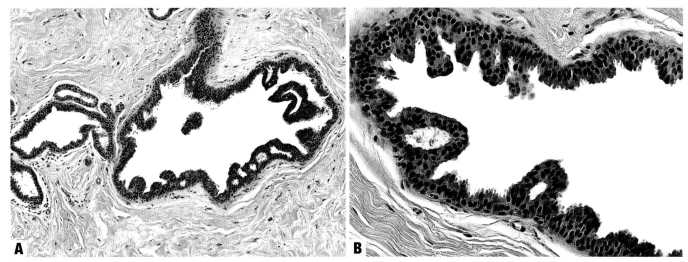

**Fig. 2.07** Atypical ductal hyperplasia. **A** An intraductal proliferation with early neoplastic architectural forms such as arches of cells and small micropapillae involving part of the duct space. **B** A higher-power view reveals the low-grade cytological monotony of the cells making up the arches and small micropapillary structures. These findings are consistent with the diagnosis of atypical ductal hyperplasia.

more-recent decades. ADH now accounts for 2–14% of diagnoses in breast biopsies within screened populations {1649,563, 38,106}.

### Etiology
Because ADH is an estrogen-driven process, the factors that are associated with the development of ER-positive invasive breast carcinomas are generally also associated with an increased risk for the development of ADH {829}.

### Pathogenesis
Studies of loss of heterozygosity in ADH and low-grade DCIS have shown similar genetic abnormalities, providing evidence that these are related clonal processes {1097}. The current model of the pathogenesis of breast cancer places many of the high-risk lesions, including ADH, in the low-grade pathway to luminal/ER-positive invasive disease {4}. ADH is thought to be a very early neoplastic step in the pathway to low-grade DCIS and ER-positive, low-grade invasive ductal carcinomas {1237}. Allelic imbalances are seen at similar frequencies in ADH and low-grade DCIS, and there are similar recurrent regions with loss of heterozygosity, including loci on 1q, 16q, and 17p {182, 254,698,1116}.

### Macroscopic appearance
ADH is not macroscopically identifiable.

### Histopathology
ADH is an intraductal proliferation with cytological and architectural features similar to those of low-grade DCIS, but with partial involvement of ductal spaces and/or uniform involvement of limited extent. Microcalcifications are often seen in association with these lesions. The cytological features include evenly spaced monotonous cells containing rounded nuclei with dense chromatin. Intermediate-grade and high-grade nuclear features are not seen, and necrosis is highly unusual. The cell borders are well defined. In some examples of ADH, the lesional cells are admixed with the non-uniform cell population of usual ductal

hyperplasia or arise in association with other benign proliferations.

The architectural features include rigid bridges, bars, and arcades of uniform thickness; bulbous micropapillations (with narrow bases and broad tips); and a cribriform pattern. Solid and pagetoid patterns of ADH are less common and can be difficult to distinguish from classic lobular carcinoma in situ. When duct spaces are uniformly involved by an intraductal proliferation with the cytological and architectural features of low-grade DCIS, the distinction between ADH and DCIS is based on size/extent criteria. Page et al. {1575} proposed a cut-off of 2 involved duct spaces with < 2 involved spaces classified as ADH. Tavassoli and Norris {2056} proposed that lesions ≤ 2 mm in contiguous extent be classified as ADH. These thresholds are arbitrary and should be used as general guidelines. Because both of these systems were developed on the basis of findings in excisional biopsies, these criteria should be applied with caution, and the

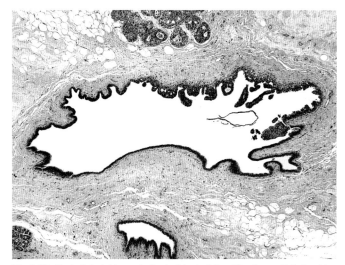

**Fig. 2.08** Atypical ductal hyperplasia. An intraductal proliferation partially involving a duct space, with formation of elongated, bulbous micropapillae. The partial involvement of a single duct by the process (if low-grade) is consistent with atypical ductal hyperplasia.

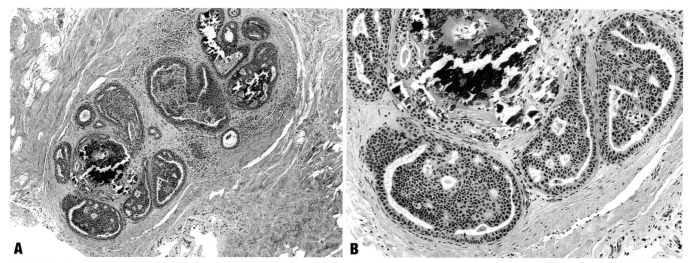

**Fig. 2.09** Atypical ductal hyperplasia. **A,B** The intraductal proliferation shows early cribriform structures containing polarized spaces and monotonous cells. The area involved is ≤ 2.0 mm and therefore consistent with atypical ductal hyperplasia.

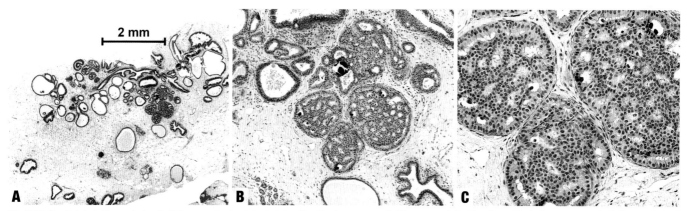

**Fig. 2.10** Atypical ductal hyperplasia. **A–C** An example of an intraductal proliferation in a core needle biopsy sample that has the cytological monotony and cribriform, polarized spaces of low-grade ductal carcinoma in situ but due to its limited extent (≤ 2.0 mm) is best classified on core needle biopsy as atypical ductal hyperplasia.

WHO Classification of Tumours Editorial Board recommends a conservative approach when lesions of limited extent are identified, particularly in core needle biopsies, in which the entire lesion may not be visualized. Clinical trial results are awaited. Because ADH represents a spectrum of atypical architectural patterns ranging from flat epithelial atypia to low-grade DCIS, its diagnosis can be problematic. Diagnostic agreement rates for biopsies with ADH are low (40–60%) compared with the much higher agreement for high-grade DCIS, invasive carcinoma, and benign breast lesions {1868,578,577}. Variability in diagnosis is frequently related to subtle differences in professional opinion and diagnostic thresholds and may be reduced when additional consensus or second reviews are sought with the assistance of immunohistochemistry {42,578,579,41,2099,748,931}.

The cells of ADH are typically strongly and diffusely positive for ER and lack staining for high-molecular-weight cytokeratins such as CK5/6. This staining pattern is similar to that seen in other lesions in the low-grade breast neoplasia pathway (including columnar cell lesions, flat epithelial atypia, and low-grade DCIS). In contrast, the cells of usual ductal hyperplasia show variable staining for both ER and high-molecular-weight cytokeratins.

### Cytology
It is not possible to diagnose ADH on cytology specimens, because the combination of cytology, architecture, and extent is required for distinguishing this lesion from low-grade DCIS.

### Diagnostic molecular pathology
Not clinically relevant

### Essential and desirable diagnostic criteria
*Essential*

*Cytological features:* low-grade monotonous cells similar to those of low-grade DCIS, with uniform, round, evenly spaced nuclei and distinct cell borders.

*Architectural features:* rigid bridges, bars, or arcades of uniform thickness; or bulbous micropapillations (with narrow bases and broad tips); or a cribriform pattern (should not be just a flat pattern).

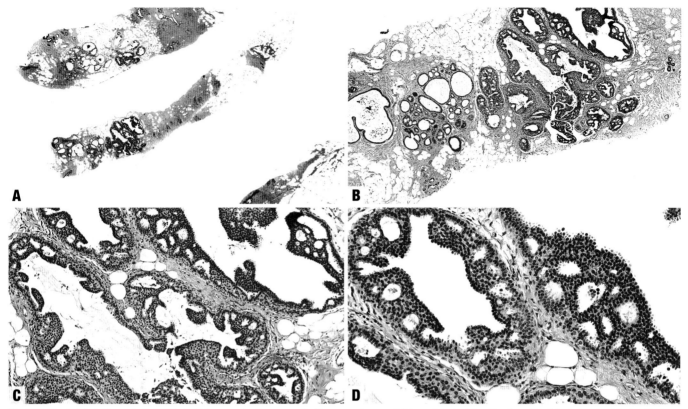

**Fig. 2.11** Atypical ductal hyperplasia (ADH). **A–D** An example of a core needle biopsy specimen containing an intraductal proliferation with cytological and architectural features of low-grade ductal carcinoma in situ, but the degree of involvement of ducts and span is borderline (close to 2 mm), at the upper end of the spectrum of ADH. On a core needle sample, the diagnosis of ADH rather than low-grade ductal carcinoma in situ is appropriate.

*Extent:* partial involvement of multiple spaces; or uniformly involved duct spaces but measuring ≤ 2 mm in contiguous extent.

*Desirable*
Cells uniformly ER-positive and CK5/6-negative.

## Staging
Not clinically relevant

## Prognosis and prediction
ADH is associated with a 3- to 5-fold increased risk of developing invasive breast carcinoma in either breast, although some studies have found the risk to be higher in the ipsilateral breast {650,1575,474,385,830}. The absolute risk of breast cancer after a diagnosis of ADH is approximately 1% per year for at least 25 years, with a mean latency period before the development of cancer of 8–12 years after diagnosis {829,828}. The risk slowly increases over several decades and has been shown (in some but not all studies) to increase with the number of ADH foci {473,384,828}. Hormonal agents such as tamoxifen significantly reduce the future risk of invasive disease {828,2236}.

For ADH identified on core needle biopsy, the reported upgrade rate to DCIS or invasive breast carcinoma has been variable; in more-contemporary series with careful radiological–pathological correlation, the rate is 10–20% {1412,1622,2271, 39,563,2256,2012,1692,613,267,1104,1688,270,1003,1000, 2212,1475,282,2153}. There are few available prospective studies that have used selective criteria to avoid excision in some patients with ADH on core needle biopsy, and although there have been minimal events, follow-up is currently limited {282, 1346,622}. Additional studies to identify patients with ADH on core needle biopsy who do not require excision are ongoing {1278}.

# Adenosis and benign sclerosing lesions: Introduction

Sahin A
Collins LC

Adenosis is defined as a relative increase in the number of acinar units in the terminal duct lobular units. It is a non-neoplastic proliferation, and the normal two-cell population and basement membrane are maintained.

Adenosis and benign sclerosing lesions (specifically radial scar and complex sclerosing lesion) are characterized by a lobulocentric proliferation of tubules and acini, with both epithelial and myoepithelial cell layers. Benign sclerosing lesions additionally have a central sclerotic and/or elastotic nidus from which the glandular structures radiate. Benign sclerosing lesions are often involved by epithelial hyperplastic processes, whereas adenosis typically has a single layer of epithelial cells lining the acini.

# Sclerosing adenosis

Sahin A
Collins LC
Yang WT

## Definition
Sclerosing adenosis is a lobulocentric proliferation of benign glandular structures distorted by fibrosis.

## ICD-O coding
None

## ICD-11 coding
GB20.Y Other specified benign breast disease

## Related terminology
None

## Subtype(s)
None

## Localization
Sclerosing adenosis shows no characteristic location or laterality.

## Clinical features
Sclerosing adenosis is a frequent incidental microscopic finding in breast specimens removed for other indications. Many lesions are associated with microcalcifications and/or architectural distortion detected mammographically, which leads to core needle biopsy {329}. On occasion, large areas of adenosis may present as a non-palpable image-detected mass lesion {1685,443,2333}.

## Epidemiology
Sclerosing adenosis occurs in a wide age group, but it most commonly occurs in women in the third or fourth decade of life {1685,2333}.

## Etiology
No specific factors have been identified that are etiologically linked to sclerosing adenosis.

## Pathogenesis
Adenosis is a non-neoplastic proliferation, and there are no known molecular or genetic abnormalities.

## Macroscopic appearance
The gross appearance depends on the size and histopathological features of the lesion. Because most adenosis lesions are small, they are usually grossly inapparent. On rare occasions, they may form a firm, rubbery, grey mass, called nodular adenosis or adenosis tumour. They can be associated with microcalcifications, which can be so abundant that they impart a gritty texture on cut surface {1685,443}.

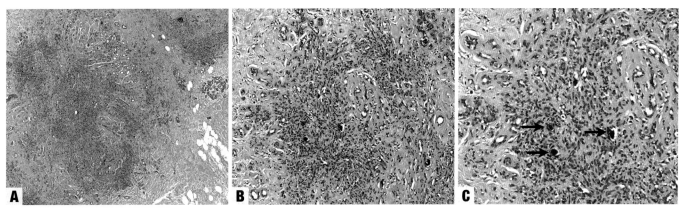

**Fig. 2.12** Sclerosing adenosis. **A** Low-power view is characterized by an increase in glandular elements and stromal proliferation that distorts and compresses glands. Lobular architecture with rounded edges is important to appreciate at this magnification. **B** The lumina of the glands are frequently compressed or obliterated by intralobular stromal fibrosis. **C** Microcalcifications (arrows) are commonly seen.

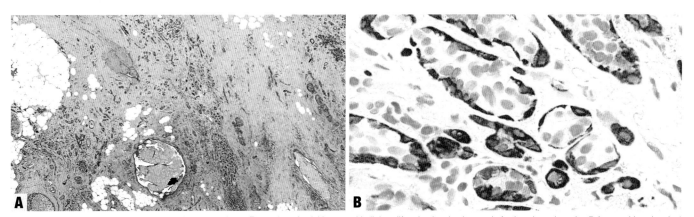

**Fig. 2.13** Ductal carcinoma in situ in sclerosing adenosis. **A** Expansion of acini by an epithelial proliferation in a background of sclerosing adenosis. **B** Immunohistochemical staining for SMM highlights intact myoepithelial cells around acini.

## Histopathology

Sclerosing adenosis is characterized by enlarged lobular units due to proliferation of small acinar or tubular structures that are compressed or distorted by stromal collagen {1685,443}. The ductules are small, round to somewhat angular, and generally uniform in size. Microcalcifications are common in sclerosing adenosis and can be present in either fibrotic stroma or glandular lumina. The epithelial cells are small and usually cuboidal to columnar, and they have centrally located nuclei. Myoepithelial cells at the periphery of the ductules are usually easily identified by their more-hyperchromatic spindle-shaped nuclei {443}. The ratio of epithelial to myoepithelial cells can vary substantially from case to case. In some cases, epithelial cells appear more atrophic, with preferential proliferation of myoepithelial cells. In others, both the epithelial and myoepithelial cell components become hyperplastic. Both the epithelial and myoepithelial components can show metaplastic changes. Variable amounts of stromal collagen can be identified in different cases. The accumulation of stromal collagen results in compression of the ductules, which may confer a growth pattern that mimics infiltration. Glandular compression and distortion are more prominent in the centre of the lesion and may completely obliterate

glandular lumina, resulting in a solid or cord-like growth pattern {443}. Sclerosing adenosis glands may extend into adipose tissue, but the lobulocentric growth pattern is maintained. The finding of this lobulocentric growth pattern on low-power microscopic examination is very useful in establishing the diagnosis.

Atypical epithelial proliferations and carcinoma in situ of both ductal and lobular types may involve sclerosing adenosis and can cause diagnostic problems. In particular, carcinoma in situ involving sclerosing adenosis may mimic invasive carcinoma, and this may be particularly problematic in small samples (e.g. core needle biopsy samples) {468,1129,741}. Identification of the lobulocentric growth pattern of the underlying sclerosing adenosis and the presence of myoepithelial cells around ducts should be useful in establishing the diagnosis. Immunohistochemical staining to highlight myoepithelial cells may be required to confirm the in situ nature of the process.

Although rare, sclerosing adenosis glands may be present around nerves, which may mimic perineural invasion by invasive carcinoma {741}. The benign cytological features and the presence of myoepithelial cells around the glandular structures are helpful to differentiate sclerosing adenosis glands from invasive carcinoma.

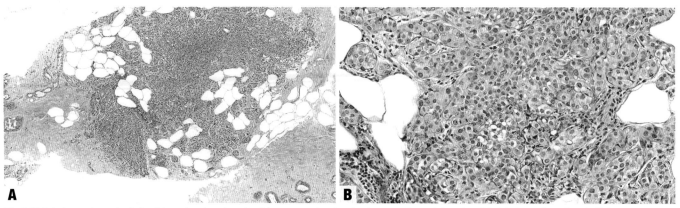

**Fig. 2.14** Lobular carcinoma in situ involving sclerosing adenosis. **A** Low-power view showing the expansion and alteration of the lobular configuration. **B** Higher power reveals that the expanded and distorted acini have closely packed epithelial cells with uniform lobular neoplasia cells.

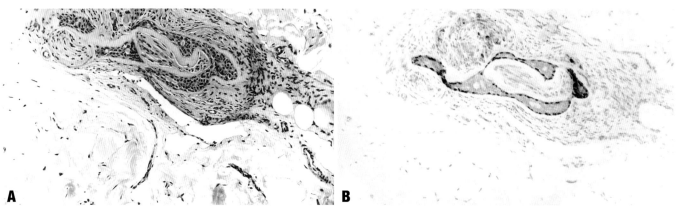

**Fig. 2.15** Sclerosing adenosis. **A** Sclerosing adenosis glands in the perineural space. **B** Immunohistochemical staining for SMA shows diffuse staining around glands, supporting the benign nature of these glands in the perineural space.

## Cytology
The epithelial cells are unremarkable and often somewhat atrophic. The myoepithelial cells may be variably prominent. Cytological atypia is absent {1078}.

## Diagnostic molecular pathology
Not clinically relevant

## Essential and desirable diagnostic criteria
*Essential:* lobulocentric architecture; proliferation of small, compressed acinar or tubular structures distorted by stromal collagen; presence of basement membrane and retained myoepithelial layer around acinar or tubular structures.
*Desirable:* immunohistochemistry (e.g. p63, calponin, SMMHC) for further identification of myoepithelial cells.

## Staging
Not clinically relevant

## Prognosis and prediction
Sclerosing adenosis is associated with a 1.5- to 2-fold increase in the risk of developing subsequent breast cancer, which is similar to the level of risk associated with other proliferative lesions without atypia {2181,1543,2281}. The diagnosis of sclerosing adenosis is not an indication for surgical excision. If there is an atypical epithelial proliferation, clinical and imaging correlation and multidisciplinary assessment is required to inform subsequent management.

# Apocrine adenosis and adenoma

Sahin A
Collins LC
Jaffer SM
Moritani S
Silva L
Waitzberg AFL

## Definition

Apocrine adenosis is a lobulocentric proliferation of benign glandular structures composed of cells with abundant granular pink cytoplasm and distorted by fibrosis. Apocrine adenoma is a well-delineated benign tumour characterized by a dense, diffuse proliferation of round and oval tubular structures composed of large epithelial cells with abundant eosinophilic cytoplasm.

## ICD-O coding

8401/0 Apocrine adenoma

## ICD-11 coding

2F30 & XH6YZ9 Benign neoplasm of breast & Apocrine adenoma

## Related terminology

*Not recommended:* sclerosing adenosis with apocrine metaplasia; nodular adenosis with apocrine metaplasia.

## Subtype(s)

None

## Localization

Apocrine adenosis and adenoma arise in the terminal duct lobular units.

## Clinical features

Apocrine adenosis is often an incidental microscopic finding, but it may be detected mammographically because of associated microcalcifications or on MRI as a non–mass-like enhancement {1549}. Apocrine adenoma may present as a solitary, painless, freely mobile, well-defined palpable nodule. In one case, the size minimally fluctuated with the menstrual cycle and was also associated with a white nipple discharge {102}. On imaging, apocrine adenoma usually presents as a well-circumscribed mass that is hypoechoic on ultrasonography. One case presented as a poorly defined calcific density. Apocrine adenoma and fibroadenoma share similar clinical and radiological findings, making the distinction difficult, but they can be definitively distinguished on histopathology.

## Epidemiology

Apocrine adenosis occurs most frequently in the third or fourth decade of life. The expected frequency on core biopsies is not well established but appears to be < 1–2% {1549,878}.

In contrast to apocrine metaplasia, which commonly occurs in the setting of fibrocystic changes, apocrine adenoma seems to be extremely rare, with only a handful of cases described in the literature. However, because there is no size criterion to discriminate a collection of apocrine metaplastic ducts from full-blown apocrine adenoma, apocrine adenoma is probably underrepresented in the literature. It predominates in females, with few case reports in males {1609}. Patient age ranges from 14 years (1 male and 1 female) to 72 years.

## Etiology

No specific factors have been identified that are etiologically linked to apocrine adenosis. It is unclear whether apocrine adenoma is a de novo tumour or a hyperplastic lesion such as nodular sclerosing adenosis with superimposed apocrine metaplasia.

## Pathogenesis

Apocrine change is the most common metaplastic change in the breast {1549}. When present in association with sclerosing adenosis, the lesion is called apocrine adenosis. Loss of heterozygosity has been identified in apocrine proliferations in several loci (1p, 3, 11q, 16, and 17q) {1893}. Comparative genomic hybridization showed losses and gains in apocrine adenosis, with accumulation through apocrine ductal carcinoma in situ and apocrine carcinoma {956}.

Given the low prevalence of apocrine adenoma in the literature, the pathogenesis of these tumours has not been well studied. However, there are theories for the origin of apocrine cells. Most agree that breast ductal cells undergo metaplasia around puberty to become apocrine cells, similar to those seen in the axilla, areola, and perineum. This is supported by a transition from normal cuboidal ductal epithelium to an intermediate form that culminates in the fully mature apocrine cell, influenced by androgens and activin (which may explain the few cases of apocrine adenoma that have been described in males). An alternative theory for the origin of the apocrine cells is embryological entrapment from cutaneous apocrine glands during development. Some authors refute both theories, arguing that apocrine cells are normal constituents of breast epithelium.

Molecularly, the few described cases are diploid, but some may be tetraploid. Studies performed on the more common entities of apocrine metaplasia and apocrine adenosis have found an elevated risk of subsequent breast cancer and possibly premalignant potential {2259A}. Abnormal oncoprotein expression and apoptosis-related protein expression associated with higher proliferation have been described in some cases, as have loss of heterozygosity and allelic imbalance, suggesting a possible oncogenic potential for some apocrine metaplastic lesions that may have genetic instability {568}.

## Macroscopic appearance

Apocrine adenosis is usually grossly inapparent. In some cases of nodular adenosis or adenosis tumour, a rubbery grey mass may be appreciated on gross examination. Because of the association of microcalcifications, the cut surface may be gritty {1549}. On gross examination, apocrine adenomas are

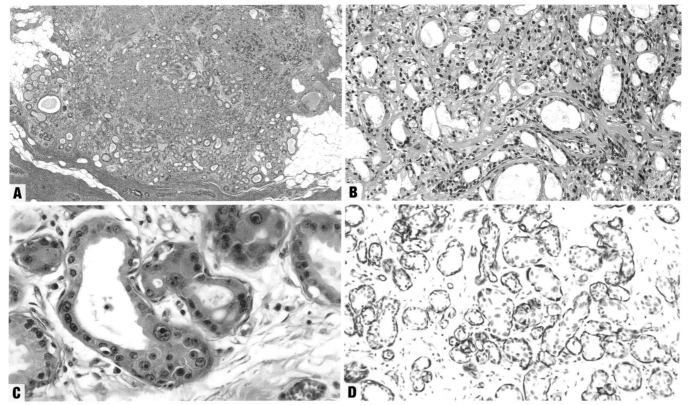

**Fig. 2.16** Apocrine adenoma and adenosis. **A** Apocrine adenoma. Low power shows a well-circumscribed compact proliferation composed of round and regular glands lined exclusively by luminal apocrine cells and an outer attenuated basal myoepithelial cell layer. **B** Apocrine adenosis. The epithelial cells have the eosinophilic cytoplasm of apocrine metaplasia. Nuclear enlargement and hyperchromasia are minimal. **C** Apocrine adenosis. The apocrine cell population may show atypical cytological features, with nuclear enlargement and prominent pleomorphic nucleoli. **D** Apocrine adenosis. Immunostaining for actin demonstrates the retained myoepithelial cell layer.

well-circumscribed nodules that may be focally cystic, with a size range of 0.3–1.7 cm.

## Histopathology

Apocrine adenosis is characterized by a lobulocentric proliferation of acini composed of an epithelial and myoepithelial cell layer and surrounded by a basement membrane. Apocrine cells are typically ER-negative and AR-positive. The cells are also positive for CK8/18, CD10, and GCDFP-15. The apocrine cell population sometimes shows atypical cytological features, with nuclear enlargement and prominent pleomorphic nucleoli {1550,685}. These lesions also express three proteins found in cyst fluid: GCDFP-15 (identical to prolactin-inducible protein), GCDFP-24 (apolipoprotein D), and GCDFP-44 (zinc-α2-glycoprotein).

Low-power histology of apocrine adenoma shows a well-circumscribed compact proliferation composed of round and regular glands lined exclusively by luminal apocrine cells and an outer attenuated basal myoepithelial cell layer. In addition to tubular forms, the glands may be cystically dilated or form delicate papillary fronds. The apocrine cells are evenly spaced and columnar or cuboidal in shape, containing abundant finely granular or brightly eosinophilic cytoplasm with apical luminal blebs (snouts) and decapitated eosinophilic secretory luminal debris. Ultrastructurally, the granularity of the cytoplasm is attributable to abundant endoplasmic reticulum, mitochondria, intermediate filaments, and secretory vesicles. The cytoplasm may also contain supranuclear golden-brown granules that

stain positively with PAS and Prussian blue (iron). The nuclei are basally located, bland-looking, and round to oval in shape, with uniformly dense chromatin containing a single punctate nucleolus. Rare calcifications and mitoses may be present. In some cases, cytological atypia may be present (atypical apocrine adenosis), defined as ≥ 3-fold variation in nuclear size with nucleolar enlargement {685}.

Complex fibroadenoma may contain apocrine metaplasia and is distinguished from apocrine adenoma by its preserved fibroepithelial architecture, prominent stroma, and focal rather than dense proliferation of apocrine cells. Tubular adenoma is similar in architecture to apocrine adenoma composed of densely packed tubules, but it lacks apocrine metaplasia. Apocrine adenoma is differentiated from ductal adenoma by the lack of a thick duct wall and diffuse rather than focal apocrine metaplasia. It is discriminated from prominent apocrine metaplasia, seen as part of the spectrum of fibrocystic changes, by its well-demarcated mass. Lastly, it is differentiated from atypical and malignant apocrine proliferations by the lack of cytological and architectural atypia and necrosis.

## Cytology

The cytological findings in apocrine adenosis include cellular smears consisting of small and compact cohesive cell clusters that occasionally form cribriform-like structures. The background contains few to rare bipolar naked nuclei. The epithelial cells have the features of apocrine metaplastic cells (i.e. abundant, granular, pink or foamy cytoplasm; round nuclei; and prominent

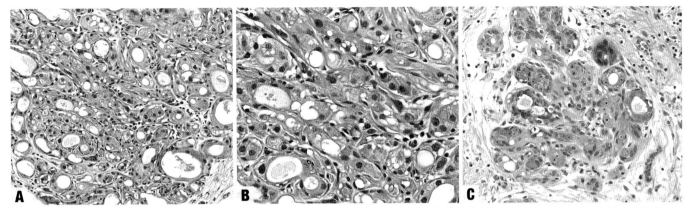

**Fig. 2.17** Apocrine adenosis with atypia. **A** Compact proliferation of small glands lined by apocrine-type epithelial cells with variation in nuclear size. **B** The nuclei of some apocrine cells are > 2–3 times the size of those seen in conventional apocrine metaplasia. **C** The lesion has nuclei with > 3-fold enlargement and prominent nucleoli.

nucleoli). A supranuclear vacuole may contain a yellowish-brown pigment consistent with iron, lipofuscin, or haemosiderin. In atypical apocrine adenosis, there is 2- to 3-fold variation in nuclear size and contour, often with particularly prominent nucleoli {1549,268,89}. The nuclear features may lead to misinterpretation of the proliferation as atypia or malignancy.

## Diagnostic molecular pathology
Not clinically relevant

## Essential and desirable diagnostic criteria
### Essential
*Apocrine adenosis:* a lobulocentric proliferation of benign glandular structures, distorted by fibrosis and lined by apocrine cells characterized by eosinophilic granular or vacuolated cytoplasm containing a prominent nucleolus.
*Apocrine adenoma:* a well-delineated benign tumour characterized by a dense, diffuse proliferation of round and oval tubular structures with luminal apocrine cells and an outer attenuated basal myoepithelial cell layer with little background stroma.

### Desirable
PASD positivity of apocrine cells and immunohistochemical expression of EMA, CK8/18, and AR, with ER and PR negativity of apocrine cells, are desirable diagnostic criteria for both adenosis and adenoma if needed to support morphological interpretation.

## Staging
Not clinically relevant

## Prognosis and prediction
The subsequent breast cancer risk associated with the diagnosis of apocrine adenosis is on the order of 1- to 2-fold. Data are limited, but atypical apocrine adenosis does not appear to behave like a high-risk precursor lesion {685}. On the basis of the handful of cases described in the literature, apocrine adenoma is considered benign and stable, a conclusion further supported by the low Ki-67 proliferation index (range: 0.7–1.3%) {568}. After core biopsy diagnosis confirmation, apocrine adenoma can be managed like fibroadenoma, with observation, annual clinical breast examination, and imaging. No recurrence or malignant transformation has been noted. However, one case of invasive ductal carcinoma associated with apocrine adenoma has been described, most likely attributable to coexistence {156}.

# Microglandular adenosis

Sahin A
Collins LC

## Definition
Microglandular adenosis is a haphazard proliferation of small round glands consisting of a single layer of epithelial cells without an accompanying myoepithelial cell layer.

## ICD-O coding
None

## ICD-11 coding
GB20.Y Other specified benign breast disease

## Related terminology
None

## Subtype(s)
None

## Localization
Microglandular adenosis occurs in the breast.

## Clinical features
Microglandular adenosis is often diagnosed incidentally in breast biopsies performed for other reasons. It may also form a mass {1008} or present as a mammographic density or occasionally as mammographically detected calcifications. Carcinomas arising in microglandular adenosis have presented with a palpable mass {2361}.

## Epidemiology
Microglandular adenosis has been reported in women over a wide age range.

## Etiology
No specific factors have been identified that are etiologically linked to microglandular adenosis.

## Pathogenesis
Several array comparative genomic hybridization–based analyses showed that progressive molecular changes were present in microglandular adenosis and associated invasive carcinomas.

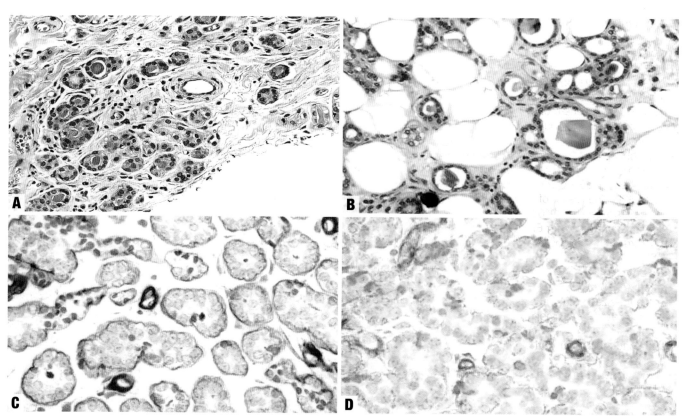

**Fig. 2.18** Microglandular adenosis. **A** Small round glands infiltrate haphazardly through the fibrous stroma. **B** The glands are lined by a single layer of cuboidal cells with uniform nuclei. Lumina contain eosinophilic secretions. **C** Immunohistochemical staining for collagen IV highlights the intact basement membrane around individual glands. **D** Immunohistochemical staining for SMA. No myoepithelial cells are identified around the microglandular adenosis glands.

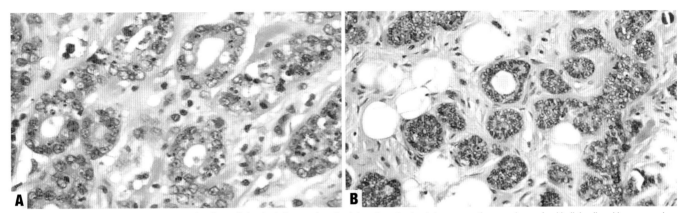

**Fig. 2.19** Atypical microglandular adenosis. **A** Small round glands similar to microglandular adenosis glands have more than one layer of epithelial cells, with some nuclear enlargement. **B** Cellular proliferation obliterates the glandular lumina.

The acquisition of genetic alterations was identified in the progression from microglandular adenosis to the synchronous invasive carcinoma component, suggesting a clonal evolution. However, these findings are preliminary and additional studies are needed {712,783,710}.

## Macroscopic appearance
Microglandular adenosis does not have a characteristic appearance on macroscopic evaluation. It can look like normal breast parenchyma or form a poorly defined nodularity or mass. In cases of carcinoma arising in a background of microglandular adenosis, a grossly evident mass lesion is usually present.

## Histopathology
Microglandular adenosis is composed of small, round, tubular structures that grow in a haphazard non-lobulocentric pattern {665}. The glands are not compressed by surrounding stroma; luminal spaces are open and often contain colloid-like eosinophilic PAS-positive diastase-resistant secretions. Microglandular adenosis glands are uniform and similar in size to or slightly larger than a normal lobular acinus. The glands are composed of a single layer of cuboidal epithelial cells with small nuclei and amphophilic cytoplasm. Myoepithelial cells are absent, but immunohistochemistry or electron microscopy can be used to demonstrate a basement membrane surrounding the glands {665,2262}. The cells of microglandular adenosis typically express cytokeratins, S100, cathepsin D, and EGFR (HER1), and they are negative for EMA, ER and PR, and ERBB2 (HER2) overexpression by immunohistochemistry {995}.

## Cytology
Cytology shows sparse cellularity and a monotonous population of medium-sized cells with uniform round nuclei, small nucleoli, and vacuolated clear cytoplasm {721}.

## Diagnostic molecular pathology
Not clinically relevant

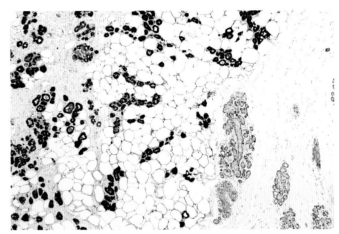

**Fig. 2.20** Microglandular adenosis. The microglandular adenosis glands are strongly positive for S100. The normal lobules/ducts show staining of the myoepithelium only; fat cells are also positive.

## Essential and desirable diagnostic criteria
*Essential:* a haphazard proliferation of small, round, and uniform glands infiltrating into the breast parenchyma and adipose tissue without destroying the pre-existing normal glands; the glands are lined by a single layer of cuboidal cells without atypia.

## Staging
Not clinically relevant

## Prognosis and prediction
Microglandular adenosis is a benign proliferation, but atypical forms and carcinomas arising in microglandular adenosis have been described {1928,10}. On the basis of molecular and cytogenetic similarities among these lesions, some investigators have suggested that microglandular adenosis is a nonobligate precursor lesion of basal-type breast carcinoma {712}. More studies are needed to establish this connection.

# Radial scar / complex sclerosing lesion

Sahin A
Collins LC

## Definition
Radial scar / complex sclerosing lesion is a benign lesion with fibroelastosis and entrapped glandular structures, with or without proliferative epithelial lesions. Radial scars are small lesions, typically with a stellate configuration, whereas complex sclerosing lesions are larger and more disorganized.

## ICD-O coding
None

## ICD-11 coding
GB20.Y Other specified benign breast disease

## Related terminology
*Acceptable:* radial scar; radial sclerosing lesion; benign sclerosing ductal proliferation.
*Not recommended:* sclerosing papillary lesion; scleroelastotic scar; stellate scar; non-encapsulated sclerosing lesion; infiltrating epitheliosis.

## Subtype(s)
None

## Localization
Not applicable

## Clinical features
On breast imaging, the irregular stellate configuration may mimic an invasive carcinoma; the presence of a radiolucent centre is reported as indicative of radial scar as opposed to carcinoma.

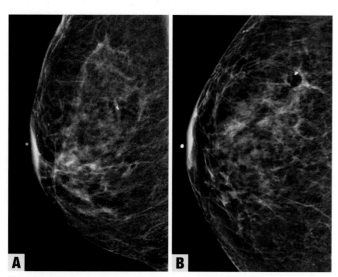

**Fig. 2.21** Radial scar / complex sclerosing lesion. **A** Right breast architectural distortion. **B** The spiculated appearance is similar to that of carcinoma, but the centre is a translucent, low-density area rather than a mass.

Very occasionally, the lesion is of sufficient size to produce a palpable mass. Radial scar / complex sclerosing lesion may be multiple and is frequently bilateral {378,1461,604}.

## Epidemiology
The reported incidence varies depending on the mode of detection. In current practice, these lesions are most often identified by mammography {798}.

## Etiology
No specific factors have been identified that are etiologically linked to radial scar / complex sclerosing lesion.

## Pathogenesis
The molecular genetics of radial scar / complex sclerosing lesion have not been described. The molecular characteristics of the various epithelial hyperplastic processes found within them, and the forms of malignancy associated with them, are as described elsewhere in the relevant sections of this volume.

## Macroscopic appearance
These lesions may be undetectable on gross examination or may be of sufficient size to produce an irregular area of firmness that can exhibit yellow streaks reflecting the elastotic stroma. The gross appearance may be indistinguishable from that of an invasive carcinoma {798,378,1461,604}.

## Histopathology
Radial scar is a lobulocentric proliferation containing benign changes that may include cysts, usual ductal hyperplasia, and sclerosing adenosis. Radial scar has a stellate configuration, whereas complex sclerosing lesions are larger and more disorganized. Central dense hyalinized collagen and elastosis (sometimes marked) are seen. Entrapped in the central fibrous tissue are small, irregular, benign tubules. A two-cell layer is retained, although this layer may not always be visible on H&E staining, because the myoepithelial cell layer is occasionally attenuated. Around the periphery of the lesion there are various degrees of ductal dilatation, usual ductal hyperplasia, and apocrine metaplasia. In larger complex sclerosing lesions, several of these components appear to combine and then converge with intermingling areas of sclerosing adenosis and small, frequently sclerosing micropapillomas and various patterns of epithelial proliferation {798,378,1461,604}.

## Cytology
The epithelial cells may show the characteristics of usual ductal hyperplasia and/or apocrine metaplasia. The myoepithelial cells may be variably prominent. Cytological atypia is absent {764}.

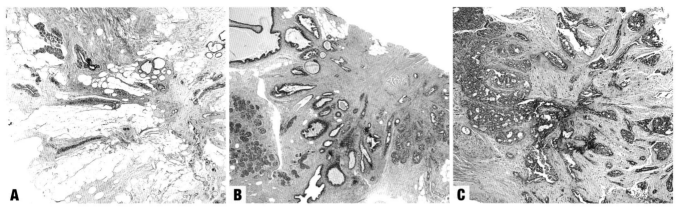

**Fig. 2.22** Radial scar / complex sclerosing lesion. **A** A small radial scar characterized by a fibroelastotic core and ducts radiating from the centre in a stellate configuration. **B** A larger radial scar with central fibroelastotic stroma. **C** A complex sclerosing lesion composed of proliferating glands associated with fibrotic stroma. The surrounding ducts show various degrees of epithelial proliferation.

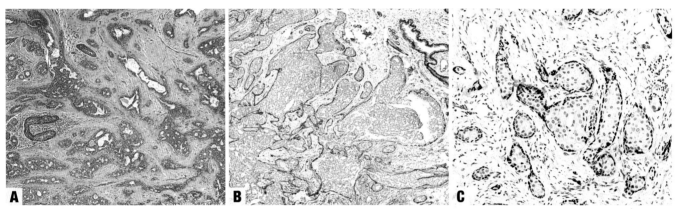

**Fig. 2.23** Ductal carcinoma in situ involving complex sclerosing lesion. **A** Irregularly proliferating glands are expanded by ductal carcinoma in situ cells. Immunohistochemical staining for SMM (**B**) and p63 (**C**) highlights the myoepithelial cells.

## Diagnostic molecular pathology
Not clinically relevant

## Essential and desirable diagnostic criteria
*Essential:* characteristic lobulocentric architecture; presence of a myoepithelial cell layer and basement membrane around the tubular structures; dense hyalinized stroma with elastosis with lack of reactive fibroblastic stroma.
*Desirable:* demonstration of myoepithelial cells by immunohisto-chemistry (e.g. p63, calponin, SMMHC) if needed.

## Staging
Not clinically relevant

## Prognosis and prediction
Despite suggestions (especially in the radiology literature) that these lesions may be premalignant, there is no evidence to support this contention. The results of two long-term follow-up studies suggest that any apparent risk is related to the various patterns of associated intraductal hyperplasia. An update analysis of one of these studies showed that radial scar is associated with an increased risk of breast cancer even after adjustment for histological category of benign breast disease (relative risk: 1.74), whereas a meta-analysis suggested that the magnitude of risk is more modest (relative risk: 1.45). Atypical hyperplasia and carcinoma (both in situ and invasive) may involve or arise in association with radial scar / complex sclerosing lesion, particularly in lesions measuring > 0.6 cm, which are more often mammographically detected and found in women aged > 50 years. The management of radial scar and complex sclerosing lesion detected by mammography remains controversial {635,350, 535,1119}. Lesions with associated epithelial atypia detected on core needle biopsy have a risk of associated malignancy and should be excised. Newer data indicate that radiological–pathological concordant lesions without atypia may not require excision. A rare association between complex sclerosing lesion and metaplastic carcinoma, in particular low-grade adenosquamous carcinoma, has been described {378,1119,1970,1562}.

# Adenomas: Introduction

Jaffer SM
Moritani S
Silva L

"Adenoma" is the generic term for a benign glandular epithelial tumour. In the breast, adenomas are derived from a proliferation of the cells in the terminal duct lobular unit, resulting in a discrete mass corresponding to a well-circumscribed mass on clinical examination and imaging. The benign breast lesions categorized under the umbrella term "adenoma" contain various proportions of glandular, fibrous, and fatty tissue. The specific terminology applied to a given adenoma depends on the dominant proliferating cell type and its ratio to other cell types. For example, fibroadenoma (the most common type of adenoma) is a fibroepithelial lesion with an admixture of stroma and glands, whereas the predominant cells in tubular adenoma are the densely packed ductal and myoepithelial cells, with little or no background stroma. Lactating adenoma is a tumour that arises during pregnancy or lactation. Ductal adenoma is considered by some to be the equivalent of sclerosed intraductal papilloma. All of these adenomas have a negligible risk of malignant transformation.

# Tubular adenoma

Jaffer SM
Moritani S
Silva L

### Definition
Tubular adenoma is a benign well-circumscribed tumour composed of a dense proliferation of closely approximated round and oval tubular structures composed of bilayered ductal and myoepithelial cells, with little background stroma.

### ICD-O coding
8211/0 Tubular adenoma NOS

### ICD-11 coding
2F30.0 & XH7SY6 Tubular adenoma of breast & Tubular adenoma NOS

### Related terminology
*Not recommended:* fibroadenoma, pericanalicular subtype (with prominent epithelial proliferation).

### Subtype(s)
None

### Localization
Tubular adenoma arises in the upper-outer quadrant of the breast.

### Clinical features
Tubular adenomas are slow-growing neoplasms that may be detected 2–12 months after inception {1897}. On physical examination, they may present as a palpable, solitary, painless, freely mobile, well-defined mass. On imaging, they usually present as a well-circumscribed mass. On ultrasonography, they are hypoechoic with mild posterior acoustic resonance. Rapid enlargement has been described in two case reports: one in a pregnant woman {889} and the other in a postmenopausal woman {1829}. Rarely, tubular adenomas may present with clinical features suggestive of malignancy, including older patient age (> 48 years), a hard consistency, restricted mobility, poorly defined margins, large size, skin ulceration, rapid enlargement (2 months) {1897}, and suspicious findings on imaging (BI-RADS 4) {565}. Less commonly, they can present as clustered high-density suspicious calcifications in postmenopausal women, necessitating core biopsy, and can be found to be associated with intraluminal secretion. Only one case report describes the presentation in a postmenopausal woman with nipple discharge. Fibroadenoma and tubular adenoma share similar clinical, radiological, cytological, and immunohistochemical findings; therefore, tubular adenomas may be mistaken for fibroadenoma preoperatively, but they can be distinguished by histopathology.

### Epidemiology
The incidence of tubular adenoma ranges from 0.13% to 2.9% {1897,1896}. These tumours usually occur in young premenopausal women of childbearing age (15–49 years), with 90% of cases occurring in women aged < 40 years {1897}. Tubular

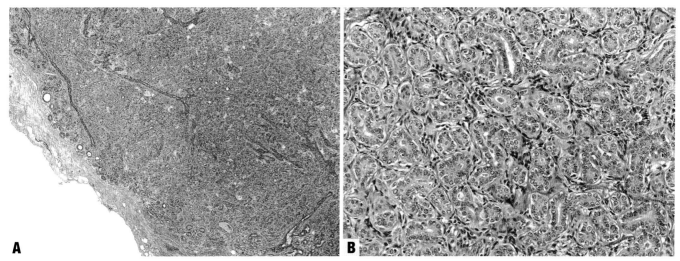

**Fig. 2.24** Tubular adenoma. **A** A well-circumscribed tumour composed of densely packed round tubules. **B** A high-power view shows tubules lined by an inner layer of ductal luminal cells and outer attenuated basal myoepithelial cells with minimal intervening stroma.

adenoma very rarely arises before menarche or after menopause.

## Etiology

Tubular adenomas arise from terminal duct lobular units. The exact etiology is unknown, but given the incidence in women of reproductive age, it is most likely related to reproductive hormones. This assumption is also supported by the close similarity and relationship of tubular adenoma to fibroadenoma, which is also influenced by hormones during the reproductive years. However, no association with pregnancy or oral contraceptive use has been described.

## Pathogenesis

The overlap in clinicopathological features between tubular adenoma and fibroadenoma, their occasional coexistence, and their combined features in an adenoma {1375} suggest that they share a common histogenetic mechanism {157}, with the stromal component dominating in fibroadenoma and the epithelial and myoepithelial cells dominating in tubular adenoma. The few cases of tubular adenoma that have been studied using next-generation sequencing showed mutations in *MET* and *FGFR3*. Despite the similarity between fibroadenoma and tubular adenoma, these studies failed to show the presence of *MED12* exon 2 mutations, a frequent finding in fibroadenoma {2189}. This discrepancy is best explained by the fact that tubular adenomas closely resemble the pericanalicular subset of fibroadenomas, which are known to have a lower prevalence of *MED12* exon 2 mutations than intracanalicular fibroadenomas. Given their similarities in clinical, radiological, cytological, and immunohistochemical findings, as well as their occasional admixture and association, tubular adenoma and fibroadenoma may be histogenetically related, despite the few cases exhibiting differences in molecular pathology {2189}.

## Macroscopic appearance

Tumour size is generally 1–7.5 cm (average: 3.0 cm), with a few giant forms (as large as 15 cm {2365}) reported in the literature. Like fibroadenomas, tubular adenomas are usually smoothly rounded, unencapsulated, firm tumours that have a solid homogeneous or micronodular rubbery cut surface. However, they tend to be softer than fibroadenomas and are yellow to tan-brown in colour rather than white like fibroadenomas.

## Histopathology

Low-power histology of tubular adenoma shows a sharply demarcated compact proliferation of small uniformly round and regular tubular structures. At high power, the tubules are noted to be lined by a double layer of inner ductal luminal cells and an outer layer of attenuated basal myoepithelial cells, similar to normal resting breast epithelium. Rare nucleoli, atypia, and mitoses are seen. The lumen is usually empty but can occasionally contain mucin or PAS-positive eosinophilic proteinaceous material, which is not immunoreactive for α-lactalbumin. Unlike in fibroadenomas, there is sparse intervening stroma, mainly consisting of a delicate fibrovascular network and possibly containing a few scattered lymphocytes. Consequently, no compression of the tubules due to fibrosis is evident. Infarction has rarely been described (in 2.4% of cases). Fibroadenoma and tubular adenoma can be definitively distinguished only on histopathology, the key features being the prominent florid adenosis-like epithelial proliferation and the minimal stroma within tubular adenoma.

## Cytology

The cytological findings of tubular adenoma have been described (in only a few retrospective series {1897}) as moderately to highly cellular smears containing numerous tight 3D ball-like clusters composed of bland-looking ductal cells with probable acinar formation. The ductal cells may also occasionally be arranged in papillary or staghorn shapes. The background contains myoepithelial cells appearing as naked nuclei, with hardly any stromal fragments. These constellations of findings may also be seen in fibroadenoma, for which tubular adenoma may therefore be easily mistaken. When excess tubular fragments are present, the diagnosis of tubular adenoma should be considered, but this diagnosis can rarely be accurately rendered preoperatively {1896}. One case in the recent literature was misinterpreted as atypical due to the high cellularity of the specimen, large size of the lesion (> 8.5 cm), and associated calcifications {1897}. Given the difficulty in recognizing tubular adenoma on cytology, histopathology remains the gold standard for definitive diagnosis.

## Diagnostic molecular pathology
Not clinically relevant

## Essential and desirable diagnostic criteria
*Essential:* a well-circumscribed tumour composed of a dense proliferation of closely approximated round and oval tubular structures with little background stroma; tubules composed of bilayered ductal and myoepithelial cells.

*Desirable:* immunohistochemical evaluation for confirmation of the dual cell population by myoepithelial markers (p63, p40, SMA, calponin) and luminal markers (EMA, CK19, CK8/18) if needed.

## Staging
Not clinically relevant

## Prognosis and prediction
Tubular adenomas are benign, stable neoplasms with no increased risk of developing into a malignancy. However, there are a few case reports in the literature that describe their association with ductal carcinoma in situ and invasive ductal carcinoma {1822,534}. In one of the two such cases reported, the two entities were histologically distinct and most likely collision tumours. In the other, the two entities were admixed, raising the possibility of malignant transformation. No recurrences have been reported in the few completely excised cases with short-term follow-up (18 months). As with fibroadenomas, it is sufficient to follow asymptomatic tubular adenomas with observation, annual clinical breast examination, and imaging. Surgical excision may be necessary in cases with worrisome clinical features, for cosmetic reasons, or for definitive diagnosis.

# Lactating adenoma

Jaffer SM
Moritani S
Silva L

## Definition
Lactating adenoma is a benign breast nodule, diagnosed during pregnancy or breastfeeding, that is composed of aggregates of glands showing lactational change.

## ICD-O coding
8204/0 Lactating adenoma

## ICD-11 coding
2F30.1 & XH0W31 Lactating adcnoma of breast & Lactating adenoma

## Related terminology
*Not recommended:* tumour of pregnancy; nodular lactational hyperplasia.

## Subtype(s)
None

## Localization
Lactating adenoma occurs predominantly in the breast (sometimes bilaterally and multifocally) and rarely along the milk line from the axilla to the groin.

## Clinical features
Lactating adenoma usually presents as a soft, painless, palpable, solid, mobile, discrete mass, without nipple or skin changes. Infarction can occur in as many as 5% of cases {2019}, due to vascular insufficiency from increased physiological demands, which may result in enlargement, pain, tenderness, and suspicious imaging findings. Lactating adenoma is usually < 5 cm, but it has the potential for rapid growth and enlargement (up to 25 cm). Termination of breastfeeding usually leads to spontaneous regression within 1–5 months, but rare antepartum {2067, 1288} and postpartum {587} enlargement has been described. Mammography usually shows a well-circumscribed tumour, but lactating adenoma can rarely present as a partially obscured or asymmetrical mass. The sonographic features include a smooth homogeneously hypoechoic solid round to oval mass with the longer axis (when there is one) parallel to the chest wall (transverse). Additionally, a microlobulated border, hypervascularization, posterior acoustic enhancement, and an echogenic pseudocapsule may be seen. Alternatively, due to the milk fat, lactating adenoma may appear hyperechoic or radiolucent. A conspicuous midline tubular structure may be seen, representing a dilated duct. Sonography is the preferred mode of diagnosis {121} due to the increased physiological density of the pregnant/lactating breast, which can interfere with the interpretation of mammography and MRI. Additionally, irradiation from mammography and the administration of contrast material for MRI are not favoured during pregnancy. Although sonography may be reliable in diagnosing lactating adenoma, the definitive distinction from fibroadenoma can be challenging. Confirmatory tissue diagnosis, which is achieved with biopsy/excision, is indicated if the mass rapidly enlarges and has worrisome sonographic findings such as posterior shadowing, irregular margins, and heterogeneity.

## Epidemiology
Despite its name, lactating adenoma occurs more frequently during the third trimester of pregnancy (and rarely in the first or second) than after childbirth, and it almost never occurs outside of gestation, accounting for approximately 70% of all core biopsies in this population. However, not all lactating adenomas

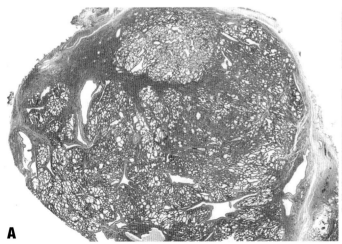
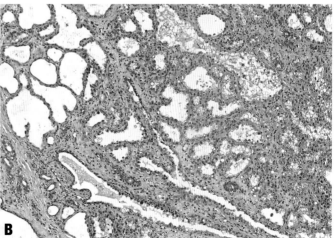

**Fig. 2.25** Lactating adenoma. **A** Low magnification shows a circumscribed nodule composed of closely packed and dilated tubules. **B** At higher magnification, the tubules are lined by single-layered cuboidal epithelial cells with vacuolated cytoplasm and occasional hobnail nuclei, with myoepithelial attenuation. Some dilated tubules contain luminal pink flocculent secretions.

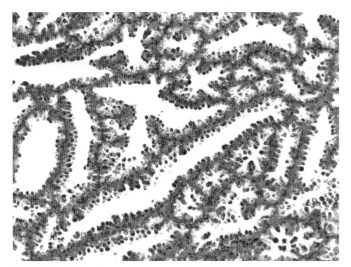

**Fig. 2.26** Lactating adenoma. High-power view showing epithelial cells arranged in a ductuloalveolar network lined by hobnail-shaped cells containing granular or vacuolated clear cytoplasm.

undergo biopsy/excision, and the true incidence is therefore unknown. Lactating adenoma usually affects women aged 19–34 years, with most cases occurring in the third decade of life.

### Etiology
Unknown

### Pathogenesis
It remains unknown whether lactating adenoma is a de novo tumour, a hyperplastic lesion, or a pre-existing fibroadenoma with superimposed induced physiological changes. Lactating adenoma and tubular adenoma are considered two ends of a spectrum, because both are characterized by florid epithelial proliferation with minimal stroma. In fact, the histological and ultrastructural changes of lactating adenoma in the first and second trimester resemble those of tubular adenoma. The few cases of lactating adenoma that have been studied using next-generation sequencing failed to show any of the mutations, including *MED12* exon 2 mutations, frequently seen in fibroadenomas {2189}.

### Macroscopic appearance
Lactating adenoma is a well-circumscribed, unencapsulated, lobulated solid mass, with a firm (but softer than fibroadenoma or tubular adenoma) to rubbery greyish-tan to yellow cut surface. Necrosis may be seen in infarcted tumours.

### Histopathology
Lactating adenoma is a well-circumscribed proliferation of closely packed hyperplastic secretory lobules separated by sparse delicate connective tissue, which may be oedematous. Lactating adenomas in the first and second trimester resemble tubular adenomas because they are composed of round to irregular oval acinar structures, but with variability in the size and shape of the glands. After the second trimester, the tumours mature and are composed of epithelial cells arranged in variably sized ductuloalveolar spaces. This network is lined by cuboidal or hobnail-shaped cells containing granular or vacuolated clear cytoplasm, as well as luminal eosinophilic secretions (milk), both of which are Oil Red O–positive and contain α-lactalbumin. The cells have small round nuclei, with no atypia and occasional mitoses. Identical cytological and ultrastructural changes are seen in surrounding breast tissue. Fibroadenoma may also show secretory activity, but it is distinguished from lactating adenoma by its preserved fibroepithelial architecture, prominent stroma, and focal rather than dense proliferation of cells with secretory activity.

### Cytology
Low power shows moderately cellular specimens with an abundant secretory proteinaceous background containing a monotonous population of dyscohesive single cells with naked nuclei, as well as large 3D acinar cell aggregates. At high power, the acinar cell aggregates are noted to have vacuolated and wispy cytoplasm, as well as smoothly contoured nuclei containing fine nuclear chromatin with prominent but uniform pinpoint nucleoli. In the absence of information regarding pregnancy and lactation, the physiological proliferative cytological features may be easily overdiagnosed as atypia. The cytological findings include atypical dyscohesive cells containing prominent macronucleoli in a granular lacy background {852}. However, false negativity may occur due to atypia being obscured by the lactational changes. Therefore, histopathology is the gold standard for definitive diagnosis.

### Diagnostic molecular pathology
Not clinically relevant

### Essential and desirable diagnostic criteria
*Essential:* a well-circumscribed proliferation of closely packed hyperplastic secretory lobules separated by sparse delicate connective tissue; bland-looking lining epithelial cells containing vacuolated or granular cytoplasm and small nuclei with pinpoint uniform nucleoli.

### Staging
Not clinically relevant

### Prognosis and prediction
Given the tumour's stable, slow growth and spontaneous regression, the management of lactating adenoma is observation, but follow-up is necessary to exclude malignancy {2067}. Enucleation may be necessary due to worrisome features, with resumption of breastfeeding after surgery. Bromocriptine treatment causes involution by suppressing prolactin, but this also leads to cessation of breastfeeding. Studies with follow-up ranging from 6 months to 14 years (average: 3.4 years) have shown no progression to cancer, but simultaneous occurrence with breast cancer has been described in some cases {1077,1817}. In one case, invasive carcinoma occurred at the site of a previously excised lactating adenoma. In another, transition from lactating adenoma to carcinoma was noted. Importantly, the hormones that prime breast development during pregnancy, such as estrogen, progesterone, and prolactin (especially progesterone and prolactin), also play a role in carcinogenesis. Therefore, it is unclear whether lactating adenoma is capable of malignant transformation, is a risk factor, or happens to coincidentally occur adjacent to malignancy.

# Ductal adenoma

Jaffer SM
Moritani S
Silva L

## Definition
Ductal adenoma is a benign tumour composed of distorted glands in a sclerotic stroma surrounded by a fibrous capsule.

## ICD-O coding
8503/0 Duct adenoma NOS

## ICD-11 coding
2F30.2 & XH4LZ4 Intraductal papilloma of breast & Intraductal papilloma

## Related terminology
*Not recommended:* sclerosing papilloma.

## Subtype(s)
None

## Localization
Ductal adenoma arises in medium-sized and small ducts of the peripheral breast.

## Clinical features
Ductal adenoma usually presents as a palpable solitary lump, but it may have an irregular appearance when multifocal. It usually arises from the small and medium-sized ducts. Rarely, it can involve the larger ducts and present with nipple discharge, similar to intraductal papilloma. Mammography shows a discrete mass, poorly defined margins, spiculation, multilobulation, and/or irregularly shaped calcifications. Sonography shows a well-defined, round hypoechoic nodule, with shadowing and posterior enhancement. Few cases of infarction have been described in pregnancy and lactation {1545}.

## Epidemiology
Ductal adenoma is a rare tumour that occurs in the sixth decade of life. It has been described in four cases to be bilateral and associated with Carney complex {291}.

## Etiology
Ductal adenoma predominantly arises from the small and medium-sized ductal lumina in the peripheral breast, but it may rarely arise from the larger ducts {1107}. In contrast, intraductal papilloma arises from both small to medium-sized peripheral ducts and predominantly larger subareolar ducts.

## Pathogenesis
It is hypothesized that ductal adenoma most likely originates from intraductal papilloma in small and medium-sized ducts. Due to a stromal repair process, intraductal papilloma may undergo sclerosis, which is manifested by a myofibroblastic proliferation and deposition of fibronectin and interstitial collagen, resulting in loss of the arborizing papillary architecture.

Overlapping features of radial scar (e.g. central elastosis) may also be seen, because radial scars in ductal adenoma are considered part of the spectrum of papillary lesions. Some authors contend that a hyperplastic process such as sclerosing adenosis, which is prevalent in ductal adenoma, may lead to ductal adenoma by direct expansion into small and medium-sized ducts or into a coexistent intraductal papilloma. The few cases of ductal adenoma that have been studied using next-generation sequencing show mutations in *PIK3CA*, *GNAS*, and *AKT1* {2189}. *AKT1* mutations have also been detected in intraductal papillomas {2106}, supporting a close relationship with (or an origin similar to that of) ductal adenomas.

## Macroscopic appearance
Ductal adenomas range in size from 0.5 to 5.0 cm (average: 0.85 cm) and present as a discrete, white, solid nodule. On cut surface, they are lobulated and granular, with central grey softening. Calcified areas may seem firm, gritty, and pseudoinvasive. Focal attachment to a dilated cyst or duct may occasionally be seen. Rarely, the tumour may have a poorly defined edge that is firmly adherent to the surrounding breast stroma, raising suspicion for an invasive carcinoma. Additionally, ductal adenoma can be multinodular due to involvement of proximal or distal parts of the same ductal system.

## Histopathology
Ductal adenoma is usually a solitary solid adenomatous proliferation surrounded by a densely thickened concentric fibroelastotic wall, but it may be multinodular at times. The adenomatous portion consists of glands arranged in organized parallel patterns, radiating outwards from the centre to the periphery. The glands range in shape from round to oval, elongated to branched; they are composed of a bilayer of luminal ductal and attenuated myoepithelial cells, with a modest amount of intervening fibrous stroma. The stroma may compress and obliterate the glands, similar to in sclerosing adenosis. The glands may cystically dilate, have luminal tufting, contain PAS-positive eosinophilic secretions, and/or contain associated laminated calcifications. At high power, the ductal cells are noted to be cuboidal, columnar, and/or spindled, with eosinophilic cytoplasm, but they lack atypia and may have rare mitoses. The capsule is laminated and hyalinized; it contains dystrophic calcifications and thus may entrap glands or protrude into surrounding tissue and appear to have a pushing or pseudoinfiltrative border. In addition to calcifications, the sclerotic wall may also show chronic inflammation, haemorrhage, myxoid change, and squamous and chondroid metaplasia. Degenerative changes with or without calcifications may be seen in the periphery or centre; degenerative changes in the centre may resemble and overlap with histological features of a radial scar. The surrounding breast may show sclerosing adenosis, apocrine metaplasia, or cystic duct ectasia. No arborizing papillary fronds (as seen in

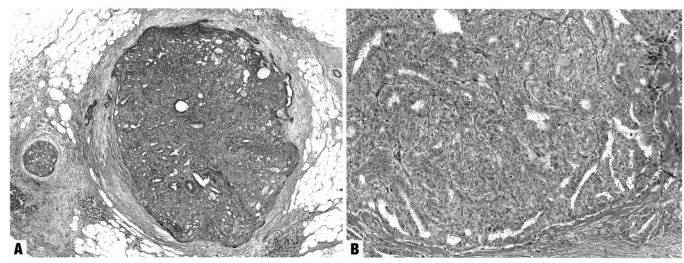

**Fig. 2.27** Ductal adenoma. **A** Low power shows a discrete solid adenomatous proliferation surrounded by a thick, concentric sclerotic wall that entraps glands, resulting in pushing or pseudoinfiltrative borders. **B** High power shows round to oval, elongated to branched glands composed of a bilayer of luminal ductal and attenuated myoepithelial cells, focally appearing pseudoinvasive.

intraductal papilloma) or myoepithelial hyperplasia (as seen in adenomyoepithelioma) is evident. Ductal adenomas show low p53 and Ki-67 labelling {2069}.

## Cytology

Aspirates of ductal adenoma are highly cellular, consisting of numerous branching monolayered sheets of regularly arranged cohesive epithelial cells with uniform nuclei, nucleoli, chromatin, and punched-out cytoplasmic vacuoles. The background consists of bipolar and oval naked nuclei, histiocytes, and apocrine cells. The unique feature is the presence of metachromatic or eosinophilic stroma that is intimately admixed with the stroma in finger-like hyaline projections or as small ovoid well-circumscribed globules {941}. These globules may mimic some features of collagenous spherulosis but lack other features. The high cellularity may prompt consideration of malignancy (in particular adenoid cystic carcinoma) in the differential, but all malignancies are easily excluded when the benign cytological details of the epithelial cells are appreciated. Fibroadenoma is differentiated by its cellular stroma, which is separate from the epithelium.

## Diagnostic molecular pathology

Not clinically relevant

## Essential and desirable diagnostic criteria

*Essential:* well-circumscribed tumour composed of an adenomatous proliferation surrounded by a laminated concentric fibrosclerotic wall; round to oval, elongated to branched glands composed of a bilayer of luminal ductal and attenuated myoepithelial cells, with a modest amount of intervening fibrous stroma; cuboidal, columnar, and/or spindled ductal cells with eosinophilic cytoplasm, lacking atypia, with rare mitoses.

## Staging

Not clinically relevant

## Prognosis and prediction

Ductal adenoma is a benign, stable neoplasm with no increased risk for recurrence or malignant development after complete excision, a finding supported by low p53 and Ki-67 labelling {2069}. Excision is often recommended due to histological and radiological mimicry of carcinoma, especially on clinical examination, imaging, and core biopsy. A few cases reported in the literature have been associated with ductal and lobular carcinoma in situ, but this association is most likely attributable to coexistence rather than malignant transformation.

# Epithelial-myoepithelial tumours: Introduction

Tan PH
Ellis IO

Epithelial-myoepithelial tumours of the breast are biphasic neoplasms composed of both epithelial and myoepithelial cells. The benign epithelial-myoepithelial tumours are pleomorphic adenoma and adenomyoepithelioma (AME). The malignant epithelial-myoepithelial tumours include adenoid cystic carcinoma and malignant AME, in which the malignant component may be derived from luminal epithelium, myoepithelium, or both. Adenoid cystic carcinoma is described in the section on rare and salivary gland–type tumours.

AME of the breast was first described by Hamperl in 1970 {817}. Its morphological resemblance to epithelial-myoepithelial carcinoma of the salivary glands was noted in previous reports {2343,1888,666,927}. For this edition of the WHO Classification of Tumours series, there was a proposal to consider harmonizing the terminology with that of the salivary glands, where no benign counterpart exists (i.e. breast AME would instead be referred to as epithelial-myoepithelial carcinoma). However, breast AMEs demonstrate a spectrum of histological patterns {2328,1338,2053}, and many display benign clinical behaviour {1419,2328,2242}, although there have been reports of local recurrence, malignant transformation, and metastasis {2328},

including rare anecdotal reports of metastasis from histologically benign tumours {1438}. The morphological heterogeneity of breast AME is also affirmed by recent genetic data, with ER-positive AMEs displaying *PIK3CA* or *AKT1* activating mutations, whereas ER-negative tumours harbour *HRAS* mutations {715}. In consideration of the usually indolent course after excision and concern for possible overtreatment if the terminology is uniformly replaced by "carcinoma" {1338}, it was decided that the term "adenomyoepithelioma" be retained, albeit acknowledging that some tumours may be accompanied by malignant change, which should be identified through careful histological examination. Such tumours should then be referred to as malignant AMEs (AMEs with carcinoma) with description of the corresponding malignant component, which will facilitate appropriate therapy.

Because myoepithelial cells in epithelial-myoepithelial tumours may be demonstrated by immunohistochemistry, it is important to be familiar with the range, sensitivity, and specificity of the antibodies that may be used for their detection. Table 2.01 shows a list of such antibodies, including their cross-reactivities. It is recommended to use a limited panel

**Table 2.01** Antibodies to detect myoepithelial cells

| Myoepithelial marker | Subcellular localization | Comments |
|---|---|---|
| High-molecular-weight (basal) cytokeratins (CK5, CK5/6, CK14, CK17) | Cytoplasmic | May stain epithelial cells of basal-like (usually high-grade) in situ and invasive carcinomas, as well as luminal cells |
| SMA | Cytoplasmic | Stains stromal myofibroblasts |
| MSA | Cytoplasmic | Stains stromal myofibroblasts |
| Calponin | Cytoplasmic | Stains stromal myofibroblasts |
| Caldesmon | Cytoplasmic | No reactivity with stromal myofibroblasts |
| SMMHC | Cytoplasmic | Stains stromal myofibroblasts |
| p63 | Nuclear | May stain epithelial cells of in situ and invasive ductal carcinomas (usually high-grade) and metaplastic carcinoma with squamous differentiation |
| p40 | Nuclear | May stain epithelial cells of in situ and invasive carcinomas (usually high-grade) and metaplastic carcinoma with squamous differentiation |
| p75 | Cytoplasmic and membranous | May decorate endothelial cells, vascular adventitia, stromal cells, and benign and malignant epithelial cells |
| CD10 | Cytoplasmic | May weakly stain stromal myofibroblasts |
| S100 | Cytoplasmic and nuclear | May stain normal, hyperplastic, and neoplastic epithelial cells |
| GFAP | Cytoplasmic | |
| Maspin | Cytoplasmic and nuclear | May stain normal, hyperplastic, and neoplastic epithelial cells |
| P-cadherin | Cytoplasmic and membranous | |
| D2-40 | Cytoplasmic | Stains endothelial cells and lymphatic channels |
| WT1 | Cytoplasmic | Stains endothelial cells |

of myoepithelial markers (e.g. SMMHC and p63), rather than relying on a single marker. Some target antigens are more labile and may be lost with suboptimal fixation. Markers such as SMA, although less myoepithelial-specific, are more robust and can be helpful in assessing myoepithelial cells in poorly fixed specimens. The choice of antibodies to myoepithelial cells may also depend on the lesion being evaluated, because some antibodies may be less helpful than others in certain cases. For example, p63 is useful for distinguishing in situ from invasive carcinoma, with myoepithelial cells being retained in the former and lost in the latter, but it is not as useful as high-molecular-weight cytokeratins for corroborating usual ductal hyperplasia. Myoepithelial cells in benign sclerosing lesions and ductal carcinoma in situ may be immunophenotypically different from normal myoepithelial cells {856,855}, and acinar myoepithelial cells with less developed myofilaments can display staining differences from ductal myoepithelial cells {1100}.

# Pleomorphic adenoma

Foschini MP
Geyer FC
Hayes MM
Marchiò C
Nishimura R

## Definition
Pleomorphic adenoma (PA) is a benign tumour with variable cytomorphological and architectural manifestations of epithelial and myoepithelial components set within a chondromyxoid stroma.

## ICD-O coding
8940/0 Pleomorphic adenoma

## ICD-11 coding
2F30.Y & XH2KC1 Other specified benign neoplasm of breast & Pleomorphic adenoma

## Related terminology
None

## Subtype(s)
None

## Localization
PA of the breast usually arises in the retroareolar region {668}.

## Clinical features
PA presents as a nodule, affecting mainly adult women {505, 668}. Rare cases affect male patients {1947}. On mammography and ultrasound examination, PA appears as a roundish lesion with well-defined borders, simulating fibroadenoma. PA with intraductal growth can present as a cystic lesion {84,505}. Radiological diagnosis is sometimes complicated by the presence of microcalcifications, which can prompt suspicion for malignancy {732}.

## Epidemiology
PA is the most frequent tumour of the salivary glands, whereas it is very rare in the breast. Our knowledge of breast PA is mainly based on single case reports or small series. Therefore, exact data on incidence are unknown.

## Etiology
Unknown

## Pathogenesis
PA arising in the salivary glands shows rearrangements on PLAG1 and HMGA2 {1632,2198,981}. No data are currently available on molecular alterations in breast PA.

## Macroscopic appearance
PA presents as a solid nodule, hard in consistency and with well-defined margins. The size is usually 1–2 cm. Longstanding nodules can reach larger sizes.

## Histopathology
PA of the breast shows histological features superimposable to those seen in the salivary glands {505,668,1138}. Specifically, it

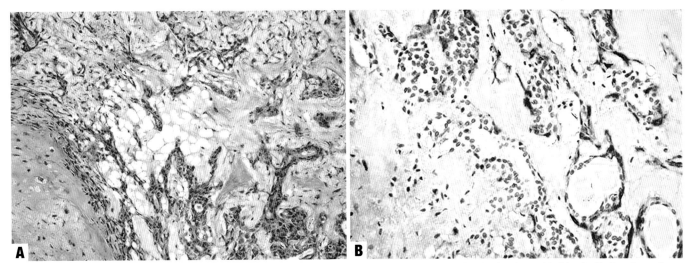

**Fig. 2.28** Pleomorphic adenoma. **A** Pleomorphic adenoma is composed of glands surrounded by epithelial cells, with a thin rim of myoepithelial cells. Single stellate cells are dispersed in the stroma. **B** Myoepithelial cell markers, such as SMA, are helpful to identify the peripheral and thin myoepithelial cell layer.

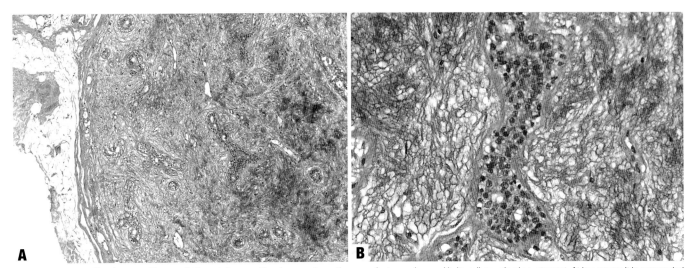

**Fig. 2.29** Pleomorphic adenoma of breast. **A** Breast pleomorphic adenoma shows the same features observed in its salivary gland counterpart. At low power, it is surrounded by a fibrous pseudocapsule and characterized by glands and cells immersed in a myxochondroid stroma. **B** Higher magnification of pleomorphic adenoma with glands and cells in a chondromyxoid stroma.

is composed of a neoplastic proliferation of epithelial and myoepithelial cells, organized in glandular structures and strands immersed in a myxochondroid stroma. In addition, single stellate cells are present. The neoplastic glands are lined by an inner layer of epithelial cells and an outer layer of myoepithelial cells. The strands of polygonal, oval, and stellate cells are mainly composed of myoepithelial cells. No cellular atypia, necrosis, or atypical mitotic figures are present. The stroma is usually myxochondroid, but cartilaginous or osseous metaplasia can be observed. PA can present as an intraductal growth {505}, sometimes similar to ductal adenoma. In some cases, PA shows a polypoid intraductal growth, resulting in a multinodular structure. In addition, some cases are associated with typical features of ductal adenoma, suggesting a relationship between the two lesions.

Immunohistochemical staining demonstrates the dual epithelial and myoepithelial cell components. Specifically, myoepithelial markers, including SMA, calponin, p63, and CK14, are usually positive in the cells composing the outer layer of the neoplastic glands and the neoplastic strands. In contrast, pure luminal cell markers, including low-molecular-weight cytokeratin and EMA, label the epithelial component.

The differential diagnosis includes tumours with mucinous and myxoid stroma (e.g. mucinous carcinoma and matrix-producing metaplastic carcinoma) and biphasic tumours such as adenomyoepithelioma. Mucinous carcinoma is easily excluded, because it is composed of neoplastic epithelial cells, lacks myoepithelium, and is immersed in a background of epithelial-type mucins. The differential diagnosis can be more subtle when matrix-producing carcinoma is considered {1699}. PA lacks cellular atypia, atypical mitotic figures, and necrosis. PA glands have a well-organized biphasic pattern, with a thin and continuous outer layer of myoepithelial cells and an inner layer of regular epithelial cells. In contrast, matrix-producing carcinoma is composed of atypical cells (with frequent atypical mitotic figures) organized in nests and aggregates, with no clearly recognizable architecture and no organized layer of myoepithelial cells around the neoplastic structures. Adenomyoepithelioma is typically composed of glands showing a double cell layer (epithelial and myoepithelial), and it may display a chondromyxoid stroma. Unlike PA, adenomyoepithelioma shows a prominent and often multistratified myoepithelial cell layer. In addition, nuclear atypia and mitoses are frequently seen in adenomyoepithelioma, whereas they are absent in PA.

## Cytology

FNA can be difficult to interpret, especially if the possibility of a salivary gland–type tumour in the breast is not taken into consideration. Specifically, smears are usually highly cellular, composed of cell aggregates and chondromyxoid material. The epithelial cells have roundish, plump cytoplasm and are typically arranged in glandular clusters, whereas the myoepithelial cells are elongated or plasmacytoid. Metachromatic chondromyxoid material can be evident with Giemsa staining {1827}. The absence of atypia, mitotic figures, and necrosis is essential to distinguish PA from matrix-producing carcinoma of the breast {2023}.

## Diagnostic molecular pathology

Not clinically relevant

## Essential and desirable diagnostic criteria

*Essential:* well-defined margins; glands lined by a double cell layer (epithelial and myoepithelial), with no atypia or mitoses, immersed in a myxochondroid background.

## Staging

Not clinically relevant

## Prognosis and prediction

PA of the breast is benign {505}. Recurrences can occur in cases characterized by extensive polypoid intraductal growth that are not completely excised at the time of surgery {952}. PA of the salivary glands can undergo malignant transformation {914}. To date, only one paper has described malignant transformation in PA of the breast: Hayes et al. reported 3 cases of in situ and invasive breast carcinoma arising in close association with PA, one of which led to the patient's death {837}.

# Adenomyoepithelioma

Foschini MP
Geyer FC
Hayes MM
Marchiò C
Nishimura R

## Definition
Adenomyoepithelioma (AME) is a biphasic neoplasm (usually benign) characterized by small epithelium-lined spaces with inner luminal ductal cells and a proliferation of variably enlarged and clearly noticeable abluminal myoepithelial cells. Malignant transformation may occur from either the luminal or myoepithelial component.

## ICD-O coding
8983/0 Adenomyoepithelioma NOS

## ICD-11 coding
2F30.Y & XH2V57 Other specified benign neoplasm of breast & Adenomyoepithelioma, benign

## Related terminology
The related lesion in the salivary glands is currently referred to as epithelial-myoepithelial carcinoma, which is histologically similar to the ER-negative form of breast AME {715}.

## Subtype(s)
None

## Localization
AME can arise in both the breast parenchyma and the retroareolar region {2328}. Nipple discharge can occur when large lactiferous ducts are involved {2366}.

## Clinical features
AME predominantly affects elderly women, with a peak age of > 60 years, but a wide age range is reported {2328}, with rare cases affecting male patients {2028,146}. AME usually presents as a palpable nodule, sometimes reaching a large size (up to 10 cm). Breast cancer screening programmes have led to the discovery of smaller lesions {1134}. On rare occasions, AME

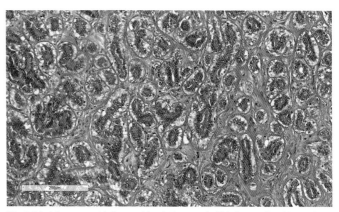

**Fig. 2.31** Adenomyoepithelioma with tubular growth. Tubules are lined by an inner layer of epithelial cells surrounded by an outer layer of prominent clear myoepithelial cells.

can be associated with genetic syndromes, such as neurofibromatosis type 1 {840}.

## Epidemiology
AME is a rare breast tumour, but its true incidence is unknown. In a series of 2078 consecutive breast tumours diagnosed by core needle biopsy, Cheung et al. found one case of AME (0.048%) {339}.

## Etiology
Unknown

## Pathogenesis
The genetic drivers of AME vary according to ER status. *PIK3CA* hotspot mutations occur across both subtypes (> 50%), whereas *AKT1* hotspot mutations may be restricted to ER-positive cases, and highly recurrent (> 60%) *HRAS* p.Gln61 hotspot mutations may be restricted to ER-negative cases. Notably, *HRAS* p.Gln61

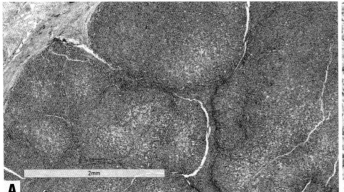

**Fig. 2.30** Adenomyoepithelioma. **A** At low power, adenomyoepithelioma can present lobulated margins. **B** Myoepithelial cells can sometimes be prominent, obscuring the epithelial component.

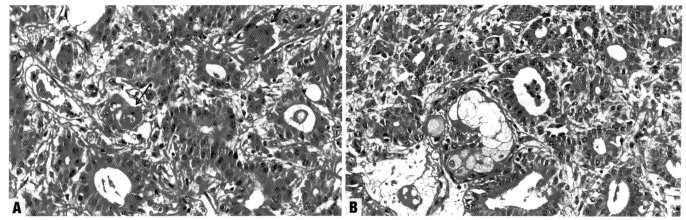

**Fig. 2.32** Adenomyoepithelioma. On rare occasions, focal squamous differentiation (**A**, arrows) or sebaceous differentiation (**B**) can be seen.

hotspot mutations are also frequently found in epithelial-myoepithelial carcinomas of the salivary glands. Homozygous deletions of *CDKN2A* are also recurrent in ER-negative AMEs and have been associated with AMEs associated with carcinoma.

## Macroscopic appearance

AME usually presents as a circumscribed nodule with pushing margins. On rare occasions, cystic or papillary areas can be present {2328}.

## Histopathology

Classic AME is composed of glandular structures surrounded by a double cell layer: epithelial cells line the glandular lumen and myoepithelial cells constitute the outer cell layer. AME presents various architectural patterns {2053,1785}, including lobulated, papillary, and tubular, frequently mixed in the same case. At low-power magnification, AME shows a multilobulated contour and contains central sclerotic areas {1338,2022,2331,1785}. Small satellite nodules can occur at the periphery of the main mass {1338,2022,2331,1785,2366}. Tubular AME is composed of a relatively uniform admixture of small ductal structures lined by a luminal layer of epithelial cells cuffed by an outer layer of conspicuous myoepithelial cells {2053,1785}. Spindle cell AME is characterized by a prominent growth of spindle myoepithelial cells surrounding and compressing glandular structures lined by epithelial cells, which can sometimes be difficult to visualize {2053,2328}. Lobulated AME shows nests of neoplastic cells predominantly of the myoepithelial type, surrounded by a dense hyaline sclerotic collagenous matrix material that probably reflects production of excessive basement membrane material {691}. The matrix may sometimes be myxoid and even chondroid, reminiscent of that seen in pleomorphic adenoma.

Limited data are available on preoperative core biopsy diagnosis {2306,303,339}. Diagnosis should be based on the classic biphasic epithelial-myoepithelial pattern, and attention should be paid to exclude other lesions, such as intraductal papilloma. Intraductal papillary growth merging with features of classic papilloma or ductal adenoma is sometimes present {1785,2328}. The papillary component may be observed in dilated ducts at the periphery of the main tumour nodule. The luminal cells show apocrine metaplasia that can be evident on H&E staining or may be corroborated by immunostaining with the GCDFP-15 antibody. On rare occasions, squamous or sebaceous differentiation can be seen {264,2053}. Myoepithelial cells in AME can present a great variety of morphological features. They often have clear glycogen-rich cytoplasm {1005} and spindle, myoid, or plasmacytoid shapes {2242}. AMEs rarely contain foci of collagenous spherulosis {1741,1537}.

AME should be differentiated from benign and malignant breast lesions. The myoepithelial cells present in AME are more numerous, plumper, and larger than those seen in normal lobules, nodular adenosis, or usual intraductal papillomas. The luminal cells may show considerable cytological atypia and may form nests and compressed cords that can simulate carcinoma. Morphological overlap between adenoid cystic carcinoma and AME may occur. Although both lesions can express MYB, the *MYB* rearrangements typically found in adenoid cystic carcinomas are not found in AMEs {116}. Mitoses are seen in both the ductal and myoepithelial components.

When a papillary architecture predominates, AME may be difficult to distinguish from intraductal papillomas with myoepithelial hyperplasia. In the tubular subtype of AME, tubular structures predominate and form a circumscribed nodular mass, in contrast to the less circumscribed tubular proliferation encountered in the adenosis of benign proliferative breast disease. The tubules are surrounded by myoepithelial cells with clear cytoplasm, giving an appearance that can be identical to that encountered in epithelial-myoepithelial carcinoma of the salivary glands. The increased number and size of myoepithelial cells allow tubular AME to be differentiated from tubular adenoma.

Immunohistochemistry can be of help in confirming the dual cell composition of the neoplasm. However, the myoepithelial cells in AME tend to stain in a variable and unpredictable pattern for the entire range of immunohistochemical markers of myoepithelial immunophenotype. High-molecular-weight cytokeratins may show a unique and characteristic paradoxical staining pattern in AME, with diffuse positivity in the inner epithelial cells and negativity in the outer myoepithelial cells {1417}.

AME can be focally positive for ER and PR on immunostaining, mainly in the epithelial cells, but the diffuse strong pattern of staining typically encountered in low-grade ductal carcinomas is not seen. In one series of 43 AMEs, a complete lack of hormone receptor expression was reported in 39% of cases and was associated with nuclear atypia, necrosis, and/or increased mitotic activity {715}.

## Cytology

FNA smears are usually highly cellular, composed of cohesive sheets of uniform ductal cells with interspersed myoepithelial cells and dispersed stripped spindle-shaped nuclei of myo-epithelial cell origin {935,1352,1815}. The cytological features should be distinguished from those of fibroadenoma, fibrocystic changes, and papilloma {935}. The identification of numerous myoepithelial cells is important for the diagnosis of AME. Atypia in myoepithelial cells, together with increased cellularity, may be an interpretive pitfall that can lead to a false positive diagnosis {1815}. Immunohistochemical analysis on cell blocks or core needle biopsy specimens can be of substantial assistance.

## Diagnostic molecular pathology

Not clinically relevant

## Essential and desirable diagnostic criteria

*Essential:* a neoplasm of biphasic appearance, with glandular structures lined by an inner layer of epithelial cells and an outer layer of prominent myoepithelial cells.

## Staging

Not clinically relevant

## Prognosis and prediction

The majority of classic breast AMEs have a benign clinical course, and complete surgical excision is curative. However, distant metastases from cases lacking histological atypia or increased proliferation are on record {1049,1438}. Molecular characterization of rare metastatic cases with benign histol-ogy is awaited. Cases showing extensive intraductal growth or satellite nodules can recur as a result of multinodular growth. Because of the few metastatic cases and the potential for malignant transformation {836,1419,1297}, AME may be bet-ter regarded as a neoplasm of low malignant potential. Cases with histological malignant transformation are termed malignant AME (see *Malignant adenomyoepithelioma*, p. 46).

# Malignant adenomyoepithelioma

Foschini MP
Geyer FC
Hayes MM
Marchiò C
Nishimura R

## Definition

Malignant adenomyoepithelioma (AME-M) is adenomyoepithelioma (AME) with carcinoma, in which the malignancy may arise from either luminal epithelial or myoepithelial components, or from both cell types. When both epithelial and myoepithelial compartments are malignant, the term "epithelial-myoepithelial carcinoma" is used.

## ICD-O coding

8983/3 Adenomyoepithelioma with carcinoma
8562/3 Epithelial-myoepithelial carcinoma

## ICD-11 coding

2C6Y & XH7TL5 Malignant neoplasms of breast & Adenomyoepithelioma with carcinoma

## Related terminology

*Acceptable:* adenomyoepithelial carcinoma.

## Subtype(s)

Adenomyoepithelioma with carcinoma; epithelial-myoepithelial carcinoma

## Localization

Like its benign counterpart, AME-M can affect any breast quadrant.

## Clinical features

AME-M most frequently affects elderly women. No cases have been reported in males or in young people. Some patients may present with a longstanding mass with recent rapid increase in size {836}. One case arising in the context of neurofibromatosis type 1 is on record {840}.

## Epidemiology

AME-M is rare, and no data on incidence have been reported {31}. Our current knowledge of this entity is mainly based on single case reports and small series.

## Etiology

Unknown

## Pathogenesis

Genetic analyses of matched classic and malignant components of AME-M suggest that it derives from malignant transformation of a pre-existing classic AME {1419,715}, but the development of de novo AME-M cannot be ruled out. Limited genetic data on AME-M are available. The common genetic drivers of AMEs, namely *PIK3CA* and *HRAS* p.Gln61 hotspot mutations, are also found in AME-M {715}. *HRAS* p.Gln61 mutations are associated with ER-negative AMEs with atypical histological

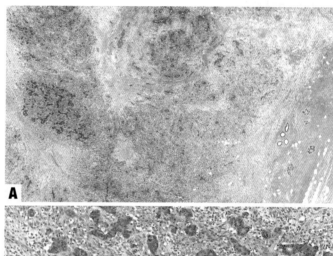

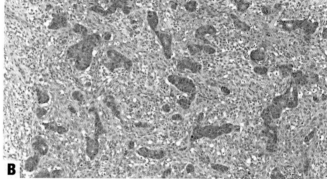

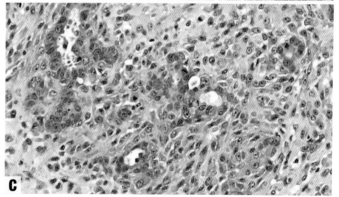

**Fig. 2.33** Malignant adenomyoepithelioma. **A** Low-power view shows irregular margins. **B** At higher power, cytological atypia is clearly evident in both epithelial and myoepithelial cells. The myoepithelial cells outnumber the epithelial cells in this case. **C** Atypical mitotic figures are seen.

features, and they are typically present in those associated with carcinoma. Homozygous *CDKN2A* deletions might be involved in the malignant transformation of ER-negative AMEs. Notably, *TP53* mutations that are typically found in conventional ER-negative breast carcinomas are not found in AME-M.

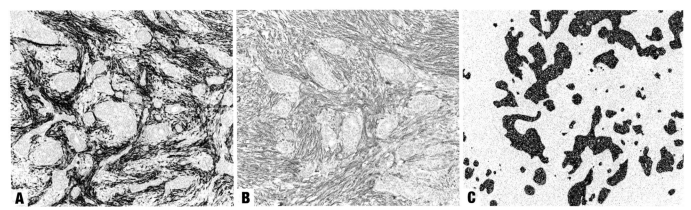

**Fig. 2.34** Malignant adenomyoepithelioma. Immunohistochemical staining is useful to demonstrate the epithelial and myoepithelial components. CK14 (**A**) and SMA (**B**) highlight the myoepithelial cells, and low-molecular-weight cytokeratin (**C**) highlights the epithelial component.

## Macroscopic appearance

When the malignant component is purely in situ {836}, AME-M can present as a multilobulated mass similar to classic AME. When an invasive malignancy is present, AME-M can show a variety of macroscopic appearances, with the mass showing infiltrative borders; a firm, rubbery, or fleshy consistency; and a grey to yellowish-white appearance. A few cases show cystic change and necrosis. The size varies, being larger in long-standing lesions.

## Histopathology

AME-M can present a wide spectrum of morphological features. In AME with malignant change of the luminal and/or myoepithelial compartment, the histological appearance of an AME is recognized, with transition to carcinoma observed as cytological atypia, increased mitoses, and necrosis in the malignant component {1419,2036,818}. When the malignant transformation involves mainly the epithelial component, it can include features of invasive breast carcinoma of no special type (NST), invasive lobular carcinoma, and carcinomas of special types {1727,669,1952}. When the malignant transformation affects mainly the myoepithelial component, features of myoepithelial cell carcinoma predominate; such cases are characterized by overgrowth of spindle or epithelioid myoepithelial cells, with clear or eosinophilic cytoplasm, nuclear atypia, and frequent mitotic figures {1366,1419,836}.

Not uncommonly, the invasive carcinoma component is of the metaplastic subtype; squamous cell carcinoma, low-grade adenosquamous carcinoma, spindle cell carcinoma, carcinosarcoma, and matrix-producing carcinoma have been reported {1727,669,836}. In these cases, an AME component should be searched for by extensive sampling of the tumour.

In rare cases, malignancy can affect both the epithelial and myoepithelial components {823,1419}, giving rise to biphasic carcinomas composed of a mixture of malignant epithelial and myoepithelial cells, with the latter often being the predominant cell type. At low-power magnification, these tumours show a multilobulated or multinodular growth pattern. Rarely, a papillary architecture can be observed. Transition between classic benign AME and AME-M features may be appreciated {599, 836}. Epithelial-myoepithelial carcinoma shows malignant changes in both the luminal and myoepithelial components.

Specifically, mitotic count is increased in the malignant areas. The biphasic epithelial-myoepithelial nature, with dual cell types, is the key feature for the differential diagnosis with metaplastic carcinoma; immunohistochemistry with markers of epithelial and myoepithelial cell lineages can be useful {836}.

Mitotically active classic AME can be difficult to distinguish from AME-M. The use of mitotic counts has been proposed {2055}; however, the validity and clinical utility of this approach have yet to be demonstrated.

## Cytology

Cytology smears from AME-M are highly cellular, with loosely cohesive neoplastic cells simulating invasive breast carcinoma NST. The presence of metachromatic matrix, highlighted by Giemsa staining, can help in the differential diagnosis. The matrix material surrounds nests of neoplastic cells (unlike in adenoid cystic carcinoma, where it is arranged in spherules) {836}.

## Diagnostic molecular pathology

AME-M may be ER-positive or ER-negative, although malignant transformation of classic AME might be more frequent in ER-negative lesions. The ER status may be concordant in both classic and malignant components, but an ER-negative carcinoma has been reported in association with an ER-positive AME. *ERBB2* (*HER2*) amplification is not detected {715}.

## Essential and desirable diagnostic criteria

*Malignant adenomyoepithelioma*

*Essential:* a malignant tumour arising in association with classic AME, with the luminal or myoepithelial component (or both) being malignant.

*Epithelial-myoepithelial carcinoma*

*Essential:* a malignant tumour with malignant changes in the luminal and myoepithelial components and high mitotic activity, irrespective of the presence of a recognizable benign AME.

## Staging

AME-M is staged according to the criteria adopted for other types of invasive breast carcinomas.

## Prognosis and prediction

The relatively low number of reported cases and short periods of follow-up limit the available information on prognostic features in AME-M. Metastases can appear several years after primary diagnosis {1049}, as well as in AMEs without atypical histological features (see *Adenomyoepithelioma*, p. 43).

The prognosis of cases with malignant transformation in both epithelial and myoepithelial components (epithelial-myoepithelial carcinoma) is difficult to assess due to the rarity of these cases. Haematogenous spread seems to be more frequent than lymphatic spread, with the lungs and brain being the most common metastatic sites {1234,669,18}.

The prognosis of AME-M with invasive carcinoma depends on the histological subtype of the invasive disease. Given that this component is most commonly metaplastic carcinoma, the prognosis may be poor, with the lungs being the most common metastatic site {836}. However, cases with adenosquamous carcinoma have shown a better outcome {669}. The genetic profile of AME-M with invasive carcinoma, and therefore its prognosis, may differ from that of invasive disease of the same subtype not associated with AME.

Lymph node metastases are rare, and there are insufficient data available to suggest axillary dissection {1419,836}. Nevertheless, management approaches based on the invasive disease present may be prudent.

# Papillary neoplasms: Introduction

Brogi E
Horii R
Mac Grogan G
Rakha EA

Troxell ML
Tse G
Yamaguchi R

Papillary neoplasms are composed predominantly of papillae, each of which consists of a fibrovascular core covered by epithelium with or without a myoepithelial layer, depending on the type of papillary neoplasm. The nature of the epithelium determines whether a papillary neoplasm is benign, atypical, or malignant. The assessment of epithelial atypia is facilitated by considering the space between adjacent fibrovascular cores as equivalent to a duct space and applying the criteria used for the interpretation of intraductal proliferations. A cut-off size of 3 mm is used to distinguish atypical ductal hyperplasia and low-grade ductal carcinoma in situ (DCIS) in a papilloma. Apocrine metaplasia commonly has papillary architecture. Usual ductal hyperplasia may also have thin papillary fronds. However, the adjective "papillary" should not be used when reporting these two lesions, because it may raise management issues. Furthermore, focal papillary usual ductal hyperplasia in the absence of a discrete papillary aggregate/nodule should not be overdiagnosed as papilloma.

Most papillary neoplasms are confined within ducts, which tend to be distended and cystic, with a thick fibrous wall. The intraductal papillary neoplasms of the breast include papilloma, papilloma with atypical ductal hyperplasia / DCIS, papillary DCIS, and solid and encapsulated papillary carcinomas in situ (see discussion in the corresponding sections that follow). All benign intraductal papillary neoplasms are surrounded by a continuous layer of myoepithelium, but the presence and distribution of myoepithelial cells along the papillae and at the periphery of malignant lesions vary according to the lesion type. Papillary lesions completely devoid of myoepithelium include invasive papillary carcinoma and most encapsulated and solid papillary carcinomas. The latter may have few scattered and focal residual myoepithelial cells (see discussion in the corresponding sections that follow). Tall cell carcinoma with

reversed polarity, which is grouped in this volume with other rare and salivary gland–type tumours (see *Tall cell carcinoma with reversed polarity*, p. 153), often has papillary areas and is devoid of myoepithelium.

Myoepithelial cells may sometimes be difficult to identify in routine H&E-stained sections, but they can be visualized with the use of immunohistochemical stains for myoepithelial antigens, such as calponin, SMA, SMMHC, and p63. These markers vary in sensitivity and specificity {2318,853}. Reactive myofibroblasts adjacent to nodules of papillary carcinoma often express myoepithelial antigens such as calponin and SMA {2107,853}. The pericytes associated with capillaries within the fibrovascular cores and at the periphery of a papillary lesion may express actin, calponin, and SMMHC, and they should not be misinterpreted as myoepithelial cells {2107}. Scattered neoplastic epithelial cells, especially in papillary carcinomas, may express p63 and should not be misinterpreted as myoepithelial cells {2264}. A panel of myoepithelial markers (e.g. calponin and p63) might be used to evaluate the myoepithelium in problematic papillary lesions. A cocktail of antibodies for myoepithelial/basal antigens (p63, CK5, CK14) and luminal cytokeratins (CK8 and CK18) is also commercially available and may be used to assess the presence and distribution of myoepithelial cells within a papillary lesion, as well as the nature of the epithelial proliferation.

Correct categorization of a papillary lesion in a core biopsy can be difficult. In this scenario, there are two important aspects to evaluate: (1) whether there are myoepithelial cells at the epithelial stroma interface and (2) whether the epithelial cell population is atypical. The presence of a myoepithelial cell layer within fibrovascular cores is evidence of an underlying papillary lesion that can be either benign or involved by neoplastic epithelium amounting to atypical ductal hyperplasia / low-grade DCIS,

**Table 2.02** Myoepithelial antigens

| Antigen(s) | Function | Distribution | Comments/caveats |
|---|---|---|---|
| **p63** | Transcription factor | Nuclear | p63 may stain the nuclei of the carcinoma cells, especially in papillary carcinomas {2264}. |
| **p40 (DNp63 isoform)** | Transcription factor | Nuclear | |
| **Calponin** | Contractile protein | Cytoplasmic | See SMA comment below. |
| **SMA** | Contractile protein | Cytoplasmic | SMA and to a lesser degree calponin are expressed in reactive stromal myofibroblasts, vessel pericytes, and endothelial cells associated with papillary neoplasms {2107}; similar patterns of cross-reactivity are also observed in the stroma adjacent to invasive carcinoma. |
| **SMMHC** | Contractile protein | Cytoplasmic | Expression is substantially reduced in the myoepithelial cells of sclerosing lesions {856} and in the ducts and lobules involved by ductal carcinoma in situ {855}. |
| **CK5/6 and CK14** | Intermediate filaments (basal cytokeratins) | Cytoplasmic | Although CK5/6 and CK14 are not sensitive or specific for myoepithelial cells, their use can also help in the differentiation between hyperplastic and clonal neoplastic proliferations in papillary lesions. |

**Table 2.03** Histopathological characteristics of breast papillary neoplasms

| Neoplasm | Presentation | Papillary architecture | Epithelial cells | Myoepithelial cells |
|---|---|---|---|---|
| Intraductal papilloma | Single lesion (central papilloma) or multiple lesions (peripheral papillomas) | Generally broad, blunt fronds | Heterogeneous non-neoplastic cell population: luminal cells, usual ductal hyperplasia, apocrine metaplasia and hyperplasia | Present throughout and at periphery |
| Papilloma with ADH or DCIS | Single lesion (central papilloma) or multiple lesions (peripheral papillomas) | Generally broad, blunt fronds | Focal areas of cells with architectural and cytological features of ADH or DCIS (usually low-grade); background of heterogeneous non-neoplastic cell population | Mostly present throughout and at periphery; may be attenuated in areas of ADH/DCIS |
| Papillary DCIS | Multiple lesions | Slender fronds, sometimes branching | Entire lesion occupied by a cell population with architectural and cytological features of DCIS of low, intermediate, or rarely high nuclear grade; can grow as a single layer along thin fibrovascular stalks | Absent or scant in papillae; present in attenuated form at the periphery of ducts |
| Encapsulated papillary carcinoma | Single lesion | Numerous slender fronds, sometimes branching; peripheral, typically well-developed, fibrous capsule | Entire lesion occupied by a cell population with architectural and cytological features of DCIS of low or intermediate grade; can grow as a single layer along thin fibrovascular stalks; cribriform, micropapillary, and solid patterns may be present, with fusion of adjacent papillae | Usually absent throughout and at periphery |
| Solid papillary carcinoma | Single or multiple lesions | Solid with inconspicuous delicate fibrovascular septa | Entire lesion occupied by a cell population with cytological features of low or intermediate nuclear grade, growing predominantly in a solid manner; spindle cell component; neuroendocrine and mucinous differentiation is frequent | Present or absent within the solid papillary proliferation or at the outer contours of the nodules |
| Invasive papillary carcinoma | Single lesion | Infiltrating carcinoma with papillary morphology, including fibrovascular cores | Low-, intermediate-, or rarely high-grade nuclear atypia | Absent throughout |

ADH, atypical ductal hyperplasia; DCIS, ductal carcinoma in situ.
Note: In rare cases, there are overlapping features between solid papillary carcinoma and encapsulated papillary carcinoma or between encapsulated papillary carcinoma and papillary DCIS, and it may not be possible to distinguish papillary carcinoma subtypes in every case.

**Table 2.04** Immunohistochemical characteristics of breast papillary neoplasms

| Neoplasm | Myoepithelial markers (e.g. p63, CK14, SMM, calponin) | | High-molecular-weight cytokeratins (CK5/6, CK14) | ER and PR | Other |
|---|---|---|---|---|---|
| | Papillary fronds | Periphery of the lesion | | | |
| Intraductal papilloma | Positive | Positive | *Positive:* myoepithelial cells, UDH (heterogeneous positivity) *Negative:* apocrine metaplasia | *Positive (heterogeneous):* luminal cells, UDH *Negative:* apocrine metaplasia | |
| Papilloma with ADH or DCIS | Positive in the papilloma; may be scant in the ADH/DCIS component | Positive | *Positive:* myoepithelial cells, UDH (heterogeneous positivity) *Negative:* apocrine metaplasia, ADH/DCIS | *Positive (strong and diffuse):* ADH/DCIS *Positive (heterogeneous):* luminal cells, UDH *Negative:* apocrine metaplasia | |
| Papillary DCIS[a] | Negative; attenuated layer in rare cases | Positive | *Positive:* myoepithelial cells *Negative:* neoplastic cell population | Positive (strong and diffuse) | |
| Encapsulated papillary carcinoma | Negative | Usually negative | Negative in the neoplastic cell population | Positive (strong and diffuse) | |
| Solid papillary carcinoma | Negative or positive | Negative or positive | Negative in the neoplastic cell population | Positive (strong and diffuse) | Frequent chromogranin and synaptophysin expression |
| Invasive papillary carcinoma | Negative | Negative | Negative | Positive | |

ADH, atypical ductal hyperplasia; DCIS, ductal carcinoma in situ; UDH, usual ductal hyperplasia.
[a]High-grade lesions may show a different pattern of staining.

**Table 2.05** Papillary carcinomas: diagnosis and staging, including ER, PR, and ERBB2 (HER2) status

| Papillary carcinoma subtype | Periphery of the lesion | Myoepithelial cell layer | Tumour grading | Tumour staging | Immunophenotypic characteristics |
|---|---|---|---|---|---|
| Encapsulated | Neoplastic cells surrounded by a fibrous capsule | Absent; occasionally present | The lesion should be graded according to nuclear grade | pTis (DCIS) | *For diagnostic purposes:* ER strongly and diffusely positive, PR variable, HER2 negative<br><br>*For therapeutic purposes:* receptor and HER2 status not needed |
| Encapsulated with frank invasion | Neoplastic cells with infiltrative growth beyond the fibrous capsule; invasive carcinoma NST, cribriform carcinoma, tubular carcinoma, mucinous carcinoma | Absent in the frankly invasive component | The frankly invasive component should be graded according to the Nottingham grading system | pT according to the size of the frankly invasive component | *For diagnostic purposes:* ER strongly and diffusely positive, PR variable, HER2 negative<br><br>*For therapeutic purposes:* ER, PR, and HER2 status should be assessed in the frankly invasive component |
| Solid in situ | Nodules with smooth rounded contours | Absent or present | The lesion should be graded according to nuclear grade | pTis (DCIS) | *For diagnostic purposes:* ER strongly and diffusely positive, PR variable, HER2 negative<br><br>*For therapeutic purposes:* receptor and HER2 status not needed |
| Solid with invasion | Nodules with smooth rounded contours associated with an invasive component that can take the form of either strands and cell clusters within pools of extracellular mucin corresponding to mucinous carcinoma or invasive carcinoma NST, cribriform carcinoma, tubular carcinoma | Absent in the invasive component | The invasive component should be graded according to the Nottingham grading system | pT according to the size of the invasive component | *For diagnostic purposes:* ER strongly and diffusely positive, PR variable, HER2 negative<br><br>*For therapeutic purposes:* receptor and HER2 status should be assessed in the invasive component only |
| Invasive solid | Nodules with ragged contours creating a geographical jigsaw pattern within a desmoplastic stroma | Absent | The invasive component should be graded according to the Nottingham grading system | pT according to the size of the invasive component | *For diagnostic purposes:* ER strongly and diffusely positive, PR variable, HER2 negative<br><br>*For therapeutic purposes:* receptor and HER2 status should be assessed in the invasive component only |
| Invasive | Invasive mammary carcinoma with predominantly papillary morphology (> 90%) and an infiltrative growth pattern | Absent | The lesion should be graded according to the Nottingham grading system | pT according to the size of the lesion | *For diagnostic purposes:* exclude metastatic carcinoma<br><br>*For therapeutic purposes:* ER, PR, and HER2 status should be assessed in the entire lesion |

DCIS, ductal carcinoma in situ; NST, of no special type.

intermediate-grade DCIS, or high-grade DCIS (depending on the size and degree of atypia). The complete absence of an underlying benign papillary lesion, defined as a complete lack of a myoepithelial cell layer or any residual benign hyperplastic epithelium, is suggestive of a papillary carcinoma (papillary DCIS or encysted papillary carcinoma). The neoplastic nature of the epithelial component is defined according to its morphological and immunohistochemical features. By definition, > 95% of the population in a papillary carcinoma is neoplastic, but that proportion cannot be estimated on core biopsy.

FNA cytological diagnosis of papillary lesions is difficult, with benign and malignant lesions showing overlapping features.

When a papillary lesion is suspected, prompt histological evaluation is warranted for accurate diagnosis {2115}.

Breast excision specimens that have undergone prior core needle biopsy often have displaced epithelium within the core needle biopsy site, a finding that is inversely related to the time interval between core biopsy and surgical excision {504,1443}. This phenomenon is particularly evident after core biopsy of a papillary neoplasm {1443}. Displaced epithelium within the core biopsy site should not be overdiagnosed as invasive carcinoma. Displaced epithelial cell clusters or single cells may also be found in the axillary lymph nodes sinuses, often in association with giant cells and haemosiderin-laden macrophages {294,

2147,2146}. In either setting, immunohistochemical staining for myoepithelial antigens is usually non-contributory, because the myoepithelial cells might not have been displaced with the epithelium; only a positive result can be interpreted with confidence.

Infarction of a papillary lesion may occur after FNA or core needle biopsy, or it may be secondary to torsion of the stalk. Infarction is unrelated to the type of papillary neoplasm, but it may be more common in larger tumours. In this setting, the use of myoepithelial and/or epithelial markers might sometimes be helpful to highlight the underlying architecture and cell composition, and possibly to determine the nature of the papillary neoplasm, with the understanding that any lack of staining is non-contributory and should not be interpreted as a negative result, and that limited tissue preservation often precludes a definitive interpretation.

# Intraductal papilloma

Troxell ML
Boulos F
Denkert C
Horii R
Yamaguchi R

## Definition
Intraductal papilloma is a benign breast lesion arising within a duct in a central (solitary) or peripheral (multiple) location, composed of papillary projections with fibrovascular cores, covered by an epithelial and myoepithelial layer.

## ICD-O coding
8503/0 Intraductal papilloma

## ICD-11 coding
2F30.2 & XH4LZ4 Intraductal papilloma of breast & Intraductal papilloma

## Related terminology
*Acceptable*
*Central papilloma:* large duct papilloma; major duct papilloma.
*Peripheral papilloma:* microscopic papilloma.

*Not recommended*
Papillomatosis.

## Subtype(s)
None

## Localization
Intraductal papillomas may occur centrally in large ducts near the nipple or peripherally in smaller ducts, in any quadrant.

## Clinical features
Central papillomas present most frequently with unilateral clear or serosanguineous nipple discharge. Presentation as a palpable mass is less common. Mammographic abnormalities include a benign-looking circumscribed retroareolar mass, a solitary retroareolar dilated duct, and (rarely) microcalcifications. Small central papillomas may be mammographically occult. Ultrasonography may show a well-defined, smooth-walled, solid hypoechoic nodule or a lobulated, smooth-walled cystic lesion with solid components; colour Doppler ultrasonography may highlight the vascular pedicle {237}. Galactography shows an intraluminal filling defect or duct dilatation. On MRI, small papillomas may appear as enhancing masses with smooth margins, whereas larger lesions can have irregular margins {237,450, 2218}. Ductoscopy allows for direct tissue sampling and duct excision {22}. Peripheral papillomas are usually clinically occult, but they can rarely present with nipple discharge or even less often with a mass resulting from a small cluster of papillomas. They are also relatively occult on breast imaging, but they may manifest as peripherally located microcalcifications; a nodular prominence of ducts; or multiple small, well-circumscribed masses {34,237,2218}.

## Epidemiology
Intraductal papillomas (with or without atypia) were found in 5.3% of benign breast biopsies from a cohort of > 9000 women

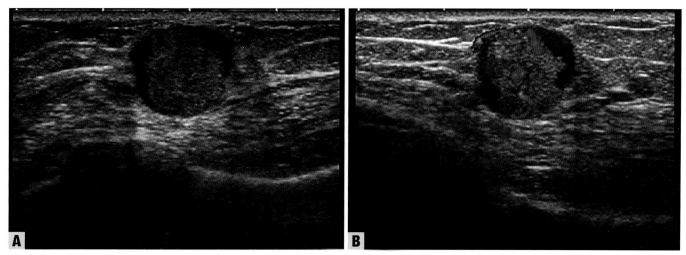

**Fig. 2.35** Intraductal papilloma. **A** Ultrasonography shows a markedly cystic dilated duct containing a large intraductal papilloma. **B** Colour Doppler indicates the vascular flow.

{1164}. Most papillomas are central. Patients present over a wide age range, but most are 30–50 years old {1164,34}.

### Etiology
Unknown

### Pathogenesis
Benign papillomas are monoclonal proliferations {1513}. Activating point mutations in the PIK3CA/AKT1 pathway have been frequently identified in benign papillomas with or without usual hyperplasia {2106,930}. Loss of heterozygosity on 16p13 was found in benign papillary lesions as well as papillary carcinomas, whereas loss of heterozygosity on 16q23 with the D16S476 marker was found only in malignant papillary lesions {494,1208}.

### Macroscopic appearance
Central papillomas may form well-circumscribed round tumours of papillary fronds attached by one or more pedicles to the wall of the dilated duct. The size of central papillomas varies from a few millimetres to > 5 cm. Focal necrosis or haemorrhage may be present, particularly in larger lesions. In contrast, peripheral papillomas are usually grossly occult unless they are associated with other findings.

### Histopathology
*Intraductal papilloma NOS*
Both central and peripheral papillomas are characterized by a cohesive but arborescent structure composed of fibrovascular cores covered by a layer of myoepithelial cells with overlying epithelial cells. The myoepithelial layer, which is always present, may be inconspicuous, and a combination of myoepithelial immunohistochemical stains such as SMMHC, calponin, CK5, CK14, and p63 can help confirm its presence (see Table 2.02, p. 49) {387}. In some lesions, the myoepithelial cells may be quite prominent or hyperplastic. The periphery of involved spaces is also surrounded by myoepithelial cells. The epithelial component may consist of one layer of cuboidal to columnar cells or may show usual ductal hyperplasia, which is typically positive for CK5/14 with non-uniform ER staining {912,769}. Apocrine change is sometimes found in the epithelium of papillomas and may be associated with diminished myoepithelium {2100}.

Squamous metaplasia may also be seen, most often in association with areas of infarction {657}, whereas mucinous, clear cell, and sebaceous metaplasia and collagenous spherulosis are rare {947}. Epithelial cell mitoses are absent or extremely rare. Ducts in the region of the papilloma often show ectasia.

Areas of haemorrhage or infarction may arise after a needling procedure or due to torsion of fibrovascular cores. Sclerosis/fibrosis is commonly seen and can be so extensive that it obscures the underlying papillary architecture of the lesion. Such lesions have been called sclerosing papillomas, a subtype of which is ductal adenoma. Epithelial nests may become entrapped in areas of fibrosis and may mimic invasive carcinoma. The epithelium retains an associated myoepithelial layer, confirming its benign nature. Similarly, displaced epithelial

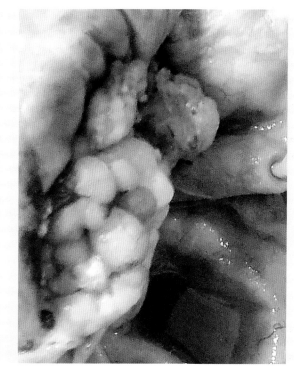

**Fig. 2.36** Intraductal papilloma. A large multinodular papillary structure projects into the lumen of a large cyst (blue colour from localization dye).

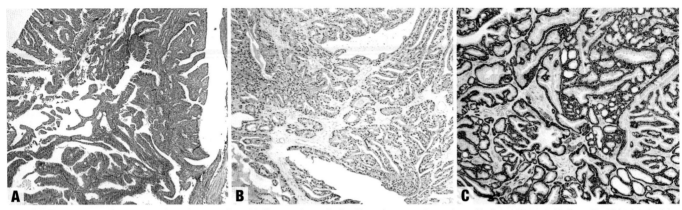

**Fig. 2.37** Intraductal papilloma. **A** Histology shows papillae with fibrovascular stalks lined by columnar and apocrine epithelium with myoepithelium. **B** p63 immunostaining demonstrates myoepithelial nuclei lining fibrovascular stalks. **C** Cytoplasmic SMMHC staining demonstrates a continuous layer of myoepithelium.

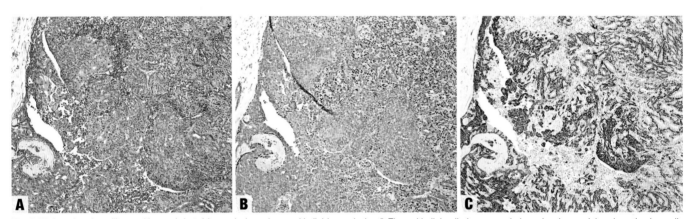

**Fig. 2.38** Intraductal papilloma with usual ductal hyperplasia and myoepithelial hyperplasia. **A** The epithelial cells have crowded overlapping nuclei and are haphazardly arranged around slit-like spaces in the centre. The prominent spindle cells in the upper right are myoepithelium. **B** p63 staining highlights the myoepithelial cells in the upper right, in addition to myoepithelial nuclei lining the fibrovascular cores. Myoepithelial cells line the edge of the involved duct at the left. **C** CK14 staining is positive in usual ductal hyperplasia at the centre, which would have a mosaic ER staining pattern (not shown). CK14 also highlights the myoepithelial cells in the upper right.

nests can be present in a healing biopsy tract; this may create an interpretive pitfall and should not be mistaken for invasive carcinoma {1443}.

On core biopsy, features of benign papilloma (as described above) are often readily recognized, even if fragmented. However, incompletely sampled papillomas may cause diagnostic difficulty, especially in the case of sclerotic papillomas or papillomas with epithelial hyperplasia or atypia. Myoepithelial immunostaining may be helpful in highlighting the underlying papillary architecture and establishing the presence or absence of myoepithelial cells. The size of a papillary lesion on core biopsy should be reported, for radiological correlation and management considerations. The management of non-atypical papillomas after core biopsy is still controversial. Although heterogeneity remains a concern, recent studies show widely variable but generally low upgrade rates {2261,767,1600}. If atypical features are seen on core biopsy (lack of myoepithelial cells, low-grade cytological or architectural atypia, or high-grade cytology), the papillary lesion should be excised.

Depending on the histopathological context, the differential diagnosis for papilloma may include the spectrum of papillary lesions – intraductal papilloma with atypical ductal hyperplasia (ADH) / ductal carcinoma in situ (DCIS), papillary DCIS / intraductal papillary carcinoma (in particular the dimorphic subtype, because globoid cells may mimic myoepithelium), encapsulated papillary carcinoma, solid papillary carcinoma, and tall cell carcinoma with reversed polarity – as well as adenomyoepithelioma or fibroepithelial tumours with polypoid stromal architecture, nipple adenoma, and sweat gland hidradenoma papilliferum. Rarely, papillomas have been described in axillary lymph nodes as a form of benign epithelial inclusion {214}.

*Intraductal papilloma with ADH and DCIS*
Foci of ADH or DCIS may be seen in papillomas, more commonly in peripheral than central papillomas {34,1540,1416}. Papillomas with ADH and DCIS are characterized by a focal population of monotonous cells with cytological and architectural features of low-grade ductal neoplasia. Myoepithelial cells may be scant or absent from these foci, and the atypical epithelial cells usually show a lack of staining for high-molecular-weight cytokeratins (CK5/14), with uniform positivity for ER (see Table 2.03 and Table 2.04, p. 50) {912,769}. Extent and proportion criteria have been used to differentiate ADH from DCIS within a papilloma. The extent cut-off point according to some authorities is 3 mm: an intraductal papilloma with ADH is diagnosed when the atypical epithelial population is < 3 mm, whereas DCIS is diagnosed when the population is ≥ 3 mm {1577,1164}. Although some authors have used a threshold of 30% {1261}, the 3 mm size criterion was adopted as a pragmatic guideline in the previous edition of the WHO classification of breast tumours {1098},

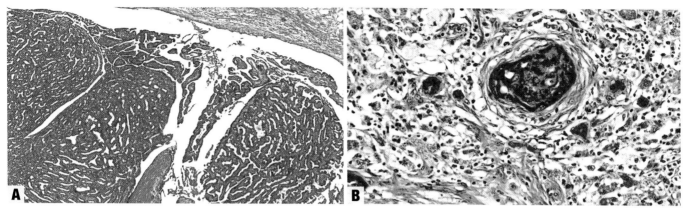

**Fig. 2.39** Intraductal papilloma with epithelial displacement. **A** Low-power view shows an intraductal papilloma. **B** At higher power. Epithelial nests may be entrapped in biopsy site granulation tissue beyond the periphery and can mimic invasion.

despite limited scientific evidence {1577,1164}. When epithelial proliferations with intermediate or high nuclear grade are seen, the diagnosis of DCIS within a papilloma should be made regardless of extent {34,2309}. Papillomas with DCIS must be distinguished from papillary DCIS and encapsulated papillary carcinoma (described in the following sections).

*Papillary DCIS*

See *Papillary ductal carcinoma in situ* (p. 57). Papillary DCIS, formerly termed intracystic papillary carcinoma, consists of DCIS lining fibrovascular cores devoid of myoepithelium but contained within a duct with preserved surrounding myoepithelium. In addition to the conventional solid, cribriform, and micropapillary patterns, papillary DCIS may appear deceptively bland with a stratified spindled, compact columnar, or dimorphic

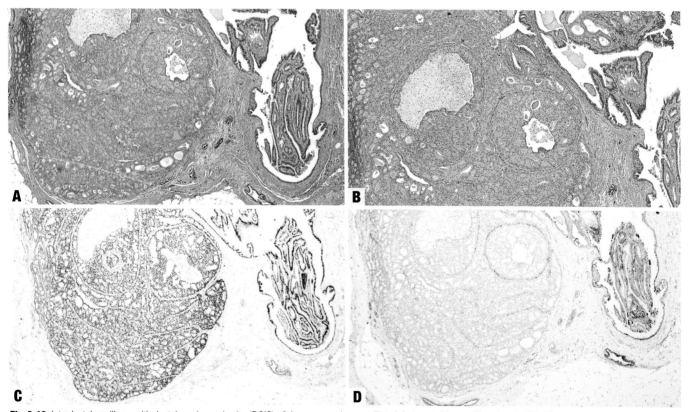

**Fig. 2.40** Intraductal papilloma with ductal carcinoma in situ (DCIS). **A** Low power shows a dilated duct containing papillary fronds (right) lined by non-atypical apocrine and columnar epithelium. The cribriform proliferation in the left portion of the lesion measures > 3 mm. **B** Medium power shows monotonous epithelial cells with low-grade nuclei in the left portion of the papillary lesion. On the basis of cytology, architecture, and size (> 3 mm), this lesion is diagnosed as intraductal papilloma with DCIS. **C** ER staining shows strong diffuse positivity in DCIS (left) but is patchy in the benign portion of the papilloma (right). **D** CK5 is negative in DCIS (left) and highlights the myoepithelial cells lining the fibrovascular cores in both portions of the papilloma. The benign epithelium is also negative for CK5 in this case, as the epithelium is apocrine and columnar. CK5 is typically positive in usual ductal hyperplasia lining papillomas.

pattern {1139}. The dimorphic pattern features a second population of epithelial cells with clear cytoplasm, which may mimic myoepithelium; this pattern can be resolved with myoepithelial immunostaining {1139}. Papillary DCIS may rarely occur in isolation. More commonly, it is one of several architectural patterns in a case of DCIS. Like all types of DCIS, papillary DCIS is graded on the basis of the nuclear atypia of the neoplastic epithelium. Solid papillary carcinoma in situ, a special subtype of papillary DCIS, is described in a dedicated section – see *Solid papillary carcinoma (in situ and invasive)*, p. 63.

*Intraductal papilloma with atypical lobular hyperplasia and lobular carcinoma in situ*
The presence of lobular neoplasia in the context of an intraductal papilloma should be reported as such.

## Cytology
The diagnosis and categorization of papillary lesions by FNA is often challenging. Smears are cellular, showing 3D papillary clusters containing myoepithelial and epithelial cells, often including columnar and apocrine cytology, with foamy histiocytes in the background. It is difficult to distinguish benign papilloma from the spectrum of more malignant papillary lesions by cytology {168}.

## Diagnostic molecular pathology
Not clinically relevant

## Essential and desirable diagnostic criteria
*Essential:* a breast lesion occurring within a duct, composed of papillary projections with fibrovascular cores, covered by an epithelial and myoepithelial layer.
*Desirable:* demonstration of myoepithelial cells within and at the periphery of the lesion immunohistochemically.

## Staging
Not clinically relevant

## Prognosis and prediction
Benign central papilloma without surrounding atypical changes is associated with a 2-fold increase in the risk of subsequent invasive breast carcinoma; this risk is 3-fold with peripheral papillomas {1164}. With atypical papillomas, the risk of subsequent invasive carcinoma was reported to be 5- to 7.5-fold, with the risk to the ipsilateral breast and bilateral breasts differing between studies {1577,1164}. The risk of subsequent carcinoma and local recurrence associated with atypical papillomas is obscured by the frequent concurrent presence of ADH or DCIS within the surrounding breast parenchyma {1577,34,1164}.

# Papillary ductal carcinoma in situ

Brogi E
Rakha EA

## Definition
Papillary ductal carcinoma in situ (DCIS) is a morphological subtype of DCIS composed of filiform arborizing fibrovascular cores lined by neoplastic ductal epithelium, devoid of myoepithelium and contained within central or peripheral ducts with retained myoepithelium at the periphery.

## ICD-O coding
8503/2 Ductal carcinoma in situ, papillary

## ICD-11 coding
2E65.2 & XH4V32 Ductal carcinoma in situ of breast & Ductal carcinoma in situ NOS

## Related terminology
*Acceptable:* papillary carcinoma in situ; intraductal papillary ductal carcinoma in situ.
*Not recommended:* intracystic papillary ductal carcinoma; encapsulated/solid papillary carcinoma.

## Subtype(s)
None

## Localization
Papillary DCIS is usually associated with DCIS having other architectural patterns, and it may involve central or peripheral ducts. Papillary DCIS in central/subareolar ducts may be associated with encapsulated papillary carcinoma.

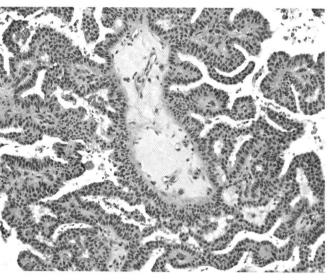

**Fig. 2.42** Papillary ductal carcinoma in situ. Delicate branching fibrovascular cores are lined by a monotonous epithelial proliferation with low nuclear grade.

## Clinical features
Papillary DCIS occurring in peripheral ducts tends to be clinically occult and is usually detected mammographically due to associated microcalcifications, or rarely as a circumscribed or scattered nodularity (see the *Clinical features* subsection of *Ductal carcinoma in situ*, p. 76). DCIS with papillary, cribriform, and micropapillary patterns often coexists with encapsulated papillary carcinoma, especially in a retroareolar location. In the past, encapsulated papillary carcinoma and DCIS near it were classified together as intracystic papillary DCIS (see also *Encapsulated*

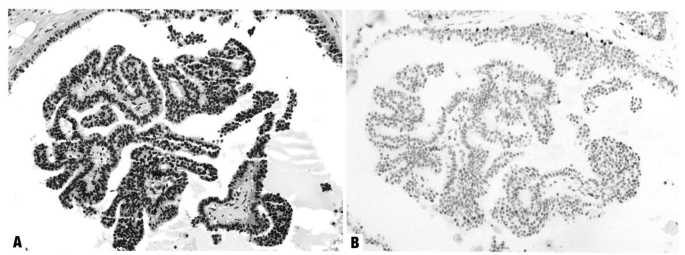

**Fig. 2.41** Papillary ductal carcinoma in situ. **A** A monotonous proliferation of ductal epithelial cells with low nuclear grade lines delicate branching fibrovascular cores within a small cystic duct. **B** p63 immunostaining shows no evidence of myoepithelium along the fibrovascular cores, but highlights the nuclei of the myoepithelial cells surrounding the duct.

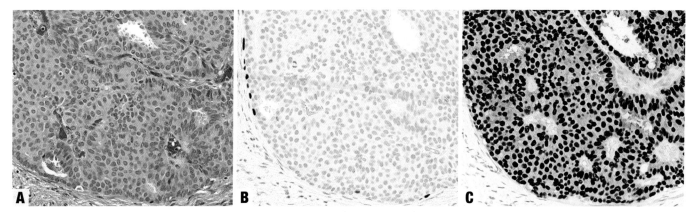

**Fig. 2.43** Solid papillary carcinoma in situ, a special subtype of papillary ductal carcinoma in situ. **A** A monotonous proliferation of ductal epithelial cells with intermediate nuclear grade fills the spaces between the delicate branching fibrovascular cores, creating a solid and focally cribriform pattern that may obscure the underlying papillary architecture. **B** p63 immunostaining shows no evidence of myoepithelium along the fibrovascular cores, but highlights the nuclei of the myoepithelial cells surrounding the duct. **C** The neoplastic cells show strong and diffuse nuclear staining for ER. The palisading arrangement of the nuclei and neoplastic cells is evident along and around the fibrovascular cores. See *Solid papillary carcinoma (in situ and invasive)*, p. 63.

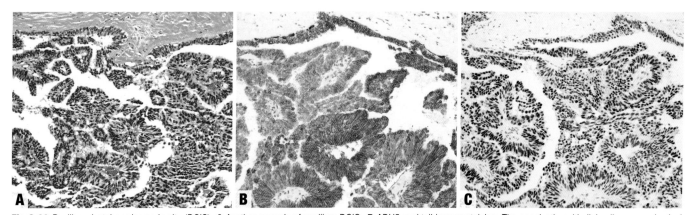

**Fig. 2.44** Papillary ductal carcinoma in situ (DCIS). **A** Another example of papillary DCIS. **B** ADH5 cocktail immunostaining. The neoplastic epithelial cells express luminal cytokeratins (CK7 and CK18: red chromogen) but are negative for basal cytokeratins (CK5, CK14, and nuclear p63: brown chromogen). Myoepithelial cells (brown chromogen) are present around the duct containing the papillary DCIS, but not along the fibrovascular cores of papillary DCIS. **C** The neoplastic cells show strong and diffuse nuclear staining for ER. The palisading arrangement of the nuclei and neoplastic cells is evident along and around the fibrovascular cores.

*papillary carcinoma*, p. 60). It has been reported that papillary DCIS accounts for approximately 3% of DCIS {1626A}.

## Epidemiology
Papillary DCIS tends to be more common in postmenopausal women. Papillary DCIS is also the most common type of DCIS in males {859}.

## Etiology
Unknown

## Pathogenesis
Papillary DCIS shows the same genetic alterations as DCIS of similar nuclear grade but different architectural patterns (see *Ductal carcinoma in situ*, p. 76).

## Macroscopic appearance
The gross appearance of papillary DCIS in a subareolar location is difficult to distinguish from that of encapsulated papillary carcinoma (see *Encapsulated papillary carcinoma*, p. 60), as the two lesions may often coexist.

## Histopathology
Papillary DCIS consists of an intraductal neoplastic epithelial proliferation lining arborizing fibrovascular cores devoid of myoepithelium. Unlike encapsulated and solid papillary carcinomas, papillary DCIS shows an intact myoepithelial layer at the epithelium–stroma interface of the periphery of the involved ducts. The epithelial proliferation may partially or completely fill the spaces between the papillae, creating solid, cribriform, micropapillary, spindled, or compact columnar patterns that may obscure the underlying papillary architecture. Papillary DCIS often constitutes one of several architectural patterns in a case of DCIS, but rarely it may be the only pattern, especially in a retroareolar location. Compared with other types of DCIS, papillary DCIS is less commonly associated with comedonecrosis {1626A}. Like all types of DCIS, papillary DCIS is graded on the basis of the nuclear atypia of the neoplastic epithelium, with some cases of high-grade papillary DCIS having been described {1626A}. Although most papillary DCIS lesions consist of a single, uniform cell population, papillary DCIS with a dimorphic pattern has also been described {1139}. In addition to neoplastic ductal cells, it features a population of cells (globoid cells) with abundant clear cytoplasm; these morphologically

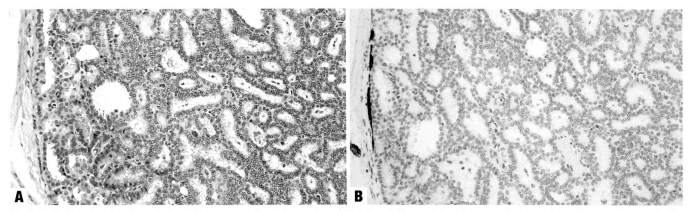

**Fig. 2.45** Papillary ductal carcinoma in situ. **A** Monotonous cells with low-grade nuclei forming cribriform and glandular spaces line inconspicuous fibrovascular cores. **B** CK5 stains the myoepithelial cells lining the peripheral duct, but not the fibrovascular cores, indicative of papillary ductal carcinoma in situ.

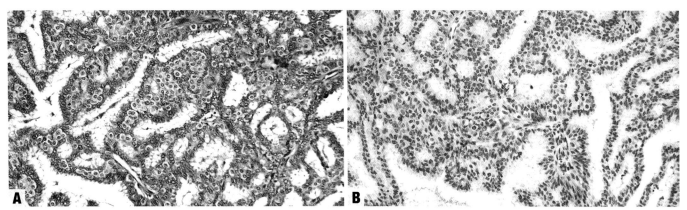

**Fig. 2.46** Papillary ductal carcinoma in situ, dimorphic. **A** H&E staining reveals two cell populations. One is luminal with apical snouts. The other, with more-abundant pale cytoplasm, mimics hyperplastic myoepithelium (also called globoid cells); however, the nuclei are large. **B** A panel of myoepithelial immunostains demonstrates the lack of myoepithelium; both cell populations in this image are epithelium (p63 immunostaining is shown here).

resemble myoepithelial cells but have nuclear features and atypia similar to those of the frankly epithelial cell component {1139}. Immunohistochemical staining for myoepithelial markers may be used to distinguish dimorphic papillary DCIS from papilloma extensively involved by DCIS (see Table 2.04, p. 50). Solid papillary carcinoma in situ, a special subtype of papillary DCIS, is described separately – see *Solid papillary carcinoma (in situ and invasive)*, p. 63.

The differential diagnosis of papillary DCIS includes papilloma, papilloma with atypia, encapsulated papillary carcinoma, and solid papillary carcinoma {2299,1706}. Immunohistochemical staining for myoepithelial antigens, high-molecular-weight cytokeratins (CK5/6 and CK14), ER, and neuroendocrine antigens may be used to distinguish between these lesions (see Table 2.04, p. 50). Low-grade and intermediate-grade lesions typically show diffuse nuclear positivity for ER and no expression of CK14 or CK5/6 in the neoplastic epithelial component; however, high-grade lesions may show a different pattern.

## Cytology

Cytological preparations are usually cellular and consist of a monomorphic population of ductal cells arranged in 3D papillary clusters, small groups, or single cells, often having columnar morphology. The nuclear grade is low to intermediate. Foamy histiocytes may be present in the background, but myoepithelial cells tend to be sparse or absent. The differential diagnosis includes papilloma, papilloma with atypia, encapsulated papillary carcinoma, and solid papillary carcinoma. In most cases, it is not possible to diagnose papillary DCIS based only on review of cytology material, in particular if the carcinoma is of low nuclear grade.

## Diagnostic molecular pathology

See *Ductal carcinoma in situ* (p. 76).

## Essential and desirable diagnostic criteria

*Essential:* a neoplastic proliferation of epithelial cells covering delicate arborizing fibrovascular cores devoid of myoepithelium but contained within a duct with a surrounding myoepithelial layer.

*Desirable:* demonstration of the absence of myoepithelium along the fibrovascular cores but presence of myoepithelium along the duct wall by immunohistochemical detection of myoepithelial antigens.

## Staging

Papillary DCIS is staged "pTis (DCIS)" in the eighth edition of the Union for International Cancer Control (UICC) TNM classification {229}.

## Prognosis and prediction

See *Ductal carcinoma in situ* (p. 76).

# Encapsulated papillary carcinoma

Mac Grogan G
Collins LC
Lerwill M
Rakha EA
Tan BY

## Definition

Encapsulated papillary carcinoma is a carcinoma characterized by fine fibrovascular stalks covered by neoplastic epithelial cells of low or intermediate nuclear grade, typically present within a cystic space and surrounded by a fibrous capsule. There are usually no myoepithelial cells along the papillae or at the periphery of the lesion.

## ICD-O coding

8504/2 Encapsulated papillary carcinoma
8504/3 Encapsulated papillary carcinoma with invasion

## ICD-11 coding

2E65.Y & XH9XV2 Other specified carcinoma in situ of breast & Encapsulated papillary carcinoma
2C6Y & XH0GT6 Other specified malignant neoplasms of breast & Encapsulated papillary carcinoma with invasion

## Related terminology

*Not recommended:* intracystic papillary carcinoma; encysted papillary carcinoma.

## Subtype(s)

None

## Localization

Most tumours are central and subareolar.

## Clinical features

This lesion presents as a circumscribed round mass, with or without nipple discharge. There are no specific imaging features that differentiate encapsulated papillary carcinoma from other papillary lesions; however, encapsulated papillary carcinomas tend to be larger at presentation, with a cystic growth pattern.

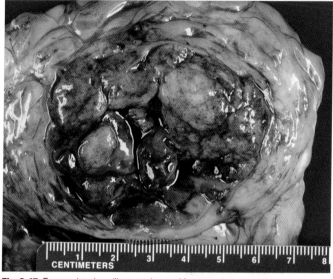

**Fig. 2.47** Encapsulated papillary carcinoma. Macroscopic appearance.

## Epidemiology

Encapsulated papillary carcinoma presents in postmenopausal women, mainly during the seventh decade of life {1706,1391}.

## Etiology

Unknown

## Pathogenesis

Encapsulated papillary carcinomas display genomic features similar to those of low-grade, ER-positive invasive breast carcinoma (IBC) of no special type (NST), for example, 16q losses, 16p gains, and 1q gains {555}. The prevalence of *PIK3CA* mutations is similar to that in ER-matched and grade-matched IBCs

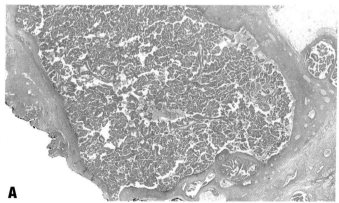
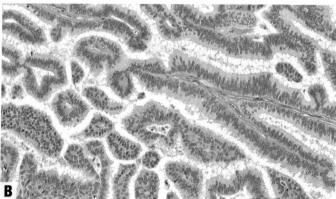

**Fig. 2.48** Encapsulated papillary carcinoma. **A** A papillary mass within a cystic space with numerous delicate fibrovascular stalks. **B** Neoplastic epithelial cells with low-grade nuclei arranged in pseudostratified cell layers covering the fibrovascular stalks.

(NST) {555}. PAM50 subtyping classifies the majority of cases as luminal A and a minority as luminal B {1658}. Compared with grade- and ER-matched IBC-NST, encapsulated papillary carcinoma displays downregulation of genes related to proliferation, cell assembly and organization, and cellular movement and migration, as well as overexpression of genes related to homeostasis and angiogenesis {1658}.

## Macroscopic appearance

Encapsulated papillary carcinoma is often observed as a friable mass within a cystic space.

## Histopathology

Encapsulated papillary carcinoma usually consists of a papillary mass within a cystic space; less often, it is composed of an aggregate of close nodules. The tumour has a rounded, pushing border and is typically surrounded by a fibrous capsule of varying thickness. The lesion consists of multiple delicate fibrovascular stalks covered by a monomorphic population of neoplastic epithelial cells with low- or intermediate-grade nuclei. The epithelial cells are arranged in single or multiple cell layers, and they can also form micropapillary or cribriform structures that fill the gaps separating adjacent papillae. There are typically no myoepithelial cells along the papillae at the epithelial stroma interface. Myoepithelial cells at the periphery of the lesion are also typically absent but can occasionally be present.

Frank invasion in this setting is defined as the presence of neoplastic elements that permeate beyond the fibrous capsule with an irregular infiltrative appearance, most often taking the form of IBC-NST. This must be differentiated from entrapment of neoplastic cells within the fibrous capsule and from epithelial displacement within the biopsy site.

The neoplastic epithelial component does not express high-molecular-weight cytokeratins. Staining for multiple myoepithelial markers demonstrates the absence of myoepithelial cells. In rare instances, an incomplete myoepithelial cell layer at the periphery of the lesion can be highlighted with these markers {2299}. Encapsulated papillary carcinomas express ER and (usually) PR, lack *ERBB2* (*HER2*) gene amplification, and demonstrate a low to occasionally moderate Ki-67 proliferation index {1391,555,2299}. The differential diagnosis includes solid papillary carcinoma, papillary ductal carcinoma in situ, invasive papillary carcinoma, and papilloma with superimposed ductal carcinoma in situ, as well as the rare cases of benign hyperplastic papillary apocrine lesions that present as papillary cystic lesions lined by benign apocrine cells, devoid of nuclear atypia or necrosis, in which a myoepithelial cell layer may be absent {414,2100}.

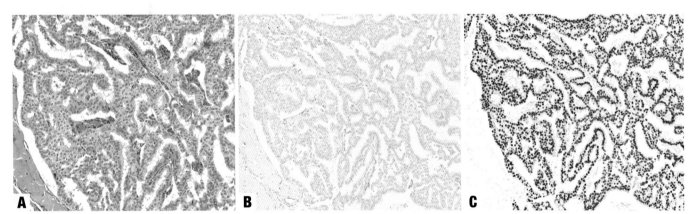

**Fig. 2.49** Encapsulated papillary carcinoma. **A** Neoplastic epithelial cells with low-grade nuclei arranged in micropapillary and cribriform structures filling the gaps between adjacent papillae. **B** CK14 staining demonstrates the absence of myoepithelial cells along the fibrovascular stalks and at the periphery (left edge of field), as well as an absence of staining in the epithelial cells. **C** Strong and diffuse staining for ER in the neoplastic cells.

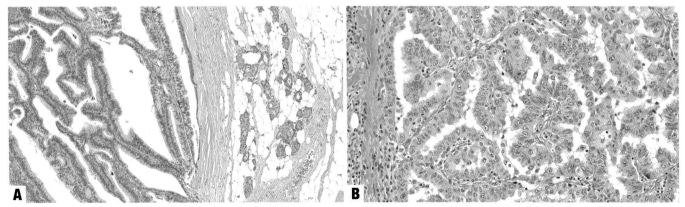

**Fig. 2.50** Encapsulated papillary carcinoma. **A** Frank invasion is defined as the presence of neoplastic elements that permeate beyond the fibrous capsule with an irregular infiltrative appearance. This most commonly takes the form of invasive carcinoma of no special type (NST). **B** Encapsulated papillary carcinomas with high-grade nuclear features should be graded, staged, and managed as invasive carcinomas.

## Cytology

Cytological diagnosis of encapsulated papillary carcinoma is difficult, with no formal cytological features that differentiate this lesion from benign papillary lesions. Cytological smears from encapsulated papillary carcinomas are characterized by high cellularity; the presence of cell balls (corresponding to rounded cohesive epithelial cell clusters of variable size, devoid of fibrovascular cores); increased numbers of single cells with mild atypia, cytoplasmic preservation, and columnar morphology; and the presence of papillae with slender fibrovascular stalks with a ramifying appearance at the edges of the fragments {2115}.

## Diagnostic molecular pathology

Not clinically relevant

## Essential and desirable diagnostic criteria

See Table 2.03 (p. 50), Table 2.04 (p. 50), and Table 2.05 (p. 51).

## Staging

Given the lack of myoepithelial cells and the rare examples of axillary lymph node metastases, the current assumption is that encapsulated papillary carcinoma is a self-confined indolent invasive carcinoma with a prognosis similar to that of carcinoma in situ {387,853,160,597}. In the absence of frank invasion beyond the fibrous capsule, encapsulated papillary carcinoma should be graded according to its nuclear grade and staged "pTis (DCIS)", in order to prevent overtreatment. In the presence of frank invasion, the Nottingham grade and tumour stage should be determined according to the morphological features and pathological size of the frankly invasive component only. ER, PR, and ERBB2 (HER2) status should also be assessed on the frankly invasive component only.

## Prognosis and prediction

In the absence of associated areas of infiltrating carcinoma, encapsulated papillary carcinoma has a very favourable prognosis with adequate local therapy {1125,1139,1706,1184,1973, 2299}. In very rare instances, lymph node metastases have been reported, with the metastases revealing typical papillary features {1425,1706}. The presence of associated ductal carcinoma in situ in the adjacent breast tissue confers a higher risk of local recurrence {297}. Complete surgical excision of the lesion, with extensive sampling of the surrounding breast tissue, is essential for treatment and for assessment of local recurrence risk. Lesions presenting with a growth pattern similar to that of encapsulated papillary carcinoma but with nuclear pleomorphism and increased mitotic activity, and/or a triple-negative or HER2-positive phenotype, should be graded, staged, and managed as IBCs {1718,1220}.

# Solid papillary carcinoma (in situ and invasive)

Mac Grogan G
Collins LC
Lerwill M
Rakha EA
Tan BY

## Definition

Solid papillary carcinomas (in situ and invasive) are tumours characterized by a solid growth pattern with delicate fibrovascular cores. They frequently show neuroendocrine differentiation and are biologically indolent.

## ICD-O coding

8509/2 Solid papillary carcinoma in situ
8509/3 Solid papillary carcinoma with invasion

## ICD-11 coding

2E65.Y & XH0134 Other specified carcinoma in situ of breast & Solid papillary carcinoma in situ
2C64 Solid papillary carcinoma of breast with evidence of invasion

## Related terminology

*Acceptable:* neuroendocrine breast carcinoma in situ; spindle cell ductal carcinoma in situ; neuroendocrine ductal carcinoma in situ; endocrine ductal carcinoma in situ.

## Subtype(s)

None

## Localization

Any part of the breast may be affected, but the central/subareolar area is affected most commonly.

## Clinical features

Solid papillary carcinoma may present as a palpable breast mass, a mammographic abnormality, and/or a bloody nipple discharge. The tumour can appear as a rounded, circumscribed mass on mammography and as a solid, well-defined hypoechoic or heterogeneous mass on ultrasonography. Coexisting stromal distortion suggests an associated invasive component.

## Epidemiology

Solid papillary carcinoma occurs primarily in postmenopausal women, mainly during the seventh decade of life or later {1284, 2112,1706}.

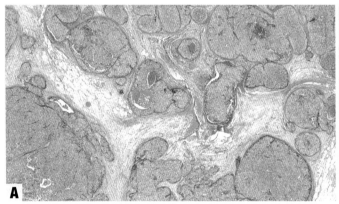
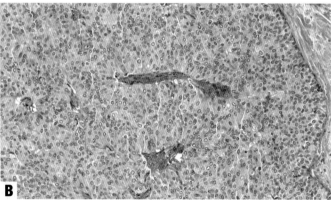

**Fig. 2.51** Solid papillary carcinoma in situ. **A** Expansile nodules with a solid growth pattern have inconspicuous, delicate fibrovascular cores, with no convincing evidence of invasion. **B** High-power view of solid nodules with inconspicuous delicate fibrovascular stalks and a monotonous population of round epithelial cells with low-grade nuclear atypia.

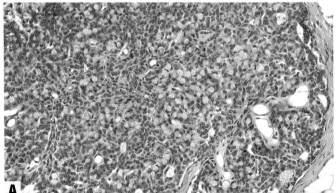
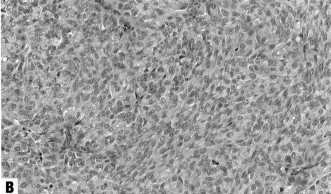

**Fig. 2.52** Solid papillary carcinoma. **A** Intracellular mucin (goblet cells) may be prominent in the neoplastic population. **B** Solid nodules composed of spindled epithelial cells.

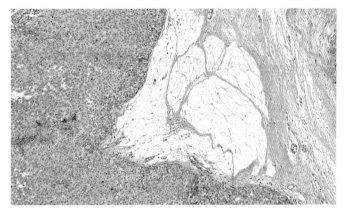

**Fig. 2.53** Solid papillary carcinoma. Extracellular mucin production can also be present, but if it is not associated with floating malignant cells, the tumour is not considered to be mucinous carcinoma.

## Etiology
Unknown

## Pathogenesis
Unknown

## Macroscopic appearance
Gross examination may show a soft, well-circumscribed, tan-pink mass.

## Histopathology
Solid papillary carcinomas are characterized by expansile nodules with a solid growth pattern and inconspicuous, delicate fibrovascular cores. The proliferation is composed of a monotonous population of round to spindle-shaped epithelial cells with (usually) mild to moderate nuclear atypia and a variable mitotic count. The cells have eosinophilic granular cytoplasm and may contain mucin vacuoles. Signet-ring cell features may be prominent. Nuclear palisading around the fibrovascular cores is common. Extracellular mucin production can also be present, but if it is prominent, mucinous carcinoma must be excluded {1284}.

Solid papillary carcinoma in situ is diagnosed when the nodules have rounded, well-circumscribed contours and a distribution pattern consistent with an in situ process, regardless of whether a myoepithelial cell layer is present around the periphery of the nodules {1502}. This tumour type is also described in the *Papillary ductal carcinoma in situ* section (p. 57). Solid papillary carcinoma with invasion is diagnosed when solid papillary carcinoma is associated with areas featuring strands or large clusters of tumour cells. This is frequently seen within pools of extracellular mucin (typically infiltrating the surrounding tissue at the periphery of the lesion), corresponding to mucinous carcinoma {1284,1565}. The invasive component may also be of a more conventional type, such as carcinoma of no special type (NST) or lobular, cribriform, or tubular carcinoma {1466}. In rare instances, solid papillary carcinoma may show features of invasive disease (invasive solid papillary carcinoma); this is diagnosed when the nodules are devoid of a myoepithelial cell layer and have ragged contours creating a geographical jigsaw pattern within a desmoplastic stroma {788,1565}. Fat infiltration by irregular solid papillary nests and vascular invasion may also be seen in these invasive cases.

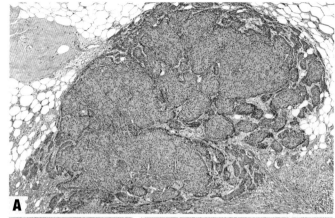

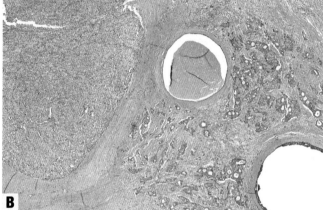

**Fig. 2.54** Solid papillary carcinoma associated with invasive carcinoma. **A** Nodules devoid of a myoepithelial cell layer with ragged contours create a geographical jigsaw pattern within a desmoplastic stroma or infiltrate the fat. **B** Irregular neoplastic glands and trabeculae infiltrate the breast parenchyma adjacent to solid papillary carcinoma.

The neoplastic cells lack expression of high-molecular-weight cytokeratins. They are strongly and diffusely positive for ER, and PR expression is variable. They do not show ERBB2 (HER2) overexpression. The Ki-67 proliferation index is usually low or intermediate {788,1466,555}. Neuroendocrine differentiation, which is demonstrated by synaptophysin and chromogranin expression, is frequent, in particular when there is an associated mucinous component {1565}.

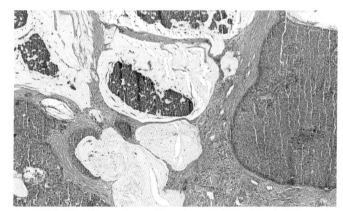

**Fig. 2.55** Solid papillary carcinoma with mucinous carcinoma. Rounded solid nodules in association with large clusters of tumour cells within pools of extracellular mucin.

Papilloma with florid usual ductal hyperplasia that completely obliterates the spaces between papillae can be mistaken for solid papillary carcinoma. In such cases, the fibrovascular cores are typically broad, with a prominent stromal component, and the proliferating cells are less monotonous and have more-irregular nuclei and less-abundant cytoplasm than those of solid papillary carcinoma. The hyperplastic epithelial cells in papilloma express high-molecular-weight cytokeratins and show heterogeneous positivity for ER, whereas the neoplastic epithelial cells of solid papillary carcinoma lack expression of high-molecular-weight cytokeratins and typically show strong ER positivity. A myoepithelial cell layer is present along the fibrovascular cores and at the periphery of the lesion.

## Cytology
Cytological smears from solid papillary carcinoma show high cellularity; highly discohesive clusters of small to large size, with many isolated cells; severe overcrowding of tumour cells; cells with round to oval, finely granular nuclei with little nuclear pleomorphism; tumour cell nuclei that are 1.5–3 times the size of the nucleus of a small lymphocyte; isolated cells with cytoplasmic preservation, a low N:C ratio, and eccentric nuclei; and no oval naked nuclei of myoepithelial cell origin {2307}.

## Diagnostic molecular pathology
Solid papillary carcinomas have relatively simple genomes with few copy-number aberrations, including 16q losses, 16p gains, and 1q gains {555}. *PIK3CA* mutations are found in 43% of cases. The rare cases that have been studied are classified as luminal B by PAM50 subtyping {1658}. Compared with invasive ductal carcinomas NST of the same grade, solid papillary carcinomas have lower expression levels of genes related to cell proliferation, adhesion, migration, and movement, suggestive of a less invasive phenotype. Genes related to neuroendocrine differentiation in human cancers, including *RET*, *ASCL1*, and *DOK7*, are expressed at substantially higher levels in solid papillary carcinomas than in encapsulated papillary carcinomas {1658}.

## Essential and desirable diagnostic criteria
See Table 2.03 (p. 50), Table 2.04 (p. 50), and Table 2.05 (p. 51).

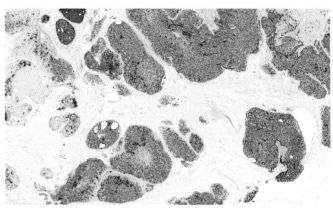

**Fig. 2.56** Solid papillary carcinoma. Neuroendocrine differentiation is frequent (chromogranin A immunostain).

## Staging
In the absence of any obvious conventional invasive component or the features of invasive solid papillary carcinoma described above, solid papillary carcinoma is staged "pTis (DCIS)", regardless of whether a myoepithelial cell layer is identified. It should be graded according to its nuclear features. Solid papillary carcinoma with invasion is staged according to the size of the invasive component only. Nottingham grading and receptor status assessment are also limited to only the invasive component. The grade and receptor status of invasive solid papillary carcinoma should be assessed as it is for other conventional-type carcinomas.

## Prognosis and prediction
Solid papillary carcinoma has an excellent prognosis. In a recent review, spread to axillary lymph nodes was reported in 0 of 76 cases without invasion and 5 of 71 cases with invasion. Distant metastases were observed in 0 of 129 cases without invasion and 7 of 135 cases with invasion {788}.

# Invasive papillary carcinoma

Mac Grogan G
Collins LC
Lerwill M
Rakha EA
Tan BY

## Definition

Invasive papillary carcinoma is an invasive carcinoma with fibrovascular cores covered by neoplastic epithelium.

## ICD-O coding

8503/3 Intraductal papillary adenocarcinoma with invasion

## ICD-11 coding

2C60 & XH8JR8 Carcinoma of breast, specialized type & Papillary carcinoma of breast

## Related terminology

None

## Subtype(s)

None

## Localization

No specific data are available.

## Clinical features

There are no specific features.

## Epidemiology

This lesion is extremely rare, and no specific epidemiological or clinical data are available. Most cases reported as invasive papillary carcinoma in the literature are in fact encapsulated papillary carcinoma or solid papillary carcinoma {2126,2241}, or metastases of carcinomas primary to other sites, especially the ovary {1734}.

## Etiology

Unknown

## Pathogenesis

Unknown

## Macroscopic appearance

Not clinically relevant

## Histopathology

Invasive papillary carcinomas display a frankly invasive growth pattern and are composed of mildly dilated ducts and microcysts containing papillary formations. Myoepithelial cells are absent at the periphery and along the papillary stalks. Invasive papillary carcinoma is graded according to the Nottingham grading system. Tubule differentiation should be assessed based on the presence of structures in which there are clearly defined central lumina surrounded by polarized tumour cells. Tumours without (or with < 10%) tubule formation are scored 3 on a scale of 3.

These tumours should be differentiated from invasive micropapillary carcinoma and metastases to the breast from other organs. Invasive micropapillary carcinomas have a distinctive growth pattern characterized by clusters of cancer cells that lack fibrovascular cores and are surrounded by clear stromal spaces. Metastases of ovarian serous carcinoma, pulmonary papillary adenocarcinoma, and thyroid papillary carcinoma can be distinguished from breast carcinoma on the basis of careful morphological assessment and, as needed, immunohistochemistry for site-of-origin markers. Invasive papillary carcinoma is

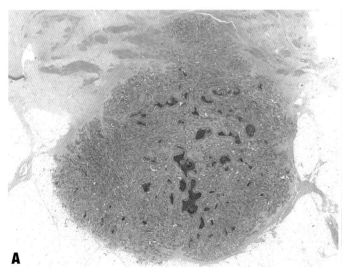
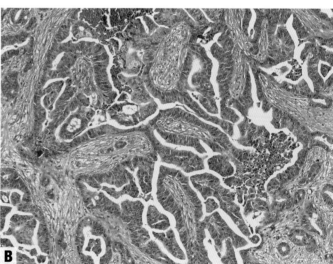

**Fig. 2.57** Invasive papillary carcinoma. **A** Low-power view of carcinoma with invasion of breast parenchyma. **B** Mildly dilated invasive ducts and glands containing papillary cores and necrotic material.

distinct from encapsulated papillary carcinoma and solid papillary carcinoma, which are classified according to their specific morphological features. Additionally, the term should not be used for non-papillary carcinomas arising in association with encapsulated papillary carcinoma or solid papillary carcinoma {2126,2241}.

## Cytology
Not clinically relevant

## Diagnostic molecular pathology
Not clinically relevant

## Essential and desirable diagnostic criteria
See Table 2.03 (p. 50), Table 2.04 (p. 50), and Table 2.05 (p. 51).

## Staging
These tumours should be staged according to their pathological size and the corresponding axillary lymph node status.

## Prognosis and prediction
No specific data are available.

# Non-invasive lobular neoplasia: Introduction

Shin SJ

The term "lobular neoplasia (LN)" refers to the entire spectrum of atypical epithelial lesions originating in the terminal duct lobular unit and characterized by a proliferation of generally small, non-cohesive monomorphic cells, with or without pagetoid involvement of terminal ducts. The designations "atypical lobular hyperplasia" and "lobular carcinoma in situ (LCIS)" are widely used to describe the variable extent of involvement of individual lobular units {1575,1576}.

The first clear clinicopathological description using the term "lobular carcinoma in situ" was published by Foote and Stewart in 1941 {662}. Foote and Stewart used this name in order to describe the morphological similarities between the cells of LCIS and those of an otherwise overt invasive lobular carcinoma. They inferred that LCIS, in a way analogous to ductal carcinoma in situ, could be an established precursor step towards the development of invasive cancer. Consequently, for the next several decades, patients with LCIS were routinely treated with mastectomy. In the late 1970s, Haagensen suggested the designation "lobular neoplasia" for the full spectrum of lesions, on the basis of his unconventional belief that LN represented a benign proliferation that should be viewed as merely a risk factor for subsequent breast carcinoma in either breast {801}. Although the term itself has not been universally adopted, the conceptual model of LN led to a paradigm shift in the way affected patients were clinically managed. By the 1990s, the practice of non-surgical management of patients with LN was fully adopted, and it continues today. Similarly, the term "lobular intraepithelial neoplasia" has also been proposed, but it has not been used widely in clinical practice {220}.

Some of the important issues with LN relate to the appropriate nomenclature, the lack of specific mammographic abnormalities, its role as a risk indicator or a non-obligate precursor, conflicting ideas in the literature regarding its biological and clinical significance, morphological variants, the risk of development of invasive carcinoma, and the best clinical approach for the management of patients diagnosed with LN by core needle biopsy.

# Atypical lobular hyperplasia

Chen YY
Decker T
King TA
Palacios J

Reis-Filho JS
Shin SJ
Simpson PT

## Definition
Atypical lobular hyperplasia (ALH) is a non-invasive neoplastic proliferation of small, dyscohesive cells, originating in the terminal duct lobular units (TDLUs), with or without pagetoid involvement of terminal ducts. Fewer than half of the acini in a TDLU are filled and expanded by the neoplastic cells.

## ICD-O coding
None

## ICD-11 coding
None

## Related terminology
*Acceptable:* lobular neoplasia.
*Not recommended:* lobular intraepithelial neoplasia.

## Subtype(s)
None

## Localization
ALH is often multicentric and bilateral {801}.

## Clinical features
ALH lacks clinical and mammographic signs. It is usually an incidental microscopic finding in breast biopsies performed for another lesion.

## Epidemiology
The true incidence of ALH in the general population is unknown. ALH is found in women over a broad age range (mean age: ~50 years), in about 0.5–1.2% of otherwise benign breast core biopsies and in 1.6–2.9% of reduction mammoplasty specimens {7,145,385,489,747,1347,1412,1504,1908}.

## Etiology
Information about risk and predisposing factors of ALH is very scant. Women with high mammographic breast density are more likely to have ALH than women without dense breasts {38,722}. The presence of columnar cell lesions in a breast biopsy is associated with higher prevalence of ALH in adjacent breast tissue, suggesting that these entities may share similar risk factors {213,1820}.

## Pathogenesis

E-cadherin inactivation, which is a hallmark of lobular lesions, is an early event already present in ALH {433,1311,1847}. By mediating cell–cell adhesion and maintaining tissue integrity, E-cadherin acts as a tumour suppressor {693}. Impaired E-cadherin function results in the characteristic non-cohesive growth of lobular cells.

Molecular studies on ALH, although sparse, have provided evidence that ALH is a clonal neoplastic proliferation. An early study reported loss of heterozygosity on 11q13 in ALH {1474}. Losses of chromosomal material from 7p, 16p, 16q, 17p, and 22q and gains of material on 2p and 6q have been identified in ALH by chromosomal comparative genomic hybridization and array comparative genomic hybridization {1246,1310}. Many of these changes were found to be shared by the associated lobular carcinoma in situ (LCIS) and/or invasive carcinoma, supporting ALH as an early lesion in the lobular carcinoma pathway and suggesting a possible non-obligate precursor role for ALH.

A recent study using whole-exome sequencing revealed that LCIS has a genomic profile similar to that of invasive lobular carcinoma, with *CDH1* mutations present in 81% of the lesions {1135}. It is likely that ALH has a genomic landscape similar to that of LCIS, including frequent *CDH1* mutations.

## Macroscopic appearance

Not clinically relevant

## Histopathology

ALH demonstrates a solid proliferation of dyscohesive monomorphic epithelial cells expanding < 50% of the acini in a TDLU, with or without pagetoid involvement of terminal ducts. Some cases of ALH may involve ducts in a pagetoid pattern in the absence of involvement of lobular acini {1574}. For practical diagnostic purposes, some authorities have applied the following two approaches as a guidepost for distension: (1) comparing the calibre of the involved acini to that of acini of adjacent uninvolved lobules – if the involved acini are larger than the uninvolved acini, they are considered distended {2055}; and (2) estimating the number of cells in the involved acini – if the involved acini have ≥ 8 cells present across the diameter of an acinus, they are considered distended {1948,1949}. However, scientific evidence for these size criteria to define distension is lacking.

The proliferation may exhibit two cell types, either singly or mixed: type A cells have scant cytoplasm and uniform, round, small to slightly enlarged nuclei (1–1.5 times the size of a lymphocyte nucleus) and inconspicuous nucleoli; type B cells have more-abundant cytoplasm and larger nuclei (2 times the

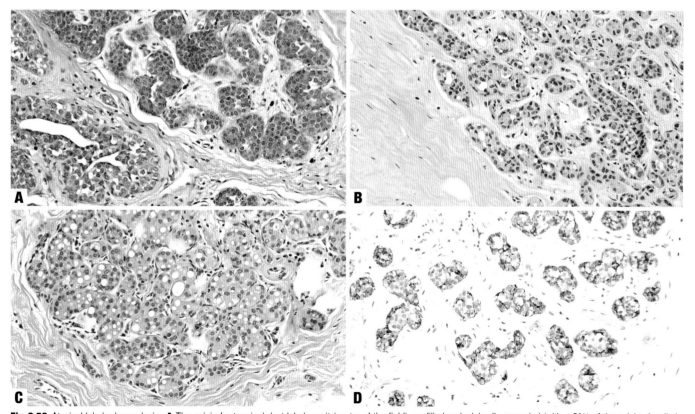

**Fig. 2.58** Atypical lobular hyperplasia. **A** The acini of a terminal duct lobular unit (centre of the field) are filled and minimally expanded (with < 50% of the acini ≥ 8 cells in diameter) by loosely cohesive, monomorphic cells displaying scant cytoplasm and small uniform nuclei with inconspicuous nucleoli. These cells are type A lobular cells. In the lower left part of the field, a duct shows pagetoid involvement by atypical lobular hyperplasia, with lobular neoplastic cells infiltrating between the duct basement membrane and an attenuated layer of residual duct epithelium. **B** The cells in this example have more-abundant cytoplasm and larger nuclei with mild to moderate variability in size and shape and more-prominent nucleoli. These are type B lobular cells. **C** Many of the neoplastic cells contain intracytoplasmic lumina, and in some cells the lumina are large enough to impart a signet-ring cell appearance. **D** E-cadherin immunostaining demonstrates a lack of E-cadherin expression in the neoplastic cells. Staining from residual ductal epithelial cells should not be interpreted to exclude a lobular phenotype.

size of a lymphocyte nucleus), with more variability in size and shape and more-prominent nucleoli {801,1966}. The distinction between type A and type B cells is of no known significance {801}. Intracytoplasmic lumina, which may impart a signet-ring cell appearance, are often present but are not specific to lobular neoplasia.

Loss of membranous E-cadherin expression is the defining immunohistochemical feature of lobular lesions, including ALH {433,1311}. β-catenin, α-catenin, and p120-catenin (proteins known to complex with E-cadherin) also demonstrate loss of membranous expression; p120-catenin is aberrantly located in the cytoplasm and is also upregulated {275,430,1421,1847}. However, approximately 15% of lobular lesions retain E-cadherin expression but with an aberrant staining pattern, which should not be interpreted to exclude a lobular phenotype {275,429, 1712}. Therefore, these immunohistochemical markers should be interpreted in conjunction with detailed histological analysis.

## Cytology
Hypocellular aspirates showing loosely cohesive groups of small, uniform cells containing clear vacuoles and eccentric minimally atypical nuclei suggest the presence of a lobular lesion (ALH, LCIS, or invasive lobular carcinoma). However, there are no reliable cytological criteria for distinguishing between ALH/LCIS and invasive lobular carcinoma {1832,1943, 2131}. Compared with core needle biopsy, FNA for non-palpable lesions (including ALH and LCIS) is characterized by lower sensitivity and specificity and a higher rate of non-diagnostic results {1654,910}.

## Diagnostic molecular pathology
Not clinically relevant

## Essential and desirable diagnostic criteria
*Essential:* small dyscohesive cells with uniform hyperchromatic nuclei (type A) to slightly larger vesicular nuclei with mild variability (type B), filling and expanding fewer than half of the acini in a TDLU.
*Desirable:* loss of membranous E-cadherin staining, if needed.

## Staging
ALH is considered a high-risk non-malignant lesion and is not staged.

## Prognosis and prediction
ALH reflects an increased constitutional breast cancer predisposition, as demonstrated by an elevated risk for subsequent cancers of different histological types in both breasts (albeit with an ipsilateral predominance) {385,398,829,1301,1575, 1578,2294}. The relative risk for breast cancer among patients with ALH is 4–5 times that expected in women without ALH. The risk associated with ductal involvement by ALH alone is lower than the risk associated with ALH involving both the lobules and ducts {1574}. The absolute risk of breast cancer associated with ALH is estimated to be about 1% per year and is fairly constant over time, with a cumulative incidence of 30% at 25 years {828}.

Younger patient age at diagnosis of ALH, histological calcifications, and less age-related lobular involution have been found to further increase the risk of breast cancer, whereas chemoprevention lowers the risk {398,474,641,828,1301}. Some (but not all) studies have demonstrated that the risk is increased with a positive family history and multiple foci of ALH {384,473, 474,828,1575}.

The management of ALH diagnosed on core needle biopsy has been controversial, due to the wide range of reported upgrade rates (0–67%) to carcinoma (including invasive carcinoma and ductal carcinoma in situ) on excision {36,81,269, 278,411,582,671,841,906,911,978,1002,1231,1274,1368,1412, 1504,1553,1709,1752,1753,1908,1925,1969,2003,2355}. However, recent studies report very low (0–4%) excisional upgrade rates of incidental cases of ALH alone or lobular neoplasia (combining ALH and LCIS cases) when concordant radiological–pathological correlation to a different target lesion has been identified {91,906,1436,1444,1447,1752,1908,2003, 2010,2355}. Therefore, patients with incidental ALH on core biopsy showing an additional benign lesion with proven radiological–pathological concordance may be safely observed. Excision should be performed if there is another lesion that by itself would warrant excision or if there is no histological correlate to the target of the biopsy.

For the purposes of risk assessment and clinical management, ALH is considered a marker of increased risk. Best practice for the care for women with ALH emphasizes close surveillance and counselling for risk reduction.

# Lobular carcinoma in situ

Chen YY
Decker T
King TA
Palacios J
Shin SJ
Simpson PT

## Definition

Lobular carcinoma in situ (LCIS) is a non-invasive neoplastic proliferation of dyscohesive cells, originating in the terminal duct lobular units (TDLUs), with or without pagetoid involvement of terminal ducts. More than half of the acini in a TDLU are filled and expanded by the neoplastic cells.

## ICD-O coding

8520/2 Lobular carcinoma in situ NOS
8519/2 Lobular carcinoma in situ, pleomorphic

## ICD-11 coding

2E65.0 & XH6EH0 Lobular carcinoma in situ of breast & Lobular carcinoma in situ NOS

## Related terminology

*Acceptable:* lobular neoplasia.
*Not recommended:* non-classic lobular carcinoma in situ; variant lobular carcinoma in situ; lobular intraepithelial neoplasia.

## Subtype(s)

Classic lobular carcinoma in situ; pleomorphic lobular carcinoma in situ; florid lobular carcinoma in situ

## Localization

LCIS is multicentric in the ipsilateral breast in as many as 80% of patients and bilateral in 30–67% {155,1488,1797,1106,1869, 800,2054}. Pleomorphic LCIS and florid LCIS have been noted to be unifocal and continuous in distribution, often colocalized with invasive lobular carcinoma (ILC) in the background of multicentric classic LCIS {105,1910}.

## Clinical features

Classic LCIS has no specific clinical features; the lesion is usually an incidental microscopic finding in breast biopsies performed for other indications {662}. Rare cases (< 2%) of classic LCIS can be targeted for biopsy due to associated imaging abnormalities, including grouped amorphous or granular calcifications on mammography or heterogeneous non–mass-like enhancement with persistent enhancement kinetics on MRI {1322,1882}. In contrast, pleomorphic LCIS and florid LCIS are usually associated with microcalcifications and detected on screening mammography {330,463,623,652,1001,1924,1966, 2004}.

## Epidemiology

LCIS is found in 0.5–3.6% of otherwise benign breast biopsies and 0.04–1.2% of reduction mammoplasty specimens {7,63, 145,155,489,1192,1412,1576,1662}. Epidemiological studies have demonstrated that the incidence rates of LCIS increased rapidly after the introduction of mammography (1978–1998) and declined sharply between 2001 and 2004, most likely due to

decreased use of menopausal hormone replacement therapy {1166,1170,2225}. Classic LCIS is predominantly diagnosed in premenopausal women (mean age: ~50 years) {155,683,801, 1021}. Pleomorphic LCIS and florid LCIS are diagnosed primarily in postmenopausal women (mean age: ~60 years) {330,789, 1910,1924}.

## Etiology

Many risk factors for LCIS are similar to those established for ductal carcinoma in situ (DCIS) and invasive breast carcinoma. Population-based studies have reported an increased risk of LCIS associated with a family history of breast cancer, a previous benign breast biopsy, nulliparity, older age at first full-term birth, older age at menopause, and high mammographic density {38,367,368,1427,2101,2255}. In postmenopausal women, hormone replacement therapy increases the risk of LCIS {1427, 1735,2101}.

CDH1 (the gene encoding the cell adhesion protein E-cadherin), localized at 16q22.1, plays an important role in the pathogenesis of lobular lesions. Germline mutations in *CDH1*, which are highly penetrant, are associated with an increased risk of hereditary diffuse gastric cancer (HDGC) and an increased risk of lobular carcinoma, including bilateral LCIS, with or without ILC {401,1639}. Of the known germline SNPs that are associated with an increased risk of ER-positive breast cancer, several have also shown an association with ILC and specifically also with LCIS {1853}.

## Pathogenesis

CDH1 inactivation, which leads to loss or impaired function of E-cadherin, is an early event and hallmark of lobular lesions {2192}. E-cadherin mediates cell–cell adhesion and plays a key role in the maintenance of lobular architecture. It can also inhibit the growth and invasion of breast cancer cells {153,305}. Defective E-cadherin results in loss of cell–cell adhesion, increased cell proliferation, and altered organization of the lobules, giving rise to the characteristic appearance of lobular neoplasia {483, 484}. *CDH1* mutation is identified in 81% of LCIS cases. Most of the mutations seen in LCIS have been found to be associated with an age-related mutation signature, consistent with mutation signatures observed in ILC and ER-positive invasive carcinoma of no special type (NST) {1135}.

Molecular analysis has demonstrated that LCIS is a clonal neoplastic proliferation and a non-obligate precursor lesion to invasive carcinoma. Studies using comparative genomic hybridization and array comparative genomic hybridization have indicated that classic LCIS, pleomorphic LCIS, and florid LCIS all harbour recurrent chromosomal gain at 1q and loss at 16q, a pattern typical of the low-grade breast neoplasia pathway {190,330,598,1246,1924}. Pleomorphic LCIS and florid LCIS exhibit greater genomic instability than classic LCIS, with increased copy-number alterations and gene amplifications,

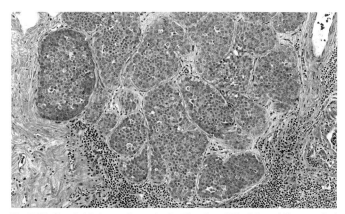

**Fig. 2.59** Classic lobular carcinoma in situ. More than 50% of the acini in a terminal duct lobular unit are filled and expanded by loosely cohesive monomorphic cells with scant cytoplasm and small uniform nuclei.

suggesting that these morphological subtypes are genetically more advanced lesions than classic LCIS {190,330,1748,1924}. Studies comparing LCIS and synchronous ILC highlight shared copy-number aberrations, indicating that LCIS is a non-obligate precursor to ILC {905,1748}.

Massively parallel sequencing studies have revealed that LCIS can be clonally related to ILC and occasionally to DCIS present in the same quadrant {1135,1825}. These studies have also demonstrated that LCIS is a genetically advanced lesion, harbouring a repertoire of copy-number alterations and somatic genetic mutations similar to that of ILCs, with the exception that *TP53* and *PTFN* mutations were found to be remarkably rare {1135}. The most frequently mutated genes in LCIS are *CDH1* (mutated in as many as 81% of cases), *PIK3CA* (41%), and *CBFB* (12%) {1135,1825,1907}. Mutation (and amplification) of *ERBB2* (*HER2*) is a frequent molecular alteration in pleomorphic ILC and pleomorphic LCIS {1193}. A recent microarray gene expression profiling study demonstrated that classic LCIS is heterogeneous at the transcriptomic level and identified potential candidate precursor genes for invasion, whose biological and clinical significance warrants further exploration {69}.

### Macroscopic appearance

LCIS is not associated with any grossly recognizable abnormalities {662,801}.

### Histopathology

Classic LCIS is characterized by dyscohesive proliferations of type A and/or type B epithelial cells. Type A cells are small cells with uniform hyperchromatic nuclei, whereas type B cells have slightly larger vesicular nuclei, with mild variability in size and shape and with small nucleoli. The cell populations may be mixed in individual proliferations. More than 50% of the acini in a TDLU must be filled and expanded by the neoplastic cells to qualify as LCIS. Glandular architecture is not observed, and mitoses and microcalcifications are uncommon. Classic LCIS may rarely show single-cell apoptosis and/or minute foci of necrosis. LCIS can show pagetoid growth in ducts and may involve other lesions, including usual ductal hyperplasia, sclerosing adenosis, radial scars, papillary lesions, fibroadenomas, and collagenous spherulosis.

The other two recognized morphological subtypes of LCIS are pleomorphic and florid. Pleomorphic LCIS is composed of larger cells with marked nuclear pleomorphism, which are > 4 times the size of a lymphocyte / equivalent to the cells of high-grade DCIS, with or without apocrine features {1966}. In florid LCIS, the LCIS cells show the cytological features of classic LCIS, but there is marked distention of TDLUs or ducts, creating a confluent mass-like architecture. Florid LCIS should have at least one of two architectural features: little to no intervening stroma between markedly distended acini of involved TDLUs and a size cut-off point at which an expanded acinus or duct fills an area equivalent to ~40–50 cells in diameter {52,1910, 1924,2260}. LCIS lesions that are borderline between classic LCIS composed of type B cells and pleomorphic LCIS should be categorized as classic LCIS composed of type B cells. Similarly, lesions with cytological features of classic LCIS that show distension of the acini borderline between classic LCIS and florid LCIS should be designated as classic LCIS, even when LCIS is extensive.

Pleomorphic LCIS and florid LCIS often demonstrate comedonecrosis and calcifications. Due to the high prevalence (as high as 87%) of associated invasive carcinoma in these morphological subtypes, with the majority (84–100%) being ILC, detection of these lesions should prompt a careful search for subtle invasion in adjacent breast tissue {610,105,1910}. Signet-ring cells may be seen in any morphological subtype. Several other terms have been used in clinical practice for these subtypes, including "non-classic LCIS" and "variant LCIS without further clarification". The WHO Classification of Tumours Editorial Board does not recommend these terms, due to lack of sufficient specificity to guide patient management.

Loss of membranous E-cadherin expression is the characteristic immunohistochemical feature for all forms of LCIS {433,694, 1311,1583}. In approximately 15% of invasive lobular lesions, the neoplastic cells have conserved but aberrant E-cadherin expression, and this is recapitulated in LCIS. Therefore, fragmented membranous and/or cytoplasmic aberrant staining should not be used to make a diagnosis of DCIS {275,429,1712}. LCIS cells exhibit strong, diffuse cytoplasmic staining for p120-catenin and loss of expression of membrane β-catenin {275, 430,1421,1847}. However, the distinction between LCIS and DCIS cannot rely solely on these immunohistochemical markers, which should be interpreted in conjunction with detailed morphological evaluation.

The classic and florid subtypes of LCIS are typically diffusely and strongly positive for ER, have a low Ki-67 proliferation index, and rarely show ERBB2 (HER2) overexpression or gene amplification, or *TP53* mutation {28,251,1588,1719,1809}. The pleomorphic subtype is more likely to be ER-negative (especially apocrine pleomorphic LCIS), may be AR-positive, may demonstrate HER2 overexpression and gene amplification or *TP53* mutation, and has a moderate to high Ki-67 proliferation index {330,1001, 1910,1924,1966}. Approximately 10% of pleomorphic cases are triple-negative {1001,1910}.

### Cytology

FNA of LCIS shows loosely cohesive groups of small, uniform cells with occasional intracytoplasmic lumina, eccentric regular nuclei, and minimal nuclear atypia {1832,1943,2131}. However, > 50% of aspirates from LCIS have been determined to be

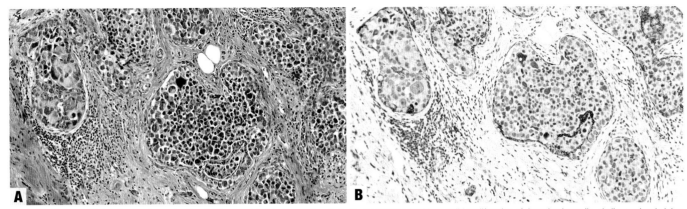

**Fig. 2.60** Pleomorphic lobular carcinoma in situ. **A** Pleomorphic lobular carcinoma in situ is characterized by a solid proliferation of dyscohesive cells, similar to classic lobular carcinoma in situ, but with marked nuclear pleomorphism equivalent to high-grade ductal carcinoma in situ. **B** Pleomorphic lobular carcinoma in situ lacks membranous E-cadherin expression.

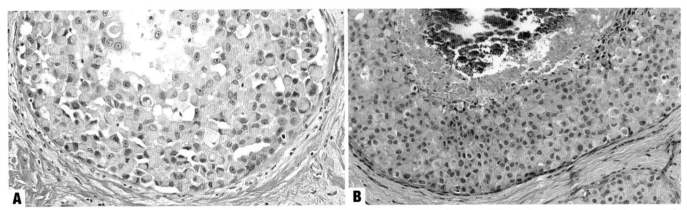

**Fig. 2.61** Apocrine pleomorphic lobular carcinoma in situ. **A** A subset of pleomorphic lobular carcinoma in situ is further categorized as apocrine type, based on large cells with abundant eosinophilic granular cytoplasm and round to oval nuclei containing prominent nucleoli. **B** Pleomorphic lobular carcinoma in situ is often associated with comedonecrosis and calcifications, leading to mammographic detection.

benign or non-diagnostic {2131}. There are no reliable cytological criteria for distinguishing between LCIS and ILC {1943,2131}.

### Diagnostic molecular pathology
Not clinically relevant

### Essential and desirable diagnostic criteria
*Classic LCIS*
*Essential:* small dyscohesive cells with uniform hyperchromatic nuclei (type A) to slightly larger vesicular nuclei with mild variability (type B), filling and expanding more than half of the acini in a TDLU.
*Desirable:* loss of E-cadherin membrane staining.

*Pleomorphic LCIS*
*Essential:* large dyscohesive cells with marked nuclear pleomorphism, > 4 times the size of a lymphocyte / equivalent to the cells of high-grade DCIS, with or without apocrine features.
*Desirable:* loss of E-cadherin membrane staining.

*Florid LCIS*
*Essential:* classic LCIS creating a confluent mass-like architecture; little to no intervening stroma between markedly distended acini of involved TDLUs, and/or a size cut-off point at which an expanded acinus or duct fills an area equivalent to ~40–50 cells in diameter.
*Desirable:* loss of E-cadherin membrane staining.

### Staging
The eighth edition of the Union for International Cancer Control (UICC) TNM classification {229} recommends that LCIS be staged as pTis. However, the eighth edition of the American Joint Committee on Cancer (AJCC) cancer staging manual {61} considers LCIS to be a benign disease and therefore does not include it in staging.

### Prognosis and prediction
LCIS is both a risk factor for and a non-obligate precursor of invasive breast carcinoma. The relative risk of subsequent breast cancer in patients with classic LCIS is 8–10 times the risk in the general population {63,180,648,801,1576,1795}. The absolute risk of breast cancer is in the range of 1–2% per year, with a cumulative long-term rate of > 20% at 20 years and a lifetime risk of 30–40% {646,648,1021,2086}. The risk is bilateral and the invasive carcinoma can be either lobular or ductal {71, 356}. However, ipsilateral cancers predominate, with an over-representation of ILC; LCIS is therefore also considered a non-obligate precursor lesion, albeit with a low risk of progression to invasive cancer {71,398,1021,1172}. This is further supported by molecular studies.

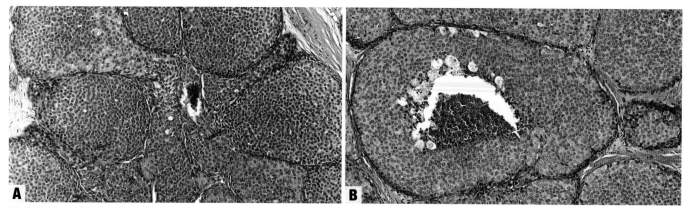

**Fig. 2.62** Florid lobular carcinoma in situ. **A** Florid lobular carcinoma in situ has cytological features similar to those of classic lobular carcinoma in situ (type A and/or type B cells) but is distinguished by marked expansion of terminal duct lobular units with little to no intervening stroma between markedly distended acini of involved terminal duct lobular units. **B** In florid lobular carcinoma in situ, the acini or ducts are markedly expanded (filling at least one high-power field, equivalent to > 40–50 cells in diameter) and often associated with central necrosis.

Current management for classic LCIS includes active surveillance and risk-reduction strategies for both breasts. The American Society of Clinical Oncology (ASCO) guidelines include recommendations for antiestrogen therapy as chemoprevention to reduce breast cancer risk in women with LCIS {2182}. The management of classic LCIS diagnosed on core needle biopsy has been controversial due to the wide range of reported upgrade rates (0–60%) to carcinoma (including invasive carcinoma and DCIS) on excision {145,269,444,490,582,671,696, 906,911,978,1002,1192,1231,1274,1368,1412,1436,1504,1553, 1691,1752,1753,1908,1925,2003,2355}. In these studies, the upgrade rates are higher when radiological–pathological correlation is not addressed or when LCIS represents the radiological target, and the rates are even higher (as high as 66%) in cases with biopsy for mass lesions and those with imaging–histological discordance {444,582,906,978,1368,1436,1504}. However, recent studies with concordant imaging findings have reported very low (~1–4%) excisional upgrade rates of incidental classic LCIS (and atypical lobular hyperplasia) to carcinoma {91,906, 1436,1444,1447,1752,1753,1908,2010}. Therefore, patients with incidental classic LCIS on core biopsy showing concordant imaging–histological findings can be spared surgical excision. There is no indication that excision of classic LCIS to negative margins is useful, and it is not necessary to assess or report the status of excision margins for classic LCIS, even in the setting of coexistent pleomorphic LCIS, florid LCIS, and/or ILC.

Information about the natural history of pleomorphic LCIS and florid LCIS is extremely limited, and the optimal treatment for patients with these excised morphological LCIS subtypes remains unclear – including whether to achieve negative margins and whether there is any potential benefit of adjuvant radiation {178}. The reported recurrence rates of pleomorphic LCIS treated with conservative surgery with or without antiestrogen therapy vary from 0% to as high as 57%, and the recurrent lesions may be pleomorphic LCIS, DCIS, ILC, or invasive ductal carcinoma {463,539,652,1001,1448,1966}. It is unclear whether positive margin status affects the likelihood of recurrence, but results from these studies generally support the practical utility of surgical excision to negative margins for pleomorphic LCIS if possible. It is recommended that margin status be reported for pleomorphic LCIS and florid LCIS to help inform further management decisions.

Approximately 25–60% of cases with pleomorphic LCIS and florid LCIS on core biopsy are upgraded to carcinoma on excision {444,623,652,789,1448,1910,2004}. Although there are limitations to the data derived from such studies, the WHO Classification of Tumours Editorial Board recommends excision for pleomorphic LCIS and florid LCIS diagnosed on core needle biopsy.

# Ductal carcinoma in situ: Introduction

Fox SB
Pinder SE

Ductal carcinoma in situ (DCIS) is a clinically, radiologically, and histologically heterogeneous non-obligate precursor of invasive breast carcinoma. DCIS is a segmental disease originating in the terminal duct lobular unit and progressing within the duct system towards the nipple and into adjacent branches of a given segment of the duct system. The rare lesions that develop within the lactiferous ducts may progress towards the nipple, resulting in Paget disease {1538,1539,1541}. However, it should be noted that the term "ductal carcinoma in situ" encompasses a highly heterogeneous group of lesions that differ with regard to their mode of presentation, histopathological features, biological markers, genetic and molecular abnormalities, and risk for progression to invasive cancer. Heterogeneity may exist even within a given DCIS lesion {44}.

Historically, DCIS presented as a mass, but most cases are now identified through screening programmes. Approximately 20% of screen-detected breast cancer is DCIS {1885,2237}. Mammographically, DCIS can be characterized by clustered microcalcifications (62–98%) with linear branching or a casting pattern, or it can present as a mass (2–23%). However, most changes are indeterminate; similar microcalcifications are common in benign conditions, and core biopsy is required for definitive diagnosis.

Our understanding of the natural history of DCIS is poor and largely based on histological review of small numbers of cases initially interpreted as benign. Although the proportion of cases developing invasive disease is similar, high-grade DCIS progresses more rapidly (average: 5 years) than low-grade disease, which may present with invasive carcinoma many decades later {391,1838}. These data are supported by recent series showing that high cytonuclear grade is a risk factor for progression of non-resected DCIS to invasive cancer, as are presentation as mammographic microcalcifications, young patient age, and lack of endocrine therapy {1323}. Because of the paucity of natural history data, prediction of the likely behaviour of DCIS is largely extrapolated from analyses of recurrent disease; about 50% of lesions that initially present as DCIS recur as such, and about 50% recur as invasive carcinoma.

The breast cancer–specific survival of women with DCIS, even those with recurrent cases, is extremely good {2075}, although patients who develop invasive recurrence have a worse outcome {2222,2075}. The current standard of care for patients with DCIS is either breast-conserving surgery and radiotherapy or mastectomy. The definition of complete excision (clear margins) in DCIS is controversial, but current guidelines (based on meta-analyses and large datasets) recommend a 2 mm tumour-free margin {2098,1423}. The use of adjuvant radiotherapy after breast-conserving surgery reduces recurrence by approximately half. This appears to be irrespective of age at diagnosis, tamoxifen use, method of DCIS detection, margin status, grade, presence of comedonecrosis, architecture, and lesion size {559}. Ongoing randomized clinical trials aim to identify low-risk disease, which can be managed conservatively with surveillance imaging {676,584}. Similarly, sentinel lymph node biopsy, previously undertaken for some patients with DCIS (e.g. large and high-grade disease or in patients receiving mastectomy) is no longer invariably performed {2234}, although there is wide variation even when national guidelines exist {867}. Tumour cells may be found in the axillary lymph nodes of patients with DCIS; in some cases, this undoubtedly represents spread from unidentified foci of invasive carcinoma, and extensive and thorough histological examination of the breast tissue is mandatory. However, mechanical displacement of epithelial cells from a previous needling procedure may explain other cases {1413}. Overall, there is wide variation in the treatment recommended for patients with DCIS {2075,1501}, especially in the use of adjuvant hormone therapy, and better prognostic and predictive markers are needed.

# Ductal carcinoma in situ

Pinder SE
Collins LC
Fox SB
Schnitt SJ

van Deurzen CHM
Weaver DL
Wesseling J

## Definition
Ductal carcinoma in situ (DCIS) is a non-invasive proliferation of cohesive neoplastic epithelial cells confined to the mammary ductal-lobular system, exhibiting a range of architectural patterns and nuclear grades.

## ICD-O coding
8500/2 Intraductal carcinoma, non-infiltrating, NOS

## ICD-11 coding
2E65.2 & XH4V32 Ductal carcinoma in situ of breast & Ductal carcinoma in situ NOS

## Related terminology
*Acceptable:* intraductal carcinoma.

## Subtype(s)
DCIS of low nuclear grade; DCIS of intermediate nuclear grade; DCIS of high nuclear grade

## Localization
DCIS can arise either in the breast or in accessory breast parenchyma in the axillary tail.

## Clinical features
Historically, DCIS presented as a palpable mass, nipple discharge, or Paget disease of the nipple. Although these presentations still occur, as many as 85% of DCIS cases are now detected mammographically, typically as calcifications, and are impalpable. The mean patient age at diagnosis is 50–59 years. The disease is most often unilateral, but about 22% of women with DCIS in one breast develop either in situ or invasive carcinoma in the contralateral breast {2224}. High-grade DCIS classically presents with linear, pleomorphic, or branching

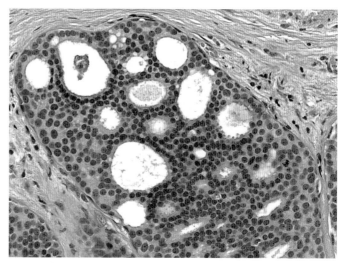

**Fig. 2.64** Cribriform ductal carcinoma in situ of low nuclear grade. Note the low-grade nuclei and the cribriform architecture.

calcifications, whereas low-grade disease has granular and amorphous patterns. On MRI, DCIS (in particular high-grade disease) may appear as a non–mass-like enhancement with delayed peak enhancement profiles. However, the sensitivity of MRI for DCIS is lower than that for invasive breast carcinoma (IBC); therefore, this technique is not widely used. Ultrasound changes are often subtle and nonspecific, unless an associated mass is present.

## Epidemiology
Before mammographic screening programmes, DCIS was infrequently identified, amounting to only 2–3% of palpable breast cancers. Because DCIS is now a predominantly radiologically identified lesion, it is most common in geographical areas with

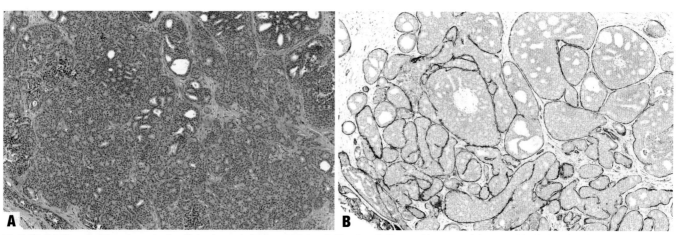

**Fig. 2.63** Cribriform ductal carcinoma in situ with involvement of adjacent lobules. **A** Note the cribriform architecture and the area of involvement. **B** Retained myoepithelial cells around the lobules are highlighted by SMMHC immunostaining.

population-based breast cancer screening programmes. As a result of mammographic diagnosis, the apparent incidence of DCIS has increased from 1.87 cases per 100 000 person-years in 1973–1975 to 32.5 cases per 100 000 person-years in 2005, and DCIS is most commonly diagnosed in women aged > 50 years {2180}, with one case identified per 1000 screening mammograms {2237}.

## Etiology

The risk factors for DCIS and IBC are similar, indicating a common etiology; germline mutations in hereditary breast cancer predisposition genes, family history, nulliparity, late age at first childbirth, late menopause, and elevated body mass index after menopause are all associated with an increased risk of DCIS, as are postmenopausal hormone replacement therapy and high mammographic breast density {992}.

## Pathogenesis

The prevalence of germline *BRCA1* and *BRCA2* mutations among women diagnosed with DCIS is similar to that among women diagnosed with IBC {366}. The increase in lifetime risk of DCIS for a BRCA mutation carrier versus a non-carrier is estimated to be about 6-fold {1325}. Consistent with a shared genetic susceptibility for DCIS and IBC, an analysis of 38 genotype studies including 5067 cases of DCIS, 24 584 cases of invasive ductal carcinoma (by previous terminology), and 37 467 controls indicated that most (67%) of the 76 known IBC predisposition loci showed a similar association with DCIS {1638}.

The evidence for DCIS as a precursor of IBC includes series demonstrating high genomic concordance between synchronous DCIS and IBC {524}. Of note, the three-tiered grading system for DCIS does not indicate progression from low, through intermediate, to high nuclear grade (although an admixture of the grades may uncommonly be seen). There is evidence that DCIS lesions of low and high nuclear grade follow different pathways, have different molecular and genetic profiles, and show different rates of progression to IBC. High levels of genomic instability are seen in DCIS of high nuclear grade, whereas DCIS of low nuclear grade shows fewer genomic alterations {575}. Distinctive chromosomal changes, similar to those observed in grade 1 and grade 3 IBCs, respectively, are seen in DCIS of low and high nuclear grade. Cases with low nuclear grade are characterized by frequent 16q loss and 1q gain, whereas cases with high nuclear grade often show gains of 5p, 8q, 17q, and 20q; amplifications of 11q13, 17q12, and 17q22-q24; and loss of 8p, 11q, 13q, and 14q {247,904}. Methylation of genes seen in IBC is also reported in DCIS and is associated with features such as high nuclear grade, *ERBB2* (*HER2*) amplification, and negative ER and PR status {1591,1390}, and the same is true for genomic gains and losses {1389}. However, none of the genomic changes identified have yet been consistently associated with invasive progression or recurrence risk, and therefore none have proven clinical utility {1592}. There is some evidence that progression of DCIS to IBC may involve an altered relationship between DCIS cell copy number and the immune microenvironment (e.g. as assessed by quantification of tumour-infiltrating lymphocytes) {842}.

## Macroscopic appearance

DCIS is now rarely identified clinically or macroscopically as a mass, except for some papillary subtypes, which may be identified as well-defined, pale, soft masses. Most DCIS detected by mammography cannot be detected visually, and there is no consistent macroscopic appearance. Identification may require specimen (and specimen slice) X-ray for localization and tissue sampling. On cut sections, DCIS with prominent comedo-type necrosis may exude pale material from the ducts within poorly defined fibrous areas. A small proportion of high-grade DCIS may be extensive enough and have such an abundance of intraluminal necrosis or associated stromal reaction that it presents as multiple areas of round, pale comedonecrosis or a firm, gritty mass.

## Histopathology

DCIS is characteristically a unifocal disease limited to a single duct system, but it can extend into the lobules (lobular involvement). Reports of high frequencies of multifocality may represent misinterpretation of the 3D duct structures when examined histologically in two dimensions. High-grade DCIS grows in a continuous pattern; however, skip lesions as large as 10 mm may be seen in low-grade disease {625}, adding to the difficulty of interpretation of assessment of focality, lesion size, and distance to surgical margins.

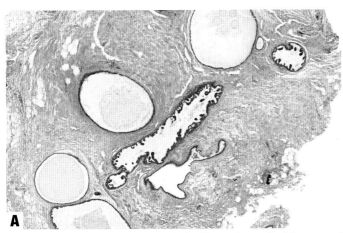 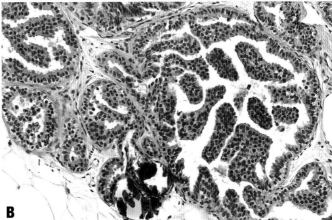

**Fig. 2.65** Micropapillary ductal carcinoma in situ of low nuclear grade. **A** Low-power view. **B** Note the low-grade nuclei and the micropapillary architecture. Microcalcifications are also present.

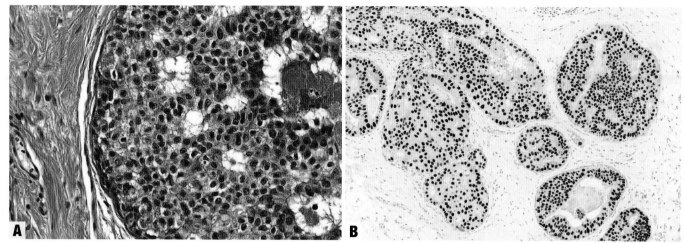

**Fig. 2.66** Ductal carcinoma in situ of intermediate nuclear grade. **A** The tumour cell nuclei are of intermediate grade. **B** ER positivity is seen in this example.

DCIS is highly heterogeneous histologically, biologically, genetically, and clinically (in terms of both diagnosis and behaviour). Classification systems have varied over time. Historically, DCIS was classified according to architectural pattern and categorized as solid, cribriform, micropapillary, or papillary types (for more information on the papillary type, see *Papillary ductal carcinoma in situ*, p. 57). Some systems also included comedo DCIS as an architectural type, whereas others use the presence or absence of comedonecrosis in combination with nuclear grade for categorization. Comedonecrosis is seen as sheets of granular eosinophilic material within the duct lumen with associated karyorrhectic/nuclear debris. It should be noted that comedonecrosis can be seen in association with a range of architectural patterns.

The use of cytonuclear morphology is recommended for histological grading of DCIS {1155,1807}. DCIS is categorized as being of low, intermediate, or high nuclear grade. In general, there is greater homogeneity of nuclear grade than of architectural pattern {1684}; however, it is not unusual to observe grade variation within DCIS, a reflection of intratumoural genetic heterogeneity {409}.

DCIS of low nuclear grade is composed of small, monomorphic cells, typically growing in a cribriform, micropapillary, or (less often) solid pattern involving more than two complete spaces (or measuring > 2 mm; see *Atypical ductal hyperplasia*,

p. 18). Low-grade solid DCIS may have microrosettes with small luminal spaces. Micropapillary and cribriform patterns are commonly admixed, but micropapillary DCIS in particular may be extensive {1880}. The nuclei are uniform in size and shape, with regular chromatin and inconspicuous nucleoli. The nuclei in DCIS of low nuclear grade are 1.5–2 times the size of an erythrocyte {1155}. Mitotic figures are rare. Microcalcification is commonly seen in secretions within the luminal spaces and may be psammomatous. Necrosis is uncommonly present in low-grade DCIS, but it does not preclude the diagnosis.

DCIS of intermediate nuclear grade is composed of cells that show moderate variability in size, shape, and polarization. The nuclei have variably coarse chromatin and sometimes have prominent nucleoli. Mitoses may be present. Necrosis (either punctate or comedo) may be seen. Microcalcifications may be present in secretions and/or in necrotic material.

DCIS of high nuclear grade is formed of large, atypical cells, most commonly with a solid architecture. However, cribriform and micropapillary patterns may be seen. Uncommonly, a single layer of large, highly atypical cells lines spaces in flat DCIS of high nuclear grade (previously sometimes called the pleomorphic subtype of clinging DCIS). Polarization around luminal spaces is minimal. The nuclei are large and typically pleomorphic, with irregular contours, coarse chromatin, and often prominent nucleoli. In high-grade DCIS, the nuclei are > 2.5 times the size of an erythrocyte in diameter {1155}. Mitoses are usually conspicuous. Central comedonecrosis bearing microcalcification is often present but is not mandatory for the diagnosis.

Histological reports of DCIS should note the cytonuclear grade, the presence/absence of necrosis (which may be subclassified as either punctate or comedo), the architectural pattern, the size of the lesion, and the distance to margins. Information about the presence and site of microcalcifications (in DCIS, a benign lesion, or both) is valuable for pathological–radiological correlation.

*Paget disease*
High-grade DCIS may present as Paget disease of the nipple, when it extends from the subareolar ducts along the basement membrane into the basal layers of the epidermis. Underlying high-grade DCIS is virtually always identified if carefully sought; occasionally invasive carcinoma is also identified, although less

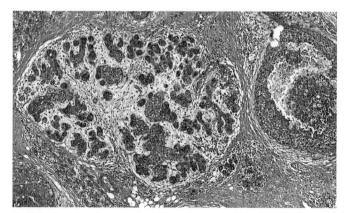

**Fig. 2.67** Ductal carcinoma in situ of high nuclear grade with involvement of adjacent lobules.

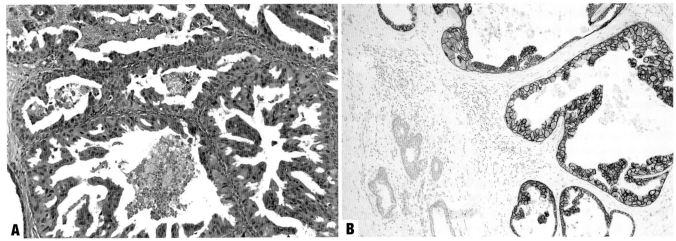

**Fig. 2.68** Apocrine ductal carcinoma in situ of high nuclear grade. **A** Cellular apocrine differentiation is seen. **B** ERBB2 (HER2) is positive.

frequently now than in the historical literature. The epidermis, which may be hyperkeratotic and parakeratotic, contains an infiltrate of single (or clusters of) large pleomorphic high-grade DCIS cells. Occasionally some acinar structures may be seen. Immunohistochemistry can be helpful for confirmation of the diagnosis; the DCIS cells are positive for CK7, ERBB2 (HER2), and GATA3 {1567,271}.

### Other subtypes

Uncommonly, DCIS is composed of apocrine, neuroendocrine, signet-ring, or clear cells. The neuroendocrine form often has a spindled cell pattern, at least focally. Squamous forms are described but are rare. There are few data on the prognostic impact of unusual types, but these are generally graded and reported histologically like the common subtypes.

### Differential diagnosis

The differential diagnosis for DCIS includes usual epithelial hyperplasia / usual ductal hyperplasia (UDH) and atypical ductal hyperplasia at one end of the spectrum and invasive and microinvasive carcinoma at the other. DCIS of intermediate nuclear grade, in particular the neuroendocrine type, which commonly shows a spindle cell pattern, can be mistaken for florid UDH. Immunohistochemistry demonstrates a heterogeneous pattern of reactivity with basal cytokeratins (e.g. CK5 and CK14) in UDH, whereas these are uniformly negative in neuroendocrine DCIS. ER is strongly and uniformly positive in neuroendocrine DCIS, whereas hormone receptors usually show a mosaic pattern in UDH. Gynaecomastoid-type UDH may mimic low-grade micropapillary DCIS, but it is formed from more-rudimentary micropapillae. Like other UDH, the gynaecomastoid type lacks the nuclear uniformity of low-grade DCIS, and the nuclei, which may be somewhat pyknotic, are aligned along the periphery of the micropapillae.

Atypical ductal hyperplasia represents a microfocal, low-grade atypical proliferation not involving more than two complete involved membrane-bound spaces (or equivalent; i.e. ≤ 2 mm). Typically, although part of the spaces have the cytological and architectural features of low-grade DCIS, they are insufficient in extent for this diagnosis; elsewhere in the spaces, there is often admixed columnar cell change or UDH. Solid DCIS, in particular of low or intermediate nuclear grade, may be difficult

to distinguish from lobular carcinoma in situ (see *Lobular carcinoma in situ*, p. 71).

DCIS may involve the lobular units, or it may extend into sclerosing lesions (e.g. sclerosing adenosis); both presentations may mimic invasive carcinoma. An inflammatory and fibrotic reaction can be observed around ducts bearing DCIS of high nuclear grade, but it is especially common in association with lobular involvement. Careful examination for small, irregular (rather than rounded) clusters of cells should be undertaken to exclude (micro)invasion, particularly if there is a prominent lymphocytic infiltrate {136}. Myoepithelial cell markers can be helpful to demonstrate an intact myoepithelial layer around involved lobules or sclerosing adenosis, but they may be difficult to assess, particularly in some cases of high-grade DCIS with an altered immunophenotype; an absence of reactivity does not unequivocally distinguish DCIS from invasive carcinoma {855}. Therefore, the use of more than one marker is recommended. The outline of the cell clusters is a valuable feature, with small foci of invasive disease having irregular contours. Invasive

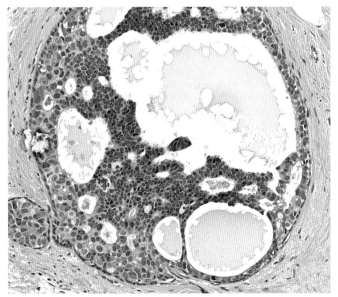

**Fig. 2.69** Mixed-grade ductal carcinoma in situ (DCIS). DCIS of high nuclear grade (left) and DCIS of low nuclear grade (right).

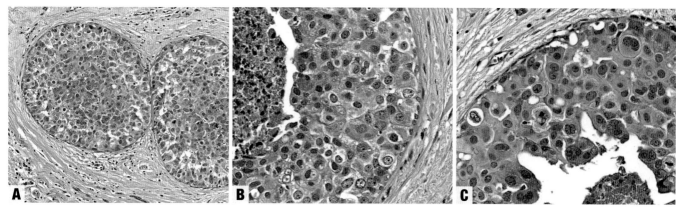

**Fig. 2.70** Ductal carcinoma in situ of high nuclear grade. Note: **A** Solid architecture. **B** Necrosis. **C** High nuclear grade.

cribriform carcinoma can potentially be mistaken for DCIS, but it has the irregular, infiltrative growth pattern of invasive disease, with desmoplastic stroma and an absent myoepithelial layer.

## Cytology
DCIS cannot be distinguished from IBC cytologically.

## Diagnostic molecular pathology
A variety of biomarkers have been assessed in DCIS. Surrogate immunoprofiles of intrinsic subtypes have been investigated; the luminal A, luminal B, HER2-enriched, and basal-like molecular subtypes are seen in DCIS. Of note, the frequency of these subtypes differs between DCIS and invasive disease; for example, HER2 overexpression is more common in DCIS than in IBC, particularly in high-grade DCIS {2027}.

### ER and PR
There is no universal agreement on the benefits of hormone receptor testing in DCIS, although there is some evidence that adjuvant hormone therapy reduces the risk of ipsilateral recurrence. Some guidelines mandate ER testing in DCIS; in others this is optional. There is little evidence regarding the optimum methodology for scoring immunohistochemical assays of hormone receptors in DCIS. In general, techniques have been extrapolated from those used for IBC, and similar cut-off points (e.g. > 1% DCIS cell nuclei) are applied, but this approach is pragmatic rather than evidence-based. The distribution of receptor expression in DCIS is similar to that in IBC; about 75% of cases are ER-positive {2027}. However, there is insufficient evidence to determine whether there is an association between levels of receptor expression and response to hormone therapy in DCIS.

## Essential and desirable diagnostic criteria
*Essential:* proliferating, cohesive neoplastic epithelial cells, confined to the mammary ductal-lobular system, exhibiting a range of architectural patterns and nuclear grades.
*Desirable:* in difficult cases, pragmatic interpretation of multiple myoepithelial markers for diagnosis.

## Staging
DCIS is staged "Tis (DCIS)" in the eighth edition of the Union for International Cancer Control (UICC) TNM classification {229}.

## Prognosis and prediction
The breast cancer–specific survival of women with DCIS is extremely good {2075,2151}. Recent reports highlight that DCIS patients aged > 50 years have a risk of dying from all causes comparable to that of the general female population {583}. The grade of DCIS is associated with breast cancer–specific survival {2151}. Breast cancer deaths after a diagnosis of DCIS may be due either to undetected invasive carcinoma at the time of diagnosis or to recurrence as invasive disease; approximately 50% of recurrences after breast-conserving surgery occur as invasive carcinoma, and women who develop recurrence as invasive disease have a significantly worse outcome than those with recurrence as pure DCIS (which does not affect breast cancer–specific survival) {2222,2075}.

A variety of factors have been associated with increased risk of recurrence after breast-conserving surgery, including younger patient age, large lesion size, high-grade disease, certain architectural patterns, comedonecrosis, and positive margins. However, the relative importance of these factors (and their possible interactions) remains unclear; algorithms for the incorporation of a number of features to predict local recurrence risk have been proposed but are not very widely used {383}. To date, no individual molecular prognostic marker has been consistently demonstrated to be of clinical value in predicting the

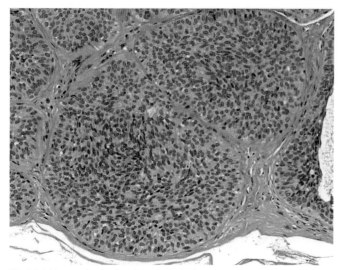

**Fig. 2.71** Neuroendocrine ductal carcinoma in situ.

behaviour of DCIS – in particular in identifying cases at risk of development of recurrence as clinically significant (i.e. invasive) disease {2075}.

No globally accepted predictive factors have been identified. Randomized clinical trials have assessed the benefits of adjuvant hormone therapy in the management of patients with DCIS {427,642}, but there is also real-world evidence that such treatment reduces the risk of ipsilateral recurrence {2075}. In the National Surgical Adjuvant Breast and Bowel Project (NSABP) B-24 study of patients treated with wide local excision and radiotherapy, this benefit was restricted to ER-positive disease {43}. Adjuvant hormone therapy also reduces the risk of contralateral breast cancer {427,43}. Results for PR are generally similar, but less significant, and the role of PR testing in DCIS is unclear.

Randomized clinical trials and large national databases consistently show an approximately 50% reduction in local ipsilateral recurrence in patients receiving breast radiotherapy. No established predictive factors for radiotherapy benefit have been identified. Even when small (≤ 25 mm), DCIS lesions of low or intermediate nuclear grade are managed with complete excision without radiotherapy; there remains a steady increase in local recurrence rate over time (14.4% at 12 years; 7.5% invasive disease) {1972}. Therefore, the selection of patients who may not require breast radiotherapy is currently done largely on a case-by-case basis rather than on the basis of a guideline or protocol. Molecular assays for the prediction of radiotherapy response have been proposed but are not yet widely used globally {1287}.

# Invasive breast carcinoma: General overview

Rakha EA
Allison KH
Ellis IO
Horii R
Masuda S
Penault-Llorca F
Tsuda H
Vincent-Salomon A

## Definition
The term "invasive breast carcinoma (IBC)" refers to a large and heterogeneous group of malignant epithelial neoplasms of the glandular elements of the breast.

## ICD-O coding
None

## ICD-11 coding
None

## Related terminology
None

## Subtype(s)
IBCs are categorized into morphologically defined subtypes in the subsequent sections. It is important to note that all IBCs are grouped into the following biomarker-defined subtypes/groups for treatment purposes on the basis of ER and ERBB2 (HER2) status:

- ER-positive, HER2-negative
- ER-positive, HER2-positive
- ER-negative, HER2-positive
- ER-negative, HER2-negative.

Despite their overlapping morphological features, these biomarker-defined subtypes show distinct outcomes and responses to therapy, as well as differences in their global genomic and transcriptomic profiles.

## Localization
The majority of breast cancers (~90%) are unifocal and can occur in any quadrant of the breast, with higher frequency in the upper-outer quadrant {230}. A synchronous contralateral tumour is found in approximately 2% of patients. About 0.1% of breast cancers present as an axillary metastasis with no clear breast primary {2208}.

## Clinical features
In non-screened populations, a palpable mass is the most common clinical sign of IBC, although skin retraction, nipple inversion, nipple discharge, and (less commonly) a change in the size or shape of the breast or a change in the colour or texture of the skin may be seen. In extreme cases, skin ulceration may occur. Inflammatory breast carcinoma is a clinical presentation of breast cancer defined by diffuse erythema and oedema involving a third or more of the skin of the breast. All the symptoms of breast cancer may also be caused by benign breast disease, so evaluation with imaging and histological sampling with core biopsy or FNA are indicated to establish a definitive diagnosis.

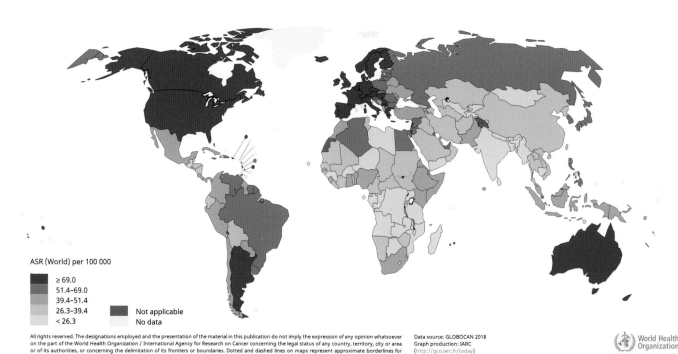

ASR (World) per 100 000

- ≥ 69.0
- 51.4–69.0
- 39.4–51.4
- 26.3–39.4
- < 26.3
- Not applicable
- No data

Data source: GLOBOCAN 2018
Graph production: IARC
(http://gco.iarc.fr/today)
World Health Organization

World Health Organization
© International Agency for Research on Cancer 2018

**Fig. 2.72** Estimated age-standardized incidence rates (ASRs; World), per 100 000 person-years, of breast cancer in 2018.

In screened populations, a spiculated mass with or without associated calcifications is the classic appearance of cancer, but cancers may also be visualized as architectural distortion, well-circumscribed masses, or calcifications alone. About 5–15% of palpable cancers are not seen on mammogram, and the majority of these can be identified with targeted ultrasonography. Ultrasonography can also be added to improve sensitivity in women with mammographically dense breasts, and it is the method of choice for imaging the breast in women aged < 40 years. The false negative rate of combined mammography and ultrasonography is quite low, ranging from 0% to 3% {1424, 1976}. Unless the presence of an unequivocally benign diagnosis such as a cyst is established on the basis of imaging, tissue sampling is usually necessary to determine that carcinoma is not present.

MRI is the most sensitive (but not the most specific) method for detecting breast cancer; therefore, its use is restricted to screening women at very high risk (e.g. carriers of *BRCA1* or *BRCA2* mutations) and in some centres after an initial diagnosis of lobular carcinoma or as part of the staging work-up for breast cancer.

When the results of the physical examination, imaging, and needle biopsy/cytology are all benign and concordant, the risk of missing a cancer is extremely low. However, when any one of these modalities is non-concordant or cannot be evaluated, repeat biopsy or surgical diagnostic biopsy is indicated.

### Epidemiology

Breast cancer is the most commonly diagnosed cancer in females (accounting for 24% of all female cancers) and the leading cause of female cancer death worldwide {221}. Breast cancer accounts for 11.6% of cancers in both sexes combined, making it the second most common cancer overall {221,2293, 1174}. Incidence rates of IBC have been increasing in most low- and middle-income countries in recent decades. In high-income countries such as the USA, Canada, the United Kingdom, France, and Australia, incidence rates decreased in the early 2000s, which was partly attributable to decreased use of postmenopausal hormone treatment after publication of the Women's Health Initiative trial linking postmenopausal hormone use to increased breast cancer risk {222,485,1804}. However, with ageing populations, the global burden increased overall. In 2018, 2.1 million new cases of breast cancer and 627 000 deaths were estimated worldwide {221}. Incidence also varies by more than 10-fold geographically. The groups at highest risk are the affluent populations of Australia, Europe, and North America, where 8–9% of women are diagnosed with an IBC before the age of 75 years {631}. Geographical variations, time trends, and studies of populations migrating from low- to high-risk areas show that the risk in migrant populations approaches that of the host country within one or two generations; this suggests an important role for environmental factors in the etiology of this cancer. Studies of variations in breast cancer subtypes in the USA have shown that the frequencies of the clinical/biomarker subtypes vary by population characteristics. In screened populations, hormone receptor–positive cancer is the most common subtype, with HER2-positive cancers constituting 10–15% and ER-negative/HER2-negative cancers accounting for 13–17%; in unscreened populations the frequency is different, with higher

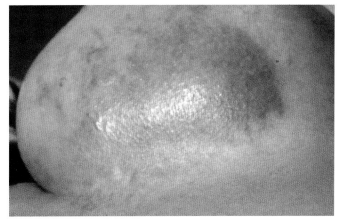

**Fig. 2.73** Inflammatory breast carcinoma. Clinically, inflammatory breast carcinoma shows diffuse erythema and oedema involving a third or more of the skin of the breast.

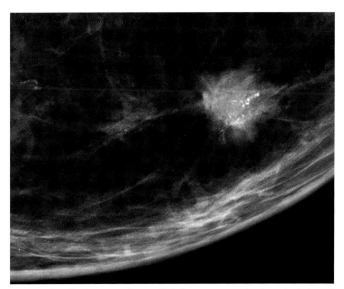

**Fig. 2.74** Invasive breast carcinoma. Digital mammogram showing a typical small spiculated breast cancer with associated calcifications.

proportions of ER-negative/HER2-negative cancers (20–40%) and HER2-positive cancers (15–25%) {1604,287}.

### Etiology

The origin of breast cancer is multifactorial. Most studies point to hormones, diet, reproductive factors, and genetics as general risk factors. From descriptive epidemiological data it has clearly emerged that breast cancer is a diagnosis of affluent societies that have acquired the so-called Western lifestyle, characterized by a high-calorie diet rich in animal fat and proteins, combined with a lack of physical exercise and obesity, older age at first childbirth, lower parity, and decreased duration of lactation. The disease occurs more frequently among women who have an early menarche, remain nulliparous, or have few children and an older age at first delivery {1486,1736}. There is also overwhelming evidence from epidemiological studies that exogenous sex steroids (estrogens and progestogens) play an important role in the development of breast carcinomas {908}. Breast cancer incidence rates increase more steeply with age before menopause (by ~8% per year) than after (~2% per year) {380}, when ovarian synthesis of estrogen and progesterone ceases and ovarian production of androgens gradually diminishes.

The consumption of alcohol has been consistently associated with a moderate increase in the risk of breast cancer, particularly hormone receptor–positive cancers {1964,2013}. Current evidence suggests no causal relationship between active smoking and breast cancer {1254}; however, one large meta-analysis has reported a link between active smoking and increased breast cancer risk for women who initiate smoking before first childbirth, and it suggested that smoking might play a role in breast cancer initiation {704}. The relationship between physical activity and risk of breast cancer has been assessed by the International Agency for Research on Cancer (IARC), which concluded that higher levels of activity are associated with a reduction in risk {2135}.

More than most other human neoplasms, breast cancer shows familial clustering. Two high-penetrance genes have been identified (BRCA1 and BRCA2) that greatly increase the risk of developing breast cancer. Additional polymorphisms and genes have recently been identified (primarily via genome-wide association studies), which are of medium or low penetrance

and confer lower risks. The evidence suggests a polygenic origin for this disease (see *Diagnostic molecular pathology*, below).

Specific etiological risk factors are suggested to contribute differently to the risks of developing the various biomarker/ clinical subtypes of IBC {2314,325,572}. Germline *BRCA1* mutations are associated with risk for triple-negative (ER-negative, PR-negative, and HER2-negative) cancers, whereas germline *BRCA2* mutations are associated with hormone receptor–positive breast cancers {403,754}. Early menarche, late menopause, postmenopausal hormone replacement therapy, nulliparity, and older age at first childbirth are associated with increases in the risk of hormone receptor–positive breast cancer {66,126, 1105}. Parity may be associated with an increased risk of triple-negative tumours {325,126}. Longer duration of breastfeeding is associated with a decrease in the risk of all subtypes. A positive association between body mass index and breast cancer risk among postmenopausal women is stronger for hormone receptor–positive cancers. A weak inverse association has been suggested among premenopausal women, in whom higher body mass index is possibly associated with decreased

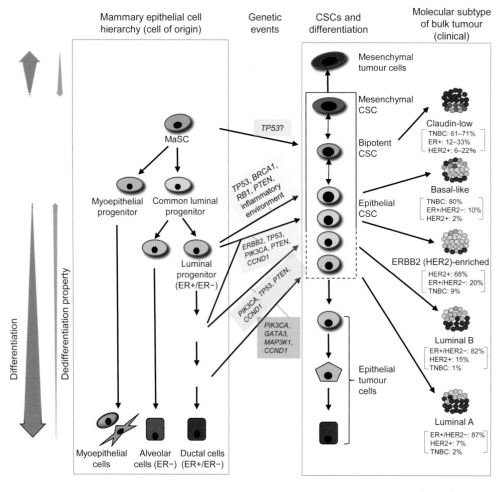

**Fig. 2.75** A schematic diagram of the presentation of pathogenesis of breast carcinoma deduced from the combination of a model of mammary epithelial cell hierarchy as cell of origin, relationships between the hierarchy and molecular subtype of bulky tumour based on gene expression profiling, genetic events that are frequent or characteristic in each subtype, and a model of varying proportions of cancer stem cells (CSCs) in mesenchymal versus epithelial status, as well as differential blocks in the differentiation hierarchy seen in normal mammary development in the various subtypes of breast carcinoma {1674,574A,2181A,237A,1223A,2204A}. MaSC, mammary stem cell; TNBC, triple-negative breast cancer.

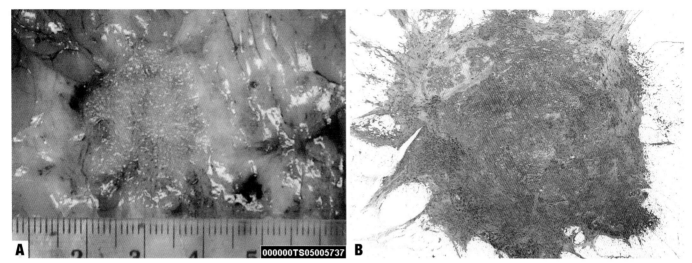

**Fig. 2.76** Breast carcinoma. **A** Gross appearance. **B** Invasive breast carcinoma of no special type (NST). Note the irregular stellate outline and the central scar.

risk of hormone receptor–positive cancers but increased risk of triple-negative cancers {126,2314}. There is some evidence that alcohol, smoking, and physical activity are associated with risk of hormone receptor–positive cancers {571}. However, studies in specific ethnic populations reveal that there may be population/ethnicity-based differences in risk factors for developing specific biomarker/clinical subtypes of breast cancer {1178}.

## Pathogenesis

The pathogenesis of breast cancer follows several pathways. Multiple linear models of breast cancer initiation, transformation, and progression have been described that are based largely on hormone receptor status and morphology. The ER-positive model recognizes flat epithelial atypia, atypical ductal hyperplasia, and ER-positive ductal carcinoma in situ (DCIS) as the non-obligate precursors of invasive and metastatic breast carcinoma. The ER-negative model recognizes ER-negative DCIS and microglandular adenosis as precursors of ER-negative cancers {192}.

At the cell-of-origin level, two leading models accounting for breast carcinogenesis have been described: the sporadic clonal evolution model and the cancer stem cell model. At the molecular level, there is evidence that strongly suggests that breast cancer evolves along two divergent molecular pathways of progression, mainly related to hormone receptors. Molecular data have also demonstrated that ER-positive and ER-negative breast cancers are fundamentally distinct diseases, and that within ER-positive cancers, histological grade and proliferation are strongly associated with the extent, complexity, and type of genetic aberrations {1237,68}. The first pathway (the ER-positive pathway) is characterized by gains of 1q, loss of 16q, infrequent amplification of 17q12, and a gene expression signature that is predominantly populated with genes associated with the ER-positive phenotype. These lesions express hormone receptors, lack HER2 overexpression and expression of basal markers, and have relatively simple diploid or near-diploid karyotypes. In general, this pathway consists of neoplastic lesions predominantly of the low- to intermediate-grade phenotype, in addition to a small subset (~9%) of morphologically defined high-grade tumours. The second pathway, designated the ER-negative pathway, is most commonly characterized by loss of

13q, gain of chromosomal region 11q13, amplification of 17q12, and a gene expression signature populated by genes associated with cellular proliferation and cell-cycle processes. This pathway consists predominantly of morphologically defined intermediate- and high-grade tumours {1237}. *PIK3CA* mutations commonly occur in both pathways, and *TP53* mutations are frequent in the ER-negative pathway {277}. Published data also suggest that the progression of a low-grade tumour to a high-grade tumour may preferentially occur in breast cancers of the luminal phenotype {1470}. The ER-negative breast cancers include both HER2-positive and HER2-negative groups. In these groups (all of which are mostly high-grade, genetically unstable, and mostly aneuploid), *TP53* mutations are common. In the ER-negative, HER2-positive group, *PIK3CA* mutations are also very frequent, in addition to 17q12 amplification. Important elements of ER-negative, HER2-negative breast cancer biology include high proliferative activity, an increased immunological infiltrate, a basal-like and a mesenchymal phenotype, and deficiency in homologous recombination.

## Macroscopic appearance

Most IBCs can be visualized or palpated as a grossly evident mass, with an irregular, stellate outline or nodular configuration. The tumour edge is usually moderately or poorly defined and lacks sharp circumscription. Classically, IBCs are firm or even hard on palpation, and they may have a gritty feel when cut with a knife (although some types of DCIS, such as the comedo type, can have a similar gritty texture and cannot always be easily distinguished grossly from invasion). However, some IBCs, including neoadjuvant-treated cases, may be grossly inapparent and require careful correlation with imaging at the time of gross examination and tissue sampling. Gross evaluation should include review of imaging findings (if performed), so that the number of lesions, expected size of lesions, and expected clips/markers and their location can inform appropriate tissue sampling {40}. Radiography of larger specimens can be helpful in identifying clips, calcifications, and other clues to guide macroscopic examination {1033,132,1643}. Ideally, surgical specimens should be differentially inked and serially sectioned into approximately 0.5 cm thick slices to ensure adequate fixation and detection of smaller invasive cancers {1965,1156}. Tissue sampling should be performed such that the T stage of the cancer can be accurately established {1965,1156,573}. Sampling between closely related gross lesions is also important so that the pathologist can document whether they are truly multiple or one larger cancer, for staging purposes. A cassette map of larger lesions is often required when the extent or size is not macroscopically obvious {768,1867,434}. This is especially true after neoadjuvant therapy, because residual cancers can become softer and more difficult to palpate, and only a fibrous scarred area may be present (except in cases of absent or minimal response) {204,1677,2017}. Another setting that requires extensive tissue sampling is cases of extensive DCIS, so that any foci of invasion can be identified {1155}.

Macroscopic assessment of skin ulceration, nipple changes, and separate skin nodules (if present) are also important for staging. Distances of grossly apparent cancers from the resection margins should be recorded and close margins sampled for microscopic analysis. Lastly, tissue handling parameters such as the time the specimen was removed by the surgeon, the time it was placed in fixative, and the amount of time between fixation and tissue sample processing should be recorded so that the cold ischaemia time (the amount of time between removal from the body and placement in fixative) and the time in fixative

before processing are clear, because these parameters can affect receptor (ER/PR and HER2) testing, grading, and lymphovascular invasion assessment {573,783A}.

### Histopathology

IBC has a broad spectrum of histological appearances. Four histological features are described to further characterize the biology: (1) histological subtype based on tumour architecture, cytonuclear features, and stromal features; (2) Nottingham grade (detailed below); (3) the presence or absence of spread in the angiolymphatic spaces (only peritumoural lymphovascular invasion is assessed in breast cancer, and this should be differentiated from tissue retraction); and (4) an associated in situ component. Other features of importance in the classification include tumour size, distance to margins, stromal changes, and tumour-infiltrating lymphocytes (TILs). It is also important to recognize when the histological features of a breast carcinoma are unusual or discordant with the hormone receptor or HER2 status {37}. For example, a low-grade cancer with either a negative ER status or a positive HER2 status would be highly unusual/discordant, and further work-up would be recommended to ensure accurate histological typing, grading, and biomarker status. In the subsequent sections of this chapter, IBCs are

## Nottingham Grading Examples: Nuclear Pleomorphism

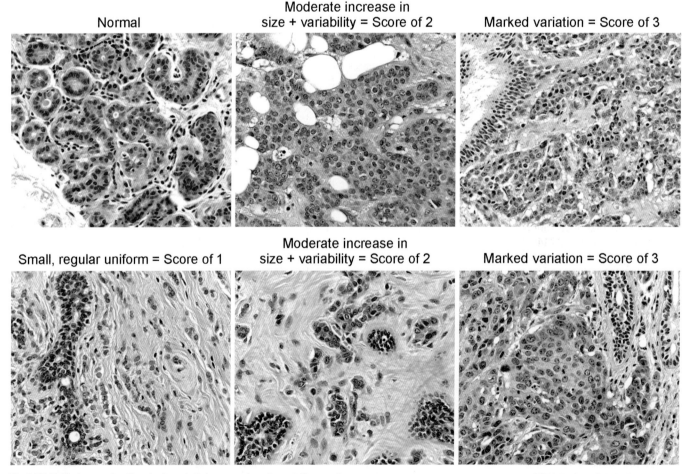

**Fig. 2.77** Nottingham grade of invasive breast carcinoma: nuclear pleomorphism scoring.

# Nottingham Grading Examples: Tubule Formation

| Majority (>75%) = Score of 1 | Moderate (10-75%) = Score of 2 | Little or none (<10%) = Score of 3 |

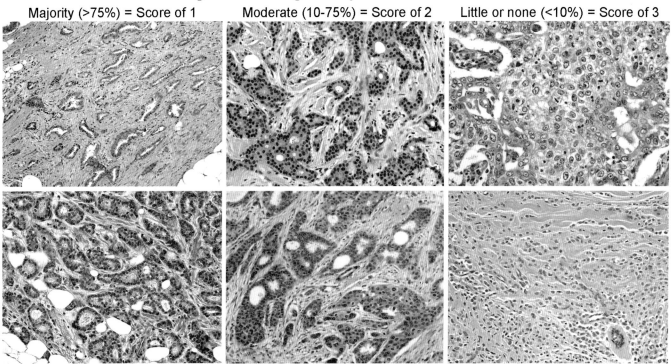

**Fig. 2.78** Nottingham grade of invasive breast carcinoma: tubule formation scoring.

organized by their morphological subtypes, although the majority of cases are of no special type (NST).

## Histological type

Breast carcinomas showing a special histological pattern in ≥ 90% of the tumour are designated as a pure special tumour type, such as lobular, mucinous, and tubular carcinomas. Tumours lacking such specific features are designated as invasive carcinoma NST, which accounts for the majority of cases, including those with mixed patterns.

## Histological grading

Three characteristics are evaluated: tubule formation as an expression of glandular differentiation, nuclear pleomorphism, and mitotic count {585,1714}. A numerical scoring system from 1 to 3 is used to ensure that each factor is assessed independently (see Table 2.06).

Tubules and glandular/acini formation are assessed throughout the whole tumour at low magnification; only structures exhibiting clear central lumina surrounded by polarized neoplastic cells are counted. Cut-off points of 75% and 10% of glandular/tumour area are used to determine the score (see Fig. 2.78).

Nuclear pleomorphism is assessed in the area showing the highest degree of pleomorphism in comparison with the regularity of the nuclear size and shape of normal epithelial cells in adjacent breast tissue (see Fig. 2.77). Increasing irregularity of nuclear outlines and the number and size of nucleoli are useful additional features in allocating scores for pleomorphism. Score 1 nuclei are very similar in size to the nuclei of benign pre-existing epithelial cells (< 1.5 times the size), and they show minimal pleomorphism, an even chromatin pattern,

and nucleoli that are either not visible or very inconspicuous. Score 2 nuclei are larger (1.5–2 times the size of benign epithelial cell nuclei), with mild to moderate pleomorphism and visible but small and inconspicuous nucleoli. Score 3 nuclei are even

**Table 2.06** Semiqualitative method for assessing histological grade in breast tumours {585}

| Feature | Score |
|---|---|
| **Tubule and gland formation** | |
| Majority of tumour (> 75%) | 1 |
| Moderate degree (10–75%) | 2 |
| Little or none (< 10%) | 3 |
| **Nuclear pleomorphism** | |
| Small, regular, uniform cells | 1 |
| Moderate increase in size and variability | 2 |
| Marked variation | 3 |
| **Mitotic count** | |
| Dependent on microscope field area[a] | 1–3 |

| Total score | Final grading |
|---|---|
| Add the scores for gland formation, nuclear polymorphism, and mitotic count: | |
| 3–5 | Grade 1 |
| 6 or 7 | Grade 2 |
| 8 or 9 | Grade 3 |

[a]See Table 1.01 (p. 6).

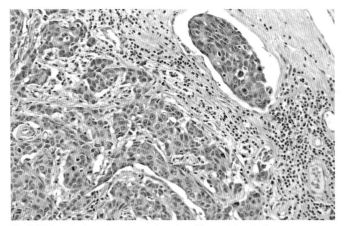

**Fig. 2.79** Invasive breast carcinoma. Invasion of the angiolymphatic space.

larger (> 2 times the size of benign epithelial cell nuclei), with vesicular chromatin; they vary markedly in size and shape and often show prominent nucleoli. The preferred magnification for nuclear scoring is 40× objective.

The evaluation of mitotic figures requires care and relies on optimal tissue fixation and good preparation of sections. Observers must count only definite mitotic figures; hyperchromatic and pyknotic nuclei should be ignored because they are more likely to represent apoptosis rather than cells in mitosis. Mitotic counts

require standardization to a fixed field area, because field area varies between microscopes. The total number of mitoses per 10 high-power fields is recorded. The cut-off points for scoring depend on the field area size, and the microscope used should be calibrated by measuring the diameter of the high-power field (40× objective) (see Table 1.01, p. 6). Scoring is performed on the area exhibiting the highest frequency of mitotic figures (the hotspot method), typically the peripheral leading edge of the tumour. If there is heterogeneity, regions exhibiting a higher frequency of mitoses should be chosen. Once the hotspot is chosen and the first field is considered, subsequent field selection is by random meander through the chosen area, but only fields with a representative tumour cell burden should be assessed.

The three values are added together to produce a score of 3–9, to which grades are assigned as follows: 3–5 points = grade 1, well differentiated; 6–7 points = grade 2, moderately differentiated; and 8–9 points = grade 3, poorly differentiated. For the purpose of quality assurance, it is recommended that the individual score components be reported in addition to the calculated grade. The grading of small tissue samples such as core needle biopsy (CNB) specimens is possible and often necessary in the era of neoadjuvant treatment, but it should be recognized to have limitations, in particular due to the inherent reduced ability to accurately assess mitotic frequency. This may lead to underestimation of the true grade in such specimens.

## Hormone receptor staining interpretation (ER and PR)
### Evaluate overall percentage of cancer in sample with nuclear staining and intensity of stain

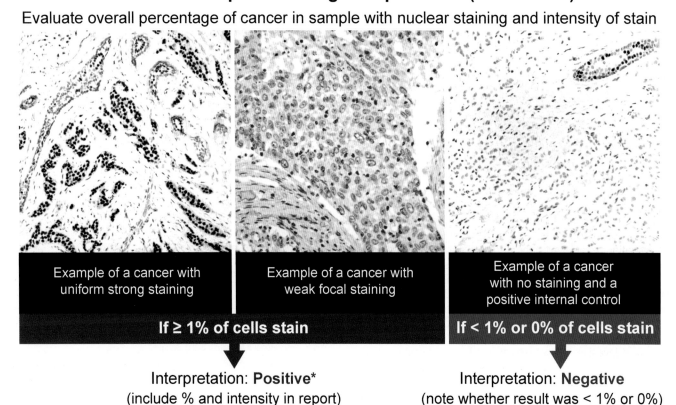

Example of a cancer with uniform strong staining

Example of a cancer with weak focal staining

Example of a cancer with no staining and a positive internal control

**If ≥ 1% of cells stain**

**If < 1% or 0% of cells stain**

Interpretation: **Positive***
(include % and intensity in report)
*Report as low positive if 1–10% of cells stain

Interpretation: **Negative**
(note whether result was < 1% or 0%)

**Fig. 2.80** Invasive breast carcinoma. Hormone receptor staining interpretation (ER and PR).

## Immunohistochemistry

IBC cells are generally positive for low-molecular-weight cyto-keratins (CK7, CK8/18, CK19), EMA, E-cadherin, BCL2, and GATA3 (however, poorly differentiated forms may lose expression of one or more of these markers). A proportion of IBCs (typically the better-differentiated forms) are also positive for GCDFP-15, mammaglobin, milk fat globule, lactalbumin, CEA, and B72.3. Approximately 30% of breast cancers express one or more basal markers, including high-molecular-weight cytokeratins (CK5/6, CK14, CK17) and EGFR (HER1), and these markers are more frequently positive in ER-negative tumours. S100 is expressed in a proportion of breast cancers but also in the myoepithelial cells. Breast cancers are negative for CD34 and typically negative for CK20 and p63 (although exceptions occur, such as p63 expression in metaplastic and salivary gland–like carcinomas). Most breast cancers are negative for other tissue-specific markers, such as CDX2, PAX8, WT1, TTF1, HMB45, melan-A, CD20, and CD3, but may be positive for CD138.

**Hormone receptors:** Nuclear ER expression should be evaluated in IBC because of its utility in predicting clinical benefit from endocrine therapy and its use in various clinical treatment algorithms for ER-positive versus ER-negative cancers (see Fig. 2.80). PR expression tends to vary more than ER expression, and this helps account for the effectiveness of PR to further stratify ER-positive cases into prognostic categories, although specific PR thresholds for this purpose are not well validated (see *Prognosis and prediction*, below) {1081}. The 2010 American Society of Clinical Oncology (ASCO) / College of American Pathologists (CAP) guideline recommendations for immunohistochemical testing of ER and PR in breast cancer state that breast cancers with as few as 1% of cells with weak intensity of ER staining should be considered positive, because of evidence of potential benefit from endocrine therapy, and the 2019 update to these guidelines has maintained this threshold {831,1394,815,816}. However, invasive cancers with 1–10% ER positivity should be reported as ER low positive, with additional interpretation and reporting recommendations. There are more-limited data on the benefit of endocrine therapies in this group, but they suggest possible benefit from endocrine therapies, so patients are considered eligible for this treatment. However, this group is noted to be heterogeneous, and the biological behaviour of ER low positive cancers may be more similar to that of ER-negative cancers. This should be considered in decision-making for other adjuvant therapy and overall treatment pathway/classification. An external control should always be evaluated (with appropriately positive and negative tissues), and internal controls should also stain as expected when present. See the most recent version of the guidelines for up-to-date information about test interpretation {60A}. There can be regional variability in hormone receptor expression, and the percentage reported should reflect the percentage of positive cells in the entire sample of the invasive cancer tested (not just the area of highest expression). When the intensity is variable, it can be reported as a range or an average intensity, with many systems using a range of 0, 1+, 2+, and 3+. Different scoring systems can be used to combine the intensity and percentage information for an overall score (e.g. the H-score or Allred score). In addition to percentage and intensity results, an interpretation as ER/

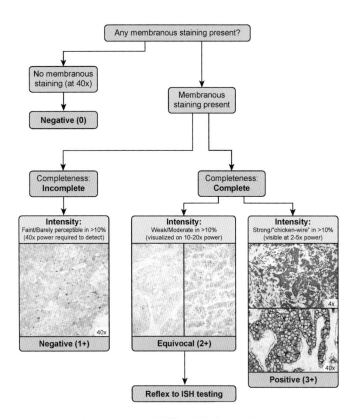

**Fig. 2.81** Algorithm for interpreting ERBB2 (HER2) immunohistochemical staining in invasive breast carcinoma. ISH, in situ hybridization.

PR-positive or -negative should also be included in the report. Low-power scanning is often insufficient for the detection of focal or weak levels of hormone receptor expression; therefore, in cases that appear negative on low power, a higher-power scan of the slide is also appropriate, to rule out weak hormone receptor positivity.

**HER2:** HER2 is a member of a family of growth factor receptors – also including EGFR (HER1), ERBB3 (HER3), and ERBB4 (HER4) – that regulate normal cell proliferation, development, and survival. HER2 is located on the cell surface at low levels in normal breast epithelium. In 10–20% of IBCs, the *ERBB2* (*HER2*) gene is amplified, resulting in overexpression of the HER2 protein at the cell surface. This protein overexpression can then result in the promotion of more-aggressive cancer biology due to increases in cancer proliferation, cell motility, and angiogenesis. There are a number of HER2-targeted therapies available today, some of which are used in combination with the first (and still standard) anti-HER2 biologic therapy, trastuzumab (Herceptin) {1564A,1627}. HER2 testing is required on any new IBC-NST, because positive cases can be treated with HER2-targeted therapies in addition to chemotherapy, with significant increases in survival. HER2 protein overexpression can be assessed using immunohistochemistry, or *ERBB2* amplification can be identified by in situ hybridization. Detailed test performance and interpretation recommendations are available in country-specific guidelines, for example those published by ASCO/CAP {2285,2284}. Because immunohistochemistry is readily available, with a lower cost, many

**Table 2.07** Standard required biomarkers in invasive breast cancer: purpose, reporting, and scoring criteria {2285,2284}

| Biomarker & purpose | Test type | Reporting categories | Scoring criteria (ASCO/CAP) |
|---|---|---|---|
| **ER**<br>*Validated for:*<br>Prediction of benefit from hormone therapies if positive | IHC | Positive | ≥ 1% of invasive cancer has nuclear staining of any intensity |
| *Other uses:*<br>Categorization for overall treatment pathways<br>Characterization as the IHC luminal group if positive<br>Poor prognostic marker if negative | | Negative | < 1% or 0% of invasive cancer has nuclear staining (follow proper QA and most-recent guidelines to ensure not a false negative result) |
| **PR**<br>*Validated for:*<br>Primarily prognostic in ER-positive cancers (not well-validated for prediction of endocrine therapy benefit) | IHC | Positive | ≥ 1% of invasive cancer has nuclear staining of any intensity |
| *Other uses:*<br>Poor prognostic marker if negative (in ER-positive cancers)<br>Further characterization of the IHC group subtype | | Negative | < 1% or 0% of invasive cancer has nuclear staining (follow proper QA and most-recent guidelines to ensure not a false negative result) |

ASCO, American Society of Clinical Oncology; CAP, College of American Pathologists; IHC, immunohistochemistry; QA, quality assurance.

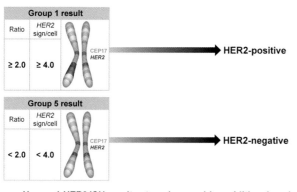

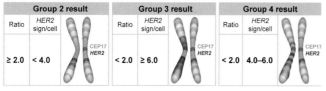

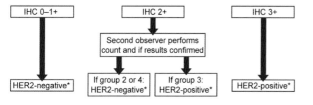

**Fig. 2.82** Dual-probe *ERBB2* (*HER2*) in situ hybridization (ISH) test interpretation. CEP17, chromosome enumeration probe 17; IHC, immunohistochemistry. *As determined by concurrent IHC and ISH. Report comments recommended; see American Society of Clinical Oncology (ASCO) / College of American Pathologists (CAP) guidelines for details {2284}.

laboratories use immunohistochemistry as the first test performed; if there is an equivocal result (2+ staining), the case is automatically referred for in situ hybridization (either in-house or at a reference laboratory). The 2018 update of the ASCO/CAP HER2 testing guidelines recommend greater emphasis on using immunohistochemistry to guide interpretation and testing of unusual in situ hybridization categories (so-called groups 2, 3, and 4). See Fig. 2.81 (p. 89), Fig. 2.82, and Table 2.07 for the interpretation criteria for HER2 immunohistochemistry and in situ hybridization. The evaluation of stain intensity is also critical to the appropriate determination of HER2 immunohistochemical status, with overinterpretation of stain intensity being one of the most common causes of discordance between HER2 immunohistochemistry (positive) and in situ hybridization (negative) {766}. The comparison of stain intensity with negative (0–1+) and positive (3+) controls should serve as a reference for intensity measures. A practical approach is to use the magnification rule, which takes into account the magnification of the lens required to assess the staining, as follows: using a 10× ocular, if staining is noted with a 2–5× objective, it can be considered strong intensity; staining detected using a 10–20× objective is considered weak to moderate; and staining detectable only on 40× is considered faint / barely perceptible. Interpreters should be aware of unusual staining patterns (e.g. clustered heterogeneity) and discordant results (e.g. a grade 1 cancer with 3+ HER2 staining) {37}. Laboratories and pathologists assessing HER2 immunohistochemistry and/or *ERBB2* in situ hybridization should participate in external quality assurance processes to ensure the accuracy of results.

**Histology of hormone receptor–positive cancers:** Hormone receptor–positive breast cancers have a spectrum of morphologies and grades. They range from well-differentiated cancers composed of bland cells forming tubular/ductal structures to poorly differentiated cancers composed of cells with substantial

**Table 2.07** Standard required biomarkers in invasive breast cancer: purpose, reporting, and scoring criteria {2285,2284} (continued)

| Biomarker & purpose | Test type | Reporting categories | Scoring criteria (ASCO/CAP) |
|---|---|---|---|
| ERBB2 (HER2)<br><br>*Validated for:*<br>Prediction of benefit from HER2-targeted therapy if positive (administered with chemotherapy)<br><br>*Other uses:*<br>Categorization for overall treatment pathways<br>Characterization as the HER2-enriched IHC subtype (if ER-negative) or luminal B (if ER-positive)<br>Marker of aggressive biology | IHC | Positive | **3+:** Circumferential membrane staining that is complete, intense, and in > 10% of tumour cells |
| | | Equivocal | **2+:** Weak to moderate complete membrane staining observed in > 10% of tumour cells |
| | | Negative | **1+:** Incomplete membrane staining that is faint / barely perceptible and in > 10% of tumour cells<br>**0:** No staining is observed, or incomplete membrane staining that is faint / barely perceptible and in ≤ 10% of tumour cells |
| | Dual-probe ISH | Negative | ERBB2 (HER2)/CEP17 ratio < 2.0 AND average ERBB2 (HER2) copy number < 4.0 signals per cell (group 5) |
| | | Negative[a] | ERBB2 (HER2)/CEP17 ratio ≥ 2.0 AND average ERBB2 (HER2) copy number < 4.0 signals per cell (group 2) **and concurrent IHC 0, 1+, or 2+**; or<br>ERBB2 (HER2)/CEP17 ratio < 2.0 AND average ERBB2 (HER2) copy number ≥ 6.0 signals per cell (group 3) **and concurrent IHC 0 or 1+**; or<br>ERBB2 (HER2)/CEP17 ratio < 2.0 AND average ERBB2 (HER2) copy number ≥ 4.0 but < 6.0 signals per cell (group 4) **and concurrent IHC 0, 1+, or 2+** |
| | | Positive[a] | ERBB2 (HER2)/CEP17 ratio ≥ 2.0 AND average ERBB2 (HER2) copy number < 4.0 signals per cell (group 2) **and concurrent IHC 3+**; or<br>ERBB2 (HER2)/CEP17 ratio < 2.0 AND average ERBB2 (HER2) copy number ≥ 6.0 signals per cell (group 3) **and concurrent IHC 2+ or 3+**; or<br>ERBB2 (HER2)/CEP17 ratio < 2.0 AND average ERBB2 (HER2) copy number ≥ 4.0 but < 6.0 signals per cell (group 4) **and concurrent IHC 3+** |
| | | Positive | ERBB2 (HER2)/CEP17 ratio ≥ 2.0 AND average ERBB2 (HER2) copy number ≥ 4.0 signals per cell (group 1) |
| | Single-probe ISH[b] | Negative | Average ERBB2 (HER2) copy number < 4.0 signals per cell; or<br>Average ERBB2 (HER2) copy number ≥ 4.0 but < 6.0 signals per cell **and concurrent IHC 0 or 1+**; or<br>Average ERBB2 (HER2) copy number ≥ 4.0 but < 6.0 signals per cell **and concurrent dual-probe ISH group 5** |
| | | Positive | Average ERBB2 (HER2) copy number ≥ 6.0 signals per cell; or<br>Average ERBB2 (HER2) copy number ≥ 4.0 but < 6.0 signals per cell **and concurrent IHC 3+**; or<br>Average ERBB2 (HER2) copy number ≥ 4.0 but < 6.0 signals per cell **and concurrent dual-probe ISH group 1** |

ASCO, American Society of Clinical Oncology; CAP, College of American Pathologists; IHC, immunohistochemistry; ISH, in situ hybridization.

[a]For dual-probe groups 2–4, the final ISH results are based on concurrent review of IHC, with recounting of the ISH test by a second reviewer if IHC is 2+ (per the updated 2018 ASCO/CAP recommendations {2285,2284}).

**Comment for group 2 negative result:** "Evidence is limited on the efficacy of HER2-targeted therapy in the small subset of cases with a *HER2*/CEP17 ratio ≥ 2.0 and an average *HER2* copy number of < 4.0 per cell. In the first generation of adjuvant trastuzumab trials, patients in this subgroup who were randomly assigned to the trastuzumab arm did not seem to derive an improvement in disease-free or overall survival, but there were too few such cases to draw definitive conclusions. IHC expression of HER2 should be used to complement ISH and define HER2 status. If IHC result is not 3+ positive, it is recommended that the specimen be considered HER2-negative because of the low *HER2* copy number by ISH and the lack of protein overexpression."

**Comment for group 3 negative result:** "There are insufficient data on the efficacy of HER2-targeted therapy in cases with a *HER2*/CEP17 ratio of < 2.0 in the absence of protein overexpression because such patients were not eligible for the first generation of adjuvant trastuzumab clinical trials. When concurrent IHC results are negative (0 or 1+), it is recommended that the specimen be considered HER2-negative."

**Comment for group 4 negative result:** "It is uncertain whether patients with an average of ≥ 4.0 and < 6.0 HER2 signals per cell and a *HER2*/CEP17 ratio of < 2.0 benefit from HER2-targeted therapy in the absence of protein overexpression (IHC 3+). If the specimen test result is close to the ISH ratio threshold for positive, there is a higher likelihood that repeat testing will result in different results by chance alone. Therefore, when IHC results are not 3+ positive, it is recommended that the sample be considered HER2-negative without additional testing on the same specimen."

[b]For single-probe ISH: It is recommended that concomitant IHC review become part of the interpretation of single-probe ISH results. ASCO/CAP also preferentially recommends the use of dual-probe rather than single-probe ISH assays.

nuclear pleomorphism and more sheet-like growth. However, most breast cancers that are strongly ER-positive and HER2-negative are in the low- to intermediate-grade spectrum. Of note, cancers with low percentages of ER-positive cells (and HER2 negativity) frequently have histological features more similar to those of high-grade triple-negative cancers {1913}. Because the pathway to typical strongly ER-positive breast cancers includes other non-obligate precursor/risk lesions with high ER expression, such as DCIS (predominantly of low to intermediate nuclear grade), atypical ductal hyperplasia, and flat epithelial atypia, as well as lobular in situ lesions, these lesions are frequently identified in the background of ER-positive IBC-NSTs, and they sometimes account for a large proportion of the initial imaging findings. Cancers associated with germline *BRCA2* mutations are often ER-positive {1099,1057}.

**Histology of triple-negative cancers:** Although triple-negative (hormone receptor–negative, HER2-negative) breast cancers can also have a spectrum of morphologies (including special types such as adenoid cystic carcinoma and metaplastic

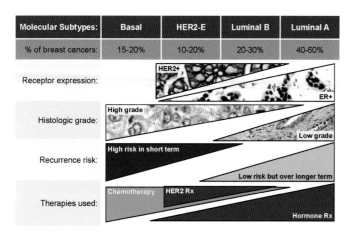

| Molecular Subtypes: | Basal | HER2-E | Luminal B | Luminal A |
|---|---|---|---|---|
| % of breast cancers: | 15-20% | 10-20% | 20-30% | 40-60% |

Receptor expression: HER2+ ... ER+

Histologic grade: High grade ... Low grade

Recurrence risk: High risk in short term ... Low risk but over longer term

Therapies used: Chemotherapy ... HER2 Rx ... Hormone Rx

**Fig. 2.83** Correlation of breast cancer molecular subtypes with clinicopathological features.

carcinoma), the majority of these IBCs are high-grade, with tumour cells displaying high N:C ratios, a solid growth pattern, frequently pushing borders, and geographical necrosis {266, 1222}. Mitotic counts are typically very high (with proliferation often > 80%). The lesions can have a central scar and/or a large central acellular zone, and some triple-negative cancers have a dense lymphocytic stromal infiltrate, which is associated with better response to treatment. DCIS is less frequently identified in the background of triple-negative cancers than in hormone receptor–positive cases {1702,1713}. Cancers associated with germline *BRCA1* mutations are frequently of this morphology {1099}. As noted above, cancers with low percentages of ER-positive cells (and HER2 negativity) frequently have histological features more similar to those of high-grade triple-negative cancers {1913}.

**Histology of HER2-positive cancers:** These breast cancers are typically of high histological grade, and they are frequently associated with background high-grade comedo DCIS. HER2-positive cancers usually have very pleomorphic nuclei and more-abundant eosinophilic cytoplasm than triple-negative cancers, sometimes giving cells a vaguely apocrine appearance. Proliferation is high, but lower on average than in triple-negative cancers (in the 20–60% range). The typical growth patterns are infiltrative cords or solid nests of cells, but single-file patterns are occasionally seen.

*Stromal response patterns and tumour microenvironment*
The stromal component is extremely variable. There may be a highly cellular fibroblastic proliferation, a scant element of connective tissue, or marked hyalinization. Foci of elastosis may also be present in a periductal or perivenous distribution. Some IBC-NSTs show a fibrotic focus, defined as an area of exaggerated reactive tumour stroma formation > 1 mm within the tumour {832,1276,2143}, with or without coagulative necrosis {2143,1276}, and these cases have been reported to show more-aggressive behaviour {832,833}, independent of other variables {1276,2169}.

The immune infiltrate in tumours is referred to as TILs. TILs are mononucleated lymphoid cells infiltrating the tumour and its stroma; they reflect the host immune response against the tumour cells. The extent of TILs in IBC is gaining importance as a prognostic marker, with high numbers of TILs associated with a better outcome and better response to neoadjuvant therapy in triple-negative and HER2-positive breast carcinomas (see *Prognosis and prediction*, below) {482,1227,1228,1830}.

For quantifying TILs, it is recommended to follow the international consensus scoring recommendations {1831,922}. The steps are outlined in Fig. 2.84. It is recommended that quantification is done on H&E-stained tissue sections at a magnification of 20–40× with a 10× ocular in core biopsies or surgical specimens, on the most representative tumour block. TILs should be scored in the stroma between the areas of carcinoma, and all mononuclear cells (lymphocytes and plasma cells) should be included. Stromal TILs should be scored as a percentage of the stromal areas alone – the carcinoma cells should not be included in the total assessed surface area. Peritumoural follicular aggregates and tertiary lymphoid structures with germinal centres are indicative of an active immune response, but they should not be included in the stromal TIL assessment. TIL quantification should be reported as a percentage – a mean score based on the available tissue analysed. If the TILs appear to be heterogeneously distributed, an average should be reported, disregarding hotspots {1831}. The development of computational pathology methods is likely to make automated counting an option in the future.

*Morphological characteristics after neoadjuvant treatment*
The residual carcinoma or tumour bed in the breast and the response in the lymph nodes can serve as measures of response to neoadjuvant treatment and can provide valuable prognostic information, so these should be evaluated and reported {204,203}. Multidisciplinary collaboration and correlation of clinical, imaging, gross, and microscopic findings are essential for accurately sampling and histologically quantifying response to treatment. The residual cancer burden index is a clinically validated, standardized reporting system that incorporates response in the breast and response in the lymph nodes into a score that can be combined with other emerging prognostic factors.

Changes in the residual tumour cells, if present, are extremely variable in degree. In therapy-resistant cancers, no morphological alteration may be detected. More commonly, carcinomas become less cellular and are often present as scattered small nests across the tumour bed. The size and cellularity of foci of the overall residual cancer should be recorded, because the extent of residual invasive carcinoma, together with lymph node status, is a powerful predictor of long-term survival {286}. In a few cases, the remaining cancer cells become bizarre, with large and irregular nuclei. The cytoplasm of the residual tumour cells may become vacuolated (in ~40% of cases) {1400}. In some cases, the only residual cancer is in lymphatic spaces, and this finding has been associated with recurrence after neoadjuvant therapy {320}. The mitotic count is often lower in the residual carcinoma. Nevertheless, histological grade remains a prognostic factor after neoadjuvant therapy and therefore may be relevant to report (this is not standard) {218}. After a complete response, only a loose, oedematous, vascularized fibroelastotic area of connective tissue with chronic inflammatory cells and macrophages may mark the tumour bed. When only small foci of atypical cells are present, immunohistochemical studies may

# Evaluation of tumour-infiltrating lymphocytes (TILs)

## Step 1: Define the area for evaluation

Large areas of central necrosis or fibrosis are not included in the evaluation.

## Step 2: Focus only on stromal TILs

## Step 3: Determine the type of inflammatory infiltrate

Include only mononuclear infiltrate (lymphocytes and plasma cells).

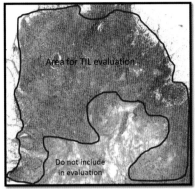

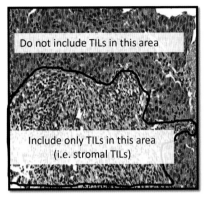

Do not include TILs in this area

Include only TILs in this area (i.e. stromal TILs)

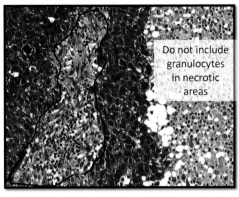

Do not include granulocytes in necrotic areas

## Steps 4 & 5: Assess and report the percentage of the stromal area involved by TILs

Report the average of the stromal area; do not focus on hotspots.

For more detail, visit: www.tilsinbreastcancer.org

**Fig. 2.84** Evaluation of tumour-infiltrating lymphocytes (TILs) in breast cancer.

be helpful for distinguishing cancer cells from benign histiocytic cells and invasive carcinoma from carcinoma in situ. DCIS may be present in the absence of residual invasive carcinoma. This finding does not exclude pathological complete response, and these patients have a good prognosis {194,649}. Primary neoadjuvant endocrine therapy is sometimes administered, but it rarely results in pathological complete response. Treated cancers may have a central area of fibrous scarring {2074}.

Normal breast epithelial structures may show atypia, in the form of enlarged and occasionally pleomorphic nuclei, after neoadjuvant therapy. These may be present at some distance from the site of the invasive tumour and can be present throughout the specimen rather than only in the vicinity of the tumour bed; care should be taken not to overdiagnose these as in situ disease. Radiation can cause the stroma to be dense and hypocellular. The epithelial cells of ducts and lobules may show slightly irregular and hyperchromatic nuclei, and lobules may become sclerotic. Radiation fibroblasts may be seen, and bizarre stromal cells may also be present.

### Differential diagnosis

IBC should be differentiated from malignant breast in situ lesions (carcinoma in situ) and benign infiltrative lesions such as sclerosing lesions and microglandular adenosis. Although most IBCs

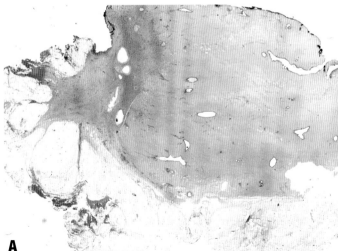

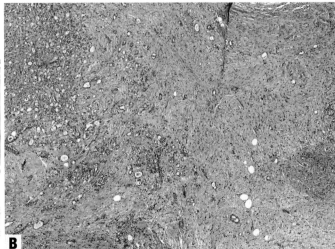

**A**

**B**

**Fig. 2.85** Breast carcinoma. **A** Low-power view of breast carcinoma after neoadjuvant chemotherapy, featuring partial response with areas of fibrosis without residual tumour representing tumour bed. Residual invasive tumour is seen in part of the tumour bed. **B** Higher-power view shows residual breast carcinoma after neoadjuvant treatment. There is a decrease of tumour cellularity compared with cellularity in the core biopsy.

have an infiltrative growth pattern, more-nested patterns can mimic in situ lesions, such as DCIS. Conversely, DCIS involving a sclerosing lesion can mimic invasive carcinoma. Benign sclerosing lesions such as sclerosing adenosis and radial scar can mimic the infiltrative pattern of an invasive lesion. Myoepithelial stains are essential for distinguishing between these lesions, with invasive lesions lacking myoepithelial cells at their periphery. However, the correct interpretation of myoepithelial staining is important, because stromal or vascular staining can mimic a myoepithelial cell layer in some cases. A nuclear myoepithelial stain (e.g. p63) in addition to a cytoplasmic stain (e.g. calponin or SMMHC) can be useful to help avoid pitfalls in interpretation.

Rare breast lesions that can mimic primary IBC include microglandular adenosis (which can mimic a well-differentiated invasive cancer) and primary breast melanoma and lymphoma (which can mimic a poorly differentiated breast cancer). In addition, primary breast sarcomas resemble IBCs, often with metaplastic features but sometimes also IBC-NST. Diagnostic difficulties can also be encountered with malignant phyllodes tumour (especially when the lesion lacks characteristic epithelial areas of phyllodes tumour), primary breast sarcoma NOS, and primary or secondary breast angiosarcoma (with epithelioid subtypes being a problematic mimic of carcinoma).

Although rare, metastatic carcinoma to the breast should be considered when unusual growth patterns are present or there is a previous history or a clinical concern {2104}. Among the most common metastatic cancers to the breast are lung adenocarcinomas and ovarian, uterine, and renal cell carcinomas {2104,1128,707}. Clinical history and immunohistochemistry are essential for making the correct diagnosis. IBC should also be distinguished from primary or metastatic cutaneous carcinomas, including squamous cell carcinoma (differential diagnosis with metaplastic squamous breast carcinoma), skin adnexal carcinomas, and cutaneous melanoma. Rarely, primary breast salivary gland–like carcinomas may need to be distinguished from metastatic salivary gland carcinomas, in particular if there is a clinical history of salivary gland carcinoma of similar type.

## Cytology

Because it is not possible to distinguish between in situ and invasive carcinomas cytologically, CNB has largely replaced breast FNA, except in settings where access to image-guided biopsy is limited {1460}. However, cytological preparations from FNA samples of suspicious axillary lymph nodes or other sites of suspected metastasis are commonly used to rule out metastatic breast cancer and have reasonable sensitivity and high specificity {110}. The analysis of ER/PR and HER2 on FNA material should be limited to cases of metastasis, to avoid testing non-cancerous breast tissue {2089,1031,1906,1991}.

Cytological preparations of IBC are often characterized by highly cellular, loosely cohesive groups and single atypical cells with syncytial arrangement and loss of polarity. The cells have hyperchromatic nuclei; irregular, thickened nuclear membranes; nucleoli; and increased N:C ratios. Cells are often arranged in 3D clusters or syncytial groups, or occasionally in acinar or gland-like patterns. The malignant cells are usually larger than lymphocytes or benign ductal cells, but they can be less obviously enlarged in well-differentiated cancers. The nuclei can be eccentrically located, with a plasmacytoid appearance. Bipolar naked nuclei are not a feature. Occasionally, cytoplasmic

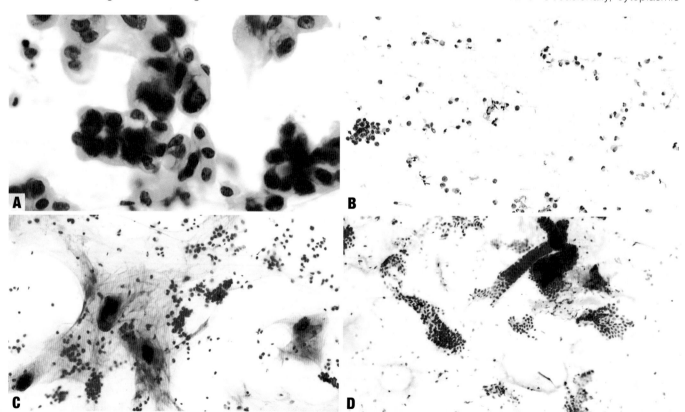

**Fig. 2.86** Morphological aspects on FNA (Papanicolaou staining). **A** Invasive carcinoma of no special type (NST). **B** Invasive lobular carcinoma, classic type. **C** Invasive mucinous carcinoma. **D** Tubular carcinoma.

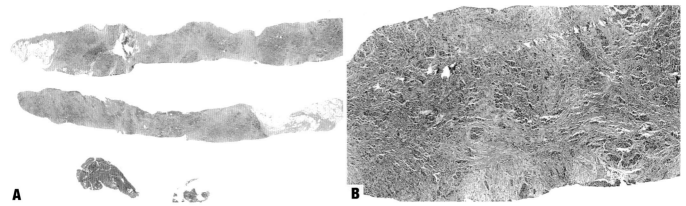

**Fig. 2.87** Invasive breast carcinoma of no special type (NST). **A** Core biopsy of a breast tumour reveals an invasive carcinoma NST. **B** At medium magnification, invasive carcinoma NST shows irregular malignant tumour cords amid chronic inflammatory cells on core biopsy.

vacuolization, signet-ring cells, or intracellular lumina can be seen. Smears of poorly differentiated carcinoma may contain pleomorphic, bizarre cells and multinucleated malignant cells.

### Core needle biopsy

CNB for the initial evaluation of a breast lesion has been used extensively for years as a non-surgical approach that allows for more-rapid diagnosis of palpable and non-palpable imaging-detected findings than excision (open) biopsy. With imaging guidance, CNB is highly sensitive and specific for the diagnosis and initial classification of breast cancer {233}. There is excellent correlation between the findings on CNB and those on open excisional biopsy {2287}, and diagnostic agreement on CNB is also high {389}. Sometimes a definitive diagnosis of invasive cancer is not possible on the limited sampling of a CNB. If there is not 100% certainty in the diagnosis of invasion on CNB, an equivocal classification of a lesion as "suspicious", "indeterminate", "cannot rule out invasion", or "uncertain malignant potential" may be most appropriate, with deferral to a surgical specimen for definitive classification {1707,513}. When the diagnosis of invasion is made on CNB, a preliminary histological grade should be reported, and ER/PR and HER2 testing can be performed if there is sufficient invasive cancer for testing. Because of the limited cold ischaemic time and excellent fixation of CNB samples, as well as the ability to make treatment decisions about possible neoadjuvant therapy before surgery, core needle biopsies are the preferred sample type for these ancillary tests. Therefore, all breast core needle biopsies should be performed per the recommendations for adequate total fixation time in formalin (a minimum of 6 hours) before processing and should not be rush processed {2285,2284,831,1394,815, 816}.

### Diagnostic molecular pathology

*Molecular classification of breast cancer*

Breast cancer is heterogeneous at the molecular level, with different patterns of gene expression leading to differences in behaviour and prognosis {277}. Over the past few years, there has been considerable effort to characterize and classify breast cancer at the molecular level in order to effectively tailor treatment. However, due to time and cost constraints, in the great majority of health care systems, surrogate molecular breast cancer classification is still largely based on immunohistochemical assessment of biomarkers (ER, PR, HER2, and Ki-67). Nevertheless, the examination of global gene expression patterns (especially of genes involved in the regulation of cell growth and other important aspects of cell behaviour, such as invasion) has resulted in the identification of intrinsic molecular subtypes of biological and clinical relevance and of gene signatures predictive of outcome or response to therapy.

*Intrinsic subtype classification*

Hierarchical cluster analysis of the genes that vary more between tumours than between repeated samples of the same tumour (i.e. intrinsic genes) has revealed the existence of four major breast cancer intrinsic subtypes (luminal A, luminal B, HER2-enriched, and basal-like), as well as a normal breast-like group {277,1630}. Other rare subtypes, such as the claudin-low class, which mostly comprises triple-negative tumours and shows a poor prognosis, have also been added. Subclassification of the major subtypes has also been attempted, including HER2-enriched and triple-negative subtypes. In order to improve the standardization and reproducibility of the intrinsic subtype classification, a quantitative RT-PCR–based test with a curated list of 50 genes (the PAM50 gene signature) was proposed. These genes were selected to classify IBCs into luminal A, luminal B, HER2-enriched, and basal-like subtypes {1608}. Because high-throughput transcriptomic analysis is expensive and by no means widespread, a classification based on the above-mentioned immunohistochemical biomarkers was further developed, classifying tumours into the five subtypes shown in Box 2.01 (p. 96) {745}.

**Box 2.01** The clinicopathological surrogate definitions of early invasive breast carcinoma subtypes adopted by the 13th St. Gallen International Breast Cancer Conference (2013) Expert Panel, based on immunohistochemical measurements of ER, PR, ERBB2 (HER2), and Ki-67 with in situ hybridization confirmation where appropriate {745}

**Luminal A–like**
- ER: positive
- PR: positive
- HER2: negative
- Ki-67 proliferation index: low

**Luminal B–like (HER2-negative)**
- ER: positive
- HER2: negative
- At least one of the following:
  - Ki-67 proliferation index: high
  - PR: negative or low

**Luminal B–like (HER2-positive)**
- ER: positive
- HER2: overexpressed or amplified
- Ki-67 proliferation index: any
- PR: any

**HER2-positive (non-luminal)**
- HER2: overexpressed or amplified
- ER: absent
- PR: absent

**Triple-negative**
- ER: absent
- PR: absent
- HER2: negative

*Integrative cluster classification*

This classification divides breast cancer into 10 integrative cluster subgroups (IntClusters) based on the integration of genomic and transcriptomic data {423}. Each subgroup has a distinct pattern of copy-number aberrations and is associated with different clinical outcomes and response to therapy. Six of the subgroups (IntClusters 1, 2, 3, 6, 7, and 8) comprise predominantly ER-positive tumours and the PAM50 subtypes luminal A and luminal B, but with distinct genomic alterations. IntCluster 10 comprises mostly ER-negative tumours, with high genomic instability and a worse prognosis. IntCluster 4 comprises mostly tumours with extensive intratumoural lymphocytic infiltration.

*Triple-negative breast cancer molecular subclassification*

Triple-negative breast cancer (TNBC) is defined by the absence of expression of ER, PR, and HER2 by immunohistochemistry, which results in limited targeted therapeutic options. This is a heterogeneous group of tumours with different molecular drivers and prognoses {1702,1360}. Using gene expression data, a classification of TNBC into the following four tumour-specific subtypes (TNBCtype-4) has been developed {1140}: basal-like 1 and basal-like 2 (which differ in immune response), mesenchymal, and luminal AR. These subtypes present distinct survival patterns and sensitivity to neoadjuvant chemotherapy {1140A}. Combining RNA and DNA profiling analyses also produces four distinct subtypes: luminal AR, mesenchymal, basal-like immunosuppressed, and basal-like immune-activated {256}. Each subtype presents specific targets for treatment (e.g. AR and the cell surface mucin EMA [MUC1] in the luminal AR subtype) and a different prognosis (e.g. the basal-like immune-activated

subtype has a better prognosis than the basal-like immunosuppressed subtype). However, despite multiple efforts, there is not yet an established or clinically verified diagnostic assay for the classification of TNBC.

*Mutation profiles of IBC*

Breast cancer subtypes present different mutation patterns, which influence response to treatment and prognosis. Luminal A tumours have a high prevalence of *PIK3CA* mutations (49%), whereas basal-like tumours have mostly *TP53* mutations (84%). In the setting of early disease, *PIK3CA* mutations have an overall prevalence of 32%, and they are associated with older patient age; histologically well-differentiated and smaller tumours; and ER-positive, HER2-negative tumour status {2344}. Recently, there was approval for using a *PIK3CA* mutation testing method (by RT-PCR) to determine whether patients with advanced ER-positive breast cancer are eligible for treatment with alpelisib (a PI3K inhibitor) {69A}.

Characterization of the genomic drivers of the various molecular subtypes of TNBC has been attempted {122}. The basal-like 1 subtype was the most genomically unstable, with a high *TP53* mutation rate (92%) and copy-number deletions in genes involved in DNA repair (*BRCA2*, *MDM2*, *PTEN*, *RB1*, and *TP53*). Luminal AR tumours were also found to be associated with a higher mutation burden, with significantly enriched mutations in *PIK3CA* (55%), *AKT1* (13%), and *CDH1* (13%).

With the wider availability of next-generation sequencing, breast tumours are increasingly being tested for multiple mutations and/or other genetic alterations, such as mutations in *PIK3CA*, *ERBB2* (*HER2*), and *ESR1*. Recently, the use of whole-genome sequencing has led to the identification of mutation signatures. These signatures can reflect etiology or biology, for example, damage due to ultraviolet (UV) radiation or defective DNA repair pathways. In breast cancer, it is known that inherited mutations in *BRCA1* or *BRCA2* (present in ~1–5% of breast tumours) result in homologous recombination deficiency, and the characteristic signature can be identified using whole-genome sequencing. The signature can also be identified in patients without germline *BRCA1/2* mutations with tumours showing BRCA1/2 dysfunction, such as sporadic basal-like/triple-negative cancers. This has led to the development of tools to detect homologous recombination deficiency (e.g. the HRDetect assay). As of recently, patients who have recurrent or stage 4 HER2-negative cancer and a known *BRCA1* or *BRCA2* germline mutation are now considered candidates for therapies that target this deficiency – namely, poly (ADP-ribose) polymerase (PARP) inhibitors {1773A,1773B}.

Using next-generation sequencing, it is also possible to quantify a tumour's total mutation burden, which is associated with therapeutic response to immunotherapy. Breast cancer does not have as high a total mutation burden as melanoma, but the total mutation burden tends to be higher in TNBC (at 1.68 mutations/Mb) than in luminal tumours (0.84–1.38 mutations/Mb) {277,246}. Among the TNBCs, the luminal AR subtype seems to have a higher total mutation burden than the mesenchymal stem-like subtype {122}. Therefore, immunotherapy may be useful in some subsets of breast cancers, especially subsets of TNBC.

### Essential and desirable diagnostic criteria

*Essential:* an invasive malignant process of breast epithelium lacking a peripheral myoepithelial cell layer (immunohistochemistry may be required), with or without carcinoma in situ; ER, PR, and HER2 immunohistochemistry to guide classification, treatment, and prognosis.

### Staging

The most widely used system for staging breast carcinoma is the TNM system published by the Union for International Cancer Control (UICC) {229} and the American Joint Committee on Cancer (AJCC) {61}. This system captures information about the extent of cancer at the primary site (Tumour, T), the regional lymph nodes (Node, N), and spread to distant metastatic sites (Metastasis, M). Special techniques for classification are not required, and comparable information can therefore be collected across time and in different locations. The T, N, and M information is combined to define five stages (0, I, II, III, and IV) that summarize information about the extent of regional disease (tumour size, skin or chest-wall invasion, and nodal involvement) and metastasis to distant sites. In individual cases, this information is important for making decisions concerning the control of local disease, as well as to determine the value of systemic therapy. Determining tumour stage is also essential for organizing groups of similar patients for comparison in clinical trials, epidemiological studies, or other types of investigations.

Both clinical staging and pathological staging are used for patients with breast cancer. Clinical stage depends on physical examination and imaging studies, with or without confirmation by FNA or CNB. Pathological classification of T and N primarily relies on the gross and microscopic examination of surgically excised specimens. In most patients, T is based on the size of the invasive carcinoma. If multiple areas of invasion are present, T classification is based on the largest focus. A small cancer is sometimes best evaluated by measuring its size on glass slides. Correlation of gross, microscopic, and imaging findings is often necessary to determine the best T category. Lymph nodes should be evaluated in 2 mm slices, to identify all macrometastases (metastases > 2 mm). Metastatic deposits ≤ 2 mm but > 0.2 mm (or > 200 cells) in a lymph node are known as micrometastases and define the case as node-positive (pN1mi), whereas cases with only isolated tumour cells (< 0.2 mm) are considered node-negative (pN0i+) for staging purposes. M classification is primarily determined by the results of radiological studies, with pathological confirmation after biopsy in some cases. Approximately 48% of breast cancers present as stage I disease, 34% as stage II, 13% as stage III, and 5% as stage IV {925}. However, the stage distribution is dependent on several variables, including race/ethnicity; patient age; ER status {925,2051,2232}; and the existence of population-based breast cancer screening, which is associated with earlier stage at presentation. There is also a correlation between the components of the stage; for example, only 19% of pT1 tumours are associated with nodal metastasis and only 1% are associated with distant metastasis, compared with as many as 40% and 10%, respectively, of pT3 tumours {925}.

Most breast carcinomas first metastasize to regional lymph nodes via the lymphatics draining the tumour. The first draining

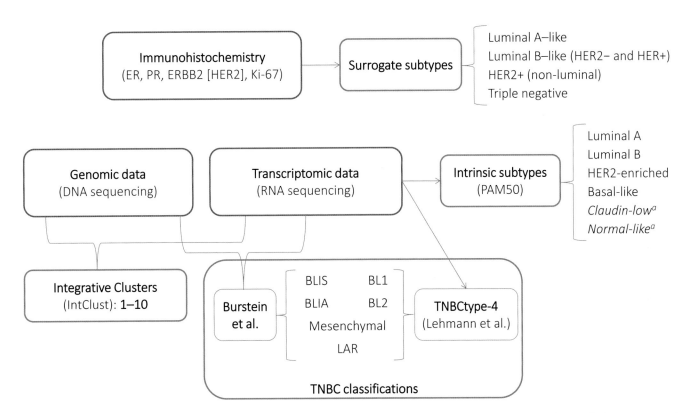

**Fig. 2.88** Classification of breast cancer of no special type (NST). BL1, basal-like 1; BL2, basal-like 2; BLIA, basal-like immune-activated; BLIS, basal-like immunosuppressed; LAR, luminal androgen receptor; TNBC, triple-negative breast cancer. [a]Not included in the PAM50 signature's classification.

node is known as the sentinel lymph node. There is level 1 evidence that sampling this node for assessment results in accurate staging, and this approach can be used to obviate the need for axillary dissection and the associated risk of lymphoedema in patients without metastases {421}. The sentinel lymph node can be identified preoperatively by injection of blue dye and a radioactive marker into the tissue around the tumour. Axillary dissection is usually unnecessary in patients with metastatic foci totalling ≤ 2.0 mm. Immunohistochemistry is not usually required, but it may be used to clarify the nature of suspicious or atypical cells in some cases (e.g. lobular carcinoma or postneoadjuvant cases). Intraoperative molecular testing (e.g. one-step nucleic acid amplification) is highly sensitive but not widespread {315,495,2363,2020,1614,1821}, whereas frozen section or imprint cytology is less sensitive but more commonly performed {1198,638,424,1614,1641}. However, assessment of nodes by high-resolution ultrasonography can provide similar benefits without the need for intraoperative assessment {846}. In the neoadjuvant setting, the value of sentinel node examination and the clinical significance of residual isolated tumour cells are unknown, pending the results of ongoing clinical trials.

Biological tests, such as receptor status and gene expression profiling, may complement staging information by estimating the risk of future metastasis or recurrence or by predicting the likely response to treatment. In a major departure from traditional anatomical staging, the eighth edition of the AJCC cancer staging manual {61} TNM staging system has introduced a breast cancer prognostic stage that incorporates anatomical TNM information with tumour-intrinsic biology: namely, histological tumour grade {735,62} and predictive biomarkers (ER, PR, and HER2 expression), in addition to multigene assays in a subgroup of patients. The proposed prognostic stage incorporating these seven variables (T, N, M, ER, PR, HER2, and grade) aims to improve stratification of patients with respect to outcome.

The increasingly common practice of initiating therapy before definitive surgical treatment (i.e. neoadjuvant or presurgical therapy) requires a combination of information from clinical examination, imaging, and pathological examination to determine the most likely T, N, and M classifications in addition to tumour grade and receptor status before treatment. Posttreatment yT and yN classifications are determined after definitive surgery. Determining stage both before and after treatment provides important prognostic information {286,943}.

## Prognosis and prediction
The prognosis of IBC is profoundly influenced by the standard variables discussed below. Some prognostic markers are also predictors of therapeutic response, such as ER and HER2 status {1703,925,1710}. The management of breast carcinoma is influenced by both prognostic and predictive characteristics.

### Standard clinicopathological prognostic factors
Standard prognostic factors include patient age, disease stage, tumour grade, tumour type, margin status, and lymphovascular status. Breast cancer in individuals aged < 35 years at diagnosis is rare (< 5%) and potentially more aggressive, leading to more chemotherapy. However, one study found that patients who were older at the time of diagnosis experienced a 17% higher disease-specific mortality rate than younger

patients {2052}. The 10-year breast cancer–specific mortality rate associated with small, early-stage breast cancer (TNM stage T1a/bN0M0) has been reported to be as low as 4% {819}. The 5-year relative survival rate of patients with localized breast cancer (~60% of patients) is > 95%, which decreases to 85% when regional lymph nodes are involved and to about 25% with metastatic disease. Completeness of excision is also an important factor affecting local recurrence, but the only margin status proven to have a significant effect on local recurrence after conservation surgery is a positive margin (0 mm, tumour at ink) {881,1954}. Therefore, most guidelines endorse the adequacy of a "no invasive tumour at ink" margin for IBC and a 2 mm margin for DCIS (when DCIS is not associated with invasion) {1423,1414}. Lymphovascular invasion (tumour emboli in blood or lymphatic peritumoural vessels) should be reported when present, because it is associated with risk of local recurrence (for which radiation may be offered even in the mastectomy setting) and distant recurrence, especially for node-negative patients {1710}.

### Standard required prognostic/predictive markers
**Hormone receptor and HER2 status:** Hormone receptor (ER and PR) status and HER2 status of IBC cells are recognized as indispensable predictive and prognostic factors for IBC therapy decision-making by international guidelines such as those published by the St. Gallen International Breast Cancer Expert Panel {422,421}, the European Society for Medical Oncology (ESMO) {1899}, ASCO {815,2283}, and the National Comprehensive Cancer Network (NCCN) {759,1469}. Assessment of hormone receptor and HER2 status is obligatory and usually reflex for all IBC.

**Hormone receptors:** The primary role of ER status is as a predictive marker: patients with cancers expressing ≥ 1% nuclear ER are significantly more likely to benefit from endocrine therapies than patients with cancers showing < 1% ER expression (who do not benefit.) Most ER-positive cancers have high levels of ER expression. ER is also prognostic: strongly ER-positive breast cancers have a better prognosis over the short term (5 years) than ER-negative breast cancers, but this is modified by grade and stage, and late recurrences can occur decades after initial diagnosis. Cancers with low levels of ER (most often defined as 1–10% ER staining) are uncommon but appear to have a worse prognosis than those with high ER expression levels. Within the group of cancers that are ER-positive, PR expression levels (the percentage of stained cells) are considered a prognostic marker: cases with lower PR expression levels are associated with worse outcomes, but patients still receive benefit from endocrine therapy {1030,1519,1737}.

**HER2:** HER2 is both a predictive and prognostic marker. A positive HER2 test is predictive of survival benefit when HER2-targeted therapies are added to chemotherapy regimens. Therefore, a HER2-positive test makes a patient a candidate for both chemotherapy and HER2-targeted therapies. HER2 is also a marker of aggressive biology and poor prognosis in the absence of appropriate targeted therapies.

### Additional prognostic/predictive markers
**Single markers of proliferation / Ki-67:** Breast cancer proliferation is an important parameter to consider in the evaluation of disease aggressiveness and therefore in therapeutic

decision-making, especially concerning chemotherapy. Ki-67 is not universally used or officially recommended, due to a lack of international consensus about scoring and cut-off values {542}, as well as a potential lack of reproducibility. Nevertheless, it could be of clinical value (if available and accurately scored) as a supplement to grade in determining prognosis and potential chemotherapy benefit {542}. Because ER-negative, HER2-positive cancers and ER-negative, HER2-negative cancers are highly proliferative (Ki-67 proliferation index: 30–100%), these cancers are more rapidly growing and are more often treated with chemotherapy. ER-positive cancers have a wider range of proliferation, with highly proliferative forms correlated with more-aggressive behaviour, although most cases have a Ki-67 proliferation index < 20%. A threshold of 14% or 15% has been proposed for helping to discriminate between cases likely to correlate with the more aggressive luminal B molecular subtype (Ki-67 proliferation index ≥ 14% or 15%) versus the less aggressive luminal A subtype (Ki-67 proliferation index < 14% or 15%) {316A,1971}. However, this threshold has not been validated for the purpose of predicting response to chemotherapy. Panel-based gene expression assays that are largely proliferation-driven, such as the 21-gene recurrence score (RS; see below), have been validated for this purpose in ER-positive cancers.

Of note, IHC4 is an immunohistochemistry-based assay of four markers, including Ki-67, that was shown to predict residual risk of distant recurrence in patients on adjuvant endocrine therapy in the ATAC trial as robustly as the 21-gene RS {426}, although it has not gained regulatory acceptance. Most often, Ki-67 is used as a preliminary, inexpensive but non-predictive marker of proliferation. Correlating a Ki-67 result with other findings, such as grade, ER status, or HER2 status, can also be useful to ensure the findings all correlate well with each other and to accurately characterize the biology of the cancer for prognostic purposes.

**AR status:** Recent systematic review and meta-analysis data have shown that AR expression by immunohistochemistry {2164,217} and high AR mRNA levels by pooled gene analysis {217} are associated with improved disease-free survival and better overall survival in patients with early-stage breast cancer. However, AR's function in ER-positive and ER-negative breast cancers appears to be complex, and data on AR as a predictor of response to hormone/androgen-targeted therapies are currently somewhat limited and still under investigation {991,734}. Therefore, AR testing is not currently performed as standard practice on all breast cancer cases, although it may be requested in certain clinical settings.

**Table 2.08** Gene expression signatures used for chemotherapy decision-making in ER-positive, ERBB2 (HER2)-negative breast cancer

| | MammaPrint | Oncotype DX | Prosigna (PAM50) | EndoPredict | Breast Cancer Index | Genomic Grade Index |
|---|---|---|---|---|---|---|
| Number of genes | 70 | 21 | 50 | 11 | 7 | 97 |
| Method | DNA microarray | RT-PCR | NanoString | RT-PCR | RT-PCR | RT-PCR |
| Tissue sample type | Frozen/FFPE | FFPE | FFPE | FFPE | FFPE | FFPE |
| Location | Central[a] | Central | Local | Local | Central | Central |
| Test results | High or low risk + subtype | High, intermediate, or low risk | High, intermediate, or low risk + subtype | High or low risk | High or low risk, high or low benefit | High or low risk |
| Clinical indication (according to EGTM) | Predicting prognosis and guiding decision-making regarding chemotherapy for women with **ER+/HER2– EBC, LN– or LN+ (1–3)** | Predicting prognosis and guiding decision-making regarding chemotherapy for women with **ER+/HER2– EBC, LN– or LN+ (1–3)** | Predicting prognosis and guiding decision-making regarding chemotherapy for women with **ER+/HER2– EBC, LN– or LN+ (1–3)** | Predicting prognosis and guiding decision-making regarding chemotherapy for women with **ER+/HER2– EBC, LN– or LN+ (1–3)** | Predicting prognosis and guiding decision-making regarding chemotherapy for women with **ER+/HER2– EBC, LN–** | No recommendation |
| Prospective validation trial(s) | MINDACT (positive) | TAILORx (positive) and RxPONDER (ongoing) | OPTIMA (ongoing) | None | None | ASTER70 (ongoing) |
| Regulatory approval | EMA, FDA | EMA, FDA | EMA, FDA | EMA, FDA | Not approved | Not approved |
| Original validation set | Developed in young patients (aged < 55 years) who had not received systemic therapy after surgery | Developed in patients who had received tamoxifen only in the NSABP B-20 and B-14 trials | Postmenopausal patients in the training and development sets received heterogeneous treatment | Developed in postmenopausal patients who had received endocrine therapy only in the ABCSG-6 and -8 trials | Initially developed in patients treated with tamoxifen only and then further refined in heterogeneously treated patients | Developed in a heterogeneous patient population (62% aged ≤ 50 years), in order to permit the measurement of histological grade via gene expression profile |

EBC, early breast cancer; EGTM, European Group on Tumor Markers; EMA, European Medicines Agency; FDA, United States Food and Drug Administration; FFPE, formalin-fixed, paraffin-embedded; LN, lymph node; NSABP, National Surgical Adjuvant Breast and Bowel Project; RT-PCR, reverse transcriptase PCR.
[a]Descentralization, to allow for local testing, is ongoing.

**Assessment of response to neoadjuvant therapy:** Achievement of pathological complete response after neoadjuvant therapy is highly prognostic for HER2-positive and triple-negative breast cancers {1623}. The residual cancer burden index can be used to establish risk classes associated with recurrence in cases with residual disease. The parameters to be quantified and reported, as well as a calculator, are available online {2128B,2017}.

**Gene expression signatures:** Gene expression signatures may be used in clinical practice in some countries (when available and/or reimbursed) for chemotherapy decision-making in ER-positive, HER2-negative breast cancer. Low-risk patients as defined by a gene expression signature can be spared chemotherapy, whereas high-risk patients should benefit from chemotherapy. Several signature assays are available (see Table 2.08, p. 99). First-generation signatures (the 21-gene RS and 70-gene signature) are centrally performed, and their prognostic value is supported by level 1a evidence {285,1982,1981}. The use of these assays is endorsed by ASCO, ESMO, the European Group on Tumor Markers (EGTM), and the St. Gallen Panel in certain clinical situations {824,1898,421}. Consensus opinion is that patients with a low genomic risk score result can safely be spared the use of adjuvant chemotherapy in the setting of ER-positive, HER2-negative, node-negative early breast cancer (which is considered to have a high clinical risk of relapse according to traditional criteria). The use of these signatures in patients with 1–3 positive lymph nodes is more debatable.

*21-gene RS:* The 21-gene RS is a quantitative RT-PCR–based signature based on the expression of 21 genes (16 cancer-related and 5 reference genes) that can be applied to RNA extracted from formalin-fixed, paraffin-embedded tissue samples {1579}. The score is a mathematical function developed to predict the risk of distant relapse at 10 years for patients with ER-positive, HER2-negative, lymph node–negative breast cancer {1579}. It is a continuous variable (ranging from 0 to 100) associated with the risk of distant relapse within 10 years, as well as an independent prognostic factor for ER-positive, node-negative patients with breast cancer treated with adjuvant endocrine therapy (i.e. tamoxifen and aromatase inhibitors) {1579,541}. On the basis of the 21-gene RS, cases were initially classified into three categories: low-risk (score: < 18), intermediate-risk (score: 18–31), and high-risk (score: > 31), which equate with 10-year relapse rates of 7%, 14%, and 30%, respectively. The 21-gene RS also correlates with benefit from chemotherapy in ER-positive, HER2-negative breast cancers {1580}. Its use has been prospectively tested in a randomized trial, supported by level 1a evidence using new RS thresholds that stratify the benefit of adding chemotherapy on the basis of a combination of RS and patient age {1982,1981}. The 21-gene RS is also endorsed by NCCN, ASCO, ESMO, the EGTM, and the St. Gallen Panel for ER-positive, HER2-negative, node-negative breast cancer {824,1898,421}. A trial regarding its use in patients with as many as 3 positive lymph nodes is ongoing {753}. Both the 21-gene RS and the 70-gene signature have been incorporated in the eighth edition of the AJCC cancer staging manual for the classification of breast cancer {61}. A low genomic risk result downstages selected ER-positive, HER2-negative, node-negative tumours into the same prognostic category as T1a–bN0M0 {735}.

*70-gene signature:* A 70-gene prognostic signature was developed as a microarray-based test that can be used to determine the prognosis of patients with stage I or II, node-negative IBC of tumour size < 5.0 cm {2152}. It was later tested in patients with as many as 3 positive lymph nodes {285}. This dichotomous test classifies tumours as having either a good or a poor prognosis, which is an independent predictor of distant metastasis {2141}. The prognostic information provided by the 70-gene signature largely stems from the expression levels of ER-related and proliferation-related genes {486}; therefore, it is useful for ER-positive, HER2-negative breast carcinomas, although its utility is limited or non-existent for the other breast carcinoma subtypes. The test can currently be performed in formalin-fixed, paraffin-embedded tissue with analytical validity equivalent to fresh frozen tissue {1845}. The 70-gene signature's prognostic value is supported by level 1a evidence {285}, and its use is endorsed by ASCO, ESMO, the EGTM, and the St. Gallen Panel {1065,1898,550,740}. Consensus opinion is that patients with a 70-gene signature result associated with low genomic risk can safely be spared the use of adjuvant chemotherapy in the setting of ER-positive, HER2-negative, node-negative early breast cancer (which is considered to have a high clinical risk of relapse according to traditional criteria). The use of this test in patients with 1–3 positive lymph nodes is more debatable. High genomic risk as defined by the signature has been shown to be associated with higher sensitivity to neoadjuvant chemotherapy {1999}. Therefore, the 70-gene signature has also been used as a selection factor in clinical trials in the neoadjuvant setting {1812}. Second-generation signatures can be assessed using dedicated instruments. They have level 1b evidence for prognostic value in ER-positive, HER2-negative patients treated with hormone therapy. High-risk second-generation signatures predict late recurrence, but the clinical value of this information is low, because patients with a high-risk signature nowadays receive chemotherapy in the adjuvant setting. Therefore, the data generated from retrospective trials are not valid in this setting, because the trial participants were only treated with hormone therapy.

*Prognostic scoring systems*

Prognostic scoring systems such as the Nottingham Prognostic Index (NPI) {1703} and Adjuvant! Online (www.adjuvantonline.com) incorporate the clinical parameters of patient age, disease stage, ER status, and tumour grade, but not HER2 status. Another prognostic algorithm, Predict (https://breast.predict.nhs.uk/), does include HER2 status. These algorithms can guide treatment decisions. The Magee equation–based RS is a noncommercial predictive tool based on tumour pathological characteristics (Scarff–Bloom–Richardson grade, H-scores for ER and PR, HER2 status, Ki-67 proliferation index, and tumour size) that can be used to estimate the 21-gene RS using the Magee equation {2128A}. The Magee method may be used instead of the actual 21-gene RS if the estimated Magee score is clearly high or low {1026}.

*Tumour-infiltrating lymphocytes*

TIL assessment is gaining importance as a prognostic marker. High numbers of TILs are associated with better outcome and better response to neoadjuvant therapy in triple-negative and HER2-positive breast carcinomas (level 1b evidence) {482,1227,

1228,1830}. TILs have a strong prognostic value in improving estimates of distant recurrence–free survival, disease-free survival, and overall survival in early-stage TNBCs treated with standard adjuvant/neoadjuvant chemotherapy (level 1b evidence). This finding is based on an evaluation by pathologists using H&E-stained glass slides at the time of diagnosis (before treatment) and in the residual disease after neoadjuvant chemotherapy. The presence and extent of TILs in IBC vary greatly from tumour to tumour. The quantification of TILs is feasible on H&E-stained tissue sections during the diagnostic procedure and follows international recommendations {1831}. The development of computational pathology methods is likely to make automated counting an option within the next few years. Clinical utility (for treatment allocation) is under investigation. TILs should be considered as a stratification factor in clinical trials and should be included in studies involving or evaluating prognosis. It is recommended to follow the international consensus scoring recommendations for quantifying TILs {1831,922}.

## Markers relevant to immune-checkpoint therapy (PDL1 testing)

Clinical trial evidence regarding immune-checkpoint blockade therapies in a variety of tumour types (including breast tumours) is rapidly evolving. Monoclonal antibodies targeting the PD1/PDL1 pathway or CTLA-4 are thought to function by removing the inhibition of the antitumour immune response {1598}. Data from the phase III IMpassion130 clinical trial have shown that immunohistochemical PDL1 expression on > 1% of immune cells in metastatic TNBC is predictive of improvements in progression-free survival and overall survival when first-line atezolizumab is added to protein-bound paclitaxel (nab-paclitaxel) {1859}. The use of approved and validated antibodies and their corresponding organ-specific scoring systems is recommended if testing is performed. However, the field is rapidly evolving and other biomarkers may emerge that prove to be important for prediction of response to checkpoint inhibitors.

# Invasive breast carcinoma of no special type

Rakha EA
Allison KH
Bu H
Ellis IO
Foschini MP
Horii R
Masuda S
Penault-Llorca F
Schnitt SJ
Tsuda H
Vincent-Salomon A
Yang WT

## Definition

The term "invasive breast carcinoma (IBC) of no special type (NST)" refers to a large and heterogeneous group of IBCs that cannot be classified morphologically as any of the special histological types.

## ICD-O coding

8500/3 Infiltrating duct carcinoma NOS
8290/3 Oncocytic carcinoma
8314/3 Lipid-rich carcinoma
8315/3 Glycogen-rich carcinoma
8410/3 Sebaceous carcinoma

## ICD-11 coding

2C61.0 & XH7KH3 Invasive carcinoma of breast NOS & Infiltrating duct carcinoma NOS

## Related terminology

*Acceptable:* invasive breast carcinoma NOS; invasive ductal carcinoma; infiltrating ductal carcinoma.
*Not recommended:* invasive mammary carcinoma of no special type.

## Subtype(s)

There is a wide spectrum of histological patterns seen in IBC-NST, including some special morphological patterns (see *Histopathology*, below), but these are not considered clinically distinct subtypes. For management purposes, IBC-NSTs are further divided into the following biomarker-defined subtypes/groups on the basis of ER and ERBB2 (HER2) status: ER-positive, HER2-negative; ER-positive, HER2-positive; ER-negative, HER2-positive; and ER-negative, HER2-negative.

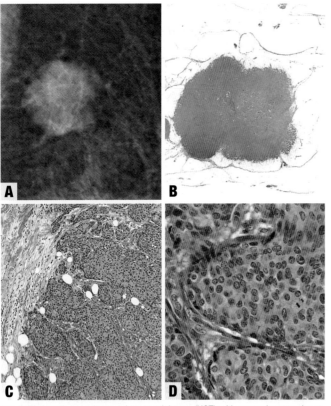

**Fig. 2.89** Invasive carcinoma of no special type (NST) with expansive growth pattern. **A** A polygonal mass with microlobulated margins on mammography. **B** A whole-mount histological section of the tumour. **C** The tumour consists of solid and large invasive cancer nests. **D** The tumour is of histological grade 2. It is moderately differentiated and ER-positive, PR-positive, and ERBB2 (HER2)-negative.

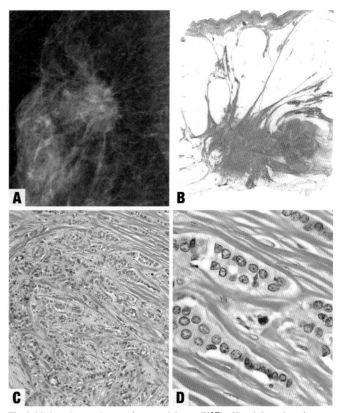

**Fig. 2.90** Invasive carcinoma of no special type (NST) with scirrhous invasive pattern. **A** An irregularly shaped spiculated mass on mammography. **B** A whole-mount histological section of the stellate tumour. **C** Although a trabecular pattern and single-file infiltration with marked fibrosis were seen, the cytomorphological characteristics of an invasive lobular carcinoma were absent. **D** The tumour is of histological grade 2. It is moderately differentiated and ER-positive, PR-positive, and ERBB2 (HER2)-negative.

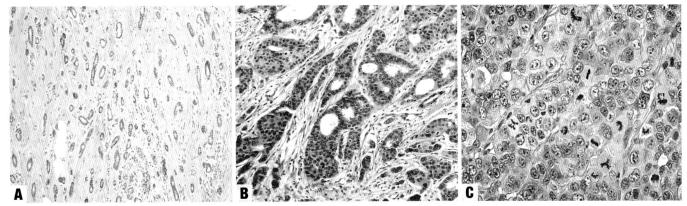

**Fig. 2.91** Invasive breast carcinoma of no special type (NST). **A** Nottingham grade 1. **B** Grade 2. **C** Grade 3.

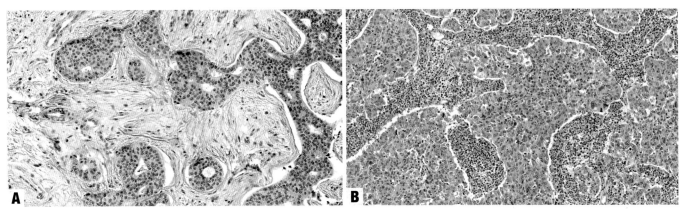

**Fig. 2.92** Invasive breast carcinoma of no special type (NST). **A** Note the sparse tumour-infiltrating lymphocytes (~1%). **B** This tumour is rich in tumour-infiltrating lymphocytes (~95%).

## Localization

IBC-NST has no unique localization features beyond those of all IBCs (see *Invasive breast carcinoma: General overview*, p. 82).

## Clinical features

See *Invasive breast carcinoma: General overview* (p. 82).

## Epidemiology

See *Invasive breast carcinoma: General overview* (p. 82).

## Etiology

There are no well-recognized differences between the known risk factors for breast cancer in general (see *Invasive breast carcinoma: General overview*, p. 82) and for IBC-NST in particular.

## Pathogenesis

See *Invasive breast carcinoma: General overview* (p. 82).

## Macroscopic appearance

See *Invasive breast carcinoma: General overview* (p. 82).

## Histopathology

### General histological features

The histopathological features of IBC-NST vary considerably from case to case and can even vary within the same case. All types of tumour margins can be observed, from highly infiltrative (permeating the surrounding stroma and disrupting the normal lobular units) to continuous pushing margins with an expansive pattern of growth. Architecturally, the tumour cells may be arranged in cords, clusters, and trabeculae, and some tumours are characterized by a predominantly solid or syncytial infiltrative pattern with little associated stroma. In a proportion of cases, glandular differentiation may be apparent as tubular structures with central lumina in tumour-cell groups. Occasionally, areas with single-file infiltration or targetoid features are seen, but these lack the cytomorphological characteristics of invasive lobular carcinoma; the tumour cells are typically more pleomorphic than in lobular carcinoma and they typically show membrane E-cadherin expression. A wide range of mitotic and apoptotic activity, as well as necrosis, can be seen. Similarly, a spectrum of Nottingham grades is observed (see *Invasive breast carcinoma: General overview*, p. 82, for detailed information on grading).

The stromal component is extremely variable. There may be a highly cellular fibroblastic proliferation, a scant element of connective tissue, or marked hyalinization. Some IBC-NSTs are accompanied by marked fibrosis in a scirrhous pattern, with diffuse infiltration of the surrounding tissue as an irregularly

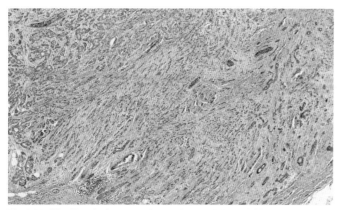

**Fig. 2.93** Mixed invasive breast carcinoma of no special type (NST) with special subtype. Invasive breast carcinoma NST (upper left) mixed with invasive lobular carcinoma (lower left).

shaped spiculated mass. Foci of elastosis may also be present in a periductal or perivenous distribution. Focal necrosis may be present and is occasionally extensive with secondary formation of cyst-like cavities. In a minority of cases, a distinct tumour-associated lymphoplasmacytoid infiltrate can be identified.

In as many as 80% of cases, foci of associated ductal carcinoma in situ are present, and in some cases ductal carcinoma in situ is extensive. Coexistent ductal carcinoma in situ is usually of the same nuclear grade as the invasive carcinoma. Approximately 20–30% of IBC-NSTs show lymphovascular invasion or perineural invasion. Lymphovascular emboli are typically seen within lymphatic spaces and rarely in vascular spaces. Vascular tumour emboli can be observed throughout the tumour, but only extratumoural lymphovascular invasion is routinely assessed in breast cancer, and this should be differentiated from tissue retraction.

### Mixed IBC-NST and special subtypes

Some IBCs can contain a mixture of both IBC-NST and a special subtype. If the special subtype makes up 10–90% of the cancer, the term "mixed IBC-NST and special subtype carcinoma" may be used. For this type of mixed IBC-NST and special subtype, it is recommended to report both elements present, as well as the overall percentage of the special subtype – for example, "mixed IBC-NST and invasive lobular carcinoma (30% lobular)". The grade and biomarker status of both components should be reported, because they can be distinct. Cancers with < 10% special subtype should be classified as IBC-NST, with the focal specialized subtype optionally described in the report comment. Cancers with > 90% specialized subtype should be classified as the special subtype.

### Special morphological patterns

Oncocytic, lipid-rich, glycogen-rich clear cell, and sebaceous carcinomas are rare tumours without sufficient clinical evidence available for their designation as special tumour subtypes, and their specific pattern is considered part of the spectrum of differentiation seen in IBC-NST. Similarly, carcinoma with medullary pattern, invasive carcinoma with neuroendocrine differentiation, carcinomas with pleomorphic and choriocarcinomatous patterns, and tumours with melanocytic features are currently considered to be special morphological patterns of IBC-NST. These tumours are considered morphological patterns of IBC-NST regardless of the extent of differentiation/pattern, and the 90% rule for special subtype is not applied to tumours showing any of these patterns (see below).

**Medullary pattern:** Cancers historically described as medullary carcinoma, atypical medullary carcinoma, or carcinoma with medullary features were previously recognized as a specific special type of well-circumscribed breast cancer with high histological grade, pushing margins, syncytial architecture with no glandular structures, regions of necrosis, a prominent tumour-infiltrating lymphocyte (TIL) infiltrate, and a better clinical outcome than other stage-matched high-grade cancers. These tumours are most often negative for hormone receptors (ER and PR) and HER2 (triple-negative), and they variably express basal markers such as CK5/6, CK14, EGFR (HER1), and p53. However, weak hormone receptor expression also occurs. Genomic instability is common in these high-grade tumours, and they are highly proliferative. As a diagnostic category, "carcinoma with medullary features" has suffered from poor interobserver reproducibility and overlap in features with carcinomas that have basal-like molecular profiles and carcinomas associated with *BRCA1* mutations. In addition, the more recent discovery of the prognostic importance of TILs in high-grade breast cancers appears to explain the good prognosis of these cancers

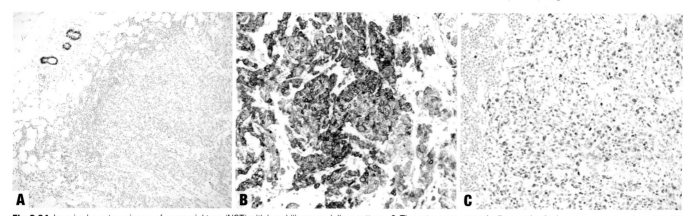

**Fig. 2.94** Invasive breast carcinoma of no special type (NST) with basal-like or medullary pattern. **A** These tumours are typically negative for hormone receptors (negative ER staining with positive internal controls is shown here). However, weak hormone receptor expression also occurs and does not exclude this diagnosis. **B** These tumours frequently have some degree of expression of basal markers such as CK5/6 (shown here), although this is not required for the diagnosis. **C** These tumours should have high proliferation, as shown here with Ki-67 antibody staining. The Ki-67 proliferation index is typically > 50%, as in this case.

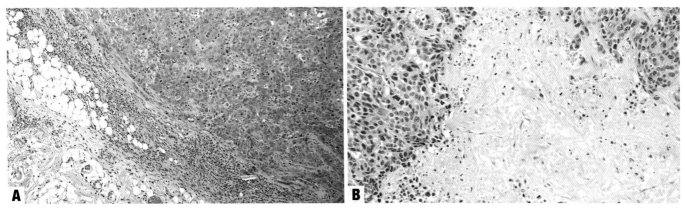

**Fig. 2.95** Invasive breast carcinoma of no special type (NST) with basal-like or medullary pattern. **A** High-grade breast cancer with features of invasive breast carcinoma NST with basal-like or medullary pattern. These cancers have a high Nottingham grade, pushing margins, and syncytial architecture, and they often have prominent tumour-associated lymphocytes at the tumour edge. **B** Regions of geographical necrosis are often seen in these tumours.

(and high-grade cancers not meeting strict medullary criteria) {1697}. Therefore, for clinical purposes, it is now proposed to consider carcinomas with medullary pattern as representing one end of the spectrum of the TIL-rich IBC-NSTs rather than a distinct morphological subtype, and to use the term "IBC-NST with medullary pattern". These cancers can be described as having histological features that correlate with the basal-like molecular profiles, with some quantification of the degree of TILs present if clinically relevant. However, they are categorized diagnostically as IBC-NST, with inclusion of descriptive modifiers referring to medullary pattern or basal-like features. Cancers with these features belong to the immunomodulatory subgroup of triple-negative carcinomas mainly characterized by a high level of expression of immune-related and inflammation genes {256,1140,1680,2176A,1780A}.

**Invasive carcinoma with neuroendocrine differentiation:** Some degree of neuroendocrine differentiation, as determined by histochemical and immunohistochemical analysis, occurs in 10–30% of carcinomas NST {2215,1764}, but it is more common in some special types, in particular mucinous carcinomas and solid papillary carcinomas (occurring in 20% and 72%, respectively). The distinction of invasive carcinoma NST with

neuroendocrine differentiation from well-differentiated neuroendocrine tumours (NETs, which appear similar to what were previously known as carcinoid-like cancers) and higher-grade forms of neuroendocrine carcinoma (NEC) of the breast (see *Neuroendocrine tumour*, p. 156, and *Neuroendocrine carcinoma*, p. 159) is based on the presence and extent of the histological features characteristic of neuroendocrine differentiation in the invasive cancer. If neuroendocrine histological features and neuroendocrine marker expression are not distinct or uniform enough to classify a cancer as one of the rare NETs or NECs of the breast, invasive carcinoma NST with neuroendocrine differentiation should be diagnosed. Although neuroendocrine marker expression is probably underrecognized in breast cancer, because there is currently no clinical relevance of neuroendocrine differentiation as a standalone feature, routine staining of IBCs for neuroendocrine markers is not recommended. These cancers are typically hormone receptor–positive and HER2-negative {1118B}.

**Carcinoma with osteoclast-like stromal giant cells:** Although osteoclastic giant cells can be found in the stroma of breast cancers of any type {849}, they are described in some detail here. Carcinomas with osteoclast-like stromal giant cells are

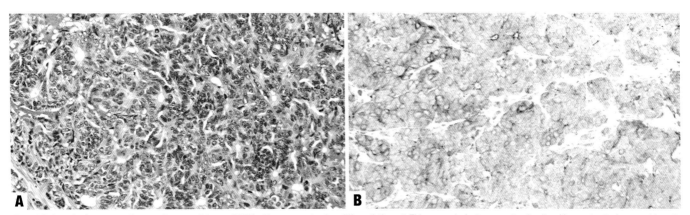

**Fig. 2.96** Invasive breast carcinoma of no special type (NST) with neuroendocrine differentiation. **A** This example features nests of cells with scant cytoplasm and low- to intermediate-grade nuclei that are polarized around abortive lumina. These cancers typically have variable expression of neuroendocrine markers by immunohistochemistry. Importantly, features of the rare high-grade forms of neuroendocrine carcinoma (NEC; e.g. small or large cell carcinoma) or of a specific special subtype (e.g. mucinous or solid papillary carcinoma) are absent. A diagnosis of the rare low-grade tumour (neuroendocrine tumour; NET) of the breast should be reserved for cancers with particularly uniform neuroendocrine features and a carcinoid-like appearance, although strict criteria to differentiate this entity from invasive carcinoma with neuroendocrine differentiation are currently lacking. **B** Variable synaptophysin expression in an invasive carcinoma with neuroendocrine differentiation.

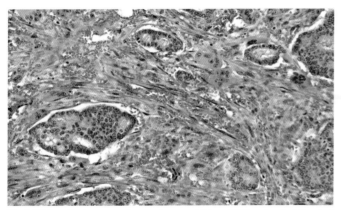

**Fig. 2.97** Invasive breast carcinoma of no special type (NST), osteoclast-like giant cell pattern. A well-differentiated invasive carcinoma with a prominent hypervascular stroma containing extravasated erythrocytes and multiple osteoclast-like giant cells. This invasive carcinoma with osteoclast-like stromal giant cells had variable regions of this pattern.

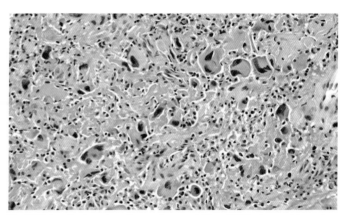

**Fig. 2.98** Invasive breast carcinoma of no special type (NST), pleomorphic carcinoma pattern. This invasive carcinoma with pleomorphic pattern has wildly pleomorphic, enlarged and bizarre cells, some with multiple nuclei.

often associated with an inflammatory, fibroblastic, hypervascular stroma, with extravasated erythrocytes, lymphocytes, and monocytes along with mononucleated and binucleated histiocytes, some containing haemosiderin. The giant cells and hypervascular reactive stroma can be observed in lymph node metastases and in recurrences {2102}. The carcinomatous part of the lesion is most frequently a well-differentiated to moderately differentiated IBC, but all the other histological subtypes have also been observed (most commonly invasive cribriform carcinoma), as have squamous and other metaplastic patterns {849,1942}. The giant cells show uniform expression of CD68 {849} and are negative for S100 and actin. They are also negative for keratin, EMA, ER, and PR. The giant cells are strongly positive for acid phosphatase, NSE, and lysozyme, but negative for alkaline phosphatase, which is indicative of morphological similarity to histiocytic cells and osteoclasts {2102,2057}. The genomic aberrations observed in invasive carcinomas with osteoclast-like stromal giant cells support its classification as IBC-NST {871}. Prognosis is related to the characteristics of the associated carcinoma and does not appear to be influenced by the presence of stromal giant cells.

**Pleomorphic pattern:** Pleomorphic carcinoma is a rare pattern of high-grade IBC-NST characterized by a proliferation of pleomorphic and bizarre (sometimes multinucleated) tumour giant cells constituting > 50% of the tumour cells in a background of adenocarcinoma or adenocarcinoma with metaplastic spindle and squamous differentiation {1941,1776}. These tumours could represent an extreme end of dedifferentiation of IBC-NST or part of the differentiation of metaplastic spindle cell carcinoma. Hormone receptor expression is usually negative, but a proportion of cases overexpress HER2 {1941}. Axillary lymph node metastases are present in 50% of cases, with involvement of ≥ 3 lymph nodes in most of these. Many patients present with advanced disease. One study reported that the presence of a spindle cell metaplastic component in these tumours is associated with poor outcome {1495}.

**Choriocarcinomatous pattern:** Patients with breast carcinoma NST may have elevated levels of serum hCG {1408}, and as many as 60% of ductal carcinomas NST have been found to contain hCG-positive cells {872,1916}. However, histological evidence of choriocarcinomatous differentiation is exceptionally rare, with only a few cases reported {2007,1392,21,1938,1755}; all were in women aged 50–70 years.

**Melanotic pattern:** A few case reports have described exceptional tumours of the mammary parenchyma that appear to represent combinations of ductal carcinoma and melanoma, and in some

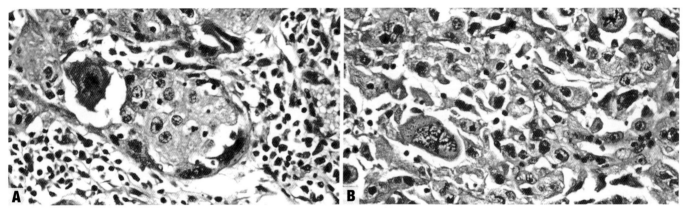

**Fig. 2.99** Invasive breast carcinoma of no special type (NST): carcinoma with choriocarcinomatous features. **A,B** Multinucleated tumour cells with smudged nuclei extend their irregular, elongated cytoplasmic processes around clusters of monocytic tumour cells, mimicking the biphasic growth pattern of choriocarcinoma. Note the abnormal mitotic figures in this high-grade carcinoma.

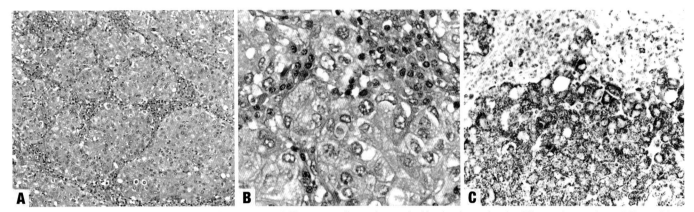

**Fig. 2.100** Invasive breast carcinoma, oncocytic carcinoma pattern. **A** The tumour cells are characterized by abundant and eosinophilic granular cytoplasm. **B** The nuclei are round, with prominent nucleoli. **C** The tumour cells are strongly positive for antimitochondrial antibody.

of these cases there appeared to be a transition from one cell type to the other {1511,1570,1811}. A genetic analysis of one such case showed loss of heterozygosity at the same chromosomal loci in all the components of the tumour, suggesting an origin from the same neoplastic clone {1511}. The mere presence of melanin in breast cancer cells should not be construed as evidence of melanocytic differentiation, because pigmentation of carcinoma cells with melanin can occur when breast cancers invade the skin and involve the dermoepidermal junction {97}. In one study, focal expression of melan-A was found in 18% of breast cancers. The presence and extent of melan-A expression showed a statistically significant association with a reduction in tumour cell differentiation but not with tumour type, size, lymph node metastasis, hormone receptor status, or HER2 expression. The expression of melanocytic markers in breast tissue also appears to be related to lineage infidelity {101}. In addition, care must be taken to distinguish tumours showing melanocytic differentiation from breast carcinomas with prominent cytoplasmic deposition of lipofuscin {1923}. Most melanotic tumours of the breast represent metastases from melanomas originating in extramammary sites. Primary melanomas may arise anywhere in the skin of the breast, but an origin in the nipple–areola complex is extremely rare {1595}. The differential diagnosis of melanoma arising in the nipple–areola region must include Paget disease, the cells of which may occasionally contain melanin pigment {1850}.

**Oncocytic pattern:** Some breast carcinomas demonstrate oncocytic differentiation, with neoplastic cells featuring eosinophilic and granular cytoplasm due to high numbers of mitochondria {926,711}. The clinical features are not distinct from those of IBC-NST; therefore, these features are primarily relevant for excluding apocrine differentiation (which is a close mimic). In one series, mitochondrion-rich features, defined as strong positive mitochondrial immunohistochemical staining of > 50% of the tumour cells, were present in 19.7% of 76 consecutive invasive carcinomas of the breast {1690}. Tumour cells in the oncocytic pattern display predominantly solid growth featuring sheets, islands, and nests with pushing borders. Papillary, plexiform, and glandular patterns are occasionally seen. The tumour cells are characterized by abundant, brightly eosinophilic, granular cytoplasm with well-defined borders. The nuclei are round and centrally located, with prominent nucleoli {668}. These cancers often display chromosomal gains of 11q13.1-q13.2 and 19p13, which are potentially relevant for mitochondrion accumulation. Changes in these chromosomal regions are frequently seen in oncocytic tumours of the kidney and thyroid {711}. ER, PR, and HER2 expression in the oncocytic pattern is variable. In the study cited above, ER was expressed in 78% of the cases, PR in 62.5%, and HER2 in 25% {1690}. Carcinoma in situ was identified in 64.4% of the cases {1690}. Because breast carcinomas with eosinophilic granular cytoplasm are not rare, the

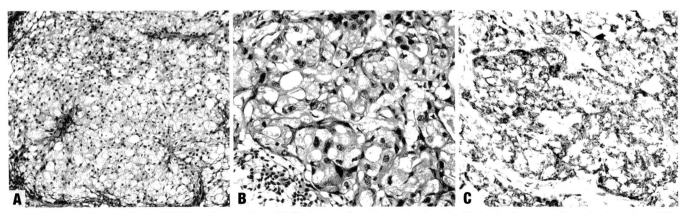

**Fig. 2.101** Invasive breast carcinoma, lipid-rich carcinoma pattern. **A,B** The tumour cells are large and polygonal, with abundant foamy or multivacuolated cytoplasm. **C** Tumour cells stain positively for adipophilin.

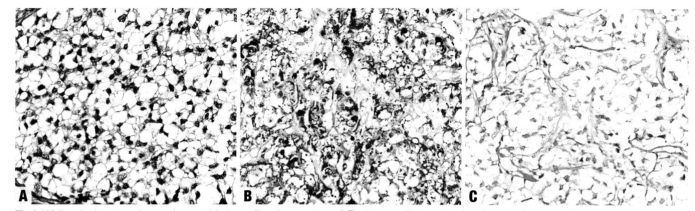

**Fig. 2.102** Invasive breast carcinoma, glycogen-rich clear cell carcinoma pattern. **A** The tumour cells have abundant clear cytoplasm, as well as round or oval nuclei with clumped chromatin. **B,C** The clear cytoplasm contains glycogen that is PAS-positive (**B**) and diastase-sensitive (**C**).

term "IBC-NST with oncocytic carcinoma pattern" should be reserved only for lesions with typical morphology and appropriate immunohistochemical and/or ultrastructural characteristics. These lesions should be distinguished from cancers with apocrine differentiation, which are typically hormone receptor–negative and AR-positive.

**Lipid-rich pattern:** In this pattern of IBC-NST, abundant cytoplasmic neutral lipids are present, creating cytoplasmic vacuoles. The vacuoles in the cytoplasm stain positively with Sudan III or Oil Red O, whereas they do not stain with PAS, Alcian blue, or mucicarmine. The nuclei are irregular, with moderate to severe atypia and one or more nucleoli. Mitotic figures are easily identified. In most cases, lipid-rich carcinoma is classified as histological grade 3. Most of the reported cases are negative for ER and PR {1917,780,1525}. There has been a tendency for HER2 positivity and high proliferation. HER2 positivity in the literature varies from 50% to 100% {20,1080, 1201,1324,1742,2119,2156,2295}. Tumour cells stain positively for α-lactalbumin {20,2119,2257,2295}, lactoferrin {2257,2295}, EMA {20,302,2156}, and adipophilin, but they do not stain for CK5/6, CK14, S100, or myoepithelial cell markers.

**Glycogen-rich clear cell pattern:** In this pattern of IBC-NST, there is abundant clear cytoplasm that contains glycogen. Most glycogen-rich clear cell carcinomas (GRCCs) have a sheet-like, nested, or corded growth pattern. However,

papillary, lobular, or tubular patterns may be seen {2055}. The tumour cells tend to have sharply defined borders and polygonal contours. The clear or finely granular cytoplasm contains PAS-positive, diastase-sensitive glycogen. The nuclei are round or oval, with clumped chromatin and prominent nucleoli. Because intracytoplasmic glycogen can be observed without a substantial clear cell appearance and because clear cell morphology can be caused by substances other than glycogen, both features are required for the diagnosis of this pattern. Lipid-rich carcinoma, sebaceous carcinoma, secretory carcinoma, histiocytoid carcinoma, and myoepithelial tumours may be in the differential. Although non-primary tumours with clear cell histology involving the breast (e.g. metastatic clear cell carcinoma of the kidney) are extremely uncommon, they should also be considered in the differential diagnosis. ER is positive in 35–50% of cases, and most cases are negative for PR {1791}. HER2 status is variable in the published literature. Some authors have reported an *ERBB2* (*HER2*) amplification rate similar to that among breast cancers generally {1016, 2158}; others have reported a lower rate {2363A}. A 2019 SEER Program database review compared the clinicopathological features of 155 cases of GRCC to non-GRCC breast cancers and found that GRCC was more likely to be high-grade, advanced-stage, and triple-negative (44.8% of cases were ER-negative and HER2-negative) {2363A}. Because of

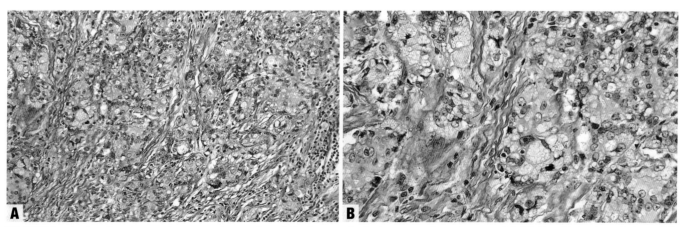

**Fig. 2.103** Invasive breast carcinoma, sebaceous carcinoma pattern. **A** The tumour cells of sebaceous carcinoma have vacuolated, lipid-containing clear cytoplasm. **B** At higher power.

the rarity of GRCC, the prognosis is still controversial. Most reports suggest that GRCC tends to follow an aggressive clinical course {2363A}, but others have concluded that the prognosis is not different from that of IBC-NST when matched for tumour size, grade, and lymph node status {1300A,1258A}.

**Sebaceous pattern:** In this rare pattern of IBC-NST, prominent sebaceous differentiation is present {858,1324,1430, 1675,1720,2155,2054}. The tumour must originate within the mammary gland parenchyma, lacking any evidence of origin from cutaneous adnexal sebaceous glands. The tumour cells are composed of sebaceous cells with abundant clear and vacuolated cytoplasm, which is positive by Oil Red O in frozen sections of fixed or fresh tissue. The nuclei of the sebaceous component vary from small, monomorphic, darkly staining small cells to pleomorphic large cells with prominent nucleoli. The nuclei are mostly eccentrically located. The second component of the tumour consists of smaller, ovoid to spindle cells with non-vacuolated eosinophilic or basophilic cytoplasm. These cells are mostly present at the periphery of the lobules, but they can also be intermixed with sebaceous cells or form separate tumour sheets. Mitotic figures can be numerous, with a range of 5–39 mitoses per 10 high-power fields (undefined) in one study {2014}. The stroma can be densely collagenous or myxoid. The tumour cells are positive for adipophilin. In the literature, ER, PR, and HER2 were positive in 7 of 12 cases, 8 of 12 cases, and 3 of 9 cases, respectively {1675,1324, 2058,2155,858,1430,1720,2014}. It is hypothesized that breast sebaceous carcinoma is a consequence of malignant transformation of local pluripotent cells capable of divergent differentiation {2058,947,264,1275}. However, genetic studies are necessary to evaluate this hypothesis.

## Cytology
See *Invasive breast carcinoma: General overview* (p. 82).

## Diagnostic molecular pathology
See *Invasive breast carcinoma: General overview* (p. 82).

## Essential and desirable diagnostic criteria
*Essential:* invasive carcinoma with evidence of mammary epithelial origin using morphology with or without immunohistochemistry; features characteristic of pure special subtypes, if present, constitute < 90% of the tumour (default diagnosis).

## Staging
See *Invasive breast carcinoma: General overview* (p. 82).

## Prognosis and prediction
IBC-NST forms the bulk of cases of breast cancer, and its prognostic characteristics and management are similar or slightly worse, with a 10-year survival rate of 65–78% {574} compared with about 80% for breast cancer overall {1173,1165,331,2289}. Prognosis is profoundly influenced by the classic variables of patient age, tumour histological grade, tumour stage, lymphovascular invasion, and TILs (see *Invasive breast carcinoma: General overview*, p. 82), as well as by predictors of therapeutic response, such as ER, PR, and HER2 status {1703,925,1710}. Ki-67 proliferation index and AR status have been shown to have prognostic value {2164,217}. Approximately 70–80% of IBC-NSTs are ER-positive, and 12–20% of cases are HER2-positive. The management of IBC-NST is also influenced by these prognostic and predictive characteristics. In one study, breast cancer patients aged ≥ 50 years at diagnosis experienced 17% higher disease-specific mortality than younger patients {2052}. In another study, middle-aged patients (aged 40–60 years) exhibited better outcome than young and elderly patients {324A}. In general, the same prognostic and predictive concepts apply as for other IBCs (see *Invasive breast carcinoma: General overview*, p. 82).

# Microinvasive carcinoma

Cserni G
Pinder SE
Koo JS
Rakha EA

## Definition

Microinvasive carcinoma of the breast is an invasive breast carcinoma ≤ 1 mm in size.

## ICD-O coding

Microinvasive carcinoma does not have an ICD-O code because it does not represent a single biological or phenotypic entity. It is best coded based on the tumour type, for example, 8500/3 (Carcinoma of no special type) or 8520/3 (Invasive lobular carcinoma).

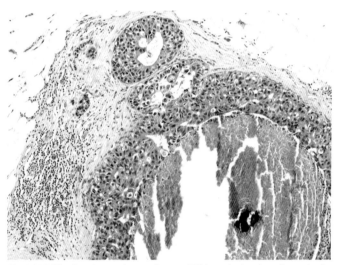

**Fig. 2.104** Microinvasive carcinoma. A case of high-grade ductal carcinoma in situ (DCIS) with scant foci of microinvasion in the adjacent tissue (< 1 mm to the margin of DCIS). The presence of single-cell infiltration as seen in this case (in the top left of the field) supports the diagnosis of microinvasion.

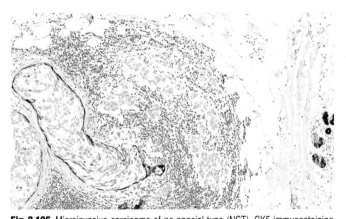

**Fig. 2.105** Microinvasive carcinoma of no special type (NST). CK5 immunostaining demonstrates myoepithelial cells surrounding intermediate-grade ductal carcinoma in situ on the left and normal acini of a lobule on the right, but staining is absent around microinvasive carcinoma in the central part. Note the lymphoid reaction.

## ICD-11 coding

2C61.0 is a code for primary invasive breast carcinoma and therefore includes microinvasive carcinoma.

## Related terminology

*Not recommended:* carcinoma in situ with microinvasion.

## Subtype(s)

Various morphological subtypes of breast carcinoma may be identified that are ≤ 1 mm in size; most often, this is invasive breast carcinoma of no special type, but other histological subtypes (e.g. invasive lobular carcinoma) may be seen less commonly {166,420}. Microinvasive carcinoma is also heterogeneous in molecular subtype, with immunohistochemically defined surrogate classifications: it can belong to the luminal A–like, luminal B–like, ERBB2 (HER2)-overexpressing (nonluminal), or triple-negative category {1561,1185}.

## Localization

Microinvasive carcinoma can be found in any part of the breast, typically in the vicinity of carcinoma in situ (generally ductal carcinoma in situ [DCIS] of high grade). Rarely, microinvasive lobular carcinoma has been described in association with classic, florid, or pleomorphic lobular carcinoma in situ {1801}.

## Clinical features

Microinvasive carcinoma has no specific clinical features. It is not palpable and is generally identified by chance during microscopic assessment of a carcinoma in situ {2175}. The clinical and/or imaging features are those of the associated in situ component.

## Epidemiology

The incidence of microinvasive carcinoma is related to the grade and size of the DCIS lesion and therefore varies widely in the literature. One series identified a 3% risk of microinvasion with DCIS lesions < 5 mm, a 6% risk with those 6–10 mm, and a risk as high as 23% with tumours ≥ 50 mm {1945}. Although some data suggest that 8–9% {2219,1978} or even > 20% {1012} of carcinoma in situ lesions may have microinvasion, most suggest that microinvasive carcinoma is much rarer. Although all carcinoma in situ progressing to invasive carcinoma theoretically passes through this stage during its evolution, the exact moment when this occurs is rarely captured histologically. Data relating to its incidence are therefore subject to bias due to variations in population breast screening, differences in definitions varying over time, and relatively common misdiagnosis.

## Etiology

The etiology of microinvasive carcinoma is the same as that of invasive breast carcinoma.

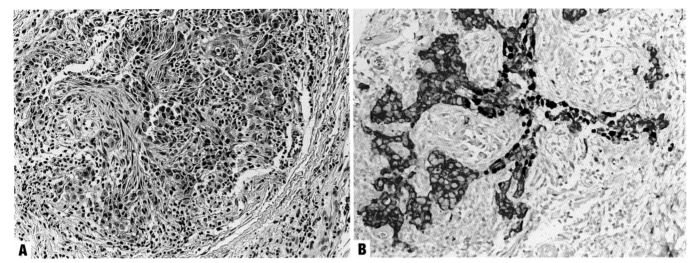

**Fig. 2.106** Microinvasive carcinoma associated with high-grade ductal carcinoma in situ. High-grade ductal carcinoma (**A**), which is identified as microinvasive carcinoma arising from high-grade ductal carcinoma in situ by dual immunostaining (**B**) for cytokeratin (red) and p63 (brown).

## Pathogenesis

The pathogenesis of microinvasive carcinoma is largely unstudied (due to the limited size and low incidence of the lesion), but it is believed to be similar to that of invasive breast carcinoma, of which microinvasive carcinoma is an early manifestation. In addition to tumour-associated factors resulting in the breakdown of the myoepithelial / basement membrane barrier, the inflammatory response may also contribute {1415A}. The molecular pathology of microinvasive carcinoma is unknown and difficult to study. It may reflect the earliest changes related to invasion. On the basis of the different molecular phenotypes seen, microinvasive carcinoma does not appear to have unique biological characteristics {1561}.

## Macroscopic appearance

Microinvasive carcinoma has the gross features of carcinoma in situ. By far the most commonly associated in situ lesion, high-grade DCIS often presents as poorly defined fibrous areas with comedo-type necrosis extruding from the surface on close inspection, but it may be undetectable to the naked eye. The rare examples without identifiable carcinoma in situ also lack macroscopic features.

## Histopathology

Microinvasive carcinoma is the earliest morphologically recognized form of invasive carcinoma with a dominant carcinoma in situ (generally DCIS of high grade, but sometimes also lower-grade DCIS, lobular carcinoma in situ, or Paget disease of the nipple). Microinvasive carcinoma should only be diagnosed when clear evidence of invasion is seen in one focus or several distinctly separate foci, none of which is > 1 mm. Some earlier definitions mandated the presence of invasion into the non-specialized stroma, but this is no longer a requirement. The distinction between intralobular and periductal (specialized) stroma and the non-specialized (interlobular) stroma can generally be made in normal breast histology but becomes less obvious when an inflammatory infiltrate and oedema obscure the boundary. Therefore, invasion in the context of microinvasive disease means invasion beyond the myoepithelium and the basement membrane of the in situ component. Small angulated

clusters of tumour cells (or less commonly, single cells) infiltrate the stroma, which typically demonstrates reactive changes (e.g. mononuclear infiltrate, oedema, and desmoplastic changes).

Whenever suspicion of microinvasion is raised, the examination of deeper levels is indicated, to exclude larger foci of invasion. This may also clarify the contours of the lesion (well-circumscribed, rounded clusters of neoplastic cells are unlikely to represent microinvasion) and help to avoid misdiagnosis of a mimic. The consistency of diagnosing microinvasive carcinoma is less than perfect: in one series, only one fifth of 109 cases in which microinvasion was diagnosed or suspected were actually found to be microinvasive carcinoma on review {1673}. In another series, experts disagreed on a considerable number of the cases, with 100% agreement for only 9 of 50 cases with H&E-stained sections {420}. Because the lesions are small, they may cut out in deeper levels or subsequent immunohistochemistry, which may also affect interobserver reproducibility. Peer review of these cases may be of value. Serial H&E-stained

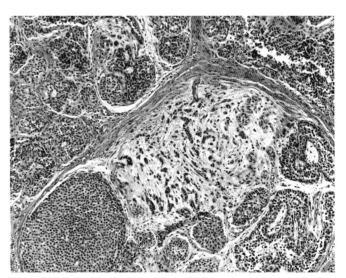

**Fig. 2.107** Microinvasive lobular carcinoma. The central area shows an invasive lobular carcinoma < 1 mm with oedematous stromal reaction; this is surrounded by lobular neoplasia (lobular carcinoma in situ).

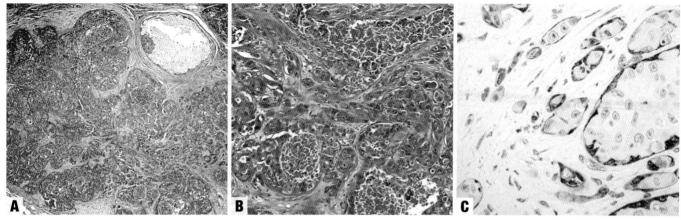

**Fig. 2.108** Ductal carcinoma in situ spreading to sclerosing adenosis. This is a frequent mimic of microinvasion. **A** At low power, the distorted but maintained lobular architecture can be appreciated. **B** At medium power, the small acini involved are suggestive of microinvasion, with the haphazardly oriented tumour cell nests. **C** Immunostaining for calponin (a cytoplasmic myoepithelial marker) reveals attenuated myoepithelium around all tumour cell clusters and nests.

slides are generally of greater value than immunohistochemistry, although the latter may help in both assessment and reproducibility of diagnosis {420}. Immunohistochemistry is generally used to demonstrate the lack of myoepithelium or a basement membrane around the microinvasive carcinoma cells. However, myoepithelial markers may be absent (or virtually absent) in some benign lesions {856,414,1711} or around DCIS {1711,855}, and incomplete basement membranes (identified by laminin or collagen IV immunohistochemistry) may be present around some invasive lesions {416}. Immunohistochemistry with cytokeratins to highlight scant infiltrating neoplastic cells may be of value.

Lesions that are prone to being overdiagnosed as microinvasive carcinoma include involvement of lobules, DCIS involving sclerosing adenosis, entrapment and distortion of epithelium in sclerosing lesions, carcinoma cell displacement by needling procedures (especially from papillary lesions), cautery or crush artefacts, and lymphocytic infiltration around ducts and lobules involved by carcinoma in situ. Of note, tertiary lymphoid structures around DCIS are more commonly found in cases with microinvasion; therefore, a particularly careful assessment for microinvasion is warranted in such instances {1007A}. When microinvasion occurs, it is not uncommonly multifocal {2312}, so searching for further foci of (micro)invasion is recommended. If any invasive focus is > 1 mm, the lesion is designated invasive carcinoma, and the other foci represent satellites or parts of a multifocal cancer.

When there is doubt about the diagnosis of microinvasion, or if the lesion of concern has been cut out of any further sections, it is recommended (in keeping with standardized TNM practice) that the case be diagnosed as an in situ lesion with no evidence of established (micro)invasion. Caution is recommended when considering this diagnosis on core needle samples. Microinvasive carcinomas carry a risk of metastasis: hormone receptor and HER2 status should be considered where possible.

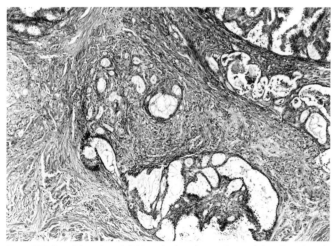

**Fig. 2.109** Pseudoinvasion mimicking microinvasive carcinoma. Sclerosing adenosis adjacent to low-grade cribriform ductal carcinoma in situ and papilloma, mimicking invasion.

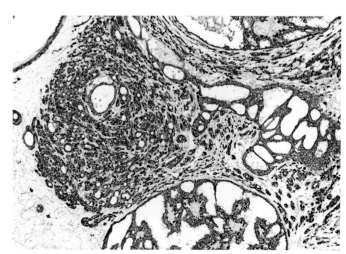

**Fig. 2.110** Pseudoinvasion mimicking microinvasive carcinoma. The presence of myoepithelial cells is clearly highlighted with dual immunostaining for cytokeratin (red) and p63 (brown).

## Cytology
Not clinically relevant

## Diagnostic molecular pathology
Not clinically relevant

## Essential and desirable diagnostic criteria
*Essential:* invasive carcinoma ≤ 1 mm in size; exclusion of the presence of larger foci by deeper sections to avoid underdiagnosis and to exclude non-invasive mimics to avoid overdiagnosis.
*Desirable:* pre-existing lesion, most often carcinoma in situ (usually high-grade ductal).

## Staging
Microinvasive carcinoma is defined as pT1mi, regardless of the number of foci of microinvasion {61,229}. The general rule of rounding tumour size to the closest millimetre does not apply at the boundary of microinvasive carcinoma; i.e. a 1.1 mm carcinoma is classified as invasive disease, pT1a {61}.

## Prognosis and prediction
The rate of nodal involvement associated with microinvasive carcinoma varies in the literature, and it is dependent on whether sentinel node biopsy was performed, whether enhanced histopathology (levels and immunohistochemistry) was applied, and how nodal positivity was defined {417}. A recent meta-analysis of 968 microinvasive carcinomas (without central review) found a sentinel node positivity rate of 3.2% for macrometastasis and 4% for micrometastasis {743}. The prognosis of microinvasive carcinoma is controversial, most likely in part because of differences in diagnosis and incidence. Microinvasive carcinoma has long been believed to be equivalent to DCIS, and some series support this {1012,1185}. Other recent publications suggest that the prognosis is closer to that of very small invasive cancers {1978,616}. There is some evidence that patients with HER2-positive microinvasive disease not receiving anti-HER2 therapy or chemotherapy have a worse outcome {616}. However, the prognosis is very good overall, with 20-year cancer-specific mortality rates of 9.65% for DCIS with microinvasion (vs 4.00% for DCIS) reported in one SEER Program dataset analysis {2219} and 6.9% for microinvasive carcinoma in another {1978}.

# Invasive lobular carcinoma

Shin SJ
Desmedt C
Kristiansen G
Reis-Filho JS
Sasano H

## Definition

Invasive lobular carcinoma (ILC) is an invasive breast carcinoma (IBC) composed of dyscohesive cells that are most often individually dispersed or arranged in a single-file linear pattern.

## ICD-O coding

8520/3 Lobular carcinoma NOS

## ICD-11 coding

2C61.1 & XH2XR3 Invasive lobular carcinoma of breast & Lobular carcinoma NOS

## Related terminology

*Not recommended:* infiltrating lobular carcinoma.

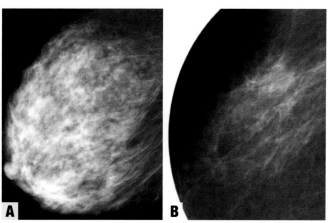

**Fig. 2.111** Invasive lobular carcinoma (mammography). **A** Architectural distortion in the axillary tail, corresponding to a palpable area of thickening. **B** Magnified view of the architectural axillary distortion.

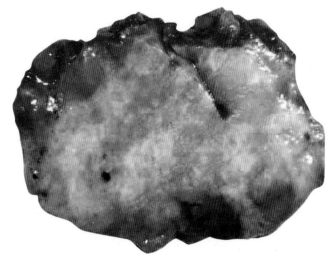

**Fig. 2.112** Invasive lobular carcinoma. Macroscopy displays a poorly defined lesion.

## Subtype(s)

None

## Localization

ILC can affect any part of the breast, although one study found that centrally located tumours were slightly more common in these cases than in IBC of no special type (NST) {2280}. A high rate of multicentric tumours has been reported in some studies {508,1152}, but this has not been found in other series based on clinical {1848} or radiological {1123} analysis. An incidence of contralateral tumours, particularly synchronous tumours, of 5–19% has been reported, which is higher than for IBC-NST {82,235,328,1757,627,1633,1944}.

## Clinical features

Most women present with a poorly defined palpable breast mass. Radiologically, the most common mammographic findings are a spiculated mass and architectural distortion. Tumours may even be subclinical by palpation and mammography/sonography, presenting with metastases. Calcification is infrequent. Mammography has a lower sensitivity for the detection of ILC (57–89%) than IBC-NST, with false negative rates as high as 19% {854,1059,1123}. Ultrasonography is more sensitive (78–95%), although the size of the tumour can be underestimated {258,306,607,1766,1894,2235}. MRI is more helpful in diagnosing ILC, in particular multifocal lesions, but it can lead to false positives and overestimation of tumour size {511,1858}. MRI in the setting of a diagnosis of ILC on core needle biopsy is therefore part of most guidelines {1289}.

## Epidemiology

ILC accounts for 5–15% of all IBCs {574,1167,1174,1848,2091, 2280}. Since the 1980s, the incidence of ILC has increased relative to that of IBC-NST {1167,1168}. This might be attributable to the increased use of hormone replacement therapy {197, 445,1167,1175,1531,1735} or increased consumption of alcohol {1169,1171}. The mean age of patients with ILC is 57–65 years, slightly higher than that of patients with IBC-NST {82,1174,1705, 1848,2091}.

## Etiology

The etiology of ILCs is multifactorial, including likely lifestyle, hormonal, and genetic components. Deleterious germline mutations affecting *CDH1* have been shown to be causative of hereditary diffuse gastric cancer (HDGC) and ILC, and they confer a risk of ILC development as high as 42% {401}.

## Pathogenesis

The vast majority of classic ILCs express ER and PR and lack *ERBB2* (*HER2*) gene amplification/overexpression. As many as 85% are classified as luminal A subtype by gene expression profiling {363,488,2247,776}. Gene expression profiling {2247,

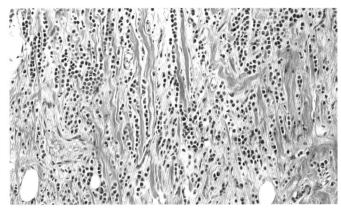

**Fig. 2.113** Invasive lobular carcinoma, classic type. Note the proliferation of discohesive small cells arranged in single-file linear cords invading the stroma. There is often little host reaction or disturbance of the background architecture.

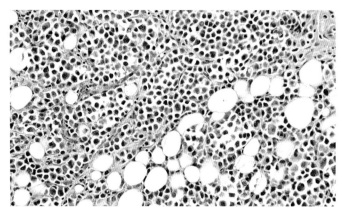

**Fig. 2.114** Invasive lobular carcinoma with solid growth pattern. Note the non-cohesive small cells of lobular morphology growing in sheets.

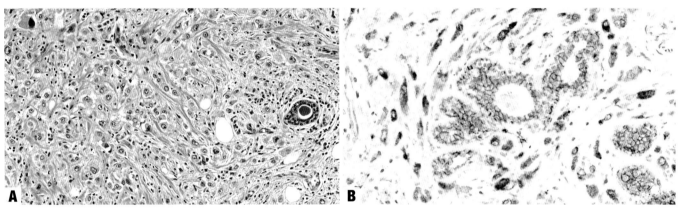

**Fig. 2.115** Invasive lobular carcinoma, pleomorphic type (pleomorphic lobular carcinoma). **A** In pleomorphic lobular carcinoma, cells are pleomorphic with or without apocrine features and a higher mitotic count than classic invasive lobular carcinoma. **B** Immunohistochemistry for p120-catenin showing cytoplasmic staining in the tumour cells.

1505,1625,363} and immunohistochemical studies {924,890, 1607,276} have additionally shown that ILCs can also be classified as luminal B and rarely as ERBB2 (HER2)-enriched or basal-like. Pleomorphic/apocrine ILCs may occasionally lack hormone receptors and overexpress HER2 {1951,2159}.

ILCs display a characteristic pattern of somatic genetic alterations, including gains of 16q and 16p and losses of 16q, which encompass the *CDH1* gene locus on 16q22.1 {694,363, 488,2247,776,1951,2159}. E-cadherin loss of function has now been shown to be causative of the characteristic lack of cohesiveness and invasiveness pattern of lobular carcinoma cells {608,187}. In fact, the vast majority of ILCs harbour deleterious mutations affecting *CDH1*, often coupled with loss of heterozygosity of the wildtype allele {363,488,2247,776}. In a minority of cases lacking *CDH1* mutations, alterations affecting α-catenin and potentially other components of the cadherin-catenin family have been reported {465}; conversely, the role of *CDH1* gene promoter methylation in the loss of E-cadherin expression in ILCs remains a matter of controversy {363,1846,547}.

Although not formally compared with each other, gene expression–based multigene classifiers of recurrence have attributed only a small proportion of ILCs to the high-risk groups {395,2108,154,1359,629,2279}. Distinct subgroups of ILC have

been identified at the gene expression level by clustering analyses, with one labelled as "immune-related" {363,1367}. However, their definition needs to be standardized. In this context, a recent study has demonstrated that ILC presents with lower levels of tumour-infiltrating lymphocytes than ER-positive, HER2-negative IBC-NST, with only 15% of cases showing > 10% of tumour-infiltrating lymphocytes {487}.

Thousands of ILCs have now been sequenced, revealing the mutation landscape of this entity. The most frequently identified somatic genomic alterations are loss of chromosomal arm 16q (seen in nearly all cases), mutations of *CDH1* (in 50–80%), and mutations of *PIK3CA* (in ~45%) {1625,363,1367,488,1507, 1802,509}. Other recurrently mutated genes include *RUNX1*, *TP53*, *TBX3*, *PTEN*, *FOXA1*, *MAP3K1*, *ERBB2* (*HER2*), and *ERBB3* (*HER3*). Compared with luminal A IBC-NSTs, ILCs more frequently harbour somatic mutations of *CDH1*, *PTEN*, *TBX3*, *ERBB2* (*HER2*), *ERBB3* (*HER3*), *ARID1A*, and *FOXA1*, and they less frequently show mutations of *GATA3*, *MAP2K4*, and *CTCF* {363,488}. Tumours with mutations of *AKT1* or *ERBB2* (*HER2*) have been associated with an increased risk of early relapse {488}. Of therapeutic interest, HER2-targeted agents could be used to treat tumours with mutations of *ERBB2* (*HER2*) and

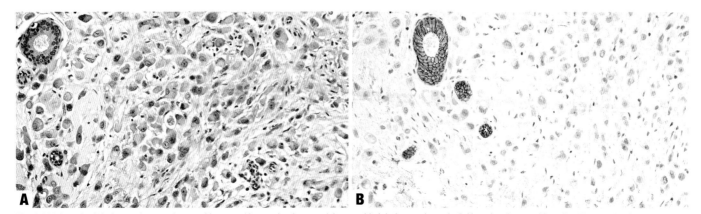

**Fig. 2.116** Invasive lobular carcinoma, pleomorphic type with apocrine features (pleomorphic lobular carcinoma). **A** Note the pleomorphic cells with apocrine features. **B** Immunohistochemistry for E-cadherin showing an absence of membranous staining in tumour cells.

possibly *ERBB3* (*HER3*), most of which lack *ERBB2* (*HER2*) amplification but present a *CDH1* mutation {1258}.

## Macroscopic appearance

ILCs frequently present as irregular and poorly delimited tumours that can be difficult to define macroscopically because of the diffuse growth pattern of the cell infiltrate {1944}. The size of ILC is also difficult to determine, although it has been reported to be slightly larger than that of IBC-NST in some series {1848, 1944,2280}.

## Histopathology

The classic pattern of ILC is characterized by a proliferation of small cells that lack cohesion and appear individually dispersed throughout a fibrous connective tissue or arranged in single-file linear cords that invade the stroma {661,1305,2233}. These infiltrating cords frequently present a concentric pattern around normal ducts. There is often little host reaction or disturbance of the background architecture. The neoplastic cells have round or notched ovoid nuclei and a thin rim of cytoplasm, with an occasional intracytoplasmic lumen {1683}, often harbouring a central mucoid inclusion. Mitoses are typically infrequent. These classic cytological features are the same as those seen in atypical lobular hyperplasia and lobular carcinoma in situ, which is associated with ILC in 58–98% of cases {3,508,521,1488}. Lymphovascular invasion is uncommon. In terms of the tissue

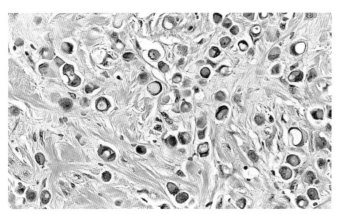

**Fig. 2.117** Invasive lobular carcinoma with signet-ring cell features. Note the tumour cells with signet-ring cell features.

microenvironment, luminal-type ILC has been reported to harbour much higher proliferation of cancer-associated fibroblasts (as defined by α-SMA immunohistochemistry) and a higher degree of tumour neovascularization, but less-mature tumour vessels, compared with luminal-type IBC-NST (after age and grade adjustment) {1445}. Therefore, despite having a gene expression profile similar to that of IBC-NST, ILC demonstrates a different status of tissue microenvironment.

A number of patterns of ILC have been described that share either the cytological pattern or the growth pattern of classic ILC, but all lack cell-to-cell cohesion. The solid pattern is characterized by the typical non-cohesive and small cells of lobular morphology, but these cells grow in sheets and have a higher frequency of mitoses than in the classic type {626}. Cells of the alveolar pattern are mainly arranged in globular aggregates of at least 20 cells {1933}. Pleomorphic lobular carcinoma (PLC) retains the distinctive growth pattern of lobular carcinoma but exhibits a greater degree of pleomorphism (defined as larger cells with marked nuclear pleomorphism, > 4 times the size of lymphocytes / equivalent to that of high-grade ductal carcinoma in situ, with or without apocrine features) {1966} and a higher mitotic count than classic ILC {603,1369,2243,1717}. This pattern is frequently associated with lobular carcinoma in situ showing the same pleomorphic cytological features. PLC may show apocrine {603} or histiocytoid {2207} differentiation and may be composed of signet-ring cells. The tubulolobular pattern is composed of the admixture of a tubular growth pattern and small uniform cells arranged in a linear pattern {647}. Lobular carcinoma in situ is observed in about one third of tubulolobular carcinomas. ILC with histiocytoid morphology can also be cytologically bland, and it can therefore be confused with histiocytes or (if additionally apocrine-appearing) with granular cell tumour {2037}.

A mixed group is composed of cases showing an admixture of the classic type with one or more of these patterns {521}. The classic ILC type and mixed patterns contribute to the majority of lobular tumours, accounting for as many as 75% of all cases {1560,1704}. In addition, both IBC-NST and lobular features of differentiation are present in about 5% of IBCs (called invasive ductulolobular carcinomas) {1174,1305}, and although these components are morphologically distinct, a recent study has shown that they arise from a common ancestor {1329}.

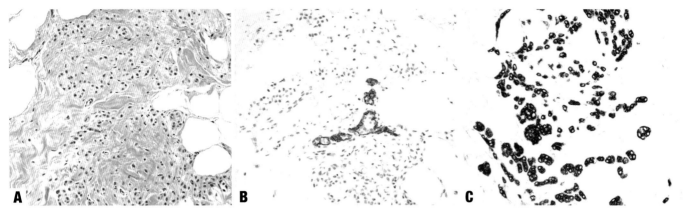

**Fig. 2.118** Histiocytoid invasive lobular carcinoma. **A** Invasive tumour cells have abundant pale eosinophilic cytoplasm, resembling histiocytes with low- to intermediate-grade nuclei. **B** The lobular subtype of this invasive breast carcinoma is confirmed by the lack of E-cadherin protein expression. **C** Cytokeratin AE1/AE3 immunohistochemical staining confirms its epithelial phenotype.

Although the literature suggests that 80–95% of ILCs are positive for ER, in current practice classic ILCs are almost invariably ER-positive. In comparison, 70–80% of IBC-NSTs are ER-positive. PR positivity is found in 60–70% of both tumour types {82,1705,1848,2339}. ER was found to be expressed in the classic form and in patterns, with the rate of positivity being highest (100%) in the alveolar pattern {1933} and lowest (10%) in PLC {1689}. *ERBB2* (*HER2*) amplification and overexpression are rare in ILC {82,1667,1705,1808,1977}, although evident in some PLCs {1369,1951}.

One of the most consistent molecular alterations in ILC and its patterns is the loss of expression of the cell–cell adhesion molecule E-cadherin, which contributes to the characteristic dyscohesive nature of lobular cells due to the disruption of the adherens complex {466,694,1399,1544,1582,1712,1726,1951}. Altered adherens complex integrity may also be due to loss of other components, such as α-catenin, β-catenin, and γ-catenin, resulting in mislocalization of p120-catenin from the cell membrane to the cytoplasm {430,1712,1847}. Analysis of the expression of E-cadherin, α-catenin, β-catenin, and p120 may help to differentiate between lobular and low-grade IBC-NSTs that are difficult to classify on the basis of morphological criteria; however, about 15% of ILCs (and most ductulolobular cancers) do express E-cadherin, so positive staining should not be used to reclassify a lobular lesion as IBC-NST {9,429,1712,581}. Inversely, tumours with NST morphology may also show loss of E-cadherin expression. The expression of p53, basal markers (CK14, CK5/6, and EGFR [HER1]), and myoepithelial markers (SMA and p63) is rare in ILC {529,611,1705}. Proliferation, measured by MIB1/Ki-67 labelling, is generally low in ILC, although higher in other morphological patterns {1510,1560}.

## Cytology

The cytomorphological features of classic ILC on FNA specimens include low cellularity, mild discohesiveness, small nuclear size, indistinct nucleoli, and mild pleomorphism, as well as the absence of apocrine change, signet-ring cell morphology, necrosis, and mitoses. In contrast, PLC is characterized by greater cellularity, nuclear pleomorphism, and hyperchromasia; prominent nucleoli; and high mitotic activity, more resembling cancers of no special type {2243,432,94,1536}.

## Diagnostic molecular pathology

Not clinically relevant

## Essential and desirable diagnostic criteria

*Classic ILC*

*Essential:* an IBC composed of dispersed or linear dyscohesive cells with low- to intermediate-nuclear-grade morphology and a low mitotic count; ER immunoreactivity is high and HER2 is negative/non-amplified.

*Desirable:* coexisting lobular neoplasia; E-cadherin loss may be useful.

*Pleomorphic ILC*

*Essential:* intermediate-high or high nuclear grade/pleomorphism.

## Staging

There are no discordances in the staging of ILC between the current (eighth) editions of the Union for International Cancer Control (UICC) TNM classification {229} and the American Joint Committee on Cancer (AJCC) cancer staging manual {61,418}.

## Prognosis and prediction

Despite the favourable prognostic features of ILC (i.e. low grade, ER positivity, HER2 negativity, and low proliferation), there remains controversy as to whether the outcome differs between patients with ILC and those with IBC-NST {351}. Several studies have reported a more favourable outcome for ILC than IBC-NST {521,548,574,1944,2091}, but others have found no significant differences {82,1040,1401,1705,2174,2186,1621, 1082} or a worse prognosis for ILC {1705,86,1633,1041}. In large series, ILCs were more likely to be of larger size (> 5 cm) and more advanced tumour stage (stage III/IV), with more lymph node positivity than IBC-NST, and they tended to occur in older patients {82,1082,1174,1229}. An important observation made in two series is that patients with ILC have an outcome better than or similar to that of patients with IBC-NST in the first 10 years after diagnosis; however, the long-term outcome associated with ILC is worse than that associated with IBC-NST {1705, 1633}. The events that show higher incidences (distant metastases, recurrences, and mortality) in ILC are long-term events after diagnosis. When the histological patterns of ILC were analysed separately, a more favourable outcome was reported for the classic type than for defined histological patterns (namely, pleomorphic and solid) {521,548,244,508,603,1560, 2243,1818}. However, tubulolobular carcinoma and alveolar ILC have been considered to be low-grade tumours {763,1933}. This correlates to the molecular subtypes of breast cancer, with classic ILCs being predominantly luminal A tumours {924}.

Most studies suggest that grade is an independent predictor of patient outcome in ILC {113,1398,1626,1704}. Most classic ILCs (~76%) are grade 2, whereas grade 3 ILCs are mostly of non-classic type {1560,2024}. Of the three components of tumour grading, mitotic count is the most useful predictor of outcome; a high mitotic count is associated with a worse prognosis {1704}. Some authors suggest that grade 2 in ILC is comparable prognostically to grade 3 IBC-NST {590}. An exploratory analysis of Ki-67 proliferation index cut-off values concluded that for ILC, a lower cut-off point (4%) better prognosticated disease progression than the 15% cut-off point used for IBC-NST {283}.

After neoadjuvant chemotherapy, lower rates of pathological complete response have been observed for ILC than for IBC-NST {2190,1637}, possibly favouring neoadjuvant hormone therapy. However, this relative resistance to cytotoxic therapy may be more related to the molecular characteristics (and especially the lower proliferation) of ILC rather than the histological pattern per se {1209}.

The metastatic pattern of ILC differs from that of IBC-NST. A lower frequency of axillary nodal metastasis in ILC than in IBC-NST has been reported, with the difference ranging from 3% to 10% {1944,2091,932,1108,1848}. Metastases of classic ILC in lymph nodes may be inconspicuous, and even an impressive number of single cells distributed in a buckshot pattern may be missed on H&E staining alone; therefore, cytokeratin immunohistochemistry increases diagnostic accuracy {1612}. A higher frequency of metastases to the bone, skin, gastrointestinal tract, uterus, meninges, and ovary, as well as of diffuse serosal involvement, is observed in ILC, whereas extension to the lung is more frequent in IBC-NST {1944,2091,82,1041,932, 1108,1848,1612,201,632,825,919}.

Immunohistochemistry using antibodies to GCDFP-15, GATA3, CK7, ER, PR, E-cadherin, and p120-catenin may help to establish an intra-abdominal tumour as a metastatic ILC {430, 1163,2263}. Concomitant expression profiling revealed three ILC molecular patterns (reactive-like, immune-related, and proliferative) with prognostic relevance; however, these patterns showed a marked lack of correlation with the widely accepted molecular subtypes of breast cancer.

Several prognostic multigene expression assays have been validated for breast cancer, but their clinical value specifically for ILC is still under investigation, because these tumours may differ in their expression profiles from IBC-NSTs. With most assays, ILCs are predominantly classified as low-risk tumours {629,395,2108,193,1025,154,2210,1505}. Some authors therefore discourage the use of genomic/transcriptional prognostic testing for ILC because of the generally good prognosis of ILC and alternatively suggest the more economical conventional immunohistochemical classification {2108,2279,880}.

# Tubular carcinoma

van Deurzen CHM
Denkert C
Purdie CA

## Definition
Tubular carcinoma (TC) is a low-grade invasive carcinoma composed of well-formed tubules with open lumina lined by a single layer of neoplastic cells.

## ICD-O coding
8211/3 Tubular carcinoma

## ICD-11 coding
2C60 & XH4TA4 Carcinoma of breast, specialized type & Tubular adenocarcinoma

## Related terminology
None

## Subtype(s)
None

## Localization
There are no specific features.

## Clinical features
There are no specific clinical features distinguishing TCs from other types of breast cancer. Nonetheless, TCs are more likely to occur in older patients and tend to be small in size {67,1708}. Most TCs are detected incidentally by mammographic screening {1708}. Mammographically, TCs may form a discrete mass, but they are most often detected as small spiculated lesions; calcifications are variably present {786,1921,2342}. On ultrasonography, TC usually appears as a hypoechoic mass with poorly defined margins and posterior acoustic shadowing {786, 1921,2342}. MRI data are limited for TCs, but these tumours have been reported as hyperintense, with or without a dark internal septation-like appearance on T2-weighted images {2323}. Approximately 10–20% of TCs are reported to be multifocal {763,1387}.

## Epidemiology
TC accounts for about 1.6% of invasive breast carcinomas (IBCs) {67,1327,501}. It is a disease of postmenopausal women (67%) {1708}, with a median patient age at presentation of 63 years; only about 17% of patients with TC are < 50 years old {67,1327,501}. In the USA, the incidence is slightly higher among white women than among black women {67}.

## Etiology
See *Invasive breast carcinoma: General overview* (p. 82).

## Pathogenesis
Gene expression profiling studies demonstrated that TC belongs to the luminal A molecular class of breast cancer {2249}, which provides a biological basis for the excellent clinical outcome.

TCs are typically positive for hormone receptors, and *ERBB2* (*HER2*) is not amplified {1524}. They also have a low frequency of genomic alterations. Loss-of-heterozygosity and comparative genomic hybridization techniques have demonstrated that the most frequent alterations detected in TC affect 16q (loss; 78–86%) and 1q (gain; 50–62%), and these usually occur concurrently. Other alterations include 16p gain, as well as loss of 8p, 3p (the *FHIT* gene locus), and 11q (the *ATM* gene locus) {95, 1285,1762,2206}. Although these chromosomal alterations are common among other low-grade breast cancers (i.e. low-grade IBC of no special type [NST] and invasive lobular carcinoma), small yet important differences have been detected at the transcriptome level {1238}.

## Macroscopic appearance
TCs are characteristically poorly defined spiculated tumours that are firm to hard in consistency and pale grey in colour. Most TCs are small, with a mean diameter of 12 mm {67,1327}. Approximately 14% of TCs are > 20 mm {501,1708}.

## Histopathology
The diagnosis of TC requires that > 90% of the tumour be composed of tubules and glands lined by a single layer of neoplastic epithelium. Tumours with 10–90% TC are classified as mixed tumours.

At low power, TC has a stellate outline and invades the adjacent normal breast parenchyma. TC is composed of small, round to ovoid or angular glands and tubules with open lumina set within a fibrous or fibroelastotic desmoplastic stroma. The cuboidal to columnar cells that line the neoplastic tubules in a single layer have relatively uniform nuclei of small or intermediate size. Apical snouts may be seen on the luminal aspect of the tubules, and secretions or calcifications may be present in the

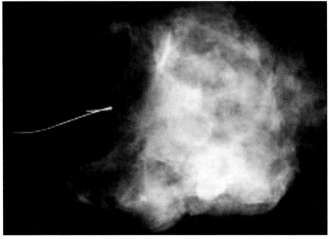

**Fig. 2.119** Tubular carcinoma. Specimen X-ray.

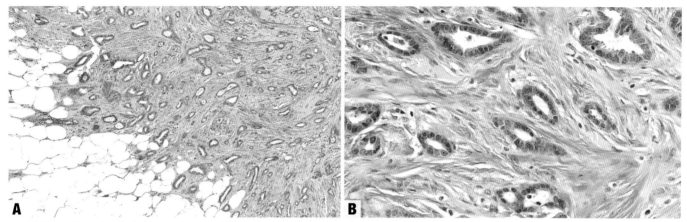

**Fig. 2.120** Tubular carcinoma. **A** There is a haphazard distribution of rounded and angulated tubules with open lumina, lined by a single layer of epithelial cells separated by abundant reactive, fibroblastic stroma. **B** The neoplastic cells lining the teardrop-shaped tubules lack substantial atypia.

lumina. TCs are by definition grade 1 carcinomas; if Nottingham grading suggests otherwise, the diagnosis of TC is precluded. Substantial cytological atypia, multilayering, or high mitotic activity excludes the diagnosis of TC.

The tubules in TC have no surrounding myoepithelium, and this is useful in differentiating them from benign conditions such as sclerosing adenosis and radial scar. In these benign conditions, the tubular structures are surrounded by myoepithelium, which can be readily demonstrated by immunohistochemistry for myoepithelial markers such as p63, SMMHC, and high-molecular-weight cytokeratins.

TC may be accompanied by precursor lesions; in a study of 147 tumours and precursor lesions, 95% of pure TCs had associated columnar cell lesions, in particular flat epithelial atypia. Atypical ductal hyperplasia / ductal carcinoma in situ was present in 89% of patients. Colocalization of columnar cell lesions, atypical ductal hyperplasia / ductal carcinoma in situ, and TC was seen in 85% patients with a similar cytological-nuclear morphology in most cases {3}. This suggests that a TC might be the result of a multistep process that starts on the level of a flat epithelial atypia.

TC is diffusely and strongly ER-positive and usually also PR-positive. TC is ERBB2 (HER2)-negative {1708}, and the diagnosis of TC should be reconsidered if a tumour is HER2-positive {2284}. The cells composing TC have a luminal phenotype (CK8/18-positive, CK5/14-negative) and a low Ki-67 proliferation index (typically < 10%). They are usually positive for E-cadherin but negative for EGFR (HER1), p53, p63, and P-cadherin. Expression of high-molecular-weight cytokeratins and/or ER negativity (especially in small diagnostic biopsies) should raise the possibility of a basal-phenotype carcinoma with tubule formation, such as adenoid cystic carcinoma or low-grade adenosquamous carcinoma. Gene expression profiling places TC into the luminal A group (ER-positive, HER2-negative, low proliferation) {2249}.

## Cytology

The cytological diagnosis of TC on FNA is problematic. FNA of TC usually yields small tubules and irregular glands lined by relatively bland and uniform epithelial cells in the absence of myoepithelial cells. Although features of malignancy (nuclear atypia, cellular dissociation, and absence of myoepithelial cells) are usually present, the findings are subtle and a definitive diagnosis of malignancy is rendered in only about 50% of cases, even in the hands of experts {195,1103,477}. Core needle biopsy is a more reliable method of preoperative diagnosis.

## Diagnostic molecular pathology

Not clinically relevant

## Essential and desirable diagnostic criteria

*Essential:* an IBC with > 90% of the tumour consisting of round to ovoid or angular tubules with open lumina, lined by a single layer of epithelial cells with low-grade nuclei and sparse mitosis (grade 1); ER-positive and HER2-negative.

## Staging

Most TCs present at a relatively early stage. Approximately 86% are T1 tumours and 85% are N0 at presentation {501,1708}. TCs are staged similarly to other types of IBCs (see *Invasive breast carcinoma: General overview*, p. 82).

## Prognosis and prediction

In large institutional series {501} and cancer registry–based studies {1240,1173,144}, women with TC had an excellent long-term outcome, with reported 5-year survival rates of 88% (overall survival) {501} to 96% (relative survival) {144}. This is supported by many retrospective cohort studies {937,1333,1634, 2185,347,628,1708,1213}. It has been shown that the prognosis of TC is better than that of grade 1 invasive ductal carcinoma {1708} and that patients' long-term outcome is similar to that of age-matched women without breast cancer {501,1240}. Recurrence after complete excision is rare. In some cohorts, axillary involvement was not associated with worse prognosis {501}. Given the consistently observed excellent prognosis, it has been suggested that adjuvant systemic therapy or axillary dissection {1708,501,967,1596,628} may not be justified for the routine management of TC.

# Cribriform carcinoma

van Deurzen CHM
Denkert C
Purdie CA

## Definition
Cribriform carcinoma is a low-grade invasive carcinoma composed of islands of tumour cells with well-defined cribriform spaces.

## ICD-O coding
8201/3 Cribriform carcinoma NOS

## ICD-11 coding
2C60 & XH1YZ3 Carcinoma of breast, specialized type & Cribriform carcinoma NOS

## Related terminology
None

## Subtype(s)
None

## Localization
There are no specific features.

## Clinical features
No specific clinical feature distinguishes invasive cribriform carcinoma (ICC) from other types of breast cancer. ICC may present as a mass, but it is frequently clinically occult. On mammography, ICC typically forms a spiculated mass, and it may harbour microcalcifications {2001}. Multifocality is observed in 10–20% of cases {1307,1573}.

## Epidemiology
Pure ICC is rare, accounting for approximately 0.4% of all invasive breast carcinomas {1573,1240,1221}. The median patient age at presentation is 63 years, and only 25% of patients are aged < 50 years {1240,1221}.

## Etiology
See *Invasive breast carcinoma: General overview* (p. 82).

## Pathogenesis
ICC has genomic and transcriptomic features similar to those of tubular carcinoma (both belong to the luminal A molecular class), with a similar immunophenotype (consistent expression of hormone receptors and lack of ERBB2 [HER2] overexpression), and both are associated with the same family of low-grade precursor lesions {2249}.

## Macroscopic appearance
No specific macroscopic features differentiate ICC from invasive (ductal) carcinoma of no special type (NST). ICC usually consists of a firm/hard spiculated mass, with a mean size of 31 mm {1573}. ICCs as large as 20 cm have been described {1307}.

## Histopathology
ICC consists of invasive epithelial islands containing well-defined, rounded spaces similar in appearance to cribriform-type ("cribriform" meaning "sieve-like" or "perforated") ductal carcinoma in situ (DCIS). The islands have an ovoid or angular outline and are set within a desmoplastic stroma. They comprise multilayered epithelial cells of small to intermediate size forming secondary glandular structures lined by cuboidal to columnar cells. Apical secretions are sometimes present and the spaces may contain mucinous secretions with or without calcification {1573,1934,2259}. Mitotic activity is sparse and there is no substantial nuclear atypia. If strict grading criteria

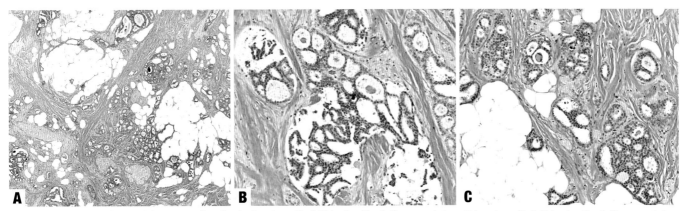

**Fig. 2.121** Cribriform carcinoma. **A** Low-power view showing invasive epithelial islands with cribriform morphology. **B** Invasive epithelial islands with cribriform morphology have an ovoid or angular outline and are set within a desmoplastic stroma. **C** Invasive epithelial islands containing well-defined, rounded spaces, similar in appearance to cribriform-type ductal carcinoma in situ. The islands comprise multilayered epithelial cells of small to intermediate size forming secondary glandular structures lined by cuboidal to columnar cells. Apical secretions are sometimes present, and the spaces may contain mucinous secretions with or without calcification. Mitotic activity is sparse and there is no substantial nuclear atypia.

are applied, ICCs should be Nottingham grade 1 tumours (with cribriform pattern given a score of 1 for tubule formation) {1714}. Stromal osteoclast-like giant cells have been described {1490}. Low- or intermediate-grade DCIS, usually with cribriform architecture, is present in 80% of cases {1573}.

Immunohistochemistry for myoepithelial markers may be used to distinguish ICC from cribriform DCIS. ICCs are typically ER-positive (95–100%) and PR-positive (69–89%) {1221,2161}. Furthermore, they are HER2-negative (94%) and form part of the low-grade breast neoplasia pathway {1221,2248}.

## Cytology
The diagnosis of ICC on FNA is problematic. Direct smears show relatively cohesive sheets and 3D clusters of somewhat bland epithelial cells. The groups of cells show a cribriform pattern. Naked bipolar nuclei and myoepithelial cells are absent {1490}. A definitive diagnosis of ICC is rarely (if ever) possible on FNA, and the differentiation from cribriform-type DCIS is not possible by cytology alone. For this reason, core needle biopsy is the preferred method of preoperative diagnosis.

## Diagnostic molecular pathology
Not clinically relevant

## Essential and desirable diagnostic criteria
*Essential:* an invasive breast carcinoma with > 90% of the tumour composed of cribriform islands of epithelial cells with low-grade nuclei and sparse mitosis (grade 1); ER-positive and HER2-negative.

## Staging
Generally, ICC presents at a relatively early stage, with 76% being T1 and 83% N0 at presentation {1221,2161}.

## Prognosis and prediction
As is seen with tubular carcinoma, the outcome for patients with ICC is favourable {1573,2161}; 10-year overall survival rates are between 90% and 100% {1573}. The outcome for patients with mixed ICC is less favourable than for patients with the pure form, but better than for patients with invasive breast carcinoma NST {1573}. The biological behaviour of ICC is similar to that of tubular carcinoma {1573}; however, many tumours have no tubular component, and the definition of ICC as a distinct clinicopathological entity appears to be justified.

# Mucinous carcinoma

Wen HY
Desmedt C
Reis-Filho JS
Schmitt F

### Definition
Mucinous carcinoma (MC) of the breast is an invasive breast carcinoma (IBC) characterized by clusters of epithelial tumour cells suspended in pools of extracellular mucin.

### ICD-O coding
8480/3 Mucinous adenocarcinoma

### ICD-11 coding
2C60 & XH1S75 Carcinoma of breast, specialized type & Mucinous carcinoma

### Related terminology
*Acceptable:* colloid carcinoma; mucinoid carcinoma; gelatinous carcinoma; mucoid carcinoma; mucinous adenocarcinoma; carcinoma with mucin production.

### Subtype(s)
None

### Localization
The localization of MC is similar to that of other types of breast carcinoma.

### Clinical features
MC appears mammographically as a well-circumscribed or lobulated mass, and it may mimic a benign process. Sonographically, most tumours are hypoechoic {1214}. MRI reveals a persistent enhancement pattern and hyperintensity on T2-weighted images {2326}.

### Epidemiology
MC accounts for approximately 2% of all breast carcinomas {517,1729,1884,1521}. It often occurs in older women {517,125}, with a median patient age of 71 years {517,501}.

### Etiology
See *Invasive breast carcinoma: General overview* (p. 82).

### Pathogenesis
MCs are of the luminal A molecular subtype {2249}, and they are transcriptionally distinct from grade- and molecular subtype–matched IBCs of no special type (NST) {2246}. The transcriptomic features of type A MC differ from those of type B MC, with the latter showing a pattern of gene expression that is similar to that of neuroendocrine carcinomas (NECs) {2246}. Pure MCs show a low level of genetic instability, less frequently harbour concurrent 1p gains and 16q losses and somatic mutations of *PIK3CA* and *AKT1* (hallmark genomic alterations of low-grade ER-positive IBC-NSTs) {1091,988,259,1602,1494}, and exhibit aberrant DNA methylation of *MUC2* {1494}. The different morphological components of mixed MCs are clonal and

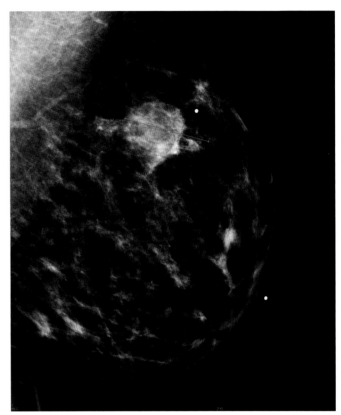

**Fig. 2.122** Mucinous carcinoma. Mammography demonstrates an irregularly shaped high-density mass associated with fine pleomorphic microcalcifications.

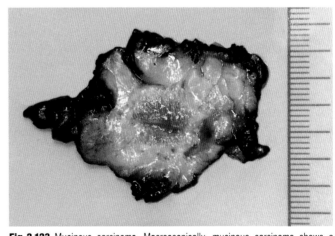

**Fig. 2.123** Mucinous carcinoma. Macroscopically, mucinous carcinoma shows a gelatinous cut surface.

display genomic profiles remarkably similar to those of pure MCs {1091}. Microsatellite instability, a common feature of colorectal MC, is exceedingly uncommon in mammary MC {1090}.

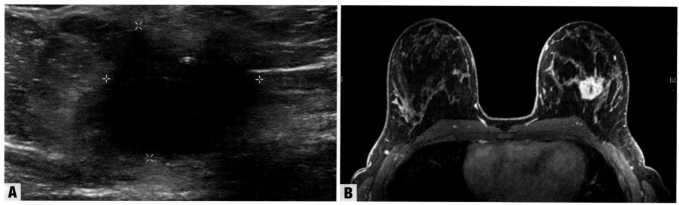

**Fig. 2.124** Mucinous carcinoma. **A** Ultrasonography shows an irregularly shaped hypoechoic mass, with angular margins. **B** MRI demonstrates an irregularly shaped heterogeneously enhancing spiculated mass.

## Macroscopic appearance

Gross examination shows a glistening and gelatinous nodule with pushing margins and a soft, viscous consistency. The tumour size ranges from < 1 cm to > 20 cm {517,125}.

## Histopathology

MC consists of clusters or sheets of neoplastic cells suspended in abundant extracellular mucin, partitioned by delicate fibrous septa containing capillary blood vessels. The tumour clusters vary in size and shape. Nuclear grade is low or intermediate. Tumours with high nuclear grade have been described {2042}, but they are best classified as IBC-NST with mucin production. As described by Capella et al. {280}, type A MCs are relatively hypocellular, with a large amount of extracellular mucin, whereas type B MCs tend to be hypercellular and consist of large epithelial clumps or sheets that often show neuroendocrine differentiation {280}. Pure MC requires a mucinous component of > 90%; mixed MC has 10–90%. A mucinous component of < 10% should be mentioned.

Occasionally, pure MCs may have foci with a micropapillary pattern consisting of morula-like clusters suspended in tight mucin pools, reminiscent of invasive micropapillary carcinoma {1491,1721,117,1212,109}. They usually exhibit more nuclear atypia than conventional MCs, and they may have hobnail cells; psammomatous calcifications may be present {1491,117}. Compared with conventional pure MC, MC with micropapillary

pattern tends to occur at a younger age and has more-frequent lymphovascular invasion and lymph node metastasis {1721, 117,1212}. One group reported significantly worse outcome for MC with > 50% micropapillary pattern compared with pure MC {1212}, but another group found no differences, although the case series was smaller {2305}.

Invasive lobular carcinoma (ILC) with abundant extracellular mucin has been described {1783,2334,807,124,749,419, 212,1953}. A non-mucinous ILC component was present in all cases. It is unknown whether these tumours represent a subtype of ILC or MC.

Carcinoma with signet-ring cell differentiation consists of cells with abundant intracellular mucin that pushes the nucleus aside, creating the characteristic signet-ring cytomorphology. Carcinomas with signet-ring cells without extracellular mucin are not classified as MCs. Signet-ring cytomorphology is most common in ILC but may also be present in IBC-NST and rarely in other special histological subtypes. Therefore, carcinomas with signet-ring cell differentiation do not represent a distinct entity, and no specific clinical or molecular features have been described. Primary carcinomas of the breast with signet-ring cell differentiation must be distinguished from metastases to the breast of signet-ring cell carcinomas from other organs, in particular from the gastrointestinal tract.

The differential diagnosis of MC includes non-neoplastic mucocoele-like lesions (MLLs) with stromal mucin and may be

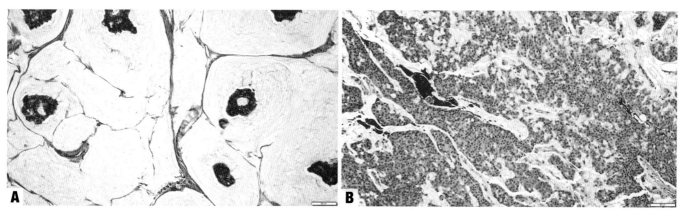

**Fig. 2.125** Mucinous carcinoma. **A** Type A mucinous carcinoma is hypocellular, with sparse clusters of tumour cells in large pools of extracellular mucin. **B** Type B mucinous carcinoma is usually hypercellular, with large sheets of tumour cells and a relatively less conspicuous amount of extracellular mucin.

challenging {2042}, especially in core biopsy material {137,564, 2042}. The absence of cytological atypia in the epithelium lining the mucin-filled ducts and the presence of myoepithelial cells adherent to the detached epithelial strips present in the mucin pools favour a non-atypical MLL over MC {2042}. The upgrade rate at excision of radiology–pathology–concordant non-atypical MLLs in a core biopsy targeting calcifications is < 3% {137, 564,797,1715,2011}. Some MLLs are associated with atypical ductal hyperplasia, ductal carcinoma in situ, or MC {811,2239, 1339,2348}; however, MLLs without atypia do not significantly increase the risk of subsequent carcinoma {1339,2348}.

MC is usually positive for ER and PR {517,125,501}, and it is positive for AR in 80% of cases {388}. ERBB2 (HER2) overexpression and/or amplification is rare in MC but is found in > 10% of MCs with micropapillary pattern {117,1212}. Pure and mixed MCs express WT1 {532,1091} and GATA3 {2263}.

## Cytology
The cytological findings include 3D epithelial clusters and single cells of small to medium size, with mild to moderate nuclear atypia and occasional intracytoplasmic vacuoles, suspended within abundant extracellular mucin containing few branching capillary vessels {2163,939,1118}.

## Diagnostic molecular pathology
Not clinically relevant

## Essential and desirable diagnostic criteria
*Essential:* Pure MC is characterized by a > 90% mucinous component, with clusters of epithelial tumour cells of low to intermediate nuclear grade, suspended in pools of extracellular mucin; usually ER/PR-positive; HER2-negative.

## Staging
MCs are staged similarly to other types of IBCs (see *Invasive breast carcinoma: General overview*, p. 82).

## Prognosis and prediction
Pure MC is generally associated with low rates of local and distant recurrence and excellent 5-year disease-free survival {517,125,501,1240}. Late distant metastases may develop {1729, 2090}. In a retrospective analysis of 11 422 pure MCs in the SEER Program database {517}, the breast cancer–specific survival rates at 5, 10, 15, and 20 years were 94%, 89%, 85%, and 81%, respectively. There is no prognostic difference between type A and type B MCs {1884,1728}. In one retrospective series, MCs with a > 50% micropapillary component had significantly worse prognosis {1212}. Mixed MCs do not have the same favourable prognosis as pure MCs {1037,1728,1520}. Most pure MCs have a low or intermediate recurrence score (RS) by the 21-gene assay. In a series of 33 pure MCs from a single institution, the median RS was 13 (range: 3–28) {2120}, and all but one

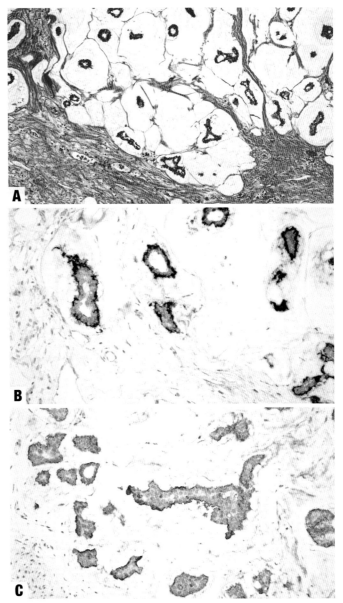

**Fig. 2.126** Mucinous carcinoma with micropapillary features. **A** The carcinoma is composed of tight morule-like epithelial clusters and ring-like structures suspended in abundant extracellular mucin parcelled by delicate fibrous bands. **B,C** EMA (MUC1) decorates the stroma-facing aspect of the cell membrane, indicating reversal of cell polarity.

case had an RS of < 25 {2120}. In a retrospective analysis of the 21-gene assay central database, 90.6% of 16 116 carcinomas classified as mucinous had an RS of ≤ 25, with a mean score of 15 {2021}.

# Mucinous cystadenocarcinoma

Wen HY
Desmedt C
Reis-Filho JS
Schmitt F

## Definition

Mucinous cystadenocarcinoma of the breast is an invasive breast carcinoma characterized by cystic structures lined by tall columnar cells with abundant intracytoplasmic mucin, resembling pancreatobiliary or ovarian mucinous cystadenocarcinoma.

## ICD-O coding

8470/3 Mucinous cystadenocarcinoma NOS

## ICD-11 coding

2C60 & XH1390 Carcinoma of breast, specialized type & Mucinous cystadenocarcinoma

## Related terminology

None

## Subtype(s)

None

## Localization

Not applicable

## Clinical features

Patients usually present with a palpable mass of 0.8–19 cm, with a median tumour size of 3 cm {1034,1052,1473}.

## Epidemiology

Fewer than 30 cases of this exceptionally rare subtype have been reported in the English-language literature (as of May 2018). Most of the reported cases affected Asian women. The tumour typically occurs in postmenopausal women, with a median patient age of 61 years (range: 41–96 years) {1034, 1052,1473}.

## Etiology

Unknown

## Pathogenesis

Unknown

## Macroscopic appearance

Mucinous cystadenocarcinoma is a well-circumscribed solid and cystic mass. The cystic spaces usually contain gelatinous material {1034}.

## Histopathology

Mucinous cystadenocarcinoma is characterized by cystic spaces lined by tall columnar cells with stratification, tufting, and papillary formations {1034}. The neoplastic cells have basally located nuclei and contain abundant intracytoplasmic mucin {1034}. Mucin is also present within the cystic spaces. The degree of cytological atypia is variable, even within the same tumour. The cystic structures have a rounded contour but lack myoepithelial cells at the periphery {1034}. Ductal carcinoma in situ (DCIS) may be present in the adjacent mammary ducts and lobules.

Mucinous cystadenocarcinoma should be differentiated from pure mucinous carcinoma (see *Mucinous carcinoma*, p. 123) and encapsulated papillary carcinoma (see *Encapsulated papillary carcinoma*, p. 60), both of which are typically strongly and diffusely positive for ER and PR. Encapsulated papillary carcinoma also lacks intracytoplasmic mucin. In the absence of DCIS, the possibility of metastatic mucinous cystadenocarcinoma of pancreatobiliary origin must be excluded.

Most mucinous cystadenocarcinomas of the breast are negative for ER, PR, and ERBB2 (HER2) {1034,1473}. Rare HER2-positive cases have been reported {1636,1071,1902}. Some tumours express CK5/6 and EGFR (HER1) {1052,1183,481}.

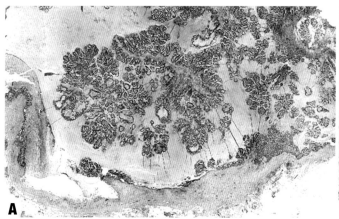
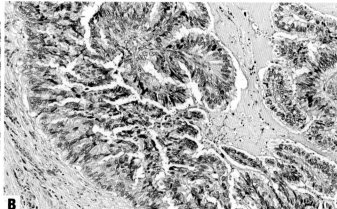

**Fig. 2.127** Mucinous cystadenocarcinoma. **A** Low-power view shows cystic tumour with intracystic papillary structures. **B** The cystic spaces and papillary structures are lined by tall columnar neoplastic cells with abundant intracytoplasmic mucin.

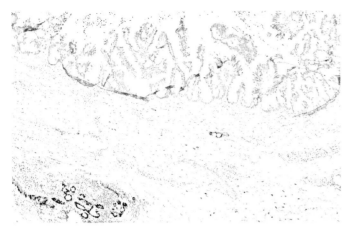

**Fig. 2.128** Mucinous cystadenocarcinoma. The internal control is positive. The mucinous cystadenocarcinoma cells do not express ER.

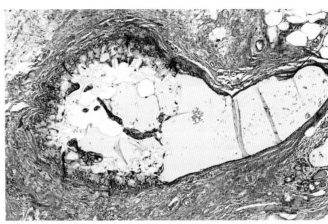

**Fig. 2.129** Ductal carcinoma in situ near a mucinous cystadenocarcinoma. Low-power view of a mammary duct partially involved by ductal carcinoma in situ (left half) in a case of mucinous cystadenocarcinoma. Focal benign breast parenchyma is also present (lower right corner).

Mucinous cystadenocarcinoma primary in the breast is CK7-positive but negative for CK20 and CDX2; these findings may help to distinguish it in particular from metastatic pancreatobiliary mucinous cystadenocarcinoma, which may also be CK7-positive but usually expresses CK20 and CDX2.

## Cytology
There are only a few descriptions of the cytological findings of this rare tumour subtype. Abundant extracellular mucin is usually present (like in cytological preparations of pure mucinous carcinoma), but the neoplastic cells within the mucin have a columnar shape and tend to be more atypical than in pure mucinous carcinoma, with coarse chromatin and prominent nucleoli; necrotic debris is also often present in the background {1017, 1900}.

## Diagnostic molecular pathology
Not clinically relevant

## Essential and desirable diagnostic criteria
*Essential:* invasive breast carcinoma with large cystic spaces containing mucin and lined by atypical columnar cells with intracytoplasmic mucin.
*Desirable:* ER-negative and PR-negative (typically); adjacent DCIS.

## Staging
Staging is based on the eighth edition of the Union for International Cancer Control (UICC) TNM classification {229} for invasive breast carcinoma.

## Prognosis and prediction
Axillary lymph node involvement is relatively uncommon, with only 4 reported patients having lymph node metastasis at presentation {1473}. Most reported cases had a relatively good prognosis. No distant metastases have been documented, but follow-up time has been limited. One case of mucinous cystadenocarcinoma arising in the background of extensive high-grade DCIS recurred locally 8 years after lumpectomy {1473}.

# Invasive micropapillary carcinoma

Marchiò C
Horlings HM
Vincent-Salomon A

## Definition

Invasive micropapillary carcinoma of the breast is an invasive breast carcinoma (IBC) composed of small, hollow, or morula-like clusters of malignant cells, surrounded by clear spaces with an inside-out growth pattern.

## ICD-O coding

8507/3 Invasive micropapillary carcinoma of breast

## ICD-11 coding

2C60 & XH9C56 Carcinoma of breast, specialized type & Invasive micropapillary carcinoma of breast

## Related terminology

*Acceptable:* micropapillary carcinoma.

## Subtype(s)

None

## Localization

Invasive micropapillary carcinomas show no predilection for a particular quadrant. Axillary lymph node metastases at diagnosis are frequent.

## Clinical features

Invasive micropapillary carcinomas usually present as a palpable mass. Mammographically, the tumour appears as a dense, irregular mass with indistinct margins. Calcifications may be present {16}. Sonographic examination shows a hypoechoic or occasionally isoechoic mass. On MRI, the tumour usually appears as an irregularly shaped mass with heterogeneous enhancement {1197}. Axillary lymph node metastases are present in more than two thirds of cases at diagnosis {2338, 49}.

## Epidemiology

Pure invasive micropapillary carcinomas are rare, accounting for 0.9–2% of all IBCs {324,1613,1212,1956}. Mixed forms are more frequent, and areas with a micropapillary pattern are found in as many as 7.4% of all IBCs {791,2346,2211}. Invasive micropapillary carcinomas may occur in female and male patients {16, 592,1294}. The mean patient age at presentation of both pure and mixed forms overlaps with the age reported for ER-positive IBCs of no special type (NST) {791,1252,1956,2211}.

## Etiology

There are no specific etiological factors for invasive micropapillary carcinomas that differ from those currently known for breast cancer in general.

## Pathogenesis

No specific pathogenetic mechanisms or highly recurrent molecular alterations have been identified. In vitro data show that increasing EMA (MUC1) expression decreases intercellular adhesion and adhesion between cells and extracellular matrix {1332,2266,2265}, suggesting that EMA expression on the stroma-facing surface of the cell membrane might account, at least in part, for the detachment of the cells from the stroma {1465}.

Invasive micropapillary carcinomas are luminal A or B carcinomas by gene expression profiling {2249}. Array comparative genomic hybridization analysis has detected recurrent gains of

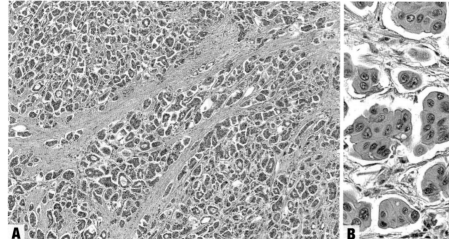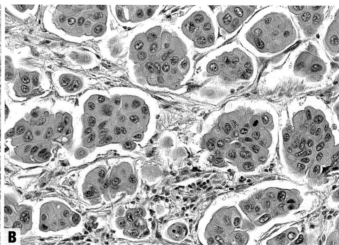

**Fig. 2.130** Invasive micropapillary carcinoma. **A** Note the morula-like and hollow clusters of cancer cells immersed in empty stromal spaces. **B** Note the cell clusters with cuboidal to columnar neoplastic cells devoid of a fibrovascular core. The cell clusters display an inside-out growth pattern and are immersed in empty stromal spaces surrounded by a delicate stromal framework composed of fibroblasts and connective tissue.

8q, 17q, and 20q; deletions of 6q and 13q {1295,2080}; and a constellation of copy-number alterations different from those of grade- and ER-matched IBC-NSTs {1295,1294}. The non-micropapillary component of mixed micropapillary carcinomas harbours genetic alterations similar to those found in the micropapillary areas {1295,1294}. *MYC*, *CCND1*, and *FGFR1* amplifications are reported in 33%, 8%, and 17% of cases, respectively {1294}. The limited data available reveal a spectrum of mutations similar to those found in luminal B IBC-NSTs, with recurrent mutations in *PIK3CA*, *TP53*, *GATA3*, *MAP2K4*, and *NBPF10* {1471,509}. Mutations in genes involved in cell polarity, cell shape, and ciliogenesis have been detected in single cases {774}. No recurrent fusion genes have been identified {1471,774}. Deregulated expression of genes related to apicobasal polarity (in particular, high levels of *LIN7A* expression), cell adhesion, and cell migration has been reported {775}.

## Macroscopic appearance
Not clinically relevant

## Histopathology
In pure invasive micropapillary carcinoma, > 90% of the tumour consists of hollow or morula-like aggregates of cuboidal to columnar neoplastic cells. These are devoid of a fibrovascular core and are immersed in a spongy stroma characterized by clear and empty spaces around the cell clusters and a delicate stromal framework composed of fibroblasts and connective tissue. The clear spaces may mimic lymphatic vessels, but they are not lined by endothelium. The epithelial clusters typically show a reversed polarity, where the apical pole of the tumour cell membrane faces outwards, towards the clear stromal space rather than towards the centre of the clusters. In H&E-stained sections, this pattern may be appreciated as secretions and blebs at the outer cell membrane; electron microscopy has revealed the presence of microvilli on the cell surface facing the stroma {1253}. The cells have a cuboidal to columnar shape; the cytoplasm is eosinophilic, dense, or finely granular. Apocrine features may be present. Nuclear grade is frequently intermediate or high, with variable pleomorphism. Some pure invasive micropapillary carcinomas may be associated with multinucleated osteoclast-like giant cells, including some as large as the micropapillary clusters {1296}. As many as 75% of invasive micropapillary carcinomas are of Nottingham histological grade 2 or 3 {1295,1294,2178,1182,2049}. A rare pattern is micropapillary mucinous carcinoma, which is described in the section on mucinous carcinoma (see *Mucinous carcinoma*, p. 123).

Most carcinomas are ER-positive and PR-positive {2049, 2178,1295,1294}, but some studies report a triple-negative phenotype in 15–20% of cases {2298,319,104,1055}. ERBB2 (HER2) overexpression and amplification are reported in a variable proportion of cases {1294,1295,2310,1669,2178}. HER2 immunoreactivity may yield intense staining that continuously lines the entire cell membrane (score: 3+) or weak to moderate staining in a U-shaped basolateral pattern that spares the luminal aspect of the cell membrane. Carcinomas with a basolateral HER2 staining pattern should be regarded as having equivocal expression (score: 2+) and reflexed to in situ hybridization testing {2285,1994}. Expression of basal antigens is uncommon {1294}.

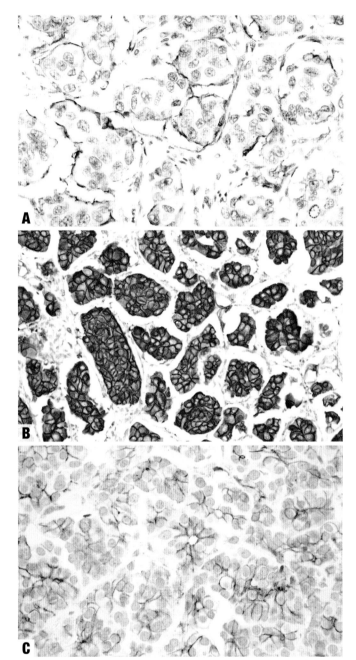

**Fig. 2.131** Invasive micropapillary carcinoma. **A** The unique pattern of polarity is best appreciated with EMA (MUC1) staining lining the peripheral cell membrane facing the stroma, confirming the inside-out growth pattern. **B** Strong and complete membranous immunohistochemical staining (score: 3+) for ERBB2 (HER2). **C** An example showing a moderate to intense but incomplete (U-shaped or basolateral) HER2 staining pattern (score: 2+). *ERBB2* (*HER2*) FISH showed *ERBB2* gene amplification (*ERBB2*/CEP17 ratio: 2.5; mean number of *ERBB2* signals/cell: > 6.0).

EMA (MUC1) is expressed on the luminal aspect of the cell membrane in well-differentiated IBC-NST, but it lines the stroma-facing surface of the membrane in invasive micropapillary carcinoma, indicating reversed polarity. Immunohistochemical staining for EMA may be used to distinguish true reversed polarity from possible artefactual stromal retraction in IBC-NST. In invasive micropapillary carcinoma, the expression of basolateral adhesion proteins (E-cadherin, p120) in a mutually exclusive pattern with EMA also indicates reversed polarity {1147,1640}. There are reports that EMA immunoreactivity also identifies reversed polarity in some mucinous carcinomas {2105}. A subset of carcinomas composed (at least in part) of micropapillary epithelial clusters suspended in abundant extracellular mucin has been described, but it is still unclear whether these tumours are genetically related to invasive micropapillary or mucinous carcinoma (see discussion in *Mucinous carcinoma*, p. 123).

## Cytology

FNA findings include numerous well-formed tumour morules and isolated malignant cells {1249,1004}.

## Diagnostic molecular pathology

FISH for *ERBB2* (*HER2*) should be performed as necessary (see *Histopathology*, above).

## Essential and desirable diagnostic criteria

*Essential:* invasive tumour clusters with micropapillary architecture with reversed cell polarity, set in clear spaces in > 90% of the tumour.

*Desirable:* clean staining for EMA (MUC1) lining the stroma-facing border of the cell clusters.

## Staging

The staging is the same as for other types of IBC.

## Prognosis and prediction

Invasive micropapillary carcinomas have peritumoural lymphovascular invasion and axillary lymph node involvement significantly more frequently than IBC-NSTs {1013,834,1463,2335, 2178}. Therefore, micropapillary morphology is associated with a worse prognosis than unselected IBC-NSTs of the same size. However, the micropapillary histological type does not seem to add independent information pertaining to risk of disease recurrence or overall survival when compared with IBCs matched for patient age, tumour size and grade, peritumoural lymphovascular invasion, immunohistochemically defined molecular subtype, and number of positive lymph nodes {2178}. A meta-analysis including 1888 micropapillary carcinomas across 14 studies revealed a higher rate of locoregional recurrence in patients with micropapillary carcinoma than in patients with IBC-NST; however, there were no statistically significant differences in overall survival, disease-specific survival, or distant metastasis–free survival {2298}.

# Carcinoma with apocrine differentiation

Provenzano E
Gatalica Z
Vranic S

## Definition
Carcinoma with apocrine differentiation is an invasive carcinoma characterized by large cells with abundant eosinophilic granular cytoplasm and enlarged nuclei with prominent nucleoli, resembling apocrine sweat glands.

## ICD-O coding
8401/3 Apocrine adenocarcinoma

## ICD-11 coding
2C61 & XH4GA3 Invasive carcinoma of breast & Adenocarcinoma with apocrine metaplasia

## Related terminology
*Acceptable:* invasive apocrine carcinoma; apocrine carcinoma.

## Subtype(s)
None

## Localization
The localization is similar to that of invasive breast carcinoma of no special type (NST).

## Clinical features
The clinical features are similar to those of invasive breast carcinoma NST. Carcinoma with apocrine differentiation usually presents as a firm, poorly circumscribed mass. Microcalcifications may be seen on mammography, in particular if associated ductal carcinoma in situ (DCIS) is present.

## Epidemiology
Apocrine carcinoma is a rare subtype, constituting about 1% of all breast carcinomas {1376}. Patients tend to be older than those with invasive carcinoma NST {1377,2351,917,478}.

## Etiology
Most carcinomas with apocrine differentiation are sporadic. Some carcinomas in patients with germline *PTEN* mutation (Cowden syndrome) may have apocrine morphology {115}.

## Pathogenesis
There is no definitive information regarding the pathogenesis of carcinoma with apocrine differentiation. The relationship between apocrine metaplasia, atypical apocrine adenosis, and carcinoma with apocrine differentiation remains controversial. One group found similar genetic alterations in papillary apocrine metaplasia and adjacent DCIS and invasive carcinoma with apocrine morphology, including loss at 1p, 16q, and 17q and gains at 2q and 13q, raising the possibility that some apocrine metaplasia might be a non-obligate precursor of a subset of carcinomas with apocrine differentiation {956}. Reports of early oncogenic events – overexpression of the ERBB2 (HER2) and MYC (c-myc) oncoproteins without alterations of the corresponding genes – in apocrine metaplasia and apocrine adenosis may also support this hypothesis {1892,1862,1891}. However, most of the genetic alterations found in carcinoma with apocrine differentiation are also present in invasive carcinoma NST. Overall, carcinomas with apocrine differentiation have heterogeneous gene expression profiles {2249}, but they constitute a more

**Table 2.09** Differential diagnosis of tumours and lesions of the breast with eosinophilic granular cells

| Diagnosis | Morphology | | Immunohistochemical profile | | | | | | |
| --- | --- | --- | --- | --- | --- | --- | --- | --- | --- |
| | Cytoplasm | Nucleus | Cytokeratin | GCDFP-15 | ER | AR | S100 | CD68 | Additional markers |
| **Invasive breast carcinoma with oncocytic pattern** | Abundant, brightly eosinophilic, and granular, with well-defined borders | Round and centrally located, with prominent nucleoli | + | –/+ | Mostly + | –/+ | – | – | Mitochondrial stains + 25% ERBB2 (HER2) + |
| **Carcinoma with apocrine differentiation** | Abundant, granular, and eosinophilic or vacuolated, with distinct cell borders | Enlarged and round to oval, with marked/ moderate atypia and prominent nucleoli | + | + | – | + | –/+ focal/ weak | – | GATA3 + 30–60% ERBB2 (HER2) + |
| **Granular cell tumour** | Abundant, granular, and eosinophilic | Lacks nuclear atypia | – | – | – | – | + | + | |
| **Histiocytic proliferation** | Pale to foamy | Lacks nuclear atypia | – | – | – | – | +/– | + | |

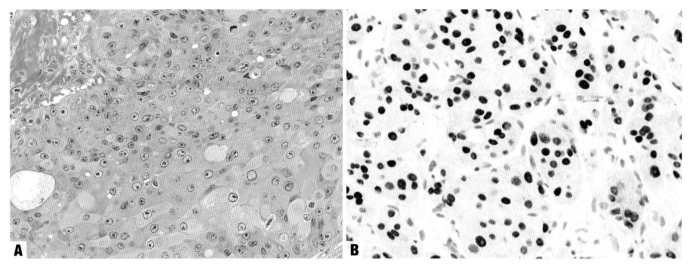

**Fig. 2.132** Carcinoma with apocrine differentiation. **A** A higher-power view illustrating the nuclear features, with large, prominent nucleoli. **B** Immunohistochemistry for AR showing strong positive nuclear staining.

homogeneous group when analysis is restricted to carcinomas with apocrine morphology and triple-negative phenotype {2254}. Carcinomas with apocrine differentiation frequently harbour mutations of *TP53* and *PIK3CA/PTEN*/AKT genes {2200, 1142,2254}. Mutations within the MAPK pathway (e.g. in *KRAS*, *NRAS*, and *BRAF*) are less common {2199,2200}.

Gene expression profiling studies have identified a molecular apocrine signature (molecular apocrine breast cancer or luminal AR) characterized by AR upregulation without ER activation {522,620,115,1497}. However, carcinomas with the molecular apocrine breast cancer / luminal AR subtypes may not be equivalent to carcinomas with apocrine differentiation as defined on the basis of morphology.

### Macroscopic appearance
The macroscopic appearance is nonspecific and similar to that of invasive carcinoma NST.

### Histopathology
The cells have abundant granular eosinophilic or vacuolated cytoplasm with distinct cell borders {605,1572}. The nuclei are enlarged and round to oval, with marked or moderate atypia and prominent nucleoli; low-grade nuclear atypia is uncommon. The predominant growth pattern is solid, but any architectural pattern may be observed. The mitotic activity is usually moderate to high. Consequently, most carcinomas with apocrine differentiation are either grade 2 or grade 3 {605,2046,2202}. DCIS with apocrine morphology usually accompanies the invasive carcinoma, and it is often of intermediate or high nuclear grade, with comedonecrosis and calcifications {2201}.

Carcinomas with apocrine differentiation express GCDFP-15 {1571}, an antigen also found in apocrine metaplasia. They also have a characteristic steroid receptor profile that is ER-negative, PR-negative, and AR-positive. AR is consistently expressed in carcinomas with apocrine differentiation {700,2202,478,1376}. AR activation is associated with HER2 overexpression and/or *ERBB2* amplification in 30–60% of cases {435,2202,53,1204}. Among triple-negative carcinomas, 50–80% of carcinomas with apocrine morphology are AR-positive {90,2202}. GATA3

is expressed in 90% of carcinomas with apocrine morphology {2263} and in > 70% of AR-positive triple-negative carcinomas {1015}.

Apocrine atypia / apocrine DCIS involving a sclerosing lesion may mimic invasive carcinoma with apocrine differentiation {1420}. Immunohistochemical staining for myoepithelial markers may be helpful in this setting. Apocrine metaplasia may have an inconspicuous to absent myoepithelial layer, but it does not show nuclear atypia {415,2100}. Granular cell tumours have abundant granular eosinophilic cytoplasm and are ER-negative, but they lack nuclear atypia, do not express any keratins, and are strongly and diffusely positive for CD68 and S100 {240}, whereas carcinomas with apocrine differentiation show only focal and weak positivity for S100. Oncocytic carcinomas of the breast are very rare and may show positivity for GCDFP-15 and HER2; they are usually ER-positive and stain positively for mitochondria {1690}. Apocrine morphology is also observed in some special subtypes of invasive carcinoma, including mucinous, micropapillary, and pleomorphic lobular carcinoma {603}. Rare carcinomas composed of apocrine cells (positive for GCDFP-15) with prominent vacuolated or foamy cytoplasm and resembling histiocytes have been described {601}. Most of these tumours show loss of E-cadherin and may represent a subtype of invasive lobular carcinoma with apocrine differentiation {792}. Carcinomas with histiocytoid apocrine cells may be confused with histiocytic proliferations, but immunohistochemical staining for cytokeratins and CD68 can be useful in distinguishing these lesions. The differential diagnosis of tumours and lesions of the breast with eosinophilic granular cells is summarized in Table 2.09 (p. 131).

### Cytology
Cytological preparations of carcinoma with apocrine differentiation consist of abundant single cells and clusters of moderately to markedly atypical epithelium with abundant vacuolated to densely eosinophilic cytoplasm. High cellularity, cell dyscohesion, and substantial nuclear atypia are required for a definitive diagnosis of malignancy, to rule out the differential diagnosis of atypical apocrine adenosis involving a mass-forming sclerosing

lesion. Degenerative changes in the epithelium of apocrine cysts may also be in the differential diagnosis.

## Diagnostic molecular pathology
No specific diagnostic molecular test is available. *ERBB2* (*HER2*) FISH testing may be performed as needed.

## Essential and desirable diagnostic criteria
*Essential:* apocrine morphology in > 90% of tumour cells.
*Desirable:* ER-negative, PR-negative, and AR-positive immuno-profile.

## Staging
Carcinoma with apocrine differentiation is staged according to the TNM classification system.

## Prognosis and prediction
The results of clinical follow-up studies are often contradictory due to the use of different criteria for the diagnosis of carcinoma with apocrine differentiation {2201}. Recent studies have reported a worse clinical outcome in patients with apocrine carcinoma than with invasive carcinoma NST {2351,478}; however, in an analysis of SEER Program population-based data, the outcome improved after adjustment for demographic and clinicopathological features {2351}. Some studies identified better overall survival and breast cancer–specific survival for patients with AR-positive apocrine triple-negative carcinomas than with other triple-negative tumours {1189,1340,1377,2357}, whereas other studies found no differences {1407,545}.

Information on the pathological response to neoadjuvant chemotherapy is very limited. One group reported partial or complete pathological response to neoadjuvant chemotherapy in about 30–50% of apocrine carcinomas {917}. However, in another series, the response of carcinomas with apocrine differentiation to neoadjuvant treatment was poor, but the patient had a good prognosis nonetheless {1439}. Similarly, in a study evaluating subtypes of triple-negative breast cancer defined by gene expression profiling, the pathological complete response rate for luminal AR cancers after neoadjuvant chemotherapy was only 10%, but the tumours behaved clinically more like ER-positive carcinomas with a favourable outcome {1314}.

# Metaplastic carcinoma

Reis-Filho JS
Gobbi H
McCart Reed AE
Rakha EA
Shin SJ
Sotiriou C
Vincent-Salomon A

## Definition
Metaplastic carcinoma is a heterogeneous group of invasive breast carcinomas (IBCs) characterized by differentiation of the neoplastic epithelium towards squamous cells and/or mesenchymal-looking elements, including but not restricted to spindle, chondroid, and osseous cells.

## ICD-O coding
8575/3 Metaplastic carcinoma NOS

## ICD-11 coding
2C6Y & XHORD4 Metaplastic carcinoma of breast & Metaplastic carcinoma NOS

## Related terminology
*Acceptable:* metaplastic carcinoma NOS.
*Not recommended:* carcinosarcoma; sarcomatoid carcinoma; carcinoma with pseudosarcomatous metaplasia; carcinoma with pseudosarcomatous stroma.

## Subtype(s)
None

## Localization
Metaplastic carcinomas can affect any anatomical area of the breast.

## Clinical features
The clinical features of metaplastic carcinoma are similar to those of ER-negative IBC of no special type (NST); however, metaplastic carcinomas are more likely to present at an advanced stage {1879}. Most cases (85%) present with a palpable lump and are detected as a mass lesion on ultrasonography (100%) or mammography (78%). Calcifications are uncommon (17%) {1113}; when present, they are often associated with ductal carcinoma in situ and/or osseous differentiation.

## Epidemiology
Metaplastic carcinomas have been reported to account for 0.2–1% of all IBCs {1879,1480,1619}. This variation in prevalence stems from the different definitions of metaplastic carcinoma used by different authors.

## Etiology
The etiology of metaplastic carcinomas is multifactorial, and it appears not to differ from that of IBC-NST (in particular of the triple-negative subtype).

## Pathogenesis
Although metaplastic carcinomas of the breast constitute a heterogeneous group of tumours with distinctive morphological characteristics and marked intertumoural and intratumoural heterogeneity, genetic studies support a monoclonal origin of the heterogeneous components of metaplastic carcinomas {717,1195,96A}, and some authors support the concept of a late-step change of tumour dedifferentiation rather than an origin from a basal-like stem cell {2148}. However, it remains unknown whether somatic mutations cause the differentiation that allows for metaplastic carcinoma subtypes {2245}, and no specific pathognomonic mutations for metaplastic carcinomas have yet been identified. The genes frequently mutated in metaplastic carcinomas include *TP53* and *PIK3CA* {2245}. Overexpression and mutations of *EGFR*, as well as p63 immunopositivity, have been reported in metaplastic carcinomas with squamous metaplasia and spindle cell morphology {1747}. Other genetic abnormalities include losses of *PTEN* and *CDKN2A* {2245}. Metaplastic carcinomas show a stem cell–like phenotype, with positivity for CD44 and negativity for CD24 {844}. Metaplastic carcinomas, as part of the group of triple-negative breast cancers, are characterized by low expression of GATA3-regulated genes and the genes that are responsible for epithelial–mesenchymal transition and cell–cell adhesion, with upregulation of vimentin and E-cadherin repressor molecules (SNAI1 [SNAIL], SNAI2 [SLUG], TWIST) and downregulation of E-cadherin. These molecular features suggest that metaplastic carcinomas arise from a breast epithelial precursor that is relatively chemoresistant {1747}.

## Macroscopic appearance
The gross appearance of metaplastic carcinoma is often not distinctive, and the tumours can either present as well-circumscribed masses or display indistinct, irregular borders. Cystic degeneration is not uncommon, in particular in metaplastic carcinomas with squamous cell carcinoma. Pearly, white-to-greyish, and glistening cut surfaces can be seen in areas of squamous and chondroid metaplasia, whereas the cut surface of areas of osseous metaplasia can be gritty and hard. Compared with IBC-NST, metaplastic carcinomas tend to be larger, with a mean size of 3.9 cm, ranging from 2 to > 10 cm. Thorough sampling of the lesion is strongly advised.

## Histopathology
Metaplastic carcinomas constitute a group of histopathologically distinct patterns with different outcomes, although there is often overlap. Given the heterogeneity of metaplastic carcinomas, the WHO Classification of Tumours Editorial Board has maintained a descriptive classification system, based on the type of the metaplastic elements. Metaplastic carcinomas can be monophasic (with only one metaplastic component) or biphasic (with two or more components). The two components can both be of metaplastic histology, such as squamous and/or spindle cells with a mesenchymal/matrix-producing component, or there can be one metaplastic component and one adenocarcinoma component (most frequently IBC-NST). If more than one component

is identified, it is suggested to note each component and its approximate percentage within the tumour. On the basis of histological pattern, metaplastic carcinomas can also be classified into epithelial-only carcinomas (with low-grade adenosquamous carcinoma [LGASC], high-grade adenosquamous carcinoma, or pure squamous cell carcinoma), pure (monophasic) sarcomatoid (spindle cell or matrix-producing) carcinomas, and biphasic epithelial and sarcomatoid carcinomas. Some IBC-NSTs may have only a very focal metaplastic component, and this should be noted in the report.

### Low-grade adenosquamous carcinoma

The LGASC pattern shows well-developed glandular and tubular formations intimately admixed with solid nests of squamous cells in a spindle cell background. The carcinomatous component is characterized by small glandular structures (with rounded rather than angulated contours) and solid cords of epithelial cells, which may contain squamous cells, squamous pearls, or squamous cyst formation. The invasive neoplastic component typically shows long, slender extensions at the periphery and infiltrates between normal breast structures. Clusters of lymphocytes are often observed at the periphery, sometimes in a cannonball pattern. Because of the favourable prognosis of this tumour {2149}, it should be differentiated from other (high-grade) adenosquamous carcinomas. It should also be distinguished from nipple (syringomatous) adenoma {186} and the early cellular phase of radial scar / complex sclerosing lesion {2276}.

### Fibromatosis-like metaplastic carcinoma

Fibromatosis-like metaplastic tumours of the breast are characterized by > 95% of the tumour being composed of bland spindle cells with pale eosinophilic cytoplasm and slender nuclei with tapered edges and finely distributed chromatin embedded in stroma with varying degrees of collagenization. High nuclear grade is not seen in this tumour, which shows only mild nuclear atypia. The spindle cells are often arranged in wavy, interlacing fascicles, or they form long fascicles with finger-like extensions infiltrating the adjacent breast parenchyma. Cords and clusters

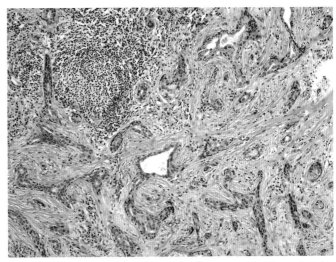

**Fig. 2.134** Metaplastic carcinoma. Low-grade adenosquamous carcinoma featuring infiltrative glands with bland cytology, focal squamoid differentiation, desmoplastic stroma, and lymphoid aggregates. Some infiltrating glands may show peripheral myoepithelial-like cells.

of plump spindled and more-epithelioid cells are often found; not uncommonly, these cells are arranged in a pattern reminiscent of a perivascular distribution {1664,742,459,1967,741A}. Focal squamous differentiation may be found. A gradual transition from plump cells to the spindle cell component is frequently observed. These tumours are almost invariably p63-positive; keratins are always expressed, occasionally focally and not uncommonly restricted to the plump spindle and epithelioid cells. Fibromatosis-like metaplastic carcinoma should always be considered as a main differential diagnosis of bland-looking spindle cell proliferations of the breast {1698,1967}. A diagnosis of fibromatosis-like metaplastic carcinoma can be rendered based on the presence of any evidence of epithelial differentiation by histopathological and/or immunohistochemical analysis (see below). Because of the relatively favourable prognosis of this tumour type, it should be differentiated from the more common high-grade spindle cell metaplastic carcinomas.

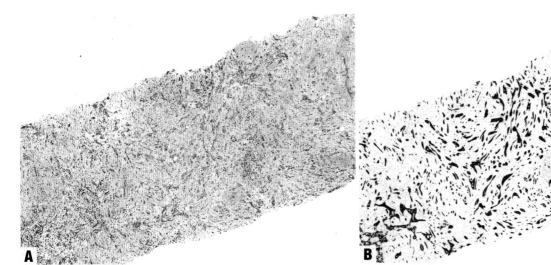

**Fig. 2.133** Metaplastic carcinoma. Low-grade adenosquamous carcinoma. **A** Core biopsy shows frankly invasive lesion on H&E section. **B** CK5/6 expression in this core biopsy is strong and diffuse. The pattern of staining is different from the mosaic pattern of the hyperplastic epithelial lesions.

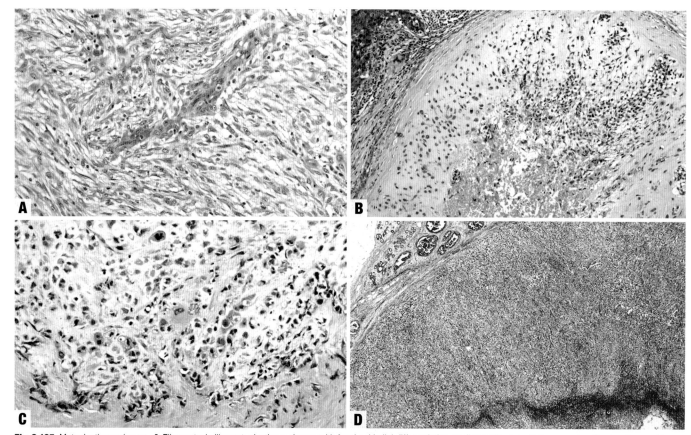

**Fig. 2.135** Metaplastic carcinoma. **A** Fibromatosis-like metaplastic carcinoma with focal epithelial differentiation as diagnostic clue. **B** An example with chondromyxoid morphology (heterologous mesenchymal differentiation). **C** A case of metaplastic matrix-producing carcinoma showing high-grade cytonuclear features, with discohesive cells in a chondroid matrix. The degree of atypia in these tumours can be variable. Although the presence of the cartilaginous/chondroid matrix is pathognomonic for these tumours, its amount and distribution can be heterogeneous. **D** High-grade spindle cell metaplastic carcinoma associated with high-grade cribriform non–spindle cell type ductal carcinoma in situ, supporting the carcinomatous nature of the invasive spindle cell component.

### Spindle cell carcinoma

Spindle cell carcinomas are characterized by atypical spindle cells arranged in a multitude of architectural patterns, ranging from long fascicles in herringbone or interwoven patterns to short fascicles in a storiform (cartwheel) pattern {298,708, 2226}. Most often, a mixture of different patterns is observed. The cytoplasm ranges from elongated to plump spindle. Nuclear pleomorphism is usually moderate to high. Inflammatory infiltrate is found in a proportion of cases, often with lymphocytes and dendritic cells percolating through the tumour bulk. Areas in which the neoplastic cells form small clusters with more-epithelioid morphology or squamous differentiation can be found. It should be noted that this group of tumours includes lesions that are likely to constitute the end of the spectrum of spindle squamous cell carcinomas on one hand and malignant myoepithelioma / myoepithelial carcinoma on the other. At present, there are no definitive criteria to differentiate these two lesions, nor are there data to suggest that these lesions display distinct clinical behaviour. Metaplastic spindle cell carcinoma should always be considered as a main differential diagnosis of atypical/malignant-looking spindle cell proliferations of the breast {1698}. A diagnosis of metaplastic spindle cell carcinoma can be rendered based on the presence of any evidence of epithelial differentiation by histopathological and/or immunohistochemical analysis (see below).

### Squamous cell carcinoma

Pure metaplastic squamous cell carcinomas usually present as a cystic lesion in which the cavity is lined by squamous cells with varying degrees of nuclear atypia and pleomorphism. The neoplastic cells infiltrate the adjacent stroma in the form of sheets, cords, and nests, with variable degrees of squamous differentiation, and they often elicit a conspicuous stromal reaction and prominent inflammatory infiltrates {2229,958}. Several patterns can be observed. The acantholytic pattern of squamous cell carcinoma, characterized by the formation of irregular spaces lined by atypical squamous cells leading to a pseudoglandular or pseudoangiosarcomatous appearance, should be considered as a potential differential diagnosis with angiosarcoma {602}. Metaplastic squamous cell carcinoma may be pure or mixed with other types of metaplastic carcinoma, usually of spindle cell carcinoma pattern, or with IBC-NST (adenosquamous carcinoma pattern). For a diagnosis of primary squamous cell carcinoma of the breast to be rendered, primary cutaneous or metastatic squamous cell carcinomas from other sites (e.g. lung and cervix) must be ruled out.

### Metaplastic carcinoma with heterologous mesenchymal differentiation

Metaplastic breast carcinomas with mesenchymal elements are often composed of an admixture of mesenchymal components (including chondroid, osseous, rhabdomyoid, and even neuroglial differentiation) with carcinomatous areas (which can be in the form of glandular differentiation, tubules, solid clusters, and/or foci of squamous differentiation) {540,1527,2228, 2227,2226}. The mesenchymal components can range from appearing differentiated with minimal atypia to exhibiting frankly malignant features that to some extent recapitulate the patterns found in true sarcomas of the soft tissues. Historically, the term "matrix-producing carcinomas" was applied to a subgroup of metaplastic carcinomas with mesenchymal elements in which an abrupt transition from the epithelial to the mesenchymal components without the presence of intervening spindle cells was found. However, some cases show a focal presence of intervening spindle cells, and this feature should not exclude the diagnosis of matrix-producing carcinoma. In such tumours, the presence of true chondroid or osteoid/osseous differentiation with chondroid or osteoid matrix is essential. Areas of epithelial differentiation can be readily found in the vast majority of cases, but in some cases, extensive sampling is required to find the carcinomatous areas and to differentiate these tumours from bone or soft tissue sarcomas. Importantly, immunohistochemical analysis also reveals the expression of epithelial markers, usually high-molecular-weight cytokeratins.

*Mixed metaplastic carcinomas*
With extensive sampling, a large proportion of metaplastic breast cancers display a mixture of different metaplastic elements, as well as metaplastic and conventional adenocarcinomatous elements. These cases should be reported as metaplastic carcinomas, and the distinct elements should be recorded in the final report.

## Cytology
The presence of biphasic tumour cells on FNA of the breast with atypical spindle cells, squamous carcinoma cells, osteoclast-like giant cells, and/or matrix with or without a component of adenocarcinoma cells may provide clues for diagnosis of metaplastic carcinomas {963,1102}. The cytology of matrix-producing metaplastic carcinoma shows abundant myxoid matrix along with cellular clusters composed of monotonous cellular populations, overlapping with the cytology of pleomorphic adenoma. Cytological diagnosis of metaplastic carcinomas may not be possible in all cases because of selective sampling of various pathological elements.

## Diagnostic molecular pathology
The vast majority (> 90%) of metaplastic carcinomas lack expression of ER, PR, and ERBB2 (HER2) {1745,1879,1701,1619}. The majority express high-molecular-weight cytokeratins (CK5/6 and CK14), p63, and EGFR (HER1) {1745,1701}; in fact, a subset of EGFR (HER1)-positive metaplastic carcinomas display *EGFR* gene amplification. However, *EGFR*-activating somatic mutations appear to be vanishingly rare in these tumours {1744,1747, 717}. The identification of epithelial differentiation in metaplastic breast carcinomas requires the use of a panel of immunohistochemical markers. The usual markers are keratins – in particular AE1/AE3 and MNF116 (positive in 75–85% of cases); 34βE12, CK5/6, and CK14 (in 70–75%); and p63 (in 77%). Low-molecular-weight cytokeratins such as CK8/18, CK7, and CK19 are positive in a lower proportion of cases (36–61%). Myoepithelial markers, including SMA, CD10, and maspin, are also frequently

positive (in 50–70% of cases). Metaplastic carcinomas are negative for CD34 (in 100% of cases) and often lack expression of desmin (in 18%) and SMMHC (in 11%) {1701}. E-cadherin may be aberrantly expressed within squamous foci {1328}; β-catenin may also be aberrantly expressed {1089}. It should be noted that metaplastic carcinoma with LGASC pattern has a biphasic composition: the epithelial layer in gland-like structures is positive for luminal and occasionally basal cytokeratins, and the myoepithelial/basal cells display varying levels of expression of basal cytokeratins and p63, with staining ranging from complete to incomplete to absent {984,714}.

Transcriptomically, these tumours are classified as being of basal-like or claudin-low subtype using the intrinsic gene classification {2249,2250,2251,1661,844,1674} or as basal-like or mesenchymal-like using the classification proposed by Lehmann et al. {1661,2251}. Whole-exome and targeted sequencing analyses of metaplastic carcinomas have demonstrated that these tumours have complex landscapes of gene copy-number alterations and a repertoire of somatic mutations including mutations affecting *TP53*, *RB1*, and chromatin-remodelling genes (i.e. *ARID1A* and *KMT2C*), as well as genes related to the PI3K pathway (i.e. *PIK3CA*, *PIK3R1*, and *PTEN*), the MAPK pathway (i.e. *NF1*, *KRAS*, and *NRAS*), and the WNT pathway (i.e. *FAT1* and *CCN6* [*WISP3*]) {1489,1062,1328}. Interestingly, there is evidence to suggest that *TP53* mutations may be less frequently found in spindle cell carcinomas than in other forms of metaplastic carcinomas {1489,1328} and in LGASC {130A}. Compared with other forms of triple-negative breast cancer, metaplastic carcinomas more frequently display mutations affecting PI3K pathway–related genes than do basal-like cancers {1489,1062,1328,130A}, but at a frequency similar to that found in luminal AR triple-negative disease. In a manner akin to phyllodes tumours, metaplastic carcinomas were reported to harbour *TERT* gene promoter mutations in 25% of cases in one study {1062}, but these mutations were not detected in others; further analysis to define the frequency of *TERT* promoter mutations in metaplastic breast cancers is needed.

## Essential and desirable diagnostic criteria
*Essential:* an IBC with atypical squamous, spindle cell, and/or mesenchymal/matrix-producing differentiation; in metaplastic carcinomas lacking ductal carcinoma in situ or conventional-type mammary carcinoma components, direct evidence of epithelial differentiation by immunohistochemistry, based on unequivocal expression of (high-molecular-weight) cytokeratins and/or p63.

## Staging
Metaplastic carcinomas are staged similarly to other types of IBCs (see *Invasive breast carcinoma: General overview*, p. 82).

## Prognosis and prediction
Lymph node metastases are found significantly less frequently in metaplastic breast cancers than in IBC-NST of similar size and grade {1619}. As for other triple-negative breast carcinomas, metaplastic carcinomas can be found to have distant metastases (preferentially affecting the brain and lungs) in the absence of lymph node metastases. There are no prognostic markers or predictive markers of therapeutic response supported by level 1 evidence for patients with metaplastic carcinoma. Retrospective

analyses have suggested that specific subtypes probably have distinct outcomes {1716,2308}. Fibromatosis-like carcinomas and LGASCs are associated with more-indolent behaviour than are other types of IBCs, despite the triple-negative phenotype {1700,1664,2149}. Among the types of metaplastic carcinoma, high-grade spindle cell, squamous cell, and high-grade adenosquamous carcinomas are associated with the worst prognosis, whereas matrix-producing carcinomas are associated with a better prognosis {1716,2308}. Higher numbers of morphologies within mixed metaplastic carcinomas correlate with a worse outcome {1328}. The prognostic value of histological grade in metaplastic breast carcinomas is uncertain.

The 3-year, 5-year, and 10-year overall survival rates for metaplastic breast cancer are 77% {1879}, 62% {1619,843}, and 53% {2118}, respectively. No difference in 5-year survival was found between hormone-positive and hormone-negative metaplastic carcinomas {1619}. There is evidence that the rare forms of HER2-positive metaplastic carcinoma may be associated with a better outcome than triple-negative metaplastic carcinomas {1879}. Radiotherapy provides a survival benefit {2118}. As a group, metaplastic breast cancers are reported to have lower response rates to conventional adjuvant chemotherapy and a worse clinical outcome after chemotherapy than other forms of triple-negative breast carcinomas {1250,965,845,843}.

# Rare and salivary gland–type tumours: Introduction

Foschini MP

Normal breast and salivary glands share a similar architecture (both are tubuloacinar glands) and a similar cellular composition (both consist of luminal epithelial cells surrounded by myoepithelial cells). Furthermore, the breast can contain lobules showing pure acinar differentiation {1315}, similar to the serous acinar cells seen in the salivary glands. The luminal epithelial cells of both glands have a similar immunoprofile, expressing low-molecular-weight cytokeratins, ER, PR, and AR. These similarities in structure result in the development of similar neoplastic lesions.

The breast can develop the entire range of tumour types encountered in the salivary glands. These salivary gland–type breast tumours share the morphological features and often the molecular alterations found in their salivary gland counterparts, but their clinical behaviour is often different. Salivary gland–type breast tumours are often triple-negative, lacking ER/PR expression and *ERBB2* (*HER2*) amplification, but they show low or intermediate aggressive potential {666,716}. Therefore, knowledge of their site-specific behaviour is important for correct management and avoidance of overtreatment.

# Acinic cell carcinoma

Foschini MP
Geyer FC
Marchiò C
Nishimura R

### Definition
Acinic cell carcinoma is a malignant epithelial neoplasm composed of clear and granular epithelial cells, some of which contain intracytoplasmic zymogen granules, arranged in microglandular and solid patterns.

### ICD-O coding
8550/3 Acinar cell carcinoma

### ICD-11 coding
2C60 & XH3PG9 Carcinoma of breast, specialized type & Acinic cell adenocarcinoma

### Related terminology
None

### Subtype(s)
None

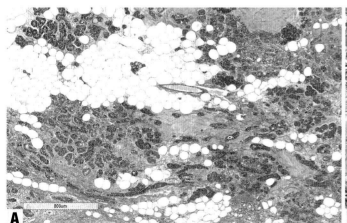
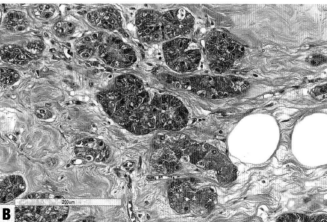

**Fig. 2.136** Acinic cell carcinoma. **A** Acinic cell carcinoma with microglandular proliferation, composed of small glands. These are irregular and lined by multiple cell layers. **B** The neoplastic cells are atypical and have granular cytoplasm. In some cells, coarse eosinophilic granules can be seen.

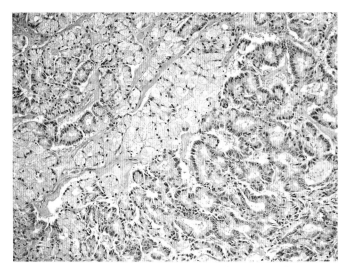

**Fig. 2.137** Acinic cell carcinoma. Neoplastic cells can show clear cytoplasm.

## Localization

Acinic cell carcinoma can affect any breast quadrant, with no site predilection.

## Clinical features

Breast acinic cell carcinoma usually affects adult women (aged 20–80 years). A single case affecting the male breast has been reported {1919}. The clinical presentation is similar to that of invasive breast carcinoma of no special type (NST).

## Epidemiology

Breast acinic cell carcinoma is a rare subtype of invasive breast carcinoma. It was originally described by Roncaroli et al. in 1996 {1781} and then subsequently better delineated by Damiani et al. in 2000 {447}. Thereafter, fewer than 50 cases have been described in the literature {668}.

## Etiology

Unknown

## Pathogenesis

Breast glands can show acinic-like differentiation {1315} that can explain the development of acinic cell carcinoma. One case arose in a *BRCA1*-mutated patient {1765}. Breast acinic cell carcinomas show a DNA copy-number and mutation landscape similar to that of triple-negative breast carcinomas of conventional histology or diagnosed in association with microglandular adenosis, harbouring mutations of *TP53*, *PIK3CA*, *KMT2D*, *ERBB4*, *ERBB3*, *NEB*, *BRCA1*, *MTOR*, *CTNNB1*, *INPP4B*, and *FGFR2* {782,1656,710}. Notably, the mutation profiles of breast acinic cell carcinomas differ from those of acinic cell carcinomas of the salivary glands, suggesting that these are not related entities, as opposed to most salivary gland–like tumours of the breast {1656}.

## Macroscopic appearance

The macroscopic appearance of acinic cell carcinoma is the same as that of invasive breast carcinoma NST, being characterized by infiltrative nodules, hard in consistency, and ranging in size from 11 to 50 mm {668}. One case arising within a fibroadenoma has been reported {1203}.

## Histopathology

At low-power view, acinic cell carcinoma can show a great variety of architectural patterns, ranging from a microglandular proliferation to solid areas often centred on necrosis. The two architectural patterns frequently merge together. Due to the high variability in architectural patterns, diagnosis is based on recognition of the cytological features. The neoplastic cells have abundant, variably eosinophilic and basophilic granular cytoplasm, imparting a variegated appearance {396}. PASD staining reveals intracellular, large, coarse eosinophilic granules. Intracytoplasmic granules are clearly evident on ultrastructural examination {447}. The cytoplasm is sometimes clear. The nucleus is centrally located and atypical, with a prominent nucleolus. The neoplastic cells show various degrees of atypia. Cellular atypia and mitotic figures are more prominent in the solid areas. Ductal carcinoma in situ of high nuclear grade can be present.

The neoplastic cells are positive for markers of serous differentiation, such as lysozyme and α1-antichymotrypsin. In addition, positivity for S100, EMA, and low-molecular-weight cytokeratins is a consistent feature. Focal positivity for GCDFP-15 can be seen.

The differential diagnosis includes a wide range of breast tumours, comprising high-grade invasive carcinomas and secretory carcinoma. Differential diagnosis is based on cell features, especially on the presence of intracytoplasmic granules and markers of serous acinar differentiation. Acinic cell

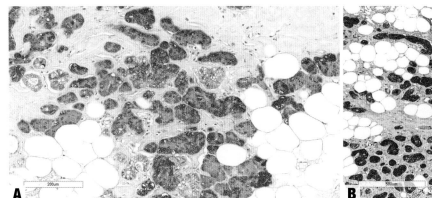

**Fig. 2.138** Acinic cell carcinoma. **A** Neoplastic cells are strongly EMA-positive. **B** Markers of serous differentiation, such as lysozyme, are strongly positive.

carcinomas with bland nuclear morphology can raise suspicion of secretory carcinoma of the breast, but acinic cell carcinoma lacks the t(12;15) *ETV6-NTRK3* translocation that is typically present in secretory carcinoma {1746}.

## Cytology

Breast acinic cell carcinoma FNA findings have been reported for a single case. The smears were hypercellular, as seen in breast carcinomas NST. Intracytoplasmic coarse granules were useful for correct diagnosis {1826}.

## Diagnostic molecular pathology

Breast acinic cell carcinoma can be included in the triple-negative breast cancer group, because it is consistently negative for ER and PR, and *ERBB2* (*HER2*) amplification has not been demonstrated. AR immunoreactivity has been documented {1202}.

## Essential and desirable diagnostic criteria

*Essential:* neoplastic cells with eosinophilic and basophilic granular cytoplasm and PASD-positive intracytoplasmic granules; immunohistochemical positivity for EMA and markers of serous acinar differentiation.

## Staging

Acinic cell carcinoma is staged according to the criteria adopted for other types of breast carcinomas.

## Prognosis and prediction

Because of the limited number of cases reported with follow-up information, our knowledge about the prognosis of acinic cell carcinoma is still limited {668}. The available data indicate that acinic cell carcinoma is a triple-negative carcinoma with intermediate aggressive potential. Axillary node metastases were present in 9 of 30 cases, and 3 patients developed metastases to the liver, bone, and lung, leading to death in 2 cases {668}. Nevertheless, most of the reported patients are alive with no evidence of recurrence 6–184 months after the diagnosis (mean: 42 months). Most of the reported patients underwent chemotherapy and radiotherapy in addition to surgery. The available molecular evidence may support the contention that acinic cell carcinoma could be the precursor of more-aggressive forms of triple-negative breast carcinomas {782}.

# Adenoid cystic carcinoma

Foschini MP
Geyer FC
Hayes MM
Marchiò C
Nishimura R

## Definition
Adenoid cystic carcinoma (AdCC) is an invasive carcinoma composed of epithelial and myoepithelial neoplastic cells arranged in tubular, cribriform, and solid patterns associated with basophilic matrix and reduplicated basement membrane material, frequently associated with *MYB-NFIB* fusion.

## ICD-O coding
8200/3 Adenoid cystic carcinoma

## ICD-11 coding
2C60 & XH4302 Carcinoma of breast, specialized type & Adenoid cystic carcinoma

## Related terminology
*Not recommended:* carcinoma adenoides cysticum; adenocystic basal cell carcinoma; cylindromatous carcinoma.

## Subtype(s)
Classic adenoid cystic carcinoma; solid-basaloid adenoid cystic carcinoma; adenoid cystic carcinoma with high-grade transformation

## Localization
AdCC can arise in any quadrant of the breast, with the retroareolar region being the most frequently affected site {211,668}.

## Clinical features
AdCC usually affects elderly women; single case reports have been reported in men {2327} and adolescents {1215}. Most of the reported cases presented as a palpable mass (mainly in elderly patients), but AdCC can present as a small nodule in younger patients and populations attending breast screening programmes {211}. AdCC is usually unifocal {211}, although a multifocal case is on record {675}.

## Epidemiology
Breast AdCC is relatively rare, accounting for 0.1–3.5% of all breast tumours {165,211}.

## Etiology
Unknown

## Pathogenesis
Most of the AdCCs investigated to date have harboured the *MYB-NFIB* fusion gene {1010}, similarly to what is observed in the salivary gland counterpart, demonstrated by FISH or PCR analysis. This fusion gene has also been detected in the solid-basaloid subtype {442}. AdCCs lacking the *MYB-NFIB* fusion gene may show *MYBL1* rearrangements or *MYB* amplification {1010}. The mutation landscape has been studied mainly in the classic subtype. The most frequently mutated genes include

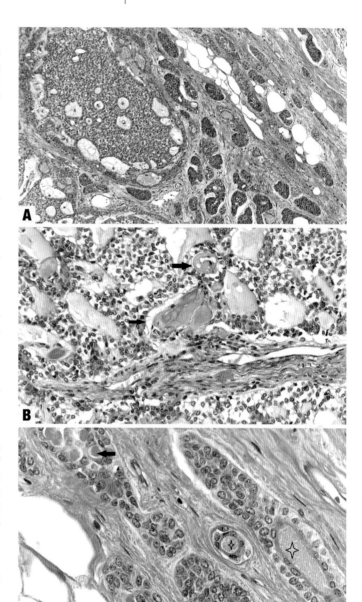

**Fig. 2.139** Adenoid cystic carcinoma. **A** An example showing cribriform and tubular architecture. **B** The cribriform subtype: glandular structures contain mucoid material. In addition, pseudoglandular spaces containing basal membrane (arrows) are seen. **C** An example with tubular architecture: at high power, it shows the same cell composition as adenoid cystic carcinoma with cribriform architecture. Glandular spaces filled with mucin (stars) and pseudoglandular spaces filled with basal membrane (arrow) are present.

*MYB*, *BRAF*, *FBXW7*, *SMARCA5*, *SF3B1*, and *FGFR2*. On rare occasions, activating mutations in RAS pathway genes have been described. AdCCs with high-grade transformation present mutations in *EP300*, *NOTCH1*, *ERBB2*, and *FGFR1* (in addition to the *MYB-NFIB* fusion gene), and they seem to lack mutations affecting common forms of triple-negative breast cancer (such as *TP53* mutations) {692}.

Recently, attention has been directed towards the microRNA expression profile in AdCC of the salivary, lacrimal, and mammary glands. In salivary and lacrimal glands, the microRNA expression profiles differ between normal tissue and AdCC neoplastic tissue. In contrast, normal breast tissue and AdCC neoplastic tissue share the same microRNA expression profile. In addition, breast AdCC shows differences from the salivary and lacrimal gland counterpart microRNA profiles {70}. These differences could help improve our understanding of the differing clinical behaviours according to the site of origin.

## Macroscopic appearance

AdCC presents as a well-circumscribed nodule with pushing borders, ranging in size from a few millimetres to as large as 12 cm {668}.

## Histopathology

Breast AdCC shows the same morphological spectrum observed in salivary gland AdCC. Three subtypes have been defined, on the basis of architectural and cytological features: classic AdCC, solid-basaloid AdCC (SB-AdCC), and AdCC with high-grade transformation {668}.

**Classic AdCC:** At low magnification, this subtype shows a central cribriform area surrounded by a peripheral area with predominant tubular architecture. Both areas show the same cellular composition, namely epithelial and myoepithelial cells. The glandular spaces in both areas are lined by epithelial-type

cells that produce mucins, evidenced by Alcian blue (pH 2.5) staining. The surrounding stroma infiltrates into the neoplastic nests, among the myoepithelial cells, forming irregular spaces called pseudolumina. Pseudolumina are filled with stromal matrix including stromal cells and basal membrane, and they often contain small capillaries and fibroblasts. Rare cases can present with sebaceous or squamous differentiation {2058}. Classic AdCC lacks marked nuclear atypia and necrosis, and the number of mitoses is very low. Perineural invasion may occasionally be present. An in situ component is rarely seen. Although these tumours are typically circumscribed grossly, the periphery of the neoplasm may be highly infiltrative, making it difficult to assess resection margins.

Immunohistochemistry is useful to confirm the different cell types. Epithelial cells are consistently positive for the low-molecular-weight cytokeratins CK7 and CK8, as well as for EMA. In some cases, the luminal cells are positive for CK5/6 {1446}. Myoepithelial cells are demonstrated with CK14, CK5/6, and p63 {1313}. The myoepithelial cell component can be additionally positive for myoepithelial markers (heavy-chain myosin, calponin, S100, and CD10). KIT (CD117) is usually strongly positive in the luminal component of AdCC, and it is sometimes used to differentiate AdCC from other breast tumours; however, it is important to remember that focal KIT positivity can be present in numerous other breast tumours, including adenomyoepithelioma {898}. Stains for the basement membrane antigens collagen IV and laminin decorate the pseudolumina.

The tubular component of classic AdCC should be differentiated from microglandular adenosis and tubular carcinoma {665}. In contrast to microglandular adenosis and tubular

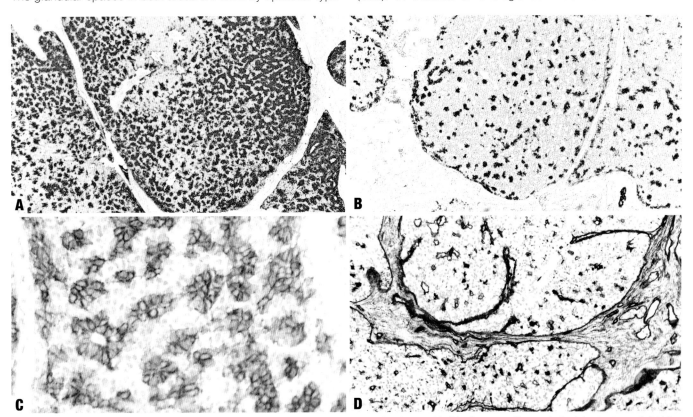

**Fig. 2.140** Adenoid cystic carcinoma. **A** CK7 highlights the epithelial component. **B** CK14 is positive in myoepithelial cells, arranged in pseudoglandular structures. **C** At higher power, KIT (CD117) is mainly positive in epithelial cells. **D** Collagen IV staining highlights pseudolumina inside the neoplastic nests.

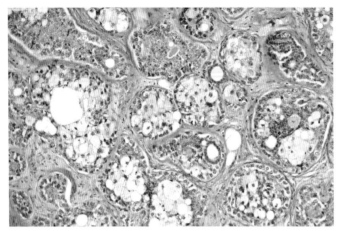

**Fig. 2.141** Adenoid cystic carcinoma. An example with sebaceous differentiation.

carcinoma, AdCC is composed of different cell types (epithelial and myoepithelial). In addition, the tubules contain mucins and basement membrane material. Tubular carcinoma shows strong positivity for ER and PR. Similarly, the cribriform areas of AdCC can raise suspicion for an invasive cribriform carcinoma, but this diagnosis can be excluded on the basis of the multilineage cellular composition of AdCC and ER and PR immunostaining, which is strongly and diffusely positive in cribriform carcinoma and negative in the vast majority of AdCCs. AdCC should also be differentiated from collagenous spherulosis, which only seldom forms a mass lesion and is characterized by basement membrane material–filled spaces in benign intraductal proliferations, such as usual duct hyperplasia. KIT and MYB immunostaining is typically negative or weak and focal in collagenous spherulosis {1686,1665}.

**SB-AdCC:** This subtype was described in 2002 by Shin and Rosen {1926}. In addition to the classic features of AdCC, SB-AdCC is characterized by solid nests composed of basaloid cells, with marked nuclear atypia, high mitotic count, and necrosis. Perineural invasion is a frequent finding in this subtype. SB-AdCC should be differentiated from carcinomas with basaloid morphology and small cell neuroendocrine carcinoma (SCNEC). Differential diagnosis, which can be difficult because these lesions share similar morphological features, is based on the finding of typical AdCC areas. Negativity for neuroendocrine markers can help to exclude neuroendocrine carcinoma (NEC).

**AdCC with high-grade transformation:** This subtype has been well delineated in the salivary glands {1887}. In the breast, rare cases of AdCC associated with high-grade carcinomas have been described. Specifically, cases of AdCC showing multiple areas of differentiation {1522}, small cell carcinoma {260}, invasive ductal carcinoma {1763}, and malignant adenomyoepithelioma {2315} are on record. In a case of AdCC described in association with an invasive ductal carcinoma (i.e. invasive breast carcinoma of no special type [NST]), similar molecular alterations were shared by the two components; in addition, mitochondrial DNA analysis demonstrated a clonal relationship between the two components, suggesting that AdCC neoplastic cells can acquire aggressive potential {1763}.

## Cytology

Preoperative diagnosis based on FNA can be difficult. FNA smears are moderately to highly cellular; the different cell types (i.e. basaloid, myoepithelial, and epithelial cells) should be recognized. In addition, hyaline cylinders are present, and these are larger and rounder than the hyaline material seen in FNA specimens from complex sclerosing lesions and collagenous spherulosis. Differential diagnosis with collagenous spherulosis can be difficult. Immunohistochemical KIT staining on cell blocks may be used to avoid misdiagnosis {1679,916}.

## Diagnostic molecular pathology

Breast AdCC usually lacks ER and PR positivity and *ERBB2* (*HER2*) amplification; it is therefore included in the group of triple-negative tumours of low malignant potential {666,718}. Focal ER and PR positivity can be seen in a minority of classic AdCC cases {83,718}. Positivity is most probably localized in the epithelial cell component.

## Essential and desirable diagnostic criteria

*Essential:* an invasive carcinoma with neoplastic cells arranged in tubular, cribriform, and solid patterns, composed of different cell types (epithelial and myoepithelial); glandular lumina filled with epithelial mucins and pseudolumina filled with stromal matrix, basal lamina, and fibroblasts.

*Desirable:* immunohistochemistry to confirm the presence of different cell types.

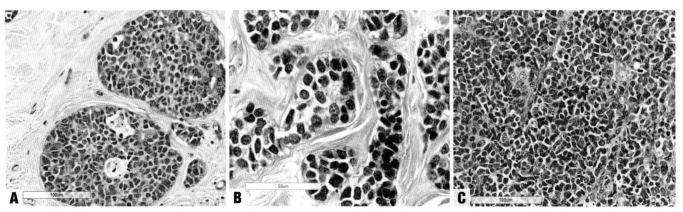

**Fig. 2.142** Adenoid cystic carcinoma, solid-basaloid subtype. **A** Focal features of adenoid cystic carcinoma are present, but the neoplastic cells are basaloid, with marked nuclear atypia. **B** At higher magnification. **C** Solid nests composed of basaloid cells, with marked nuclear atypia.

## Staging

AdCC is staged according to the criteria adopted for other types of invasive breast carcinomas.

## Prognosis and prediction

The prognostic impact of histological grade in breast AdCC has been debated, with conflicting results in the literature {1110,1769}. Histological subtype should be considered a prognostic indicator.

**Classic AdCC:** Despite the triple-negative phenotype, the classic subtype usually shows favourable behaviour. Regional and distant metastases are rare, and radical surgical excision is usually curative. In rare cases, focal positivity for ER and PR has been described {83,718}, but the therapeutic significance of this positivity is unknown. Classic AdCC constitutes the vast majority of breast AdCC and is included in large patient cohorts. It usually presents at an earlier stage, with a low rate of axillary involvement {326,718,1074}. Long-term follow-up has revealed higher survival rates than with invasive breast carcinoma NST {718,1074} in all but one study {326}. Therefore, most classic AdCCs can be cured with radical surgery alone {746}.

**SB-AdCC:** Axillary node metastases and perineural invasion can frequently be observed {442,670,690,1926}. In cases with long-term follow-up information, patients have developed local recurrences and distant metastases to lung, bone, and skin {442,670}. Patients with the basaloid subtype may survive for an extended period despite the presence of lung metastases. Scant data are available on SB-AdCC treatment. Patients with recurrent cases treated with adjuvant chemotherapy were alive and free of tumour at last follow-up {670}.

**AdCC with high-grade transformation:** These are very rare cases, most of which lead to the patient's death. Because of the small number of reported cases and the wide variety of features observed in the high-grade component, conclusions cannot be drawn about the optimal treatment strategy.

# Secretory carcinoma

Krings G
Chen YY
Sorensen PHB
Yang WT

## Definition

Secretory carcinoma is an invasive carcinoma composed of epithelial cells with intracytoplasmic secretory vacuoles and extracellular eosinophilic, bubbly secretions, arranged in a variable architecture and frequently associated with *ETV6-NTRK3* fusion.

## ICD-O coding

8502/3 Secretory carcinoma

## ICD-11 coding

2C60 & XH44J4 Carcinoma of breast, specialized type & Secretory carcinoma of breast

## Related terminology

*Not recommended:* juvenile breast carcinoma {1334}.

## Subtype(s)

None

## Localization

In women, most secretory carcinomas arise near the nipple or in the upper-outer quadrant, but any region of the breast may be involved, including ectopic breast tissue {1334,2059,1927,1177, 1063}. In men and children, most secretory carcinomas arise in the subareolar region {1334,1177,1063}.

## Clinical features

Secretory carcinoma typically presents as a slow-growing, firm, painless, mobile mass, sometimes with nipple discharge {2059, 1177}. The radiographical features of a circumscribed lobulated mass may mimic those of benign lesions such as fibroadenoma {1428}.

## Epidemiology

Secretory carcinomas account for < 0.05% of all invasive mammary carcinomas and occur predominantly in women {876,

206}. Although initially described in children, secretory carcinomas mostly occur in adults, with a mean patient age of 53 years {876}; most cases present between the fourth and seventh decades of life (range: 3–87 years) {1334,2059,1177,1063,475, 503,515,1092,1528,1790}.

## Etiology

Unknown

## Pathogenesis

Secretory carcinomas are characterized by a t(12;15)(p13;q25) translocation, which results in an *ETV6-NTRK3* fusion gene that is present in the in situ and invasive components, indicating that this is an early event in tumorigenesis {1063,1092,2088}. Among the breast carcinomas, *ETV6-NTRK3* is specific for secretory carcinoma {1279}. *ETV6-NTRK3*, which was initially identified in congenital fibrosarcoma {1028} and cellular mesoblastic nephroma {1027}, encodes a constitutively activated chimeric tyrosine kinase that signals through the RAS-MAPK and PI3K pathways to drive cellular transformation and oncogenesis {2087}. *ETV6-NTRK3* has also been identified in mammary analogue secretory carcinomas arising in other sites, such as the salivary glands, thyroid, and skin {176,526,1957}. The shared morphological, immunophenotypic, and genetic features of secretory breast carcinomas with analogous tumours at other sites suggest a common pathogenetic origin irrespective of location for these lesions. Notably, ETV6-NTRK3 expression has also been documented in other tumour types, including thyroid papillary carcinoma, leukaemia, glioma, and other carcinomas {374}. This fusion is therefore unique in being expressed in tumours derived across multiple cell lineages. Other than this alteration, these tumours are relatively quiet genomically, with very low mutation burdens and only occasional chromosomal gains and losses {1063}.

## Macroscopic appearance

Secretory carcinomas are typically solitary, firm, circumscribed masses with greyish-white or yellowish-tan cut surfaces. Multifocal tumours have been described {475,503}. The mean tumour size is about 2 cm, but size ranges from 0.5 to 16 cm {2059,1177, 1063,475,503,515,1092,1528,1058}.

## Histopathology

Secretory carcinomas are composed of polygonal tumour cells with eosinophilic granular or vacuolated cytoplasm and round to oval nuclei arranged in microcystic/honeycomb, solid, tubular, or papillary growth patterns. Microcystic areas can simulate thyroid follicles and may merge to form small solid sheets. Most tumours show mixed patterns. Intracytoplasmic and extracellular eosinophilic or amphophilic secretions are consistently present and stain positively with PAS, mucicarmine, and Alcian blue. Nuclear pleomorphism is almost always mild or moderate,

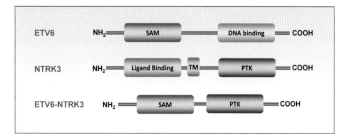

**Fig. 2.143** The ETV6-NTRK3 chimeric tyrosine kinase of secretory carcinoma. This fusion combines the sterile alpha motif dimerization domain (SAM) of the ETV6 DNA-binding domain with the protein tyrosine kinase domain (PTK) of the transmembrane (TM) NTRK3 tyrosine kinase, generating a ligand-independent constitutively active chimeric tyrosine kinase.

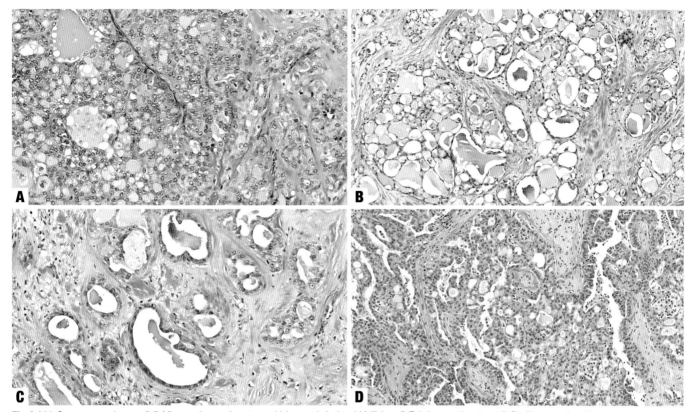

**Fig. 2.144** Secretory carcinoma. **A,B** Microcystic growth pattern, which can mimic thyroid follicles. **C** Tubular growth pattern. **D** Papillary growth pattern.

and mitotic activity is low. The vast majority of secretory carcinomas are therefore grade 1 or 2 by modified Nottingham grading, with high-grade tumours being exceptionally rare {475}. The tumour stroma is often sclerotic. An in situ component may be present; it is typically cribriform or solid with low or intermediate nuclear grade {1063,503,1092} and may be identified with the use of myoepithelial antigens.

Immunohistochemically, the tumour cells typically express CEA (polyclonal), S100, mammaglobin, SOX10, and MUC4, often in a strong and diffuse pattern {1177,1063,475,1092, 1790}. Most tumours express the basal markers CK5/6 and/ or EGFR (HER1), although this expression may be focal {1063, 1092}. GATA3, CK8/18, KIT (CD117), and vimentin may also be positive. Most cases are triple-negative for ER, PR, and ERBB2 (HER2), but weak ER/PR expression is not uncommon {1063, 475,1092}. The Ki-67 proliferation index is variable but often < 20% {1177,475,503}.

The differential diagnosis may include carcinoma with apocrine differentiation (usually AR-positive), acinic cell carcinoma {1746}, cystic hypersecretory carcinoma in situ {441}, and tall cell carcinoma with reversed polarity {342}, especially in limited biopsy material. Documentation of *ETV6-NTRK3* fusion can be used to support the diagnosis of secretory carcinoma, as needed.

## Cytology

FNA specimens are typically cellular and composed of cohesive sheets or groups of uniform tumour cells with granular or vacuolated cytoplasm, rounded nuclei with homogeneous chromatin, and few mitoses. Large intracytoplasmic vacuoles with proteinaceous material are characteristic, and similar material may be seen in the background. Signet-ring–like cells may be present {29,1496}.

## Diagnostic molecular pathology

Secretory carcinoma is characterized by pathognomonic *ETV6-NTRK3* gene fusion {2088}. Small molecule inhibitors (larotrectinib and entrectinib) that target NTRK3 and other NTRK family members have recently been developed and have shown promising efficacy in the treatment of patients with TRK fusion cancers {546,999}, including secretory breast carcinoma {1936}. This highlights the need for rapid and reliable molecular confirmation of *ETV6-NTRK3*, which has routinely been achieved by RT-PCR using *ETV6* and *NTRK3* primers,

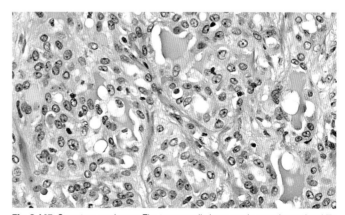

**Fig. 2.145** Secretory carcinoma. The tumour cells have ample granular eosinophilic or vacuolated cytoplasm and mild to moderate nuclear atypia. Extracellular secretions are present.

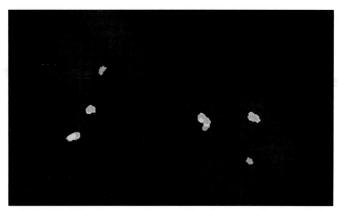

**Fig. 2.146** Secretory carcinoma. *ETV6* rearrangement can be confirmed by FISH using an *ETV6* break-apart probe. Orange: 5′ *ETV6* probe (telomeric); green: 3′ *ETV6* probe (centromeric); yellow: fused probes (normal).

including in formalin-fixed, paraffin-embedded tumour blocks {215}, and by FISH using either *ETV6* break-apart probes or 5′ *ETV6* and 3′ *NTRK3* convergence probes {1279}. The use of a pan-TRK monoclonal antibody for immunohistochemistry identified NTRK (*NTRK1*, *NTRK2*, or *NTRK3*) fusions in 20 of 21 cases in one study {839} but was less effective in detecting fusions involving *NTRK3* in a second study {701}, indicating that more-reliable NTRK antibodies will be necessary in order for immunohistochemistry to be implemented as a biomarker for NTRK3 inhibitors in secretory breast carcinoma. Next-generation sequencing methods, including hybrid-based capture for multiple specific fusions {335}, RNA-based panel sequencing for specific expressed transcripts lacking introns {2359}, and

methods that integrate RNA sequencing with whole-genome or whole-exome sequencing {2349} are likely to be combined with immunohistochemistry for routine detection of *ETV6-NTRK3* for diagnostic and therapeutic assignment.

### Essential and desirable diagnostic criteria

*Essential:* characteristic morphological and immunophenotypic features as described, especially including intracytoplasmic and extracellular secretions and an either triple-negative or weakly ER/PR-positive immunoprofile.

*Desirable:* can be confirmed by FISH showing *ETV6* rearrangement or identification of *ETV6-NTRK3* by next-generation sequencing.

### Staging

Secretory carcinoma is staged according to the guidelines for invasive carcinomas of the breast. Most secretory carcinomas present as pT1 or pT2 tumours. Axillary metastases are reported in about 20–35% and typically involve no more than three nodes {2059,1177,1063,876,475}. Distant metastases are very rare {2059,475,1058,79,850}.

### Prognosis and prediction

Secretory carcinomas generally have an indolent clinical course, especially in children and young adults, and even in patients with axillary nodal metastases {1334,2059,876,1092}. Some tumours in older adults may be more aggressive and manifest with late recurrences {1058}. Only rare deaths have been reported {2059,475,1058,79}. In a population-based study, the 5-year and 10-year cause-specific survival rates were 94% and 91%, respectively {876}.

# Mucoepidermoid carcinoma

Foschini MP
Geyer FC
Marchiò C
Nishimura R

## Definition

Mucoepidermoid carcinoma (MEC) is an invasive carcinoma composed of mixed mucinous, intermediate (transitional), and squamoid neoplastic cells arranged in solid and cystic patterns.

## ICD-O coding

8430/3 Mucoepidermoid carcinoma

## ICD-11 coding

2C60 & XH1J36 Carcinoma of breast, specialized type & Mucoepidermoid carcinoma

## Related terminology

None

## Subtype(s)

None

## Localization

MEC can affect any breast quadrant; when arising in the retroareolar region, it can cause nipple discharge {668}.

## Clinical features

Breast MEC usually arises in adult women ranging in age from 29 to 80 years {129}. One case has been described as a secondary tumour in a patient treated for lymphoma.

## Epidemiology

MEC is quite frequent in the salivary glands, but it rarely affects the breast, with < 40 cases reported to date {129}.

## Etiology

Unknown

## Pathogenesis

Unknown

## Macroscopic appearance

MEC can present as a solid nodule or a cystic lesion. The reported size ranges from 0.6 to 11 cm {129}.

## Histopathology

Similarly to its salivary gland counterpart, breast MEC can show

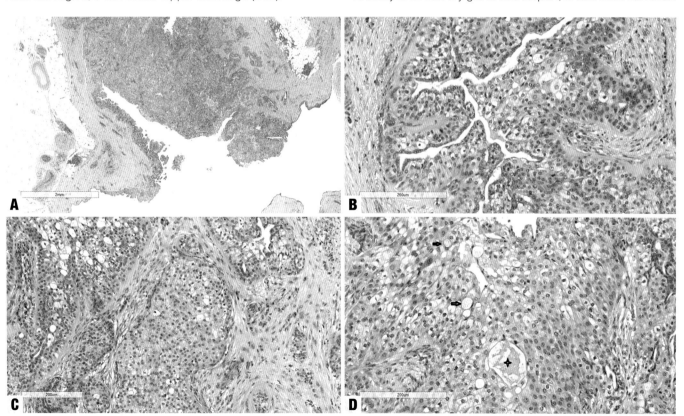

**Fig. 2.147** Mucoepidermoid carcinoma. **A** Low-grade mucoepidermoid carcinoma with polypoid and solid growth. **B** At higher power, the different cell types can be seen. Note that true keratinization is absent. **C,D** Mucoepidermoid carcinoma is composed of eosinophilic cells with epidermoid appearance, but true keratinization with squamous pearls is absent (arrows in panel D); the star in panel D indicates mucin-filled glandular structures.

a wide range of histological features, spanning from low-grade to high-grade lesions {129,499,668}. Grading can be performed by applying the salivary gland or the breast grading systems, with similar results {499}. Low-grade MEC more frequently shows a cystic component. Cystic spaces are lined by mucous cells intermingled with eosinophilic cells. Solid areas show neoplastic cell nests with a peripheral layer of basaloid cells gradually merging in groups of epidermoid cells and mucous cells. High-grade MECs are more frequently solid, and they show the same cell composition as their low-grade counterparts. In high-grade MEC, cytological atypia is present, mitotic figures are numerous, and necrosis can be present. Intermediate-grade breast MEC has been occasionally reported {499}. An intraductal component can be present {499,1585}. True keratinization with squamous pearl formation is not a feature of MEC of either low or high grade.

Immunohistochemistry is helpful in identifying the different cell types. Specifically, high-molecular-weight cytokeratins (e.g. CK14) and p63 stain basaloid and epidermoid cells, whereas low-molecular-weight cytokeratins (e.g. CK7) stain the mucous cells {499,1247,1585}. This gives rise to a peculiar zoning pattern of positivity similar to that observed in MEC of the salivary glands {499,667}. Breast MECs retain the GATA3 and mammaglobin positivity observed in other breast tumours {133}.

## Cytology
The cytological features have rarely been reported, but they seem to be similar to those observed in the corresponding salivary gland lesions; FNA specimens can show cells with abundant eosinophilic cytoplasm intermixed with mucinous and basaloid cells. In addition, mucous material can be present in the background. Diagnosis can be difficult when salivary gland–like tumours are not considered {870}.

## Diagnostic molecular pathology
Almost all reported breast MECs have been included among the triple-negative breast carcinomas, lacking ER and PR expression and ERBB2 (HER2) amplification. Recently ER, PR, and

AR positivity was described in a subpopulation of the neoplastic cells {336,133} of low- and intermediate-grade breast MEC. Few data have been reported on the molecular features of breast MEC. The t(11;19)(q21;p13) translocation, resulting in fusion of CRTC1 (MECT1) and MAML2 and considered typical of low-grade salivary gland MEC {1251,975}, has been investigated in two cases of breast MEC, which harboured partial deletion of 11q21 (MAML2) {273} and CRTC1-MAML2 fusion, respectively {133}.

## Essential and desirable diagnostic criteria
Essential: presence of basaloid, epidermoid, and mucous cells; absence of true keratinization.

## Staging
MEC is staged according to the criteria adopted for other types of breast carcinomas.

## Prognosis and prediction
Grading is the most important histopathological prognostic factor for breast MEC. Grading can be performed using the criteria usually applied to breast cancer, as well as those for MEC of the salivary glands {499,129,133}; both grading systems are based on architecture, cellular atypia, and mitotic count. Similar to its salivary gland counterpart {580}, high-grade MEC of the breast shows solid architecture, nuclear anaplasia, and a high mitotic count, often associated with necrosis and lymphovascular infiltration {129}.

According to a recent review of the literature {129} based on 26 cases with follow-up information, none of the low- or intermediate-grade MECs led to the patient's death. Only one case among the low-grade MECs recurred as high-grade disease, but the patient was alive and well 156 months later {2085}. One recent case of low-grade MEC was reported to show metastatic deposits in 3 of 18 axillary nodes, but the patient was alive and well 156 months after surgery {336}. In contrast, all high-grade MECs showing axillary and/or distant metastases lead to the patient's death {129}.

# Polymorphous adenocarcinoma

Foschini MP
Fox SB
Geyer FC

Marchiò C
McHugh JB
Nishimura R

## Definition
Polymorphous adenocarcinoma (PmA) of the breast is an infiltrative malignant epithelial neoplasm with histological features similar to those of PmA of the salivary glands, composed of a proliferation of monotonous neoplastic cells demonstrating architectural diversity, arranged in a variety of patterns including large nests surrounded by cords and single files (single-cell infiltration).

## ICD-O coding
8525/3 Polymorphous adenocarcinoma

## ICD-11 coding
2C60 & XH5SD5 Carcinoma of breast, specialized type & Polymorphous low-grade adenocarcinoma

## Related terminology
Not recommended: polymorphous low-grade adenocarcinoma.

## Subtype(s)
Unknown

## Localization
PmA arises in the breast parenchyma, with no site predilection.

## Clinical features
All three of the reported cases presented as palpable nodules affecting adult women aged 37–74 years.

## Epidemiology
PmA was originally described in the salivary glands, with a special predilection for the minor salivary glands. Only three cases of breast PmA have been reported to date {88}. Therefore, exact data on epidemiology are unavailable.

## Etiology
Unknown

## Pathogenesis
Unknown

## Macroscopic appearance
PmA presents as parenchymal nodules ranging in size from 1.5 to 4 cm.

## Histopathology
At low-power view, PmA is typically composed of a central, large, solid area surrounded by thin strands and cribriform nests of neoplastic cells. The neoplastic cells, which are uniformly small and round, harbour centrally located nucleoli with imperceptible nuclei and a thin rim of pale eosinophilic cytoplasm. Atypical mitotic figures can be detected, whereas coagulation necrosis was not present in the reported cases.

Immunohistochemistry revealed that the neoplastic cells were positive for BCL2. CK7 was only focally positive, and E-cadherin was weakly and partially positive around the cytoplasmic membrane. PmA is negative for ER, PR, and ERBB2 (HER2), with no evidence of ERBB2 amplification.

PmA should be differentiated from invasive lobular carcinoma and adenoid cystic carcinoma. PmAs were weakly and focally positive for CK7, markedly positive for BCL2, and negative for ER and PR, in contrast to invasive lobular carcinoma. PmA does not usually have the typical biphasic cellular pattern detected in adenoid cystic carcinoma. PmA is composed of a single cell type, with an absence of myoepithelial and basaloid cells.

## Cytology
Not clinically relevant

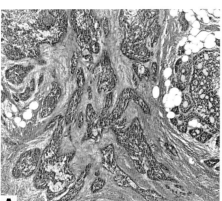 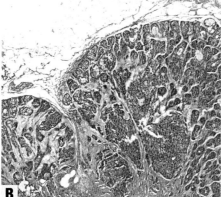 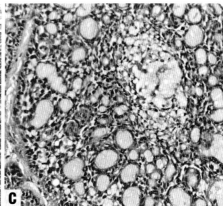

**Fig. 2.148** Polymorphous adenocarcinoma. **A** At low-power view, polymorphous adenocarcinoma is composed of solid cell nests. **B** The more-solid areas are located at the centre of the tumour. **C** This area resembles adenoid cystic carcinoma; however, in polymorphous adenocarcinoma only one cell type is present.

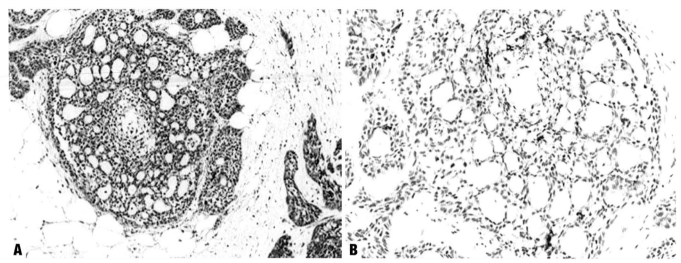

**Fig. 2.149** Polymorphous adenocarcinoma. **A** BCL2 is diffusely positive. **B** CK7 is only focally and weakly positive.

## Diagnostic molecular pathology

PmA is negative for ER, PR, and HER2, with no evidence of *ERBB2* amplification.

## Essential and desirable diagnostic criteria

*Essential:* typical architectural pattern composed of a centrally located large solid area surrounded by thin strands of uniform and monotonous neoplastic cells.

*Desirable:* focal and weak immunopositivity for CK7 and E-cadherin; negative ER, PR, and HER2.

## Staging

PmA is staged according to the criteria adopted for other types of invasive breast carcinomas.

## Prognosis and prediction

The data reported to date have been insufficient to support definitive conclusions about this tumour, but 1 of the 3 cases reported {88} had widespread metastases resulting in the patient's death 3 years after diagnosis. Therefore, as reported for similar neoplasms arising in the salivary glands {2268}, the term "low-grade" should not be used for this breast tumour.

# Tall cell carcinoma with reversed polarity

Yang WT
Bu H
Foschini MP
Schnitt SJ

## Definition
Tall cell carcinoma with reversed polarity (TCCRP) is a rare subtype of invasive breast carcinoma characterized by tall columnar cells with reversed nuclear polarity, arranged in solid and solid papillary patterns, most commonly associated with *IDH2* p.Arg172 hotspot mutations.

## ICD-O coding
8509/3 Tall cell carcinoma with reversed polarity

## ICD-11 coding
2C6Y Other specified malignant neoplasms of breast

## Related terminology
*Not recommended:* solid papillary carcinoma with reverse polarity; breast tumour resembling the tall cell variant of papillary thyroid carcinoma; solid papillary carcinoma resembling the tall cell variant of papillary thyroid carcinoma.

## Subtype(s)
None

## Localization
There is no specific predilection for location in the breast.

## Clinical features
These tumours present as a mammographic or palpable mass. Ultrasonography reveals a hypoechoic mass with or without posterior shadowing {310,1309}. Axillary lymph node metastases have been reported in 3 patients {274,2095,664,2097}.

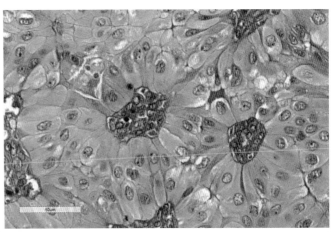

**Fig. 2.150** Tall cell carcinoma with reversed polarity. High-power view showing typical tall cells with characteristic nuclei.

## Epidemiology
No specific epidemiological data are currently available. All of the reported patients are women, with a mean age of 64 years (range: 39–89 years) {664,47,1243,2360}.

## Etiology
Unknown

## Pathogenesis
TCCRP is characterized by *IDH2* p.Arg172 hotspot mutations, which have been reported in about 84% (32 of 38) of the cases studied {161,47,1243,2360,342}. Hotspot mutations affecting

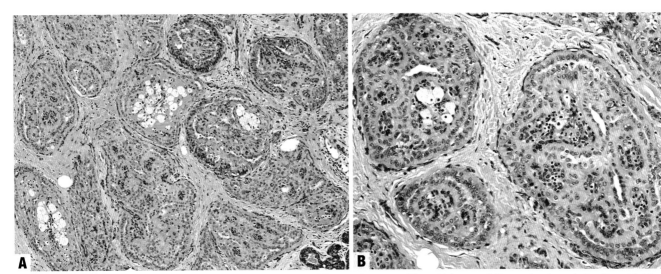

**Fig. 2.151** Tall cell carcinoma with reversed polarity. **A** Solid nests with central fibrovascular cores and foamy histiocytes. **B** Reversed nuclear polarity, with nuclei at the apical pole of the cells.

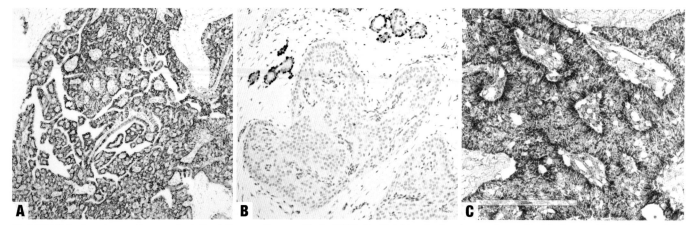

**Fig. 2.152** Tall cell carcinoma with reversed polarity. **A** Tumour cells are positive for CK5/6. **B** p63 staining showing absence of myoepithelial cells around the solid nests. **C** Immunohistochemical staining for antimitochondrial antigen demonstrates mitochondrial condensation at the basal poles of the cells.

*IDH2* have been described in glioma, acute myeloid leukaemia, chondrosarcoma, and cholangiocarcinoma, but they are extremely rare in breast carcinomas other than TCCRP {47, 342}. *PIK3CA* missense mutations have been identified in about 68% (26 of 38) of these tumours {161,47,1243,2360}, although mutations affecting PI3K pathway–related genes are quite common in breast cancer. There is no difference in the frequency of *PIK3CA* mutations in cases with and without *IDH2* mutations {161,47,1243,2360,342}. *BRAF* mutations and *RET*/PTC rearrangement, which are molecular features of papillary thyroid carcinoma, have been negative in the TCCRP cases studied {810}.

## Macroscopic appearance
TCCRP most often presents as a well-circumscribed, firm, white to grey mass {2095,381,47}. The tumours range in size from 0.6 to 5 cm, with a median size of 1.5 cm {664,47,1243,2360}.

## Histopathology
TCCRP is composed of circumscribed nests of epithelial cells, most often distributed in dense fibrous stroma. Many of the nests have delicate fibrovascular cores, imparting a solid papillary pattern. Foamy histiocytes are often present within the fibrovascular cores. True papillae and cystic structures containing colloid-like material can be observed in some cases. The neoplastic nests are surrounded by a thin rim of capillary vessels. The tumour cells are tall and columnar, with abundant eosinophilic cytoplasm. Most cases show bland, round to ovoid nuclei, with variable presence of nuclear grooves and intranuclear cytoplasmic inclusions {599A}. The most striking histological feature of TCCRP is the presence of nuclei at the apical rather than basal poles of the columnar epithelial cells. Mitotic figures are rare {664,47,2097,2360}. Although TCCRP shows some histological similarities to the tall cell variant of papillary thyroid carcinoma, immunohistochemical and molecular studies confirm the breast origin of this tumour {664,47,2097,2360}.

Most TCCRPs have a triple-negative phenotype, and the remaining cases show weak or focal hormone receptor expression {2095,342,664,1243,47,2360,2097}. Almost all reported cases are ERBB2 (HER2)-negative {664,47,1243,161}. The Ki-67 proliferation index is usually low (< 20%). These lesions characteristically express both low- and high-molecular-weight cytokeratins, as shown with CK7 and CK5/6 immunostaining, respectively. Chromogranin A and synaptophysin are consistently negative. Myoepithelial cells are not present around the tumour cell nests of TCCRP. In a study of 9 cases, all showed positive calretinin expression (with strong diffuse staining or focal staining) {47}. An origin in the breast is supported by variable staining for GCDFP-15, GATA3, and mammaglobin, along with a lack of staining for NKX2-1 (thyroid transcription factor 1) and thyroglobulin. Immunohistochemistry with antimitochondrial antigen shows condensation of mitochondria in the basal pole of the cells {664}.

## Cytology
Not clinically relevant

## Diagnostic molecular pathology
TCCRP frequently harbours *IDH2* p.Arg172 mutations {161,47, 1243,2360,342}.

## Essential and desirable diagnostic criteria
*Essential:* an invasive breast carcinoma with the neoplastic cell nests arranged in a predominantly solid papillary pattern, composed of columnar epithelial cells showing reversed polarity of the nuclei; absence of myoepithelial cells around the tumour nests.
*Desirable:* expression of both low- and high-molecular-weight cytokeratins; a triple-negative or weakly hormone receptor–positive phenotype.

## Staging
Cases should be staged according to the criteria for invasive breast carcinoma.

## Prognosis and prediction
TCCRP has an indolent clinical course, with a favourable prognosis. The majority of patients have been disease-free during the follow-up period (range: 3–132 months) {664,47,161,1663}. Only one case with aggressive clinical behaviour (bone metastases) has been reported {274}.

# Neuroendocrine neoplasms: Introduction

Rakha EA
Reis-Filho JS
Sasano H
Wu Y

Neuroendocrine differentiation in breast carcinomas was first described in mucinous carcinomas by Feyrter and Hartmann in 1963, as an invasive carcinoma morphologically similar to intestinal carcinoids based on positive silver staining. The first case series was published in 1977 under the term "primary carcinoid of the breast". Then the presence of neurosecretory granules was demonstrated using electron microscopy and modified silver staining, and these cases were referred to as argyrophilic carcinomas {98}. This was followed by demonstration of positive chromogranin A staining in 1985 {257}, which provided evidence of neuropeptide production in breast carcinomas. Neuroendocrine carcinoma (NEC) of the breast was endorsed as a distinct entity in the third edition of the WHO classification of tumours series – in the 2003 volume *Pathology and genetics of tumours of the breast and female genital organs* – and defined on the basis of the criteria of Sapino et al. {1842}. Neuroendocrine tumours (NETs) of the breast were defined as tumours of epithelial origin, with morphology similar to that of gastrointestinal and pulmonary NETs, expressing a neuroendocrine marker (specifically chromogranin or synaptophysin) in at least 50% of the total invasive tumour cell population.

In the 2012 fourth-edition volume *WHO classification of tumours of the breast*, NECs were included under the category "carcinomas with neuroendocrine features", and they were defined as tumours exhibiting morphological features similar to those of NETs of the gastrointestinal tract and lung and expressing neuroendocrine markers to any extent. In the fourth-edition volume, NETs in the breast were classified into two main categories: (1) "NETs, well-differentiated", which included low- and intermediate-grade tumours, and (2) "NECs, poorly differentiated / small cell carcinomas" – these neoplasms, based on the description, included small cell NEC (SCNEC) but not large cell NEC (LCNEC). This classification also acknowledged the existence of a third category, which comprised a subset of breast carcinomas with neuroendocrine differentiation as determined by histochemical and immunohistochemical analysis; this category included breast carcinoma of no special type (NST), as well as special types such as solid papillary carcinoma and the hypercellular subtype of mucinous carcinoma. Therefore, the distinction between NETs and grade 1 or 2 breast carcinomas of other types that show neuroendocrine differentiation was not clear. In a recent expert consensus statement by the International Agency for Research on Cancer (IARC) and WHO {1764}, it was proposed and agreed to adopt the term "neuroendocrine neoplasm (NEN)" as a term encompassing all tumour classes with predominant neuroendocrine differentiation, including both well-differentiated and poorly differentiated forms. Morphology and the expression of markers of neuroendocrine differentiation were recognized as key features defining these neoplasms at any specific anatomical site. A uniform classification framework for NENs at all anatomical locations was proposed in order to reduce inconsistencies and contradictions among the various systems currently in use. The key feature of that classification is the distinction between well-differentiated NETs and poorly differentiated NECs, as both share common expression of neuroendocrine markers. In the breast, NETs are malignant tumours by definition. It was acknowledged that NENs of the breast are rare and poorly defined. Apart from rare cases of small cell carcinoma, analogous to its pulmonary counterpart, the definition of NENs in the breast varies widely, resulting in variable incidence ranging from < 0.1% to as high as 20% {2215,1383, 188} depending on the different diagnostic criteria used. In fact, since NENs in the breast were first described, various definitions have been used and a variety of classification systems have been proposed. The overlap between NENs and other breast carcinomas showing neuroendocrine differentiation is marked, and some tumours (specifically solid papillary carcinomas and the hypercellular subtype of mucinous carcinoma) could fulfil the criteria for designation as mammary NEN. However, both of these lesions are distinct breast neoplasms that may express neuroendocrine markers, and they should not be classified as NET or NEC. Invasive carcinoma NST with neuroendocrine differentiation should be diagnosed if neuroendocrine histological features and neuroendocrine marker expression are not distinct or uniform enough to classify the tumour as a NEN. Expression of neuroendocrine markers is probably underrecognized in breast cancer, but because there is currently no clinical relevance of neuroendocrine differentiation as a standalone feature, routine staining of invasive breast carcinoma for neuroendocrine markers is not recommended. Therefore, refinement of the classification of NENs of the breast is needed in order to improve their diagnostic reproducibility, to define their clinical significance, and to follow the recent unified classification of NENs in other organs {1764}. Clinical syndromes related to hormone production are extremely rare in breast NENs, and the classic organoid features of carcinoid tumours of the lung and gastrointestinal tract (i.e. regular nests, ribbons, cords, and rosettes) are not features of primary NENs of the breast. In this volume, NENs of the breast are classified into NETs and NECs of small cell or large cell types.

Most NETs of the breast probably represent mixed NENs, with most cases showing a component of conventional-type mammary carcinoma. Similarly, the majority of primary SCNECs of the breast show a component of conventional-type mammary carcinoma {1922,1384}. If SCNEC makes up 10–90% of the tumour area, the terminology for mixed invasive (NST or other special type) and SCNEC may be used, and the NEC percentage should be reported. Cancers with < 10% NEN pattern should be classified as invasive NST or other types, with an option to describe the focal specialized neuroendocrine pattern in the report comment. Cancers with > 90% NEN pattern should be classified as NET or NEC.

# Neuroendocrine tumour

Rakha EA
Reis-Filho JS
Wu Y

## Definition

Neuroendocrine tumour (NET) is an invasive tumour characterized by low/intermediate-grade neuroendocrine morphology, supported by the presence of neurosecretory granules and a diffuse, uniform immunoreactivity for neuroendocrine markers.

## ICD-O coding

8240/3 Neuroendocrine tumour NOS
8240/3 Neuroendocrine tumour, grade 1
8249/3 Neuroendocrine tumour, grade 2

## ICD-11 coding

2C6Y & XH9LV8 Other specified malignant neoplasms of breast & Neuroendocrine tumour, grade 1

## Related terminology

*Not recommended:* endocrine carcinoma; carcinoid tumour of the breast.

## Subtype(s)

None

## Localization

No specific data are available.

## Clinical features

There are no notable or specific differences in presentation from other tumour types. NETs may present as an isolated hard breast lump with or without axillary lymphadenopathy. Clinical syndromes related to specific hormone production by breast NETs are not documented. Serological tests detecting circulating neuroendocrine markers such as chromogranin A are not sensitive or specific enough to identify breast NETs {733}.

## Epidemiology

NETs represent < 1% of breast carcinomas {1236,1174} and approximately 50% of cases designated as carcinomas with neuroendocrine differentiation as defined in the 2012 fourth-edition volume *WHO classification of tumours of the breast*. Most patients are in the sixth or seventh decade of life {1844,1842, 188}. Given that neuroendocrine markers are not routinely used in the diagnostic work-up of breast tumours with solid, alveolar, and nested patterns of growth, the true incidence is difficult to determine.

## Etiology

NETs are likely to have the same etiology as other ER-positive breast carcinomas.

## Pathogenesis

The histogenesis of primary NETs of the breast is not clearly defined. Unlike in other organs such as the lung, prostate, and gastroenteropancreatic system, neuroendocrine cells have not been consistently found in normal breast tissue, and neuroendocrine cell hyperplasia has not been identified as a precursor of neuroendocrine carcinoma (NEC). Cases of ductal carcinoma in situ with predominant neuroendocrine features have been described {412,2112}, either in the pure form or in association with an invasive component, suggesting a possible progression from in situ to invasive NET.

Primary NETs in the breast probably result from an early divergent differentiation of breast cancer stem cells into both

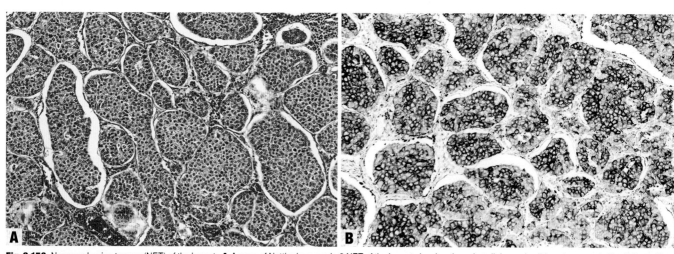

**Fig. 2.153** Neuroendocrine tumour (NET) of the breast. **A** A case of Nottingham grade 2 NET of the breast showing densely cellular and solid nests separated by delicate fibrovascular stroma (insular pattern). Cells are polygonal, with eosinophilic cytoplasm, and nuclei show moderate pleomorphism. Mitoses are rare. **B** The same case demonstrating diffuse positive staining for synaptophysin in tumour cells.

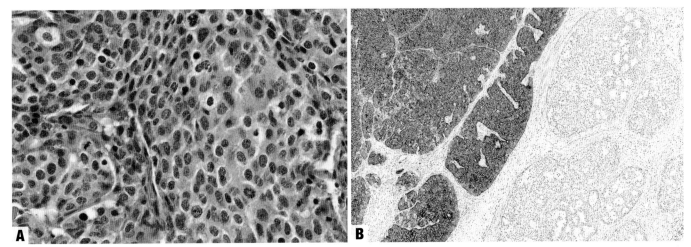

**Fig. 2.154** Neuroendocrine tumour (NET) of the breast. **A** Ovoid nuclei show typical salt-and-pepper chromatin, and mitoses are evident. **B** NET cells are widely and intensely positive for synaptophysin. Ductal carcinoma in situ at the periphery is negative.

neuroendocrine and epithelial lines. Prominent neuroendocrine differentiation is seen in distinct types of mammary carcinomas such as solid papillary carcinoma and the hypercellular subtype of mucinous carcinoma, and it is also seen in a proportion of in situ (neuroendocrine ductal carcinoma in situ) and invasive carcinomas of other histological types. Therefore, NETs probably have the same etiology as other ER-matched breast carcinomas. In addition, the transition from NET to NEC has not been reported in the breast, and NETs and NECs could develop according to different pathogenetic pathways as reported in pancreatic neuroendocrine neoplasm (PanNEN) {1764}.

The relevant gene expression studies have used genome-wide oligonucleotide microanalysis and demonstrated that solid papillary and mucinous carcinomas of the breast exhibiting neuroendocrine differentiation fall within the luminal A subgroup. No transcriptomic differences were identified between the subtypes of these tumours {2246}. NET has been reported to harbour somatic mutations affecting *PIK3CA* less frequently than ER-positive invasive breast carcinoma of no special type (NST). More frequently, they display mutations affecting chromatin-remodelling and transcription factor genes {1293}. In addition, genomic and transcriptomic similarities between NETs and mucinous carcinomas of the breast have been described {1293,1625}.

### Macroscopic appearance
NETs of the breast can grow as infiltrating or expansile tumours.

### Histopathology
NETs of the breast consist of densely cellular, solid nests and trabeculae of cells that vary from spindle cells to plasmacytoid cells to polygonal cells with eosinophilic and granular cytoplasm to large clear cells {1843} separated by delicate fibrovascular stroma. Papillary and insular patterns and alveolar-like structures may be seen {1843,2048}. The classic features of carcinoid tumours of the lung or NETs in the gastroenteropancreatic system (i.e. ribbons, cords, and rosettes) are not necessarily features of NET of the breast. In other organs, NETs are graded as G1, G2, or G3 on the basis of mitotic count and/or Ki-67 proliferation index and/or the presence of necrosis {1764}. Although this grading system is not applicable to NETs of the breast, the

number of mitoses remains the main parameter influencing grade {1843}. According to the Nottingham grading system, the majority of NETs should be G1 or G2.

Metastatic well-differentiated NETs (carcinoids) or moderately differentiated NECs, in particular those of lung or gastroenteropancreatic origin, should be excluded before making a definite diagnosis of primary NET of the breast. The presence of ductal carcinoma in situ, ER expression, axillary node metastasis, and the absence of a history of an extramammary primary neuroendocrine neoplasm (NEN) support the diagnosis of primary breast NET. Solid papillary carcinomas and the hypercellular subtype of mucinous carcinoma expressing neuroendocrine markers should not be classified as NETs, because they are distinct breast neoplasms. The distinction between well-differentiated NETs and grade 1 or 2 breast carcinomas of other histological types expressing neuroendocrine markers should be based on the presence and extent of histological features characteristic of neuroendocrine differentiation in the tumour.

Various types of dense-core granules, whose neurosecretory nature is confirmed by ultrastructural immunolocalization of chromogranin A, have been identified by electron microscopy in carcinomas with neuroendocrine differentiation {281}. The presence of clear vesicles of presynaptic type is correlated with the expression of synaptophysin.

### Cytology
FNA specimens show some features that can differentiate NETs from non-neuroendocrine breast carcinomas, but not from metastatic NETs to the breast. These features include cell clusters with rigid borders, single cells with a plasmacytoid appearance and peripheral cytoplasmic granules evident with Giemsa stain, and (importantly) immunoreactivity for synaptophysin and chromogranin A in addition to the positivity for ER {1841}.

### Diagnostic molecular pathology
Expression of chromogranin proteins and/or synaptophysin is the characteristic feature of NETs. About 50% of low- or intermediate-grade breast tumours with histological features indicative of neuroendocrine differentiation express chromogranin A

and only 16% express synaptophysin {1842}, but only tumours extensively expressing one or both of these markers should be diagnosed as NETs. ER and PR are expressed in the majority of tumour cells. NETs lack ERBB2 (HER2) expression and frequently express AR and GCDFP-15; the Ki-67 proliferation index is low {188,1843}. CD56 (NCAM) can be expressed, but the interpretation of staining may be challenging.

## Essential and desirable diagnostic criteria
*Essential:* histological features and immunoprofile characteristic of neuroendocrine differentiation; NETs are not high-grade neoplasms.
*Desirable:* coexisting ductal carcinoma in situ.

## Staging
NETs are graded according to the criteria for other types of invasive breast carcinoma.

## Prognosis and prediction
Tumour stage and histological grade, which encompass mitotic counts, are used as the main prognostic parameters. The prognostic relevance of neuroendocrine differentiation in breast carcinoma is still debated, because of the lack of specific criteria for its definition; therefore, several studies have been published with mixed results {918,1842}. Assessment of prognostic variables including mitotic count and Ki-67 proliferation index is used as a marker of aggressive behaviour, similar to in other breast carcinomas and not as a formally defined grading system for PanNENs. Unlike at most other sites, intratumoural coagulative necrosis is not used as a well-established prognostic factor in NETs of the breast.

There are no data from prospective clinical trials on the optimal management of NETs of the breast, and these tumours are usually treated with the same strategy used for other types of invasive breast carcinoma. Therefore, outside of the context of the exceedingly rare NEC of the breast, neuroendocrine differentiation in breast neoplasms is not regarded to have specific therapeutic implications.

# Neuroendocrine carcinoma

Rakha EA
Reis-Filho JS
Wu Y

## Definition
Neuroendocrine carcinoma (NEC) is an invasive carcinoma characterized by high-grade neuroendocrine morphology (small cell or large cell), supported by the presence of neuro-secretory granules and a diffuse, uniform immunoreactivity for neuroendocrine markers.

## ICD-O coding
8246/3 Neuroendocrine carcinoma NOS
8041/3 Neuroendocrine carcinoma, small cell
8013/3 Neuroendocrine carcinoma, large cell

## ICD-11 coding
2C6Y & XH0U20 Other specified malignant neoplasms of breast & Neuroendocrine carcinoma NOS
2C6Y & XH9SY0 Other specified malignant neoplasms of breast & Small cell neuroendocrine carcinoma
2C6Y & XH0NL5 Other specified malignant neoplasms of breast & Large cell neuroendocrine carcinoma

## Related terminology
*Acceptable:* small cell carcinoma; large cell neuroendocrine carcinoma.
*Not recommended:* poorly differentiated neuroendocrine carcinoma.

## Subtype(s)
Small cell neuroendocrine carcinoma; large cell neuroendocrine carcinoma

## Localization
No specific data are available.

## Clinical features
There are no notable or specific differences in presentation from other high-grade breast carcinomas. Clinical syndromes related to hormone production are not documented. Patient age ranges from 43 to 70 years {13,1922}. Tumour size ranges from 1.3 to 5.0 cm (mean: 2.6 cm) {1922}. Approximately 40% of small cell carcinomas have nodal metastasis {822}. In three population-based studies of patients with primary small cell NECs (SCNECs) of the breast {822,2291,538}, 70–81% had localized disease (local or regional) and 19–30% had distant metastasis. Lymph node positivity was reported in 41% of the cases {822}.

## Epidemiology
Primary NECs of the breast are extremely rare. SCNECs account for approximately 0.1% of all breast cancers {822} and for 3–10% of extrapulmonary small cell carcinomas {2291,538, 773}. Large cell NECs (LCNECs) are extremely rare.

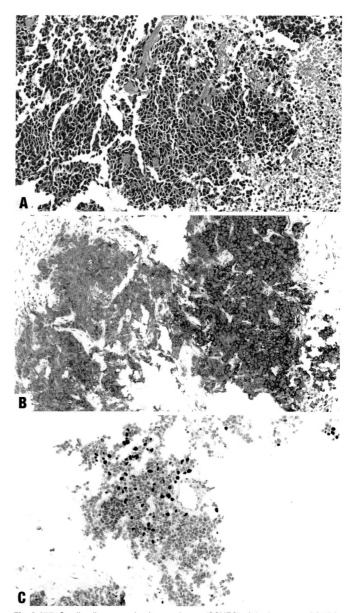

**Fig. 2.155** Small cell neuroendocrine carcinoma (SCNEC) of the breast. **A** SCNEC shows uniform small dark hyperchromatic cells with a high N:C ratio, scant cytoplasm, and necrosis. **B** Positive expression of synaptophysin. **C** Focal nuclear expression of TTF1 in primary SCNEC of the breast.

## Etiology
There are no data on the etiology of NECs, but they probably have the same etiology as other high-grade breast carcinomas. No link with cigarette smoking has been reported.

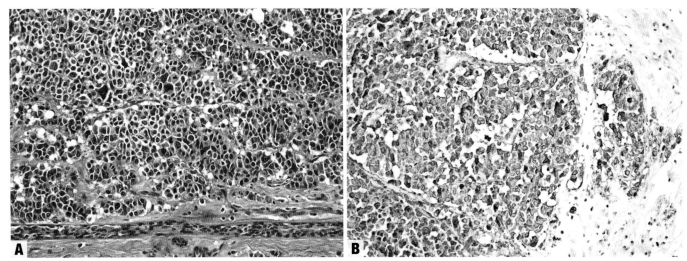

**Fig. 2.156** Large cell neuroendocrine carcinoma (LCNEC) of the breast. **A** Cells show evident cytoplasm and highly pleomorphic nuclei. **B** Chromogranin expression.

## Pathogenesis

Of the 9 SCNECs of the breast reported by Shin et al. {1922}, 3 cases were associated with invasive, poorly differentiated duct carcinoma, and ductal carcinoma in situ was seen in 7 tumours – 5 were of the small cell type in ducts and 2 were of the ductal type with high nuclear grade. These findings suggest that SCNECs result from a specific line of differentiation of mammary cancer stem cells towards neuroendocrine / small cell–type differentiation, which can take place at the in situ stage or later (at the invasive stage), rather than resulting from the malignant transformation of specific neuroendocrine cells in the normal breast tissue. In a way akin to lung SCNECs, breast SCNECs display *TP53* and *RB1* somatic genetic alterations in as many as 75% and 19% of cases, respectively {1331}. Data on the pathogenesis of LCNEC are lacking.

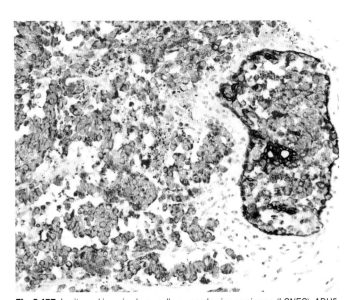

**Fig. 2.157** In situ and invasive large cell neuroendocrine carcinoma (LCNEC). ADH5, a rapid double immunostaining technique with a single cocktail of antibodies that simultaneously highlights myoepithelial cells (CK5/14 and/or p63, DAB staining) and luminal cells (CK7/CK18, Fast Red staining), highlights the carcinoma in situ associated with an LCNEC, proving the breast origin.

## Macroscopic appearance

Primary NECs have no gross features distinct from those of other types of high-grade breast cancer. They can present with poorly circumscribed, fleshy, white to tan cut surfaces and focal areas of necrosis.

## Histopathology

Histologically and immunohistochemically, NECs are morphologically indistinguishable from their counterparts in the lung {990,1749}. SCNECs display an infiltrative growth pattern and are composed of densely packed, fairly uniform, small, dark hyperchromatic cells that have a high N:C ratio, scant cytoplasm, inconspicuous nucleoli, and poorly defined cytoplasmic borders. In LCNEC, the cells show evident cytoplasm and highly pleomorphic nuclei with variably coarse chromatin. Common features of both SCNEC and LCNEC are high numbers of mitotic figures and focal areas of necrosis. An in situ component with the same cytological features may be detected. Lymphatic tumour emboli are frequently encountered {13,1922}.

The differential diagnoses of primary SCNEC include metastatic small cell carcinoma of non-mammary origin (most commonly from the lung), Merkel cell carcinoma, lymphoma, and melanoma. The presence of an associated ductal carcinoma in situ or conventional-type mammary carcinoma component confirms the primary nature of the tumour. SCNEC should also be differentiated from some forms of the high-grade solid subtype of adenoid cystic carcinoma, metaplastic carcinomas or ductal of no special type (NST) with basaloid cells and an increased N:C ratio. LCNEC should be differentiated from high-grade invasive breast carcinoma NST, by the presence of extensive neuroendocrine differentiation, and from metastatic LCNEC of non-mammary origin (i.e. from the lung).

## Cytology

FNA of SCNEC shows the presence of malignant cells with small cell phenotypes, which may display nuclear moulding, finely granular or salt-and-pepper chromatin, and scant delicate cytoplasm. Necrosis is frequently present in cytological samples of NEC.

## Diagnostic molecular pathology

Immunohistochemical analysis shows consistent staining for cytokeratin markers but variable staining for neuroendocrine markers, with more than two thirds of cases staining positively for chromogranin and synaptophysin. PGP9.5, CD56 (NCAM), and NSE are positive in the majority of cases. SCNECs are positive for BCL2 and negative for ERBB2 (HER2) {1922}. ER positivity has been reported in 30–50% of cases {1922,1331} and PR positivity in a smaller proportion, but other authors did not identify receptor expression in SCNEC {1816}. TTF1 expression in SCNEC of the breast has been reported, but not diffuse strong nuclear staining as seen in small cell carcinoma of the lung {352,595}. GATA3 expression has been reported in NEC of the breast but not in metastatic NECs, including those from the lung {1393}.

## Essential and desirable diagnostic criteria

*Essential:* histological features similar to those of SCNEC and LCNEC of the lung; high-grade tumour.
*Desirable:* coexisting ductal carcinoma in situ.

## Staging

NECs are staged similarly to other types of invasive breast carcinoma.

## Prognosis and prediction

SCNEC is significantly associated with a worse prognosis than other neuroendocrine tumours (NETs) of the breast {371}. The outcomes of patients with breast SCNEC were superior to those of patients with stage-matched small cell lung carcinoma, except in patients with distant disease {822}. It was reported that radiation therapy is not associated with a significant difference in survival for patients with either localized or regional disease {822}. Localized SCNEC is usually managed similarly to usual ductal breast cancer. In the metastatic SCNEC setting, regimens that are implemented in small cell lung cancer are usually attempted. There is some evidence that ER-positive SCNEC may respond to hormone therapy {35}. LCNECs of the breast are rare, and no clinical data on prognosis are available.

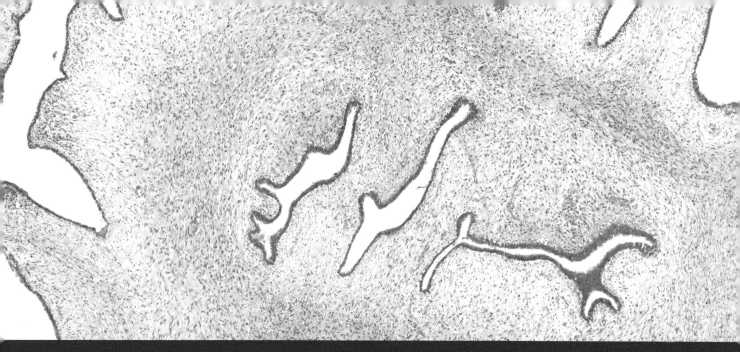

# 3

# Fibroepithelial tumours and hamartomas of the breast

Edited by: Tan PH

Hamartoma
Fibroadenoma
Phyllodes tumour

# WHO classification of fibroepithelial tumours and hamartomas of the breast

|         | Hamartoma |
|---------|-----------|
| 9010/0  | Fibroadenoma NOS |
| 9020/1  | Phyllodes tumour NOS |
|         |    Periductal stromal tumour |
| 9020/0  | Phyllodes tumour, benign |
| 9020/1  | Phyllodes tumour, borderline |
| 9020/3  | Phyllodes tumour, malignant |

These morphology codes are from the International Classification of Diseases for Oncology, third edition, second revision (ICD-O-3.2) {921}. Behaviour is coded /0 for benign tumours; /1 for unspecified, borderline, or uncertain behaviour; /2 for carcinoma in situ and grade III intraepithelial neoplasia; /3 for malignant tumours, primary site; and /6 for malignant tumours, metastatic site. Behaviour code /6 is not generally used by cancer registries.

This classification is modified from the previous WHO classification, taking into account changes in our understanding of these lesions.

Subtype labels are indented.

# Fibroepithelial tumours and hamartomas of the breast: Introduction

Tse G
Shin SJ
Val-Bernal JF

Mammary fibroepithelial tumours are biphasic neoplasms that exhibit proliferation of epithelial and stromal (mesenchymal) components. The spectrum of entities includes fibroadenomas (simple/conventional, cellular, and complex) and benign, borderline, and malignant phyllodes tumours, including periductal stromal tumour. Although hamartomas are not strictly fibroepithelial tumours, they are circumscribed lesions with lobular glands and fibroadipose stroma, with some resemblance to fibroepithelial tumours, and they are therefore discussed in this section.

Fibroepithelial tumours commonly present clinically as palpable, mobile, painless masses. Fibroadenomas occur in younger patients than phyllodes tumours, and they are generally smaller. Due to hormone sensitivity, fibroadenomas may show cyclical size change and may rarely be painful; they may also undergo a substantial increase in size during pregnancy and involute after menopause. Phyllodes tumours are often symptomatic due to their larger size and can grow rapidly over a short period of time. Hamartomas show wide age and size ranges, occurring any time after puberty. Clinically asymptomatic fibroadenomas, phyllodes tumours, and hamartomas can be detected radiologically. Fibroepithelial tumours typically appear as rounded, lobulated masses on mammography, and coarse calcifications may be observed in longstanding or involuting fibroadenomas. On ultrasonography, fibroepithelial tumours are often hypoechoic, with internal acoustic shadows being seen in phyllodes tumours. The imaging features of hamartomas are variable due to the mixture of fibrous, fatty, and glandular elements {460}.

The proliferation of the epithelial and stromal components of fibroepithelial tumours results in two histological patterns: intracanalicular, in which the compression of benign ductal elements by stroma leads to the formation of arciform slit-like, epithelium-lined luminal spaces, and pericanalicular, in which stroma grows around patent rounded tubules. These patterns often coexist and have no clinical significance. In phyllodes tumours, there is an exaggerated and accentuated intracanalicular growth pattern resulting in stromal fronds with leaf-like architecture, accompanied by stromal hypercellularity. The diagnosis of phyllodes tumour is based on the presence of expanded stromal fronds and stromal hypercellularity. Once a fibroepithelial lesion is deemed a phyllodes tumour, its grading as benign, borderline, or malignant is based on assessment of stromal characteristics – the degree of atypia and hypercellularity, mitotic activity, presence or absence of stromal overgrowth, and nature of tumour borders/contours (pushing or permeating) – and the presence of malignant heterologous elements. Because these stromal changes exist along a continuum, grade assignment is challenging, with reproducibility issues {2029}. Phyllodes tumours tend to recur locally, with malignant tumours potentially metastasizing and causing death. Some reports indicate that borderline tumours may also metastasize {2030}.

Periductal stromal tumours have histological similarities to phyllodes tumours, with the biphasic presence of hypercellular and variably atypical, mitotically active stroma hugging benign epithelium, but periductal stromal tumours do not show a distinct tumour outline or obvious fronded architecture. Instead, hypercellular stroma extends around benign epithelium of ducts and lobules in an irregular manner, between unaffected breast parenchyma. The subsequent occurrence of more-typical phyllodal patterns on recurrence suggests the close relationship and classification of periductal stromal tumour with phyllodes tumour {253,2269}. Therefore, this tumour is regarded as a subtype of phyllodes tumour.

Epithelial changes including usual ductal hyperplasia, atypical ductal hyperplasia, lobular neoplasia, and ductal carcinoma in situ can be encountered in fibroepithelial tumours {2038}. These changes are thought to occur by chance and to be unrelated pathogenetically to fibroepithelial tumorigenesis, especially in phyllodes tumours, where the stromal component is considered the biological driver of behaviour. Nevertheless, there is evidence of crosstalk between the epithelial and stromal compartments, particularly in phyllodes tumours, as exemplified by consistently higher periepithelial stromal mitotic activity {1852} and differential epithelial biomarker expression correlating to tumour grade {1855,2110}. Cytological assessment of fibroepithelial tumours was once routine, but its utility is limited by common pitfalls; therefore, preoperative core biopsies are now standard {2336,2117,1883}.

Immunohistochemistry, including for CD34 and p53 {860, 2039}, has shown variable expression among fibroepithelial tumours of different grades, potentially aiding diagnosis and grading, particularly in phyllodes tumours {980}. However, no immunohistochemical markers have proven clinical value in routine practice.

The concept that some phyllodes tumours may evolve from fibroadenoma is supported by molecular analysis {1072,865, 1655}. MED12 mutations are frequently found in all types of fibroepithelial tumours {2033}, with the MED12-mutant pathway likely to be involved in the progression of fibroadenoma to phyllodes tumour. Malignant phyllodes tumour may develop de novo through the acquisition of genetic alterations targeting other cancer genes {1601}.

Hamartomas are composed of sequestered collections of haphazardly arranged normal lobular structures, stroma, and adipose tissue (called breast in breast) {1904,2114}.

The mainstay of treatment of fibroepithelial lesions is surgery, although asymptomatic fibroadenomas may be left alone. Benign phyllodes tumours are usually excised to negative margins, but some studies suggest a low recurrence rate even if margins are positive {2031,408,1411}. For borderline and malignant phyllodes tumours, complete excision with negative margins is recommended {1014,349}. The role of adjuvant radiotherapy or chemotherapy in the treatment of malignant phyllodes tumour has not been established {2029}. Hamartomas are benign and do not require treatment.

# Hamartoma

Tse G
Koo JS
Thike AA

## Definition
A hamartoma is a well-demarcated, generally encapsulated mass composed of normal breast tissue components.

## ICD-O coding
None

## ICD-11 coding
None

## Related terminology
*Acceptable:* adenolipoma; chondrolipoma; myoid hamartoma.
*Not recommended:* fibroadenolipoma; adenolipofibroma.

## Subtype(s)
None

## Localization
There is no predilection for any breast quadrant for the development of hamartoma {847}.

## Clinical features
Hamartomas may present as soft palpable masses {847,2114} or are asymptomatic and detected by mammography {460,2205}. Imaging shows circumscribed rounded masses, sometimes with intralesional heterogeneous echogenicity on ultrasonography {177}. Owing to their well-defined borders, hamartomas are easily enucleated. Most hamartomas are sporadic; multiple hamartomas can be seen in Cowden syndrome {1878}.

## Epidemiology
Hamartomas account for < 5% of benign breast tumours {312, 1904}, occurring predominantly in women in their fifth decade of

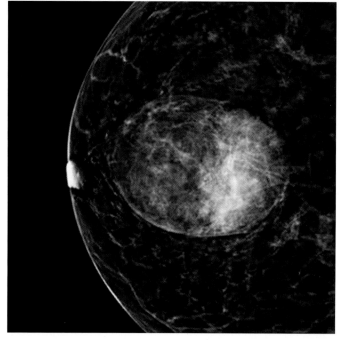

**Fig. 3.01** Hamartoma. Mammography shows a well-circumscribed mass with heterogeneous density.

life (ranging from 33.5 to 66.5 years) {1904}, although they can be found at any age.

## Etiology
Most hamartomas are sporadic, and the etiology is largely unclear, although weak evidence suggests hormonal influences {341,847}.

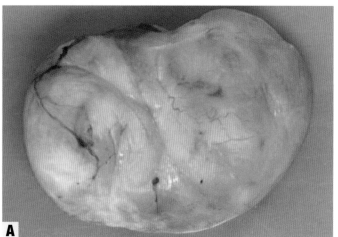
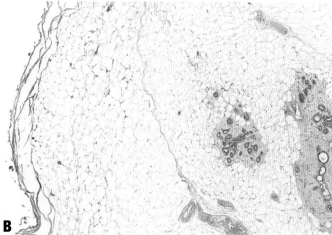

**Fig. 3.02** Breast hamartoma. **A** The gross appearance of a breast hamartoma (adenolipoma) shows a well-circumscribed adipose mass. **B** On histology, the lesion shows encapsulation by a thin fibrous layer, and it is composed of predominantly mature adipose tissue within which are benign breast lobules.

## Pathogenesis

Because some hamartomas are associated with molecular changes, different perspectives exist as to whether they are neoplasms or malformations. Genetic data are limited, but aberrations involving chromosomal regions 12q12-q15 and 6p21, as well as PTEN loss, have been described {438,1778,510}.

## Macroscopic appearance

Hamartomas are round or oval, measuring as much as 20 cm in diameter. The cut surface may resemble normal breast tissue, lipoma, or fibroadenoma.

## Histopathology

Generally encapsulated, hamartomas are lobulated and show ducts, lobules, and adipose tissue in varying proportions. Commonly there is prominent intralobular fibrosis, and the lobules have an atrophic appearance. Adipocytes may occur singly, and they are encased by dense fibrous tissue (encapsulated fat). Hamartomas may be called adenolipomas when features of normal ducts/lobules are mixed with adipose tissue {960}, myoid hamartomas when a smooth muscle component is prominent {454}, and chondrolipomas when chondroid islands exist within adipose tissue {1526}. When only limited material is available, as with core biopsy, the diagnosis may be suggested by taking into consideration the radiological and clinical findings {2114}.

## Cytology

The epithelial and stromal components of hamartomas show bland cytology. Cytological diagnosis is frequently limited by scant material and features overlapping with those of other benign lesions {2114,848}.

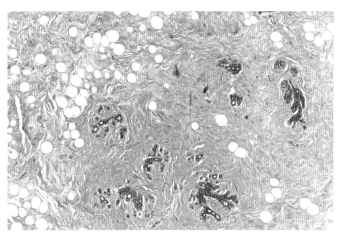

**Fig. 3.03** Hamartoma. Hamartoma shows breast tissue that is indistinguishable from normal breast parenchyma.

## Diagnostic molecular pathology

Not clinically relevant

## Essential and desirable diagnostic criteria

*Essential:* a mass lesion comprising components of normal breast tissue; correlation is required with clinical and imaging features.

## Staging

Not clinically relevant

## Prognosis and prediction

Hamartomas rarely recur. Reported recurrences probably represent incompletely excised lesions {460,309}.

# Fibroadenoma

Thike A A
Brogi E
Harada O
Oyama T
Tse G

## Definition
Fibroadenoma is a circumscribed benign neoplasm of the terminal duct lobular unit with biphasic proliferation of epithelial and stromal components.

## ICD-O coding
9010/0 Fibroadenoma NOS

## ICD-11 coding
2F30.5 & XH9HE2 Fibroadenoma of breast & Fibroadenoma NOS

## Related terminology
*Not recommended:* adenofibroma.

## Subtype(s)
None

## Localization
Fibroadenomas may occur in any region within the breast and may be multifocal and bilateral.

## Clinical features
Fibroadenomas usually present as painless, solitary, firm, slow-growing, mobile, well-defined nodules < 3 cm. Mammography shows nodular densities or calcified nodules. Multiple synchronous or metachronous fibroadenomas can be unilateral or bilateral. Symptomatic fibroadenomas are rare in older women. Giant (> 5 cm) fibroadenomas are uncommon, but may occasionally occur in adolescent girls, leading to distortion of the breast. Fibroadenomas may also develop in men with gynaecomastia {2124}. Juvenile fibroadenomas occur more commonly but not exclusively in adolescents; they can be large and grow rapidly {2240}.

## Epidemiology
Fibroadenomas are rare before menarche and are most common in adolescent girls and women aged < 35 years, except for complex fibroadenomas, which tend to occur about two decades later {1462,1958}. Juvenile fibroadenomas are relatively more common in young African-Americans {1800,621}.

## Etiology
Most fibroadenomas are sporadic. A small proportion of myxoid fibroadenomas occur in women with Carney complex {292}. Ciclosporin immunosuppression has been associated with the development of multiple large fibroadenomas in adolescent girls and young women {173,909,107,2047}; in this setting, the lesions stop growing or regress after therapy is switched to tacrolimus {909}.

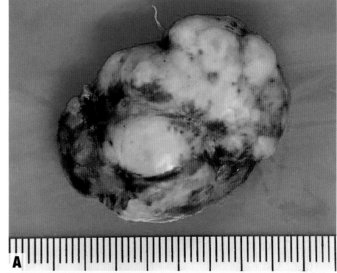

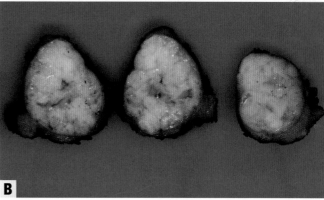

**Fig. 3.04** Fibroadenoma. **A** An excised fibroadenoma showing a smooth, lobulated yellow surface. The fibroadenoma is shelled out, with little adherent adjacent tissue. **B** The macroscopic appearance of a fibroadenoma reveals a circumscribed boundary with distinct separation from the adjacent adipose tissue. The cut surface shows whitish whorled fibrous tissue.

## Pathogenesis
Fibroadenomas are hormone-sensitive and may grow rapidly during pregnancy. The epithelium and stroma are non-clonal, but monoclonality has been demonstrated in areas of stromal expansion {1072}. Numerical abnormalities of chromosomes 16, 18, and 21 have been reported {119}, but no consistent aberrations are found {1230}.

Sequencing studies show that about 60% of fibroadenomas (except of the myxoid variety) harbour *MED12* mutations {1200, 1244} (mostly in codon 44 of exon 2 {1200,1657,1194,1385}), which are associated with dysregulated estrogen signalling and extracellular matrix organization {1200}. The spectrum of *MED12* mutations in fibroadenoma is nearly identical to that reported in uterine leiomyomas {1200}. *MED12* exon 2 mutations

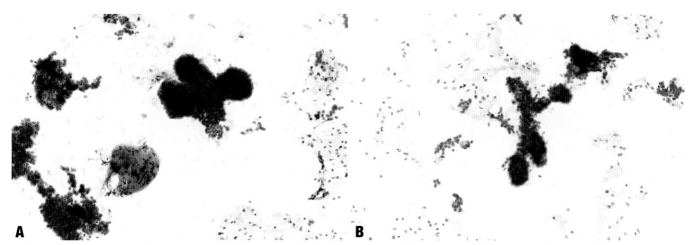

**Fig. 3.05** Fibroadenoma. **A** An FNA specimen showing fibroadenoma with benign branched epithelial fragments in small sheets. A stromal fragment is also seen. **B** Aspirate showing broad branching of the epithelium, resembling a staghorn, with bland-looking epithelial cells. The background shows naked bipolar nuclei.

are somatic and detected in stromal cells, whereas no *MED12* mutations are seen in the epithelial compartment {1200}. These mutations are more frequent in intracanalicular than pericanalicular fibroadenomas {1385}. Although some reports show that the frequency and pattern of *MED12* mutations in juvenile fibroadenomas are similar to those in conventional fibroadenomas {1194}, other authors have found a lower rate of *MED12* abnormalities in juvenile fibroadenoma, with additional differences in mutation spectrum {2063}.

Unlike in phyllodes tumour, cancer driver gene and *TERT* promoter mutations are rare in conventional and juvenile fibroadenomas {2063}. Apart from *MED12* mutations, *RARA* mutations, albeit at lower frequency, are also often found in phyllodes tumours and fibroadenomas. Mutations in other genes, such as *FLNA*, *SETD2*, *KMT2D* (*MLL2*), *BCOR*, *MAP3K1*, *NF1*, *RB1*, *PIK3CA*, *EGFR*, *TP53*, and *ERBB4*, are rare in fibroadenomas but can be found in phyllodes tumours {2033}. These genomic differences may be of potential clinical use in distinguishing fibroadenomas from phyllodes tumours.

Identical *MED12* mutations observed in fibroadenomas and phyllodes tumours from the same patient imply a clonal relationship between these two fibroepithelial lesions and suggest that some fibroadenomas may give rise to phyllodes tumours {1655, 1657}.

## Macroscopic appearance
Fibroadenomas are solid, ovoid, and well circumscribed, usually ≤ 3 cm. Sectioning reveals a uniform rubbery, lobulated, whorled, greyish-white cut surface with intervening slit-like spaces. A glistening surface or calcifications may be noticed.

## Histopathology
Fibroadenoma may show a pericanalicular pattern with stromal cells growing around open ducts in a circumferential fashion and/or an intracanalicular pattern with stromal compression of ducts into clefts. These patterns may be seen singly or in combination. The pericanalicular pattern is more common in juvenile fibroadenoma. The stromal component is usually of uniformly low cellularity and lacks atypia, but it may sometimes exhibit focal or diffuse hypercellularity (especially in women aged < 20 years), bizarre multinucleated giant cells, extensive

myxoid change {292,1244}, or hyalinization with dystrophic calcifications, and rarely ossification in postmenopausal women. Lipomatous, smooth muscle, and osteochondroid metaplasia may occur. Mitoses are uncommon but may be present in fibroadenomas in young or pregnant patients. Epithelial squamous and apocrine metaplasia, epithelial apical snouts, focal fibrocystic changes, sclerosing adenosis, usual ductal hyperplasia, and even extensive myoepithelial proliferation can occur {1073}. Atypical ductal/lobular hyperplasia and ductal/lobular carcinoma in situ may infrequently involve fibroadenomas {1073,1990}. When atypical hyperplasia is confined to the fibroadenoma, there is reportedly no increased subsequent cancer risk {295}. Invasive carcinoma may also involve fibroadenomas, often as a result of secondary involvement.

Juvenile fibroadenomas often show a pericanalicular growth pattern with a uniform mild to moderate increase in stromal cellularity, with stromal cells in fascicular arrangements and no substantial nuclear atypia, accompanied by usual ductal hyperplasia {2062,1800}, most commonly of gynaecomastoid type. Mitotic activity in the stromal component is usually low: < 2 mitoses per 10 high-power fields (< 1 mitosis/mm²) {1800,621}.

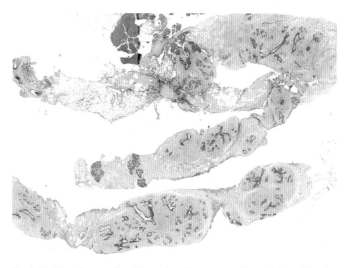

**Fig. 3.06** Fibroadenoma. Core biopsy shows tissue cores with a nodular proliferation of both the epithelial and stromal components.

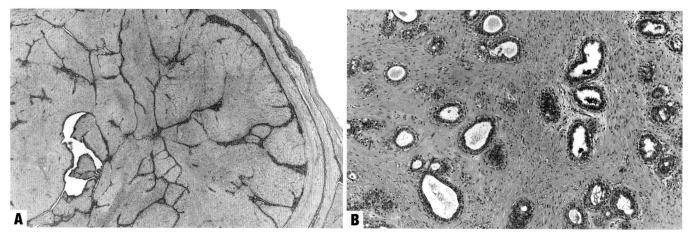

**Fig. 3.07** Fibroadenoma. **A** Predominantly intracanalicular pattern. Expansion of the stroma compresses the ductal element to form slit-like spaces. Note the rounded border. **B** Pericanalicular pattern, with stromal growth around patent ducts.

The diagnosis of fibroadenoma on core biopsy is reliable and accurate; however, the finding of a cellular fibroepithelial lesion on core biopsy may prompt consideration of phyllodes tumour. In such cases, surgical excision is usually advocated. A molecular test that may distinguish fibroadenoma from phyllodes tumour on core biopsy has been reported {2043}.

Complex fibroadenomas have one or more of the following features: cysts > 3 mm, sclerosing adenosis, epithelial calcifications, and papillary apocrine metaplasia {554}. They are present in 3–4% of benign breast biopsies {1462,966}, account for

16–23% of all fibroadenomas {554,1958}, and are smaller than other fibroadenomas {1958}. Complex fibroadenomas without atypia carry a slightly increased relative risk (2.27–3.1 times the risk in the general population) for developing subsequent breast carcinoma {1462,554,1958}.

Cellular fibroadenomas have a pericanalicular growth pattern, mildly to moderately increased stromal cellularity, and usually < 1 stromal mitosis/mm² (< 2 mitoses per 10 high-power fields), but they lack the following features: stromal nuclear atypia, exaggerated intracanalicular architecture, periductal

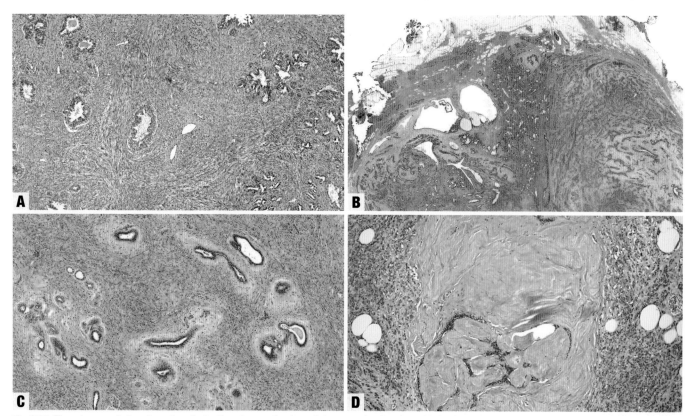

**Fig. 3.08** Fibroadenoma. **A** Juvenile pericanalicular fibroadenoma showing cellular stroma focally arranged in fascicles with slight nuclear crowding. The epithelial component shows moderate ductal hyperplasia. **B** Complex fibroadenoma showing several cysts > 3 mm in the stroma. **C** Cellular fibroadenoma showing expansion of the moderately cellular stroma. The stromal cells are devoid of nuclear atypia and mitotic activity. There is no stromal overgrowth. **D** Invasive carcinoma cells extend into the fibrotic stroma of a fibroadenoma.

subepithelial stromal condensation, and intratumoural heterogeneity {2029}.

Juvenile fibroadenomas are most common in adolescent girls or young women, and they can be very large, causing breast distortion. Stromal cellularity is mild to moderate, with fascicular arrangement and no substantial nuclear atypia. There is usually < 1 stromal mitosis/mm$^2$ (< 2 mitoses per 10 high-power fields) {2062,1800,621}. Usual ductal hyperplasia is common {2062, 1800}.

## Cytology

Cytological aspirates from fibroadenomas typically yield cellular sheets with antler- or staghorn-shaped epithelial clusters, with a clean background containing bipolar nuclei, giving an appearance of sesame seeds strewn among epithelial fragments {2030}. The epithelial clusters often show admixed myoepithelial nuclei {1280,207}. Stromal clumps can be associated with myxoid material. Rarely, multinucleated giant cells may be discerned {2134}. The presence of usual ductal hyperplasia within the fibroadenoma can result in the presence of larger branched proliferative epithelial aggregates in the aspirates. Occasionally the aspirates may show high cellularity, and isolated single epithelial cells with mild nuclear atypia may be seen, resulting in an atypical or even false positive malignant diagnosis.

## Diagnostic molecular pathology
Not clinically relevant

## Essential and desirable diagnostic criteria
*Essential:* circumscribed biphasic tumour; intracanalicular and/or pericanalicular growth pattern; no stromal overgrowth; absence of well-developed fronds; no stromal atypia; low mitotic activity in the stromal component.

## Staging
Not clinically relevant

## Prognosis and prediction
Most fibroadenomas do not recur after complete surgical excision. In adolescents, there is a tendency for one or more new lesions to develop at another site or close to the site of the previous surgical treatment {936}. Complex fibroadenomas are associated with a minimal increase in relative cancer risk {554}.

# Phyllodes tumour

Tse G
Koo JS
Thike AA

## Definition

Phyllodes tumour is a generally circumscribed fibroepithelial neoplasm showing a prominent intracanalicular architectural pattern with leaf-like stromal fronds, capped by luminal epithelial and myoepithelial cell layers, accompanied by stromal hypercellularity.

## ICD-O coding

9020/1 Phyllodes tumour NOS
9020/0 Phyllodes tumour, benign
9020/1 Phyllodes tumour, borderline
9020/3 Phyllodes tumour, malignant

## ICD-11 coding

2F30.3 & XH50P7 Benign phyllodes tumour of breast & Phyllodes tumour, benign
2F75 & XH5NK4 Neoplasms of uncertain behaviour of breast & Phyllodes tumour, borderline
2C63 & XH8HJ7 Malignant phyllodes tumour of breast & Phyllodes tumour, malignant

## Related terminology

*Not recommended:* cystosarcoma phyllodes.

## Subtype(s)

Periductal stromal tumour

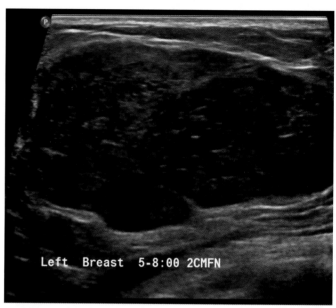

**Fig. 3.09** Phyllodes tumour. Ultrasound image of a phyllodes tumour that shows a lobulated hypoechoic mass with internal acoustic shadows.

## Localization

Phyllodes tumours may arise in any part of the breast, including the nipple {2275}, and in ectopic breast tissue {1564}.

**Table 3.01** Histological features of fibroadenoma and benign, borderline, and malignant phyllodes tumours

| Histological feature | Fibroadenoma | Phyllodes tumours | | |
| --- | --- | --- | --- | --- |
| | | Benign | Borderline | Malignant[a] |
| Tumour border | Well defined | Well defined | Well defined, may be focally permeative | Permeative |
| Stromal cellularity | Variable, scant to uncommonly cellular, usually uniform | Cellular, usually mild, may be non-uniform or diffuse | Cellular, usually moderate, may be non-uniform or diffuse | Cellular, usually marked and diffuse |
| Stromal atypia | None | Mild or none | Mild or moderate | Marked |
| Mitotic activity | Usually none, rarely low | Usually low: < 2.5 mitoses/mm$^2$ (< 5 per 10 HPFs) | Usually frequent: 2.5 to < 5 mitoses/mm$^2$ (5–9 per 10 HPFs) | Usually abundant: ≥ 5 mitoses/mm$^2$ (≥ 10 per 10 HPFs) |
| Stromal overgrowth | Absent | Absent | Absent (or very focal) | Often present |
| Malignant heterologous elements | Absent | Absent | Absent | May be present |
| Distribution relative to all breast tumours | Common | Uncommon | Rare | Rare |
| Relative proportion of all phyllodes tumours | n/a | 60–75% | 15–26% | 8–20% |

HPF, high-power field; n/a, not applicable.

[a]Although these features are often observed in combination, they may not always be present simultaneously. The presence of a malignant heterologous element (apart from liposarcoma) qualifies designation as a malignant phyllodes tumour, without requirement for other histological criteria.

## Clinical features

Phyllodes tumours usually present clinically as unilateral, firm, painless, mobile masses. Large tumours may exceed 10 cm in size, distort the breast, and ulcerate the skin. Skin ulceration does not necessarily imply malignancy; large benign or borderline phyllodes tumours may cause skin ischaemia and secondary erosion. However, tumours that fungate through the skin as fleshy polypoid outgrowths are invariably malignant. Bloody nipple discharge may be related to spontaneous tumour infarction or intraductal growth {1187}. Multifocal or bilateral lesions are unusual {2041}. Paraneoplastic syndromes such as hypoglycaemia {1569} and hypertrophic osteoarthropathy {1111} have been described.

Mammographic screening identifies smaller tumours of 2–3 cm, but the average tumour size remains at 4–5 cm. Reactive axillary lymphadenopathy due to tumour necrosis or infection is relatively common {784,2}, but lymph node metastases are infrequent {2029}. Mammography, sonography, and MRI reveal rounded, bosselated, circumscribed masses containing clefts or cysts and sometimes coarse calcifications {2032,2321}. Imaging differentiation between fibroadenomas and phyllodes tumours, as well as radiological prediction of phyllodes tumour grade, is unreliable {970,973}.

## Epidemiology

In populations of European descent, phyllodes tumours account for 0.3–1% of all primary tumours of the breast and 2.5% of all fibroepithelial neoplasms. The incidence is higher in Asian women {355,151}. Phyllodes tumours occur predominantly in older women (average age: 40–50 years), about 15–20 years later than fibroadenomas {2041,2364,372}. Malignant phyllodes tumours develop on average 2–5 years later than benign tumours, and they are more frequent among Hispanics in Central and South America {151,1651}.

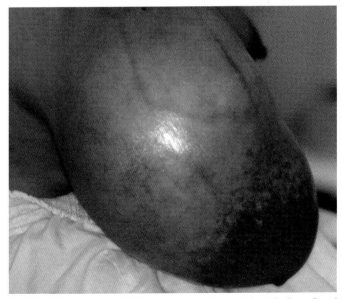

**Fig. 3.10** Phyllodes tumour. A large mass within the breast, histologically confirmed as phyllodes tumour.

## Etiology

The exact etiology of phyllodes tumours is unclear. Genetic risk factors are largely unknown, but phyllodes tumours have been described in patients with Li–Fraumeni syndrome {1061}.

## Pathogenesis

Phyllodes tumours originate from the intralobular and periductal stroma, with epithelial–stromal interactions contributing to pathogenesis {1852}. Epithelial expression of some biomarkers is associated with stromal features indicative of tumour grade and may be important in neoplastic development {980,2044, 2061}. Epithelial WNT ligand expression is correlated with stromal WNT pathway activation {1855,1854,2109}. During malignant progression, the stroma becomes independent of epithelial interactions, resulting in autonomous stromal growth {1855, 2109}. *EGFR*, *KIT* (*c-KIT*), and *TP53* overexpression / genetic aberrations are associated with malignancy in phyllodes tumours {980,1093,1216,2045}.

Recurrent *MED12* mutations in stromal cells are present in phyllodes tumours, supporting a shared pathogenesis with fibroadenomas, although malignant phyllodes tumours have a lower rate of *MED12* mutations than do benign and borderline tumours {2033,1659}. Similar mutations in fibroadenomas and synchronous/subsequent phyllodes tumours from the same patients indicate that some phyllodes tumours may arise from fibroadenomas via a *MED12*-mutant pathway {865,1514,1601, 1655}. It is reported that fibroadenoma-like areas are histologically encountered in 35.9% of phyllodes tumours, and 15.4% of phyllodes tumours are accompanied by separately occurring fibroadenomas in the ipsilateral or contralateral breast {344}. Malignant/borderline phyllodes tumours without *MED12* mutations and accompanying fibroadenomas show more alterations in cancer-related genes, indicating an additional pathogenetic mechanism (*MED12*-wildtype) independent of fibroadenomas {1601}.

Apart from *MED12* mutations, recent genomic studies have also implicated mutations in *RARA*, *TERT*, *FLNA*, *SETD2*, and *KMT2D* (*MLL2*) in driving the development of phyllodes tumours. Derangement of cancer driver genes such as *PIK3CA*, *RB1*, *TP53*, *NF1*, *PTEN*, *BRAF*, and *EGFR* promotes progression of phyllodes tumours to borderline and malignant grades {2033}. The spectrum of genetic abnormalities may be helpful in phyllodes tumour grading. One report suggested a distinct gene mutation panel that could help differentiate malignant phyllodes tumour from metaplastic carcinoma {2319}. The same panel was useful in refining phyllodes tumour grade {1034A}.

Chromosomal abnormalities increase with higher tumour grade. 1q gain and 13q loss are associated with borderline/malignant phyllodes tumours {2353,1093}. Deletion of 9p21 and loss of p16 expression were also identified {1093,360,955}.

## Macroscopic appearance

Phyllodes tumours form circumscribed, firm, bulging masses. Many benign tumours can be shelled out surgically due to their clearly defined margins. The cut surface is tan or pink to grey in colour and may be mucoid and fleshy with cystic degeneration. The characteristic whorled pattern with curved clefts resembling leaf buds is best seen in large tumours, but smaller ones may have a homogeneous appearance. Haemorrhage or necrosis may be present.

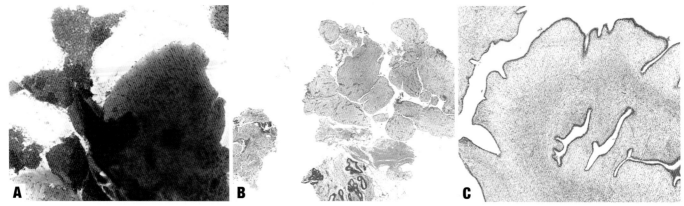

**Fig. 3.11** Benign phyllodes tumour. **A** Aspirate of a benign phyllodes tumour showing large fragments of stroma juxtaposed with large aggregates of epithelium. The cellular component forms large sheets but is composed of bland epithelial cells with interspersed scattered myoepithelial cells. **B** Core biopsy of a cellular fibroepithelial lesion, which upon subsequent excision was confirmed to be a benign phyllodes tumour. **C** Benign phyllodes tumour showing expansion of the stroma into leaf-like structures (fronds). There is variability of the stromal cellularity, but in general the cellularity is low.

## Histopathology

Phyllodes tumours typically exhibit an exaggerated intracanalicular growth pattern, with leaf-like projections extending into variably dilated elongated lumina. A pericanalicular pattern can also be seen. The epithelial component consists of luminal epithelial and myoepithelial cells stretched into arc-like clefts surmounting stromal fronds. Apocrine or squamous metaplasia and usual ductal hyperplasia can be present. Atypical ductal hyperplasia / ductal carcinoma in situ, lobular neoplasia, and invasive carcinoma can rarely occur within the tumour {373, 2038}.

In benign phyllodes tumours, the stroma is usually more cellular than in fibroadenomas. Stromal cellularity may be higher in the zone immediately adjacent to the epithelium, and it is often referred to as periepithelial or subepithelial accentuation of stromal cellularity. Areas of sparse stromal cellularity, hyalinization, or myxoid change are not uncommon {1962}, reflecting stromal heterogeneity. These areas may be mistaken for fibroadenomas in core biopsies. The spindle cell stromal nuclei are monomorphic and mitoses are rare, usually < 2.5 mitoses/mm² {2038} (corresponding to < 5 mitoses per 10 high-power fields of 0.5 mm in diameter and 0.2 mm² in area). The presence of occasional bizarre or multinucleated stromal giant cells should not be interpreted as a marker of malignancy {1670,2113}. Necrosis and benign lipomatous, cartilaginous, and osseous metaplasia have been reported. The margins of benign phyllodes tumours are usually well delimited and pushing, although very small tumour buds may protrude into the surrounding tissue, and if left behind after surgery, they may be the source of local recurrence.

Malignant phyllodes tumours are diagnosed when all of the following features are present: marked stromal nuclear pleomorphism; stromal overgrowth, defined by the absence of epithelial elements in one low-power microscopic field (40× magnification: 4× objective and 10× eyepiece) containing only stroma; increased mitoses (≥ 5 mitoses/mm²; ≥ 10 mitoses per 10 high-power fields of 0.5 mm in diameter and 0.2 mm² in area); increased stromal cellularity, which is usually diffuse; and an infiltrative border (see Table 3.01, p. 172). Because of sarcomatous overgrowth, the epithelial component may only be identified after diligent sampling of the tumour. Malignant phyllodes tumours are also diagnosed when malignant heterologous elements are present even in the absence of other features {2029}. Although liposarcoma was traditionally regarded as a malignant heterologous component, there is evidence to suggest that metastatic risk is low when well-differentiated liposarcoma occurs as the sole heterologous element in a phyllodes tumour {100}. These abnormal adipocytes

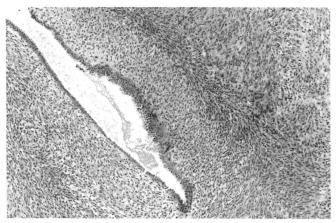

**Fig. 3.12** Borderline phyllodes tumour. Stromal hypercellularity in borderline phyllodes tumour. The epithelial component remains benign, with an intact myoepithelial cell layer.

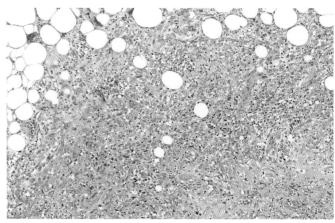

**Fig. 3.13** Malignant phyllodes tumour. Permeative margins in a malignant phyllodes tumour, featuring abnormal stromal cells percolating among adipocytes at the tumour periphery.

within phyllodes tumours lack *MDM2* or *CDK4* amplifications, in contrast to extramammary well-differentiated liposarcoma {1256, 100,923}. Therefore, it is recommended that a diagnosis of malignant phyllodes tumour is not made based purely on the finding of well-differentiated liposarcoma, but also on the basis of other stromal features. Rare pleomorphic liposarcomas in phyllodes tumours have shown more-adverse outcomes {100}. Although myxoid liposarcoma has been described in phyllodes tumours, the lack of associated characteristic molecular aberrations calls into question its true existence within phyllodes tumours.

The diagnostic criteria for benign and malignant phyllodes tumours are relatively well defined, but those for borderline phyllodes tumours are less clear. When some but not all adverse histological characteristics are seen, a diagnosis of borderline phyllodes tumour is made. Despite the known histological criteria demonstrating correlation with outcomes, their relative impact {1962,344} remains controversial. A nomogram developed to predict likely behaviour on the basis of weighted parameters {2041} has been validated in various patient populations {345,1509,344}.

Periductal stromal tumour shows a biphasic pattern of benign ductal elements in a cellular spindle stroma, with spindle cells displaying varying degrees of atypia and mitotic activity. Although periductal stromal tumour lacks the fronded architecture of typical phyllodes tumours, the finding of focal phyllodes features in recurrences {253} and the morphological coexistence of periductal stromal tumour in some phyllodes tumours favour periductal stromal tumour being regarded as a subtype of phyllodes tumour.

The main differential diagnosis for benign phyllodes tumour is fibroadenoma with a prominent intracanalicular growth pattern. Phyllodes tumours tend to have more cellular stroma and well-developed leaf-like processes. In the absence of stromal fronds, the presence of elongated, branching, and cleft-like ducts within cellular stroma may serve as a histological clue to the diagnosis of phyllodes tumour. The degree of stromal hypercellularity for benign phyllodes tumour is difficult to define, but it should be fairly uniform throughout the lesion, or closely accompanying the leafy fronds. Increased stromal cellularity adjacent to epithelium, at the epithelial–stromal interface, is often noticed. Intracanalicular fibroadenomas may also show leaf-like processes, but they are fewer and poorly formed, without increased stromal cellularity. Cellular fibroadenomas may have mitotic activity as high as 3.57 mitoses/mm² (7 mitoses per 10 high-power fields) {2063}. Although fibroadenomas and benign phyllodes tumours may present similar recurrence risks {760,1506,1556,2041}, their distinction is important in the core biopsy setting because of differences in subsequent management. In the event of uncertainty, a diagnosis of benign fibroepithelial tumour is preferable, especially in a core biopsy {2030}.

Malignant phyllodes tumours may be confused with primary or metastatic sarcomas. In such cases, the diagnosis of phyllodes tumour depends on finding residual epithelial structures by extensive sampling. However, the clinical outcomes of primary breast sarcomas and malignant phyllodes tumours appear to be similar {1199,2214}. Knowledge of the clinical history may aid in the distinction of primary versus metastatic sarcoma. Metaplastic carcinoma is another differential consideration for malignant phyllodes tumour, but immunohistochemical demonstration of

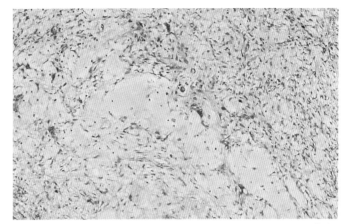

**Fig. 3.14** Malignant phyllodes tumour. Stromal overgrowth in a malignant phyllodes tumour, which displays only the stromal component on a low-power microscopic field.

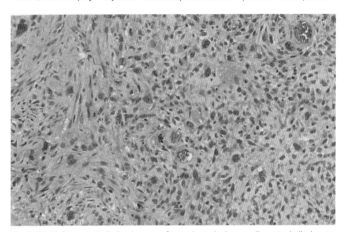

**Fig. 3.15** Malignant phyllodes tumour. Stromal atypia in a malignant phyllodes tumour, with stromal nuclei that show moderate to marked nuclear pleomorphism.

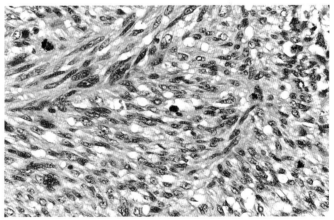

**Fig. 3.16** Malignant phyllodes tumour showing pleomorphic stromal cells with brisk mitotic activity.

diffuse epithelial differentiation in the former and distinct genetic alterations {2319} in the latter help to confirm the diagnosis. Caution must be exercised in interpreting very focal keratin expression and p63 positivity in limited samples, because positivity has been reported in phyllodes tumours (in particular the malignant ones) {340,361}.

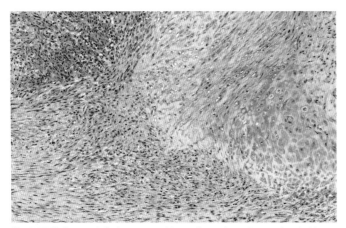 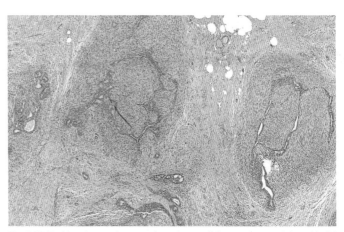

**Fig. 3.17** Malignant phyllodes tumour with a malignant heterologous chondroid component. The presence of a bona fide malignant heterologous element (apart from well-differentiated liposarcoma) justifies the diagnosis of malignant phyllodes tumour.

**Fig. 3.18** Periductal stromal tumour shows hypercellular stroma around the epithelial elements.

## Cytology

Cytological aspirates of phyllodes tumours contain cellular stromal fragments and sheets of benign epithelial and myoepithelial cells. These features overlap with those of fibroadenomas {2117,472}. The presence of large hypercellular stromal fragments, moderate to large numbers of dissociated stromal cells admixed with fibromyxoid material, a lower epithelial-to-stromal ratio, rounded epithelial fragments with mild atypia, and columnar cells with intact cytoplasm are diagnostic clues for phyllodes tumours {2116,567,1300,2030}. Cytological grading of phyllodes tumours is difficult, with malignant cases showing a higher degree of stromal nuclear atypia, mitotic activity, more atypical single cells, and sarcomatous elements {164,1883, 2184}.

## Diagnostic molecular pathology

Although not currently available as a diagnostic test, the presence of *TERT* promoter mutations favours a diagnosis of phyllodes tumour over fibroadenoma {2033,1219,2329,1659,2111}, and it is likely that this will become an adjunctive tool for distinguishing these tumours. A five-gene PCR assay has been developed into a clinical molecular test that can help distinguish phyllodes tumour from fibroadenoma on preoperative core biopsy {2043}.

## Essential and desirable diagnostic criteria

*Essential:* stromal fronds and hypercellularity; dominant intracanalicular growth pattern with stromal fronds capped by luminal/myoepithelial cell layers.

*Essential for differential diagnosis of benign versus malignant:* number of stromal mitoses – high-power field for mitotic count should be defined (40× objective and 10× eyepiece,

0.196 mm$^2$); degree of stromal cellularity; stromal atypia; stromal overgrowth: absence of epithelial elements in at least one low-power field (4× objective and 10× eyepiece, 22.9 mm$^2$); tumour borders; malignant heterologous elements (excludes well-differentiated liposarcoma).

## Staging

Because the stromal component of phyllodes tumours represents the neoplastic component, malignant phyllodes tumours may be staged as sarcomas using the eighth edition of the Union for International Cancer Control (UICC) TNM classification {229}.

## Prognosis and prediction

Most phyllodes tumours are benign. Local recurrences usually occur within 2–3 years of diagnosis, at an overall rate of 21%, with ranges of 10–17%, 14–25%, and 23–30%, respectively, for benign, borderline, and malignant tumours. Recurrences may be of similar or higher grade than the original tumour, with higher grade reported in 31.5% of cases {2041}. Margin status at excision appears to be the most reliable predictor of recurrence, except in benign tumours, where it seems to be less relevant {408,1411}. Stromal overgrowth, stromal atypia, and mitotic activity may also be important {2041}.

Axillary lymph node metastases are rare {2029}. Distant metastases occur in about 2% of tumours and are seen almost exclusively in malignant phyllodes tumours. They usually occur within 5–8 years of diagnosis. Metastases have been reported in nearly all internal organs, but the lung and skeleton are the most common sites {1881,2041}. Most metastases consist of stromal elements only. Large tumour size and malignant heterologous elements are associated with metastases {1035}.

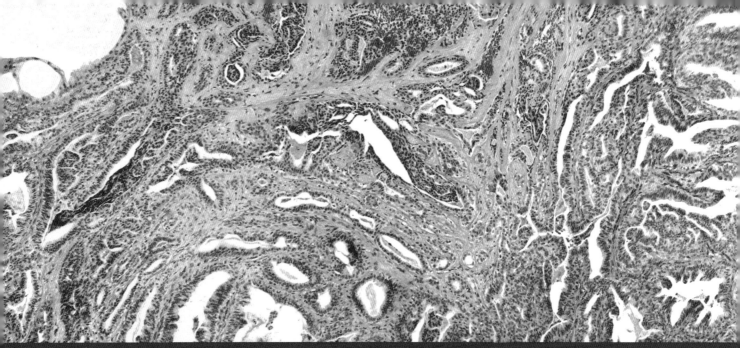

# 4

# Tumours of the nipple

Edited by: Sasano H

Epithelial tumours
    Syringomatous tumour
    Nipple adenoma
    Paget disease of the breast

# WHO classification of tumours of the nipple

**Epithelial tumours**
8407/0    Syringoma NOS
8506/0    Adenoma of nipple
8540/3    Paget disease of breast

---

These morphology codes are from the International Classification of Diseases for Oncology, third edition, second revision (ICD-O-3.2) {921}. Behaviour is coded /0 for benign tumours; /1 for unspecified, borderline, or uncertain behaviour; /2 for carcinoma in situ and grade III intraepithelial neoplasia; /3 for malignant tumours, primary site; and /6 for malignant tumours, metastatic site. Behaviour code /6 is not generally used by cancer registries.

This classification is modified from the previous WHO classification, taking into account changes in our understanding of these lesions.

# Tumours of the nipple: Introduction

Lokuhetty D

The nipple and the areola of the breast, which form the nipple–areola complex (NAC), are composed of the outlets of lactiferous ducts draining milk from mammary lobules. Large lactiferous ducts widen under the areola to form lactiferous sinuses, before narrowing down at the base of the nipple to terminate at the nipple orifice. The male breast, which does not have mammary glands, also has a nipple, but its biological significance remains unknown.

The skin lining of the nipple rests on a thin layer of smooth muscle, because the NAC lacks subcutaneous tissue. Bland cells with clear/pale cytoplasm, known as Toker cells, are present as a normal epidermal component in 10% of nipples. They usually have an immunoprofile similar to that of luminal cells, with CK7 and hormone receptor positivity {500}. The pathological relevance of these cells is presented in the section on Paget disease of the breast. The squamous epithelium of the nipple lining extends into the major ducts for 1–2 cm before being abruptly replaced by the luminal/myoepithelial cell lining of the ducts. Areola muscle comprises radial and circular fibres with a thin layer of fat including blood vessels below {2369}.

The vast majority of diseases of the nipple are non-neoplastic, including abnormal developments such as retracted or inverted nipple and various forms of acute and chronic inflammatory disorders. Normal components of the NAC can give rise to both benign and malignant tumours, including squamous cell carcinoma {557,2130}, basal cell carcinoma {48,358}, melanoma {1441}, eccrine spiradenoma {1358}, clear cell acanthoma {199},

microcystic adnexal carcinoma {2288}, haemangioma, fibroma, and leiomyoma {523,814}. A rare case of breast carcinoma recurring in the nipple is also on record {2223}.

The more frequently encountered tumours involving the NAC considered in this chapter are syringomatous tumour, nipple adenoma, and Paget disease of the breast. In this fifth-edition volume, the following information has been updated since the previous version:

**Syringomatous tumour:** Despite a very similar histological appearance to the tumour known as syringoma arising from cutaneous adnexal eccrine glands, correlation with relatively large breast ducts in the pathogenesis of syringomatous tumour with a different type of glandular differentiation is suggested {184}. This could explain why syringomatous tumour occurs only near the nipple.

**Nipple adenoma:** Although nipple adenoma is still a benign lesion, potential involvement of activating *PIK3CA* mutations and possibly *KRAS* and *BRAF* mutations is considered in the pathogenesis {1190}.

**Paget disease of the breast:** Although many studies have been conducted, no specific gene mutations have been found to be associated with the development or pathogenesis of mammary Paget disease. Gene mutations detected in Paget disease have been similar to those in underlying carcinoma in > 80% of the cases. These genetic findings reinforce the concept that mammary Paget disease reflects the cutaneous spread of underlying breast carcinoma.

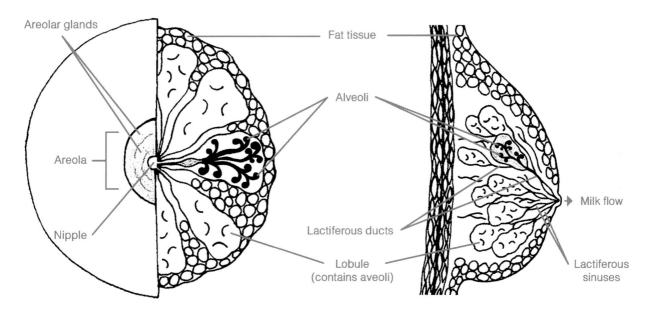

**Fig. 4.01** Anatomy of the nipple and areola.

# Syringomatous tumour

Lester SC
Lee AHS

## Definition
Syringomatous tumour (SyT) is a locally infiltrative tumour of the nipple and areolar region composed of cells with glandular and squamous morphology.

## ICD-O coding
8407/0 Syringoma NOS

## ICD-11 coding
2F30.Y & XH9GB7 Other specified benign neoplasm of breast & Syringomatous tumour of nipple

## Related terminology
*Acceptable:* syringomatous tumour of the nipple.
*Not recommended:* syringomatous adenoma of the nipple; infiltrating syringomatous adenoma of the nipple.

## Subtype(s)
None

## Localization
SyT is located in the dermis of the nipple and areola and infiltrates around lactiferous sinuses and into the areolar smooth muscle.

## Clinical features
SyT is most commonly detected as a firm mass in the dermis of the nipple and subareolar region. Tumour size is usually 0.5–4 cm, but it can be larger {1410}. Nipple discharge, tenderness, and pruritus may occur. Tumours are rarely bilateral {1410}. SyT may be difficult to detect by mammogram or ultrasound because of the superficial location and presence within dense areolar smooth muscle. If seen on imaging, the tumour can have irregular, circumscribed, or indistinct borders {50, 1009}. Calcifications in the tumour may be the only abnormal finding on imaging.

## Epidemiology
SyT is rare, with < 80 cases reported. There is a wide age range, from 11 to 76 years (average: 40–50 years). Only two cases have been reported in males {1786,913}.

## Etiology
Unknown

## Pathogenesis
Although SyT has a similar appearance to syringomas thought to arise from skin adnexal eccrine glands, SyT is reported to show a different type of glandular differentiation, suggesting a relationship to large breast ducts {184}. Origin from the lactiferous sinuses could be an explanation for the specific location of this tumour near the nipple.

## Macroscopic appearance
SyT forms a firm, poorly defined mass in the dermis.

## Histopathology
The tumour infiltrates into the dermis and smooth muscle of the nipple and areola, and it occasionally extends focally into the underlying breast parenchyma {1786,959}. SyT surrounds the lactiferous sinuses but does not invade into ducts or epidermis. There may be overlying pseudoepitheliomatous hyperplasia of the skin. The border of the tumour is usually poorly circumscribed. The surrounding stroma is either fibrous or loosely cellular and may be accentuated around tumour cell nests. No lymphovascular invasion is observed, although perineural invasion may be present, which should be distinguished from infiltration around nodular nests of areolar smooth muscle. The tumour cells form small solid nests and cords that are often tadpole-shaped with comma-like tails. There are usually multiple cell layers, although single-layered glands are also seen. The cells are cytologically bland with round to oval nuclei. Mitoses are rare and necrosis is not a feature.

The tumour consists of cells with multiple phenotypes {184, 186}. The predominant cell type has myoepithelial-like features, including a peripheral location, expression of p63, expression of high-molecular-weight cytokeratins (including CK5 and CK14), and variable expression of other myoepithelial markers. Variable numbers of squamoid cells are centrally located within tumour nests and can express CK10 and variably p63. Cysts containing keratin may be present in the superficial portion of the tumour. If these cysts rupture, there can be associated lymphoid aggregates. Calcifications may be present in keratinaceous debris. In the central portion of some tumour nests, cells with luminal-like features form glandular spaces and express low-molecular-weight cytokeratin such as CK8 and CK18. PAS-positive secretory material may be present in the lumina. Tumour cells are usually negative for hormone receptors and ERBB2 (HER2), although focal weak staining for ER may be observed.

The differential diagnosis includes low-grade adenosquamous carcinoma, tubular carcinoma, nipple adenoma, and dermal adnexal tumours {512}. SyT closely resembles low-grade adenosquamous carcinoma, as both tumours consist of multiple cell types including squamous cells {443}. However, low-grade adenosquamous carcinoma arises deeper in the breast and rarely invades into the nipple. A neoplastic spindle cell component may be present. The two lesions could be difficult to distinguish in a superficial biopsy, especially if the location of the main portion of the tumour is unknown to the pathologist. Tubular carcinoma can resemble the glandular areas of SyT, but it rarely invades the dermis. Furthermore, squamous cells are absent in tubular carcinoma, the tumour cells lack expression of high-molecular-weight cytokeratins and p63, and ER is typically positive. Although nipple adenomas occur in the same location as SyTs, they do not have an infiltrative pattern

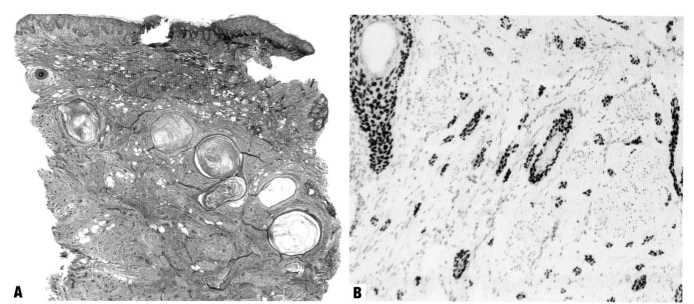

**Fig. 4.02** Syringomatous tumour of the nipple. **A** The tumour cell nests infiltrate into the dermis and smooth muscle of the nipple and areola. Cysts containing keratin are present in the superficial portion. **B** Immunostaining for p63 shows positive nuclear reactivity in small solid nests, as well as in larger nests with squamous differentiation. Centrally located p63-negative tumour cells can be seen in a cluster of tumour cells forming a tubule.

around normal structures, and a normal myoepithelial layer surrounds the involved spaces. SyT closely resembles some skin adnexal tumours, such as syringoma and microcystic adnexal carcinoma. However, its nipple location and type of glandular differentiation support that SyT is a breast-specific tumour {184}.

## Cytology
FNA of SyT shows cohesive sheets of bland ductal cells intermingled with elongated stromal cells {437}. The diagnosis can be made with more confidence by core needle biopsy or skin punch biopsy.

## Diagnostic molecular pathology
Not clinically relevant

## Essential and desirable diagnostic criteria
*Essential:* locally infiltrative tumour in the dermis and smooth muscle of the nipple and areolar region, composed of bland cells with glandular and squamous morphology with rare mitoses; tumour cells do not destructively invade into ducts or the epidermis.
*Desirable:* keratin-filled cysts may be present in a superficial location.

## Staging
SyT is not classified as a malignancy and is not staged.

## Prognosis and prediction
SyT is locally infiltrative. There is no definitive evidence that it can metastasize. In a single report of isolated tumour cells in an axillary lymph node in a case of SyT, it remains unclear whether the illustrated cells are tumour cells or displaced epithelial cells possibly related to the prior breast excision {308}. Local recurrence of SyT is possible when surgical margins are positive {959}. The optimal treatment is complete excision.

# Nipple adenoma

Lester SC
Lee AHS

## Definition

Nipple adenoma is a benign epithelial proliferative lesion of the breast featuring duct-like structures involving the superficial duct orifices of the nipple, the surrounding stroma, and often the contiguous overlying epidermis.

## ICD-O coding

8506/0 Adenoma of nipple

## ICD-11 coding

2F30.Y & XH7GN3 Other specified benign neoplasm of breast & Adenoma of nipple

## Related terminology

*Acceptable:* nipple duct adenoma.

*Not recommended:* florid papillomatosis of the nipple; erosive adenomatosis of the nipple; papillary adenoma of the nipple; papillomatosis of the nipple; superficial papillary adenomatosis.

## Subtype(s)

None

## Localization

Nipple adenomas are located in the superficial portion of the nipple and are often contiguous with the epidermis.

## Clinical features

Most nipple adenomas are clinically detected when of small size due to changes in the skin. If not excised, adenomas may evolve over many years and develop into large and pedunculated masses {686}. Sometimes the nipple appears eroded and erythematous (hence the name "erosive adenomatosis") due to replacement of the normal overlying squamous epithelium by glandular epithelium. The resulting bleeding and/or an exudative crust may cause discomfort. This finding may be described as nipple discharge. Epidermal involvement may mimic the clinical appearance of Paget disease. Careful physical examination usually reveals a small dermal nodule just below the epidermis. Mammography cannot identify the lesion in approximately one third of cases due to the lesion's superficial location and small size. Although imaging findings are nonspecific, ultrasound may detect a circumscribed mass for larger adenomas, with or without cystic components {2204,1180,1130}. MRI may show nipple enhancement {1316,1130}.

## Epidemiology

Nipple adenoma is rare. It occurs in both females and males, with a wide age range (5 months to 89 years). It is most common in women in their fifth decade of life.

## Etiology

Unknown

## Pathogenesis

Activating *PIK3CA* mutations have been reported in 12 of 24 nipple adenomas (50%), with *KRAS* and *BRAF* mutations in one and two cases, respectively {1190}.

## Macroscopic appearance

Nipple adenomas are rubbery and white to grey, ranging from 0.5 cm to > 4 cm.

## Histopathology

Nipple adenoma forms a nodular mass located in the very superficial aspect of the nipple, often in continuity with the overlying epidermis. If the glandular epithelium replaces the squamous epithelium at a duct orifice, the skin surface may be eroded, with haemorrhage and inflammation. It may arise from and incorporate lactiferous ducts, and it shows various combinations of sclerosing adenosis, papilloma, and usual ductal hyperplasia, including papillary, solid papillary, micropapillary, solid, and cribriform patterns. Superficial keratin cysts and squamous metaplasia may be seen. Rarely, ductal carcinoma in situ involving an adenoma or invasive carcinoma contiguous with an adenoma has been reported {961,1789,158,1555,252, 1723,781}.

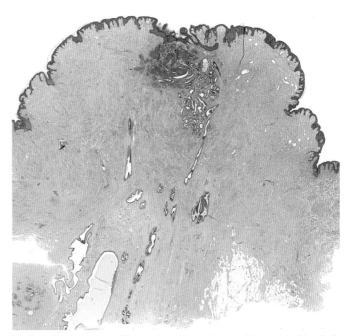

**Fig. 4.03** Nipple adenoma. These lesions arise in the superficial aspect of the nipple and present as small palpable nodules, with or without associated skin changes.

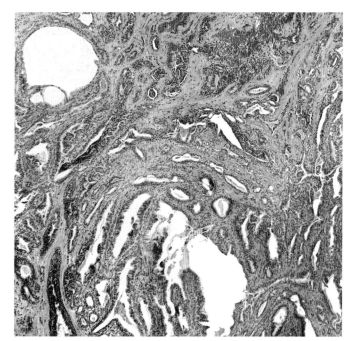

**Fig. 4.04** Nipple adenoma. The typical lesion consists of a combination of sclerosing adenosis, papilloma, and usual ductal hyperplasia.

Nipple adenoma may mimic invasive carcinoma clinically, as both may present with palpable ulcerative haemorrhagic masses {1836}, but they can be distinguished on morphological grounds. Nipple ulceration may raise clinical concern for Paget disease, but the histological features of Paget disease are absent. Usual ductal hyperplasia, which is commonly present, often makes nipple adenoma difficult to distinguish from cancer. Nipple adenoma associated with florid usual ductal hyperplasia and necrosis should be differentiated from ductal carcinoma in situ. Immunohistochemical identification of a preserved myoepithelial cell layer, as well as a heterogeneous cell population identified by CK5/14 and ER, helps in this differential diagnosis {856}. Syringomatous tumours may occur in the same location

as nipple adenomas, but unlike nipple adenomas they have an infiltrative pattern of small epithelial nests surrounding the lactiferous sinuses and involving the smooth muscle of the areola without any epidermal component. Large duct papillomas occur deeper within the lactiferous sinuses and do not involve the overlying skin.

### Cytology

Cytological specimens can be obtained by FNA or brush cytology. The reported cytological features vary, but the lesion can be recognized as benign by the presence of myoepithelial cells {1566}. The presence of coagulative necrosis and isolated epithelial cells often results in a classification of "atypical" or "suspicious" {2213,1828}.

### Diagnostic molecular pathology

Not clinically relevant

### Essential and desirable diagnostic criteria

*Essential:* an epithelial proliferative lesion featuring duct-like structures involving the superficial duct orifices of the nipple, the surrounding stroma, and often the contiguous overlying epidermis; nodular configuration on low magnification; preserved myoepithelial layer.

*Desirable:* immunohistochemical evaluation to identify a preserved myoepithelial cell layer and a heterogeneous cell population.

### Staging

Nipple adenomas are benign lesions and are not staged.

### Prognosis and prediction

Nipple adenomas can recur if not completely excised. Limited surgery, including Mohs micrographic surgery or cryosurgery, can be used to preserve the nipple {219,2213,120,1610}. The subsequent risk of developing breast cancer does not appear to be elevated beyond that associated with other proliferative breast lesions.

# Paget disease of the breast

Albarracin CT
Baldewijns M
Lester SC

## Definition

Paget disease of the breast is characterized by an intraepidermal proliferation of malignant glandular epithelial cells in the nipple areolar region.

## ICD-O coding

8540/3 Paget disease of breast

## ICD-11 coding

2E65.5 & XH3E21 Paget disease of nipple & Paget disease, mammary

## Related terminology

*Acceptable:* mammary Paget disease; ductal carcinoma in situ involving nipple skin, Paget disease of the nipple.

## Subtype(s)

None

## Localization

Paget disease is located in the nipple and/or areola region and may extend into the adjacent breast skin.

## Clinical features

A large proportion of patients (42–98%) present with eczematous or erythematous changes of the nipple with or without nipple discharge and retraction. Ulceration can be seen and is secondary to replacement of the normal squamous cells by Paget cells, which can be mistaken for ulcerating invasive carcinoma. Mammary Paget disease (MPD) rarely presents as a pigmented macule and can be mistaken for melanoma {1635}. The presence of a palpable mass in the breast usually indicates an underlying invasive carcinoma. Mammography reveals abnormalities suspicious for malignancy in 32–67% of cases {440,

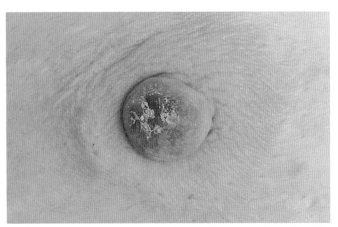

**Fig. 4.05** Mammary Paget disease. The gross appearance of a nipple affected by Paget disease shows an erythematous area with erosion, scaling, and crust formation.

1050,2341}. MPD may represent recurrence of a prior breast carcinoma {1935,1568}.

## Epidemiology

MPD represents 1–4% of all breast carcinomas {314,440}. It can be bilateral and can affect both women and men, over an age range of 27–88 years (mean: 54–63 years). Between 20% and 30% of patients are premenopausal.

## Etiology

Specific risk factors for Paget disease, beyond those recognized for breast cancer in general, have not been identified {2341}.

## Pathogenesis

Most MPD is an extension of ductal carcinoma in situ (DCIS) from the underlying ducts; invasive carcinoma may also be present. When no underlying DCIS is found, Toker cells have been hypothesized to be the precursor of this lesion {1306}.

## Macroscopic appearance

The nipple may appear normal or there may be redness or frank erosion that may extend into the areola and adjacent skin. Scaling and crusting present during physical examination can be removed during preoperative cleaning of the surgical area so that the nipple can appear grossly normal in the specimen. Pigmented MPD presents as a dark macule without the scale or crust seen in the more common type.

## Histopathology

The histological hallmark is the presence of intraepidermal large cells with abundant pale cytoplasm and pleomorphic nuclei containing prominent nucleoli with variable mitotic activity. Paget cells occur singly or in closely packed clusters and rarely form glandular structures, usually at the dermoepidermal junction {1932,2092,569}. Paget cells contain mucin in 40% of cases {2176}, and they may phagocytose melanin, mimicking melanocytes. Numerous melanophages can be seen in the adjacent dermis. Pigmented MPD is associated with a marked increase of non-neoplastic melanocytes intermingled with Paget cells {1635}.

Dermal invasion by Paget cells has been reported in 4–8% of cases of MPD {549,1837,1132,1836}. MPD with dermal invasion should be diagnosed only when clusters or isolated Paget cells can be seen to invade through the basement membrane, the cytological features of the invading cells are similar to those of the Paget cells, and there is a clear separation of the invading Paget cells from the underlying breast carcinoma {549}. An associated lymphocytic infiltrate is often present in the underlying dermis.

MPD is usually associated with an underlying carcinoma, which is most commonly high-grade invasive carcinoma of no special type (NST; 53–64%) or DCIS (24–43%). MPD without

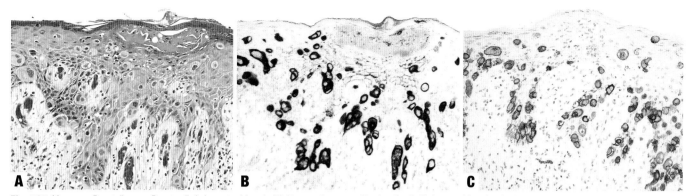

**Fig. 4.06** Mammary Paget disease. Paget cells in breast epidermis (**A**). Paget cells are readily visualized with immunohistochemical staining for CK7 (**B**) and ERBB2 (HER2) (**C**).

underlying carcinoma is rare, with a reported incidence of 0–13% {271,322,1050,1955,985}. Paget disease may also be discovered incidentally after mastectomy for invasive carcinoma; this scenario was reported to represent 15% of cases of MPD in one series {1036}. There are two reports of Paget disease associated with lobular carcinoma, but it is possible that the intraepidermal cells in those cases represent Toker cells {87,1819}.

Paget cells are usually immunohistochemically positive for low-molecular-weight cytokeratins (CK7 and CAM5.2). ERBB2 (HER2) is overexpressed in 80–90% of cases; ER and PR are positive in approximately 40% and 30% of MPD cases, respectively {271,440,159,1889}. Paget cells usually have the same immunoprofile as the underlying carcinoma {2203,65,684}. Variable expression of CEA, EMA, S100, GCDFP-15, p53, and GATA3 has been reported {1567,159,1223}.

The differential diagnoses for MPD include squamous cell carcinoma in situ (Bowen disease) and melanoma, although these diseases very rarely involve the nipple. Immunoreactivity for low-molecular-weight cytokeratins and HER2 is helpful in the diagnosis of MPD. Although squamous cell carcinoma can be positive for GATA3, it is typically positive for high-molecular-weight cytokeratins and negative for low-molecular-weight cytokeratins. Melanoma in situ is usually positive for S100, HMB45, melan-A, SOX10, and MITF, and negative for keratins. In the rare cases where Paget cells are negative for CK7, a panel

of antibodies for other low-molecular-weight cytokeratins and melanoma markers is helpful {1567}. Toker cells (and Toker cell hyperplasia) are an important diagnostic consideration, in particular when there are no clinical symptoms or in the absence of an underlying mammary carcinoma. Toker cells may resemble Paget cells in that they contain clear cytoplasm and are positive for CK7 and CAM5.2, but they differ from Paget cells in that they lack atypical or malignant nuclear features and are HER2-negative and ER-positive. Paget cells should also be differentiated from invasion of the epidermis and nipple by an underlying breast carcinoma.

### Cytology
MPD can be diagnosed in scrape preparations from the nipple, although diagnosis is challenging, especially in pigmented cases.

### Diagnostic molecular pathology
No association with a specific gene mutation has been reported. Paget cells are genetically similar to the underlying carcinoma cells in 80% of cases {1415}.

### Essential and desirable diagnostic criteria
*Essential:* large intraepidermal atypical cells with abundant pale cytoplasm and large nuclei with prominent nucleoli; typically positive for low-molecular-weight cytokeratins and HER2.

### Staging
If no underlying carcinoma is present, MPD is staged as Tis according to the eighth edition of the Union for International Cancer Control (UICC) TNM classification {229}. If underlying DCIS is present, it is also staged as Tis. If invasive carcinoma is present, it is staged on the basis of the extent of invasive carcinoma.

### Prognosis and prediction
MPD is often associated with an underlying carcinoma, and its prognosis depends on tumour stage {271,1955}. Studies suggest that invasion into the dermis by MPD is not associated with poor prognosis, with no reported recurrences or deaths {549, 1837,1132,1836}. Therefore, distinction from skin involvement by locally advanced breast cancer is important, because such involvement is associated with a poor prognosis compared with that of MPD with dermal invasion.

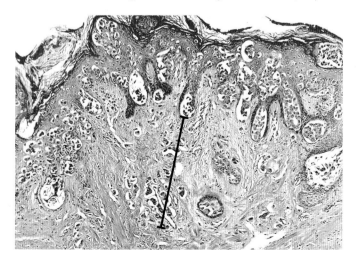

**Fig. 4.07** Invasive mammary Paget disease. A section of nipple with intraepidermal and dermal involvement.

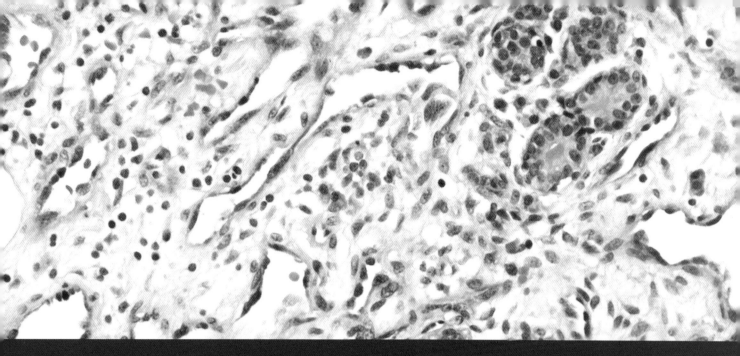

# 5

# Mesenchymal tumours of the breast

Edited by: Goldblum JR, Lazar AJ, Schnitt SJ, Tan PH

Vascular tumours
    Haemangioma
    Angiomatosis
    Atypical vascular lesions
    Postradiation angiosarcoma of the breast
    Primary angiosarcoma of the breast
Fibroblastic and myofibroblastic tumours
    Nodular fasciitis
    Myofibroblastoma
    Desmoid fibromatosis
    Inflammatory myofibroblastic tumour
Peripheral nerve sheath tumours
    Schwannoma
    Neurofibroma
    Granular cell tumour

Smooth muscle tumours
    Leiomyoma
    Leiomyosarcoma
Adipocytic tumours
    Lipoma
    Angiolipoma
    Liposarcoma
Other mesenchymal tumours and tumour-like
    conditions
    Pseudoangiomatous stromal hyperplasia

# WHO classification of mesenchymal tumours of the breast

**Vascular tumours**
9120/0    Haemangioma NOS
        Perilobular haemangioma
        Venous haemangioma
        Cavernous haemangioma
        Capillary haemangioma
        Angiomatosis
        Usual angiomatosis
        Capillary angiomatosis
9126/0    Atypical vascular lesion
        Lymphatic atypical vascular lesion, resembling lymphangioma
        Vascular atypical vascular lesion, resembling haemangioma or hobnail haemangioma
9120/3    Postradiation angiosarcoma
        Epithelioid angiosarcoma
9120/3    Angiosarcoma
        Epithelioid angiosarcoma

**Fibroblastic and myofibroblastic tumours**
8828/0    Nodular fasciitis
8825/0    Myofibroblastoma
8821/1    Desmoid-type fibromatosis
8825/1    Inflammatory myofibroblastic tumour
        Epithelioid inflammatory myofibroblastic sarcoma

**Peripheral nerve sheath tumours**
9560/0    Schwannoma NOS
        Cellular schwannoma
        Epithelioid schwannoma
        Plexiform schwannoma
        Melanotic schwannoma
9540/0    Neurofibroma NOS
        Diffuse neurofibroma
        Atypical neurofibroma
        Plexiform neurofibroma
9580/0    Granular cell tumour NOS
9580/3    Granular cell tumour, malignant

**Smooth muscle tumours**
8890/0    Leiomyoma NOS
        Cutaneous (pilar) leiomyoma
        Leiomyoma of the nipple/areola (muscularis mamillae and areolae)
        Leiomyoma of the breast parenchyma
8890/3    Leiomyosarcoma NOS

**Adipocytic tumours**
8850/0    Lipoma NOS
8861/0    Angiolipoma NOS
8850/3    Liposarcoma NOS

**Other mesenchymal tumours and tumour-like conditions**
        Pseudoangiomatous stromal hyperplasia

---

These morphology codes are from the International Classification of Diseases for Oncology, third edition, second revision (ICD-O-3.2) {921}. Behaviour is coded /0 for benign tumours; /1 for unspecified, borderline, or uncertain behaviour; /2 for carcinoma in situ and grade III intraepithelial neoplasia; /3 for malignant tumours, primary site; and /6 for malignant tumours, metastatic site. Behaviour code /6 is not generally used by cancer registries.

This classification is modified from the previous WHO classification, taking into account changes in our understanding of these lesions.

Subtype labels are indented.

# Mesenchymal tumours of the breast: Introduction

Hornick JL
Lazar AJ

Although this chapter on mesenchymal tumours is restricted to the entities most relevant to the breast, a more general introduction to soft tissue pathology is presented here. Indeed, although characteristic patterns exist, virtually any soft tissue tumour can arise at any site on at least rare occasions.

## Incidence

The incidence of soft tissue sarcomas is fairly consistent, at 30–50 cases per 1 million person-years {702,794,1312,630}. Benign soft tissue neoplasms as a group show an incidence at least 100-fold higher. Individual benign mesenchymal entities range from frequent (e.g. lipoma) to rare (e.g. spindle cell haemangioma) {1437}. Sarcomas are an exceptionally rare subset of primary breast tumours, far outnumbered by carcinomas, fibroepithelial neoplasms, and benign mesenchymal tumours.

Excluding haemangiomas, the most common benign, intermediate, and malignant primary mesenchymal neoplasms of the breast are myofibroblastoma, desmoid fibromatosis, and mammary angiosarcoma, respectively. Other mesenchymal tumour types arise only rarely within breast parenchyma, although a range of mesenchymal tumour types arise in the skin or subcutaneous tissue overlying the breast; some of these neoplasms are also covered in this chapter. The full breadth of deep soft tissue tumours is covered in the *WHO classification of tumours of soft tissue and bone* {654}, which will be updated in the fifth edition volume to be released soon after this breast tumour classification book. More-numerous sarcomas and more sarcoma types are seen in adults than in children, but sarcomas constitute only 1% of malignancies in adults {1940}. They arise mainly in the extremities (in particular the thighs), trunk, head and neck, and retroperitoneum. Sarcomas account for about 10–15% of paediatric malignancies, but their overall incidence rate is much lower in children than in adults, and fewer distinct entities are encountered {802,2273}.

## Etiology and pathogenesis

Most soft tissue neoplasms arise spontaneously, with an unknown pathogenesis, but for some cases a clear etiology can be discerned. Viruses associated with soft tissue tumours include EBV (associated with some smooth muscle tumours in immunosuppressed patients) {493} and HHV8 (associated with Kaposi sarcoma) {307}. Angiosarcoma can complicate long-standing lymphoedema, in particular after radical mastectomy (as seen in Stewart–Treves syndrome). Sarcomas can also arise in fields of prior therapeutic irradiation {1603}. Postradiation cutaneous angiosarcoma after treatment for breast carcinoma is an important complication; a small subset of such secondary angiosarcomas arise in mammary parenchyma {1780,1388}. Atypical vascular lesions also arise in the skin of the breast after radiation therapy {224,674}. Associations with chemical exposure, immunosuppression/transplant, and chronic tissue irritation have been described in a subset of sarcoma cases {1094}.

Soft tissue tumours (both benign and malignant) are also associated with several inherited syndromes, including Maffucci syndrome (associated with chondroid and vascular tumours), tuberous sclerosis (associated with angiomyolipomas of kidney and liver), and Cowden syndrome (associated with lipomas and haemangiomas). These syndromes are discussed in more detail in the *WHO classification of tumours of soft tissue and bone* volume {654}. The cell of origin of most sarcomas is unknown, and precursor or in situ lesions are not recognized. Whether some postradiation atypical vascular lesions represent precursors to (or a risk factor for) cutaneous angiosarcoma remains uncertain {658}. Somatic genetic factors such as recurrent chromosomal translocations drive the pathogenesis of some sarcomas, but how and in what cell these somatic genetic factors arise remains unknown.

## Clinical features

Benign and malignant soft tissue and neural tumours typically present as painless masses, and their growth rates vary. The vast majority of benign soft tissue tumours are < 5 cm {543}. Sarcomas can grow to be much larger. Because of their rarity, breast tumours thought to be mesenchymal should be referred to a specialist multidisciplinary centre before biopsy or surgery for optimal management {449}. The majority of suspected mesenchymal tumours of the breast in fact represent metaplastic carcinomas or malignant phyllodes tumours. Of note, alveolar rhabdomyosarcoma has a predilection for metastasizing to the breast {448}.

## Histopathology

Malignant soft tissue neoplasms sometimes exhibit nuclear pleomorphism, mitotic activity, and necrosis, although translocation-associated sarcomas may be cytologically uniform. Some benign tumours can also show one or more of these features; for example, nuclear atypia can be seen in schwannoma with ancient change. Metaplastic breast carcinomas (specifically spindle cell carcinomas) and malignant phyllodes tumours (with or without heterologous mesenchymal elements) can mimic sarcomas. Phyllodes tumours may show adipocytic differentiation and thereby mimic atypical lipomatous tumour (well-differentiated liposarcoma), myxoid liposarcoma, or pleomorphic liposarcoma; primary liposarcomas of the breast are exceptionally rare {1256}. Fibromatosis-like metaplastic carcinoma is a close histological mimic of desmoid fibromatosis. Immunohistochemistry is generally needed to confirm the tumour cell lineage and diagnosis {1967}.

## Genetics

Benign soft tissue tumours feature simple genetic properties, with diploid karyotypes perhaps adorned by a single characteristic chromosomal rearrangement. In malignancy, two genetic classes exist: simple-karyotype sarcomas associated with a recurrent mutation or translocation (e.g. synovial sarcoma) and complex-karyotype sarcomas with numerous chromosomal aberrations but generally lacking recurrent mutations (e.g. leiomyosarcoma) other than in *TP53* {200}.

As an intermediate tumour that locally recurs but does not metastasize, desmoid fibromatosis is generally associated with a single somatic mutation in *CTNNB1* or much less commonly *APC* {1959,982}.

## Diagnostic procedures

Investigation includes clinical assessment of the size and depth of the tumour, the use of imaging modalities (CT and MRI), and biopsy. Imaging can be used to assess the extent of a primary tumour, to determine its relationship to anatomical structures, and to identify metastases. Virtually all suspicious breast lesions necessitate diagnostic sampling. Core needle biopsy (often image-guided and preferably using a larger-bore needle) can provide diagnostic information on malignancy, subtype, and grade, with high sensitivity and specificity {851,2122}. Open biopsy and cytology are less commonly used.

## Tumour behaviour

The *WHO classification of tumours of soft tissue and bone* {654} recognizes four tumour behavioural categories: benign, intermediate (locally aggressive), intermediate (rarely metastasizing), and malignant. Benign tumours are usually cured by local excision and rarely recur locally (and any recurrences are non-destructive). Intermediate tumours can be either locally aggressive (e.g. desmoid fibromatosis, which locally infiltrates surrounding tissues) or rarely metastasizing (tumours with a very low [< 2%] but definite risk of metastasis; e.g. inflammatory myofibroblastic tumour). Malignant tumours such as angiosarcoma and leiomyosarcoma infiltrate, recur locally, and commonly metastasize (i.e. in > 20% of cases).

## Grading

Grading is an attempt to predict clinical behaviour on the basis of histological variables, but it can only be performed using material from primary untreated neoplasms. It is not applicable to all sarcomas; for example, angiosarcomas, clear cell sarcomas, and epithelioid sarcomas are always considered to be high-grade. The most widely used system for grading soft tissue sarcomas is the three-tiered system developed by the French Fédération Nationale des Centres de Lutte Contre le Cancer (FNCLCC) {379,1484}. It uses a combination of tumour differentiation, mitotic activity, and necrosis to categorize tumours as being of low, intermediate, or high grade. More-broadly applicable molecular approaches are currently in development {343, 1151}.

## Staging

The American Joint Committee on Cancer (AJCC) and the Union for International Cancer Control (UICC) TNM staging systems are widely used {61,229}. Sarcoma staging incorporates histological grading and site of involvement along with histological type, tumour size, extent of lymph node involvement, and presence or absence of distant metastasis. Alternative staging and risk assessment approaches incorporating non-anatomical variables such as age and sex are also under consideration {225,1731}.

## Prognosis and predictive factors

Complete excision is the most important factor in preventing local recurrence {2103,2340}. Some sarcomas (notably epithelioid sarcoma) are relentlessly recurrent, often with late metastases {1824,1984}. Factors generally associated with a greater risk of metastasis are larger tumour size and higher grade. In some instances, histological subtype alone is predictive, but one of the principal factors in assessing prognosis and determining management is histological grade. Site is also important, because low-grade sarcomas in sites where complete surgical excision is difficult (e.g. the retroperitoneum or the head and neck) generally have a worse outcome than do similarly staged tumours in the extremities {771}.

# Haemangioma

Calhoun BC
Calonje JE
Flucke U
Val-Bernal JF

## Definition
Haemangioma is a benign proliferation of mature blood vessels.

## ICD-O coding
9120/0 Haemangioma NOS

## ICD-11 coding
2F30.Y & XH5AW4 Other specified benign neoplasm of breast & Haemangioma NOS

## Related terminology
*Acceptable:* angioma.

## Subtype(s)
Perilobular haemangioma; venous haemangioma; cavernous haemangioma; capillary haemangioma

## Localization
Haemangiomas may occur in the mammary parenchyma or subcutaneous tissue.

## Clinical features
In most cases, haemangiomas are non-palpable and are found on imaging (MRI or mammography). Occasional palpable breast lesions have been described {1018,2197}. Mammary haemangiomas do not have pathognomonic imaging features. Mammography may show lobular-shaped masses with circumscribed or microlobulated margins and densities equal to that of breast parenchyma {1357}. Round calcifications are seldom associated {1357}. Most parenchymal and non-parenchymal haemangiomas measure < 2.0 cm (range: 0.3–6.0 cm) {964, 1788,1039,1038}.

## Epidemiology
Haemangiomas have been reported in patients ranging in age from 18 months to 82 years {1440,2082}. The majority of breast haemangiomas that come to clinical attention are in females {293,1038}. The most common type of haemangioma in the breast is perilobular haemangioma, which is estimated to be present in 1.2–11% of breast specimens {1796,1157}.

## Etiology
These lesions most likely represent non-neoplastic vascular malformations.

## Pathogenesis
Unknown

## Macroscopic appearance
Macroscopic examination reveals a circumscribed red or dark-brown spongy lesion {1793}.

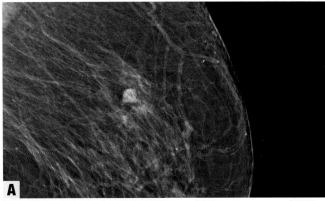

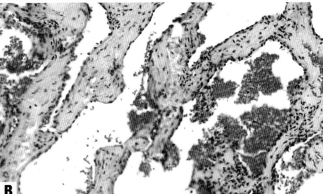

**Fig. 5.01** Cavernous haemangioma of the breast. **A** Mammography of a case in a 73-year-old woman shows a lobulated nodule of defined limits and high density, with heterogeneous calcifications (BI-RADS 4). **B** Large, cavernous, blood-filled vascular spaces separated by connective tissue stroma.

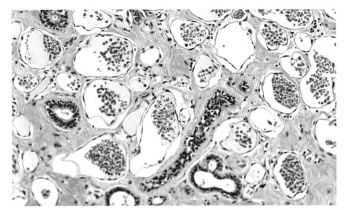

**Fig. 5.02** Perilobular haemangioma of the breast. A circumscribed aggregate of capillary-sized blood vessels in association with a lobule.

## Histopathology
Breast haemangiomas are characterized by the proliferation of well-differentiated vessels of varying sizes. The vascular channels can be interconnecting but are most often

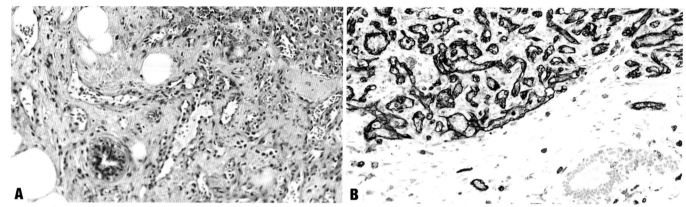

**Fig. 5.03** Capillary haemangioma (parenchymal) of the breast. **A** Parenchymal capillary haemangioma. **B** The lesion is CD31-positive.

non-anastomosing, a feature distinguishing haemangioma from low-grade angiosarcoma. The vessels are lined by endothelial cells showing neither substantial nuclear atypia nor mitotic activity. Occasional hyperchromatic nuclei may be seen, with no adverse clinical implication. The vascular channels are found within the interlobular stroma, with the notable exception of perilobular haemangiomas, in which the intralobular stroma is also involved. A larger feeding vessel may be found within the lesion or in close proximity. The lesions are more or less well circumscribed, with isolated small vessels found in the surrounding breast tissue in the periphery of the lesion. Haemorrhage with disruption of the vascular channels is typical after FNA or core needle biopsy. Thrombosis with secondary endothelial hyperplasia can occur. Microcalcifications can be found within thrombotic channels or in surrounding fibrous stroma.

Perilobular haemangiomas/angiomas are incidental microscopic vascular lesions, measuring < 2 mm, located primarily in the intralobular stroma or surrounding breast tissue. They are composed of a more or less well-circumscribed conglomerate of small, thin-walled, congested capillary vessels containing erythrocytes {964}. Other types of haemangiomas (cavernous, capillary, venous {1793,1788}) can be encountered, similar to in other anatomical sites.

## Cytology
Most aspiration biopsies result in the obtainment of blood but few if any cells. Smears are usually not diagnostic.

## Diagnostic molecular pathology
Not clinically relevant

## Essential and desirable diagnostic criteria
*Essential:* well-differentiated vascular spaces lined by a single layer of benign endothelial cells; a layer of pericytes around individual vascular channels.

## Staging
Not clinically relevant

## Prognosis and prediction
In the past, the discovery of a vascular lesion with features of a haemangioma on a breast core biopsy prompted surgical excision to exclude the diagnosis of well-differentiated angiosarcoma. More-recent data suggest that, especially in cases with radiological–pathological correlation, excision may not be mandatory for benign vascular lesions of the breast identified in core needle biopsy specimens {1291,1886}.

# Angiomatosis

Val-Bernal JF
Antonescu CR
Schnitt SJ

## Definition
Angiomatosis is a histologically benign vascular proliferation that affects a large segment of the breast.

## ICD-O coding
None

## ICD-11 coding
2E81.0Z Haemangiomatosis involving single site

## Related terminology
*Acceptable:* diffuse angioma; giant vascular tumour {688}.

## Subtype(s)
Usual angiomatosis; capillary angiomatosis

## Localization
In all cases, angiomatosis involves the interlobular stroma of the breast. The intralobular stroma is spared. Occasionally, the lesion may extend into the subcutaneous tissue and the skin.

## Clinical features
Most patients present with painless, slow enlargement of the breast. Angiomatosis may form large palpable masses, ranging in size from 9 to 22 cm {1787,1422}. The lesion is usually entirely within the breast parenchyma. Massive enlargement during pregnancy has been reported {1422}. One case showed a vertical manner of growth involving the breast parenchyma, subcutaneous tissue, and skin {1472}. Overlying skin may show hyperpigmentation, faint blue discolouration, or papules {1422, 1472}. The lesion may be transilluminated {1422}. Imaging studies can be helpful in identifying the tumour as being vascular in nature, but they are not helpful in differentiating a benign from a malignant vascular tumour. Sonography shows multiple irregular anechoic spaces separated by thin septa. Moderate blood flow can be demonstrated with colour Doppler. MRI reveals a multiseptated cystic mass, with T2-weighted imaging showing hyperintense tubular structures {1472,364,1343}.

## Epidemiology
Angiomatosis is a very rare vascular lesion, with only a few case reports published {357,1343}. It can be congenital or acquired. Cases have been described in patients from birth up to 59 years of age {1787,1472,1343}. Most cases have been observed in young women (< 40 years old). One case in a male patient, a 7-year-old boy, has been reported {1931}

## Etiology
Unknown

## Pathogenesis
Unknown

## Macroscopic appearance
Angiomatosis presents as a cystic, red, spongy, extensive lesion simulating an angiosarcoma. The cystic spaces contain haemorrhagic or serosanguineous material {1787,1422}. One case showed a large, central, unilocular cystic space filled with serosanguineous fluid {1422}.

## Histopathology
In the usual form, the process consists of a proliferation of vascular channels with wide variation in calibre, diffusely growing throughout the breast parenchyma and showing some degree of anastomosis {1787}. Vascular structures are uniformly distributed and surround the ducts and lobules. Invasion of the intralobular stroma is absent. The lesions are unencapsulated, with poorly defined infiltrative borders. The vessels are lined by flat inconspicuous endothelium without atypia or mitosis. They show sparse supporting mural tissue that is virtually free of smooth muscle. Blood vessels may contain erythrocytes in their lumina. Lymphatic vessels, empty or with aggregates of

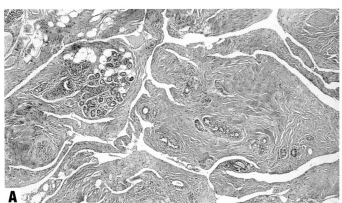 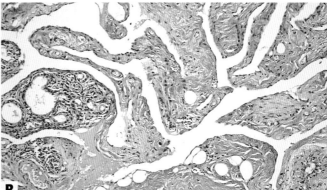

**Fig. 5.04** Angiomatosis, usual type. **A** Anastomosing vascular spaces dissect through the mammary stroma. **B** The endothelial cells are relatively inconspicuous.

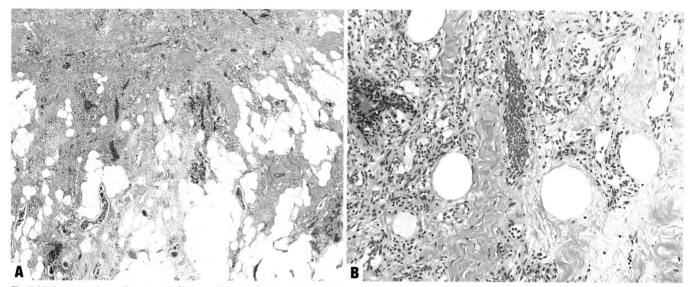

**Fig. 5.05** Angiomatosis, capillary type. **A** Clusters of histologically benign capillaries are scattered throughout the fibrous stroma and adipose tissue of the breast. **B** High-power view shows the ectatic capillary vessels with inconspicuous endothelial cells.

lymphocytes, can be present {1787,162}. Occasional foci of capillary-sized vessels can be observed within the wall of large venous structures or in the vicinity {1724,882}. A considerable part of the tumour is composed of breast parenchyma incorporated among the vascular structures {1787}. The lesion may extend to the overlying skin {1472} or to the underlying pectoralis muscle. If the lesion is observed on core biopsy, complete excision and examination are required for a definitive diagnosis. An uncommon form of angiomatosis is the capillary subtype. It consists predominantly of collections of benign, small, capillary-sized vessels arranged in nodules, often showing a larger vessel in the centre. These structures are dispersed throughout the fibrous stroma and adipose tissue {1724}.

Immunohistochemical study with CD31 and D2-40 highlights the endothelial cells lining the vascular channels of the lesion {730}. Endothelial cell proliferation as measured by the Ki-67 proliferation index is low (< 2%) {1343}.

A critical matter is the distinction from low-grade angiosarcoma, which can histologically show areas with a benign appearance. Unlike angiosarcoma, angiomatosis exhibits a uniform pattern of vessel distribution, and the endothelial nuclei are bland, without hyperchromasia. There are no papillae, endothelial tufting, blood lakes, or necrosis. Endothelial cell mitoses are rare or absent {730}. Dissection of vessels into lobules with disruption of the lobules is not observed {108}.

Diffuse dermal angiomatosis of the breast is a different disorder. It is a rare reactive angioproliferation in the skin, recognized as a distinct subtype of cutaneous reactive angioendotheliomatosis {1756}.

### Cytology
Aspiration smears do not usually provide diagnostic data. Most of them reveal erythrocytes and some lymphocytes.

### Diagnostic molecular pathology
Not clinically relevant

### Essential and desirable diagnostic criteria
*Essential:* anastomosing vascular spaces of varying calibre; diffuse growth within breast parenchyma without invading lobules; regularly distributed, flat, inconspicuous endothelial cells lacking hyperchromasia.

### Staging
Not clinically relevant

### Prognosis and prediction
Incompletely excised angiomatosis has a high risk of local recurrence, but metastasis and malignant transformation have not been described {1422,1343,357}. Complete surgical excision is commonly performed. In some cases, mastectomy may be necessary to control a bulky lesion, but whenever possible it is preferable not to perform such extensive surgery. Preoperative irradiation in one large case allowed breast-conserving surgery {357}.

# Atypical vascular lesions

Brenn T
Antonescu CR
Billings SD

## Definition
Atypical vascular lesions are atypical vascular proliferations on irradiated skin that are often small and multiple.

## ICD-O coding
9126/0 Atypical vascular lesion

## ICD-11 coding
None

## Related terminology
*Acceptable:* atypical vascular proliferation.
*Not recommended:* benign lymphangiomatous papules {507}.

## Subtype(s)
Lymphatic atypical vascular lesion, resembling lymphangioma; vascular atypical vascular lesion, resembling haemangioma or hobnail haemangioma

## Localization
The localization is strictly limited to previously irradiated skin. There is a strong predilection for the breast or the anterior chest wall after radiation treatment in the setting of breast-conserving therapy or as an adjunct to mastectomy for breast cancer {639,224,706,1616,674}. Any anatomical site may be affected, depending on the underlying reason for irradiation and the area to which radiation has been administered {1754,224}.

## Clinical features
Atypical vascular lesions present as small, brown to erythematous papules and rarely plaques measuring about 0.5 cm {224, 1616}. They are frequently multiple at presentation and typically occur within 3–4 years after radiation treatment. The postradiation latency period may be as short as 1 year.

## Epidemiology
The epidemiology is dictated by the underlying reason for radiation treatment. The vast majority of patients are women in their late sixth to early seventh decade of life who have received radiation treatment for breast cancer {224,706,1616}.

## Etiology
Atypical vascular lesions are directly associated with radiation treatment. The median total administered radiation dose is 50 Gy {224}.

## Pathogenesis
Atypical vascular lesions occur secondary to irradiation, but their precise pathogenesis is unknown.

## Macroscopic appearance
Atypical vascular lesions are papular and often erythematous.

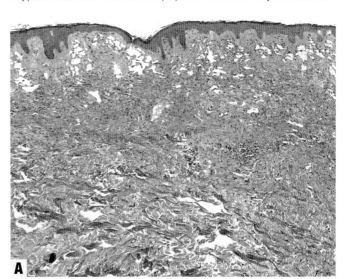

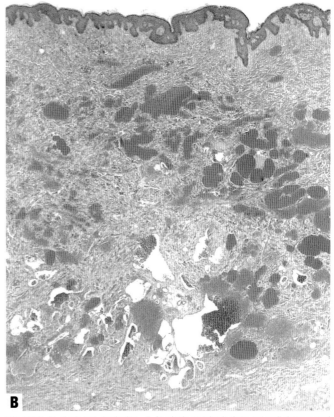

**Fig. 5.06** Atypical vascular lesion. **A** Atypical vascular lesions are well demarcated and centred in the superficial to middle dermis. **B** Occasionally, atypical vascular lesions are composed of dilated vascular channels extending into the deep dermis.

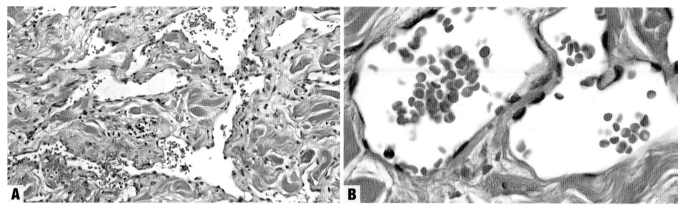

**Fig. 5.07** Atypical vascular lesion. **A** An anastomosing growth pattern of irregular vascular channels within the dermis is a characteristic feature. **B** The vascular channels are lined by a single layer of hyperchromatic endothelial cells. Cytological atypia and endothelial cell multilayering are not observed.

## Histopathology

Atypical vascular lesions are relatively circumscribed, often with somewhat wedge-shaped outlines. The proliferation is typically centred in the superficial dermis to mid-dermis, with rare extension into the deep dermis, but the subcutaneous tissues are typically spared. There are two histopathological subtypes with overlapping histological features. The more common lymphatic subtype is composed of irregularly shaped, thin-walled vascular channels with a branching and anastomosing growth. Lymphatic valve-like structures may be evident. The vessels are lined by a single layer of endothelial cells, which may show hobnailing and nuclear hyperchromasia. True cytological atypia or endothelial cell multilayering is not observed. Rare examples are characterized by more-dilated vascular spaces or focal dissecting growth through the dermal collagen bundles. Histologically, the vascular subtype resembles microvenular haemangioma or hobnail haemangioma with thin capillary channels lined by flattened to hobnail endothelium and lacking a lobular growth pattern. Individual lesions may show composite features of both vascular-type and lymphatic-type atypical vascular lesions.

The endothelial cells express the endothelial cell marker CD31 and variably CD34. The lymphatic type of atypical vascular lesion also usually expresses podoplanin. In contrast, the vascular type is typically negative for podoplanin, but there is a layer of surrounding pericytes as highlighted by SMA staining {1616}.

## Cytology

Not clinically relevant

## Diagnostic molecular pathology

Unlike most secondary cutaneous angiosarcomas, atypical vascular lesions lack *MYC* amplification as demonstrated by FISH, and there is no MYC overexpression by immunohistochemistry {790,1351,633,731}. These are important ancillary tools in diagnostically challenging cases.

## Essential and desirable diagnostic criteria

*Essential:* superficial dermal-based growth; lesional circumscription parallel to the epidermis; narrow vascular spaces lined by a single layer of hobnail endothelial cells; lack of infiltrative growth, cytological atypia, and multilayering; no *MYC* amplification by FISH; no MYC overexpression by immunohistochemistry.

## Staging

Not clinically relevant

## Prognosis and prediction

The disease may be complicated by local recurrences or the development of further atypical vascular lesions in the radiation field over time. Progression to angiosarcoma is exceedingly rare and remains controversial, because the vast majority of atypical vascular lesions have a benign clinical course {224, 1616,674}. The diagnostic biopsy must be representative of the underlying lesion to avoid missing an underlying angiosarcoma due to sampling error {1318}.

# Postradiation angiosarcoma of the breast

Antonescu CR
Billings SD
Rowe JJ
Thway K

## Definition
Postradiation angiosarcoma of the breast is a malignant neoplasm occurring secondary to irradiation in the skin or breast parenchyma.

## ICD-O coding
9120/3 Postradiation angiosarcoma

## ICD-11 coding
2B56.2 & XH6264 Angiosarcoma of breast & Angiosarcoma

## Related terminology
*Acceptable:* postradiation haemangiosarcoma; postradiation lymphangiosarcoma.

## Subtype(s)
Epithelioid angiosarcoma

## Localization
Lesions occur in the skin of the chest wall or scar of residual breast tissue in the irradiation field of previously treated breast carcinoma {171,2191}.

## Clinical features
Because postradiation angiosarcomas occur in patients treated for breast cancer, the age range at diagnosis reflects that specific cohort. Tumours arise in the radiation field with a mean latency period of 5–6 years {171,224}, with rare cases presenting after a shorter latency period of 1–2 years. They typically present as solitary or multiple cutaneous erythematous to violaceous patches, plaques, papules, or nodules {224,643}. Rarely, they may present as subtle skin thickening. Angiosarcoma may also arise in the setting of chronic lymphoedema (Stewart–Treves syndrome).

## Epidemiology
Postradiation angiosarcoma presents at an older patient age than primary angiosarcoma of the breast (at a median of 70 years vs 40 years) {1456,2191}.

## Etiology
Developing secondary to irradiation, this type of chest wall or breast angiosarcoma is most commonly seen in the setting of breast-conserving surgery with radiation therapy {171,224}. Less frequently, it occurs in the setting of mastectomy and adjuvant radiation therapy. Angiosarcoma is the most common radiation-induced sarcoma of the breast {2316,1022}.

## Pathogenesis
The gene signature of angiosarcomas, which is distinct from those of other sarcoma types, is characterized by upregulation of vascular-specific receptor tyrosine kinases, including *TIE1*,

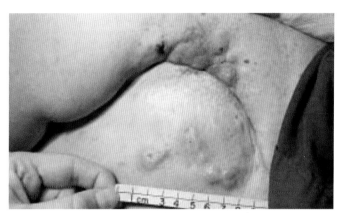

**Fig. 5.08** Postradiation angiosarcoma. Multiple cutaneous nodules in a patient with a prior history of irradiation in this area for breast cancer.

*KDR*, *TEK*, and *FLT1* {74}. A subset of radiation-induced angiosarcomas harbour mutations in genes involved in the regulation of vascular growth factor tyrosine kinases, such as *KDR* (also known as *VEGFR2*), *PLCG1*, and *PTPRB* {888,138}. *KDR* and *PLCG1* mutations are mutually exclusive; both genes are involved in the VEGFR2 signalling pathway. Truncating mutations in *PTPRB*, a tyrosine phosphatase specific to vascular endothelium that inhibits angiogenesis, have been reported in 26% of angiosarcomas, all occurring in secondary or radiation-induced tumours {138}. An alternative mechanism of VEGFR activation in secondary angiosarcoma is the presence of *FLT4* (also known as *VEGFR3*) gene amplifications at the 5q35 locus, which is coamplified with *MYC* in 5% of radiation-induced angiosarcomas {888}. *FLT4* gene abnormalities are mutually exclusive with *PLCG1*/*KDR* mutations.

## Macroscopic appearance
On cut surface, the lesions vary from haemangioma-like to solid masses, showing haemorrhagic and necrotic central areas and more spongy, vascular features towards the periphery. The extent of the tumours cannot be reliably determined on gross examination.

## Histopathology
Postradiation and postlymphoedema angiosarcomas can be diffuse or multifocal, and they are predominantly dermal-based tumours with variable infiltration into the subcutaneous tissues {639}. Infrequently, tumours extend into the deeper breast parenchyma. Although these tumours display a heterogeneous morphology, most have a vasoformative growth pattern. Well-differentiated neoplasms are composed of irregular, angulated, and variably dilated vascular channels, often with a sieve-like morphology {171}. The neoplastic channels are lined by ovoid cells with hyperchromatic or vesicular nuclei and often prominent small nucleoli. Lesions with intermediate morphology show

Chapter 5

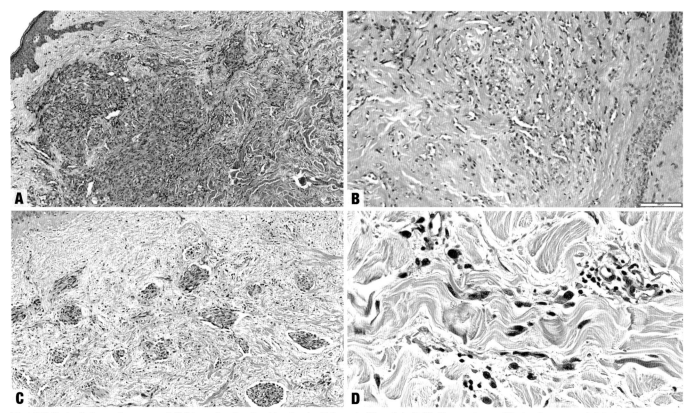

**Fig. 5.09** Postradiation angiosarcoma. **A** Solid growth pattern involving dermis. **B** A poorly differentiated infiltrative neoplasm within dermis composed of single cells and cords, as well as poorly formed slit-like spaces. The tumour cells have scant amphophilic cytoplasm and enlarged nuclei with vesicular chromatin and prominent nucleoli. **C** An unusual example of radiation-associated angiosarcoma displaying a lobular capillary pattern. **D** Radiation dermatitis pattern of angiosarcoma.

intraluminal papillary growth or multilayering, with enlarged hyperchromatic nuclei and increased mitotic figures. Poorly differentiated tumours show a solid growth pattern, either composed of sheets of epithelioid cells or short fascicles of spindle cells {1901,171}, associated with prominent mitoses, blood lakes, and necrosis. Less common patterns include the capillary lobule pattern and the radiation dermatitis–like pattern

{520,451}. The former consists of a lobular proliferation of atypical endothelial cells architecturally resembling haemangioma, but with an infiltrative growth pattern. The latter consists of scattered hyperchromatic cells associated with haemorrhage to thin, worm-like vascular channels lined by atypical endothelial cells. Despite heterogeneous morphology, the use of grading is not recommended; all cases are considered high-grade, with most following a highly aggressive course {1456}.

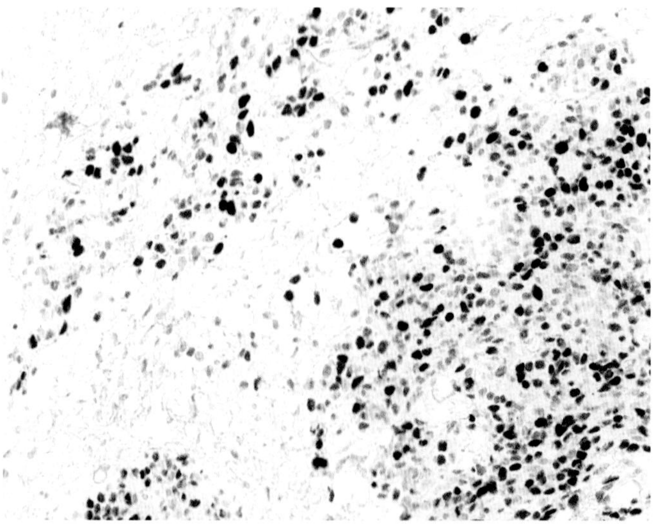

Diffuse and strong immunoreactivity is seen with both CD31 and ERG, along with variable expression of CD34, FLI1 {659}, and podoplanin (D2-40) – a marker of lymphatic endothelium. Focal keratin and rarely EMA expression can be seen, especially in epithelioid subtypes {1722}. An outer layer of SMA-positive pericytic cells is often lacking around the lesional vessels. Tumours also show strong nuclear expression of MYC, due to the consistent *MYC* gene amplifications {731,1351,633}. Radiation-associated angiosarcomas may demonstrate loss of H3K27me3 {1350}, whereas this marker is retained in the endothelial cells of benign and atypical vascular lesions.

Angiosarcomas may be associated with preceding or synchronous postradiation atypical vascular lesions in the skin and subcutis of the breast. In challenging cases, immunohistochemistry or FISH can be performed, because postradiation atypical vascular lesions are MYC-negative {1351}.

**Fig. 5.10** Postradiation angiosarcoma. MYC protein overexpression is a reliable surrogate marker of *MYC* gene amplification.

## Cytology

Not clinically relevant

## Diagnostic molecular pathology

High-level amplification of *MYC* at 8q24 is a consistent hallmark of radiation-induced and lymphoedema-associated angiosarcomas of the breast, present in > 90% of cases {1290,790,888}. In contrast, radiation-induced angiosarcomas occurring at other sites and/or after radiotherapy for other disease types show a less frequent pattern of *MYC* amplification {888}. The high-level amplification of *MYC*, typically defined as > 100 copies of *MYC*, in the form of homogeneously staining regions or multiple focal amplicons by FISH, can be used as a powerful ancillary test in excluding challenging atypical vascular lesions {790,1351}.

## Essential and desirable diagnostic criteria

*Essential:* previous irradiation of the field, usually after a time interval of > 3 years; predominantly dermal to subcutaneous growth, with rarer involvement of breast parenchyma; infiltrative growth pattern, with dissection of adipose tissue and lobular stroma; vasoformative growth with at least focal cytological atypia.

*Desirable:* MYC overexpression by immunohistochemistry; *MYC* amplification by FISH.

## Staging

Not clinically relevant

## Prognosis and prediction

There is a high rate of locoregional recurrence, which occurred in about half of the cases in one study {171}. Multiple recurrences

**Fig. 5.11** Postradiation angiosarcoma. FISH showing a high level of *MYC* gene amplification (red signals) in the form of homogeneously staining regions.

are common. Common metastatic sites include the lungs, contralateral breast and skin, liver, and bone {171}. Axillary lymph node metastases are uncommon. The median recurrence-free survival time is < 3 years and the median overall survival time < 5 years {171,224}.

# Primary angiosarcoma of the breast

Antonescu CR
Hunt KK
Rowe JJ
Thway K

## Definition
Primary angiosarcoma of the breast is a malignant primary endothelial neoplasm of mammary parenchyma, not associated with radiation exposure.

## ICD-O coding
9120/3 Angiosarcoma

## ICD-11 coding
2B56.2 & XH6264 Angiosarcoma of breast & Angiosarcoma

## Related terminology
Acceptable: haemangiosarcoma; lymphangiosarcoma.
Not recommended: malignant haemangioendothelioma.

## Subtype(s)
Epithelioid angiosarcoma

## Localization
The localization is usually parenchymal rather than cutaneous.

## Clinical features
Patients have a median age of 40 years at diagnosis {1456, 2191}, compared with the median age of 70 years for secondary angiosarcoma. Most patients present with a poorly defined, rapidly growing mass; swelling; or asymmetry of the breast {2313}. Two thirds of the neoplasms measure > 5 cm {709}. Mammography most often shows a non-calcified mass or focal asymmetry. Ultrasonography reveals either a hyperechoic mass or a mixed hyper- and hypoechogenicity with architectural distortion. Dynamic contrast-enhanced MRI reveals typical malignant enhancement characteristics. Core needle biopsy is the preferred diagnostic technique, because FNA is associated with a false negative rate as high as 40%. About 20% of patients present with regional disease at diagnosis {2324}, with 3.5% having either clinical or pathological nodal involvement {994}. The most frequent sites of distant metastatic disease are the lungs, liver, bones, and CNS.

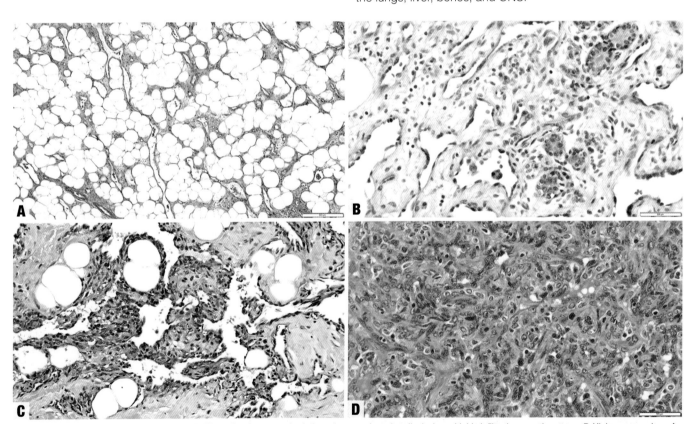

**Fig. 5.12** Primary breast angiosarcoma. **A** Well-differentiated tumour, simulating a haemangioma but displaying a highly infiltrative growth pattern. **B** Higher-power view of a well-differentiated tumour showing infiltrating and dissecting growth encasing mammary lobules. **C** Tumour with an intermediate differentiation showing vasoformation with multi-layering and intravascular papillary projections of the proliferating endothelial cells. **D** Poorly differentiated tumour composed mainly of solid growth with only focal vasoformation. High mitotic activity and substantial cytological atypia are present.

## Epidemiology

Angiosarcomas have been estimated to account for a quarter of all primary breast sarcomas {14}.

## Etiology

There is no clear etiology, although potential environmental factors have been implicated {279}.

## Pathogenesis

A small subset shows mutations in *PLCG1* and *KDR*, which are involved in the VEGFR2 signalling pathway {888}. Only rare cases show evidence of *MYC* gene amplification.

## Macroscopic appearance

The tumours are haemorrhagic, diffuse or multinodular masses that vary in size from 0.7 to 25 cm (mean: 6.7 cm, median: 5 cm) {1456}. They can be either circumscribed or poorly defined. Better-differentiated tumours often have a haemorrhagic, spongy appearance. Poorly differentiated tumours are more solid and fleshy, consisting of firm greyish-white tissue with areas of necrosis, and they may show areas of cystic, spongy, haemorrhagic vascular tissue peripherally.

## Histopathology

The tumours are typically located deep within breast parenchyma, with or without cutaneous involvement, showing an infiltrative or poorly defined border {1456,72}. A wide morphological spectrum is encountered, generally with a predominant vasoformative or solid component identified. In contrast to secondary angiosarcomas, primary lesions more often show well-formed, small to medium-sized anastomosing vessels that dissect through fibroadipose tissue {72}.

The neoplastic vascular channels in angiosarcoma have dilated, compressed, or angulated lumina. The lining endothelial cells range from bland to variably atypical, usually spindled, hyperchromatic nuclei that may be plump or flattened. Well-differentiated angiosarcomas are composed of well-formed vessels lined by flattened endothelial cells with minimal atypia. Dissection of irregular, angulated vascular channels through adipose tissue and mammary lobules indicates malignancy. A lobular-type growth pattern, typically seen in haemangioma, is not present. Lesions with an intermediate appearance show endothelial multilayering, hobnailing, or papillary-like projections. Poorly differentiated angiosarcomas have solid, cellular foci comprising sheets of spindled to epithelioid cells intermingled with variably formed anastomosing vascular channels, associated with prominent blood lakes, mitotic figures, and areas of necrosis. The vascular channels may be poorly formed, with complex dissecting patterns, or they may be compressed with subtle cleft-like spaces suggesting vascular differentiation. Epithelioid angiosarcomas have a solid appearance, with sheets of large atypical epithelioid to polygonal cells with ovoid vesicular nuclei, large nucleoli, and relatively abundant cytoplasm. Because vasoformation can be limited, epithelioid angiosarcoma may be confused with carcinoma. There are often prominent mitotic figures and necrosis.

Angiosarcomas express endothelial markers, with strong, membranous CD31 staining and nuclear ERG immunoexpression noted. Variable CD34, FLI1 {659}, and D2-40 positivity can be seen. Angiosarcomas, in particular of the epithelioid subtype, may also express epithelial markers, leading to erroneous interpretation as carcinoma {23,653}. Aberrant expression of KIT, synaptophysin, chromogranin, and CD30 can be seen {2070, 874}. Most tumours lack expression of MYC protein.

## Cytology

Not clinically relevant

## Diagnostic molecular pathology

Not clinically relevant

## Essential and desirable diagnostic criteria

*Essential:* no history of radiation exposure; malignant vascular proliferation (typically well differentiated); deep location within the breast parenchyma.
*Desirable:* diffuse infiltrative growth pattern, with dissection of adipose tissue and breast stroma.

## Staging

Not clinically relevant

## Prognosis and prediction

Total mastectomy has been the mainstay of therapy, with or without radiation therapy; however, locoregional recurrences are reported in half of all patients {1915}. There have been no randomized clinical trials assessing the outcomes with breast-conserving surgery versus mastectomy, or assessing the appropriate margin width after surgical resection. The type of local therapy is largely dependent on the tumour-to-breast size ratio. Breast-conserving surgery is considered if the tumour is small, allowing for surgical excision with negative margins and a favourable cosmetic reconstruction. In the SEER Program data, patients treated with breast-conserving surgery had better overall survival than patients who underwent mastectomy {2324}. This is probably due to the need for mastectomy in patients with larger and more-extensive tumours. Because the incidence of nodal metastasis is low overall, axillary lymph node dissection is not routinely performed unless there is pathological confirmation of nodal involvement. The role for radiation after resection has not been well established. Many series combine primary breast angiosarcomas with secondary (radiation-associated) angiosarcomas with varying combinations of radiation therapy and systemic therapy in the adjuvant or neoadjuvant setting.

Anthracycline and taxane-based regimens have been the frontline chemotherapy for angiosarcomas {2332}. Patients with locally advanced or metastatic angiosarcoma had a complete or partial response rate of 25% (vs 21% for patients with other sarcoma histologies). Better progression-free and overall survival was noted with a combination of doxorubicin and ifosfamide than with single-agent anthracycline chemotherapy.

A three-tiered grading system has been used for primary breast angiosarcomas in the past {536,1794}; however, as has been observed with angiosarcomas in other locations, grade does not seem to correlate with prognosis, because morphologically better-differentiated tumours can metastasize {1456}.

# Nodular fasciitis

Karim RZ
Brogi E
Liegl-Atzwanger B
Shin SJ

## Definition
Nodular fasciitis is a self-limited, benign clonal proliferation of fibroblastic/myofibroblastic cells.

## ICD-O coding
8828/0 Nodular fasciitis

## ICD-11 coding
2F30.Y & XH5LM1 Other specified benign neoplasm of breast & Nodular fasciitis

## Related terminology
*Not recommended:* pseudosarcomatous fasciitis.

## Subtype(s)
None

## Localization
Nodular fasciitis has been described in both the subcutis and parenchyma of the breast, occurring most frequently in the upper-outer quadrant {1586}.

## Clinical features
Nodular fasciitis in the breast presents clinically as a relatively rapidly growing mass that may be tender/painful or painless {1586}. It typically enlarges over several weeks, then regresses over several months. Skin retraction or nipple–areolar distortion has been reported {1586}. Most cases are < 5 cm in diameter, but the reported range is 0.6–6 cm {1586}.

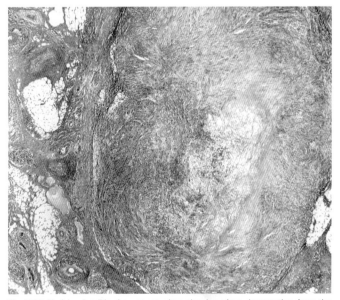

**Fig. 5.13** Nodular fasciitis. Low-power view showing clear demarcation from the breast ductular and lobular elements.

## Epidemiology
Nodular fasciitis is rare in the breast. It occurs over a broad age range, with a peak incidence in the third and fourth decades of life. In contrast to the equal sex distribution seen in soft tissues, in the breast there is a marked female predominance {1586}.

## Etiology
Unknown

## Pathogenesis
Nodular fasciitis shows fibroblastic/myofibroblastic differentiation and may arise from this lineage. It may be viewed as a form of transient neoplasia that consistently regresses {593}.

## Macroscopic appearance
Nodular fasciitis in the breast forms a well-circumscribed, unencapsulated mass. The gross appearance depends on the proportion of myxoid stroma, collagen, and cellularity within the lesion {1866}.

## Histopathology
Nodular fasciitis has the same morphology in the breast as elsewhere in the body. Microscopically, it is composed of fibroblasts and/or myofibroblasts without overt cytological atypia or pleomorphism. The stroma can be myxoid and/or collagenous {1064}. Cellularity varies between and within lesions. Early lesions are typically more cellular, and more-mature lesions tend to have more collagen {1064}. Mitotic activity can be brisk, but atypical forms are not seen {1866}. Feathery tissue culture–like areas are typical of the entity, but more-cellular areas can contain fascicles. The vasculature is rich and fine and can resemble granulation tissue. Lymphocytes and extravasated red blood cells are commonly seen {1866}. The lesions tend to be partially infiltrative, but nodular fasciitis within breast parenchyma does not entrap mammary ducts and lobules {1813}.

Immunohistochemically, the cells are positive for SMA; can have focal desmin expression; and are negative for cytokeratins, CD34, S100, and β-catenin (nuclear) {1064}.

Due to its rapid growth and infiltrative mass-like appearance on imaging, nodular fasciitis in the breast can raise concern for malignancy {594}. The diagnosis may be suspected on FNA and/or core biopsy, but excisional biopsy is often required for histological confirmation, because the differential diagnosis includes several aggressive entities that can contain fasciitis-like areas, and the histology of nodular fasciitis is variable {594}.

The differential diagnosis includes metaplastic / spindle cell carcinoma, the stromal component of phyllodes tumours, fibromatosis, pseudoangiomatous stromal hyperplasia, myofibroblastic tumours, reactive postbiopsy spindle cell nodules, and myxoid sarcomas.

Adequate sampling to confirm the absence of an epithelial component, along with negative keratin staining, assists in the

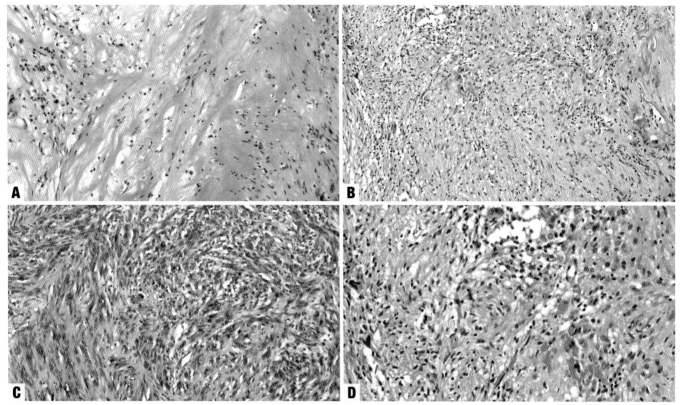

**Fig. 5.14** Nodular fasciitis. **A** Paucicellular sclerotic area. **B** Tissue culture–like areas. **C** Cellular area. **D** Feathery tissue culture–like areas with extravasated red blood cells and inflammatory cells.

differential with metaplastic carcinoma {1813}. Nodular fasciitis lacks the biphasic composition of phyllodes tumours, but again this requires sampling. Stromal overgrowth in phyllodes typically shows greater cytological atypia than seen in nodular fasciitis. Fibromatosis in the breast is more infiltrative, entraps mammary ducts and lobules, and shows nuclear staining for β-catenin {1866}. CD34 is positive in pseudoangiomatous stromal hyperplasia. Myxoid subtypes of nodular fasciitis may be mistaken for myxofibrosarcoma (primary or secondary) but do not show cytological atypia or atypical mitoses. Myofibroblastomas are typically slow-growing and uniform and lack inflammation {1866}.

## Cytology
Cytology is variable, depending on the age, cellular composition, and sampling of the lesion. It can show the spindle cells, extravasated red blood cells, and lymphocytes that would be suggestive of the diagnosis in the appropriate clinical setting. However, it can show myxoid material, clumps of collagen, blood, or nonspecific spindle cells, leading to a broad differential list, hence the usual need for histology {974}.

## Diagnostic molecular pathology
Cases of nodular fasciitis of the soft tissues have been shown to harbour a translocation between chromosomes 17 and 22 – t(17;22)(p13;q13) – in about 85% of cases {1920,1349}. *USP6* rearrangement has been demonstrated in a breast nodular fasciitis by FISH studies {974}. The fusion of the *MYH9* promoter and the *USP6* gene results in subsequent overexpression

of *USP6*. A variety of other genes can also be substituted for *MYH9* {1076}.

## Essential and desirable diagnostic criteria
*Essential:* fibroblastic/myofibroblastic proliferation without substantial atypia; admixed collagen and/or myxoid stroma with fine vasculature; does not entrap ducts and lobules in the breast; no epithelial/biphasic component on sampling.
*Desirable:* rapid growth (weeks); small size (< 5 cm); *USP6* gene rearrangement.

## Staging
Not clinically relevant

## Prognosis and prediction
Complete surgical excision is curative. Nodular fasciitis can regress spontaneously. Local recurrence is very infrequent even if there are positive surgical margins.

# Myofibroblastoma

Magro G
Charville GW
Fletcher CDM
Liegl-Atzwanger B
van de Rijn M

## Definition

Myofibroblastoma is a benign tumour of the mammary stroma composed of fibroblasts and myofibroblasts.

## ICD-O coding

8825/0 Myofibroblastoma

## ICD-11 coding

2F30.Y & XH8JB0 Other specified benign neoplasm of breast & Myofibroblastoma, mammary type

## Related terminology

None

## Subtype(s)

None

## Localization

Myofibroblastoma occurs most commonly in the breast parenchyma, but it can also occur in extramammary sites ( so-called mammary-type myofibroblastoma), especially in the inguinal/groin area, vulva, perineum, and scrotum.

## Clinical features

Myofibroblastoma usually presents as a slow-growing, painless, non-tender mass {1268,1269}. The imaging features are not specific, showing a well-circumscribed, lobulated, homogeneous, solid mass lacking microcalcifications {393,2322}. Rarely, bilateral or multicentric lesions have been reported {812}.

## Epidemiology

Although females and males are equally affected (patient age range: 1–87 years), most cases are seen in elderly men and postmenopausal women {1268}.

## Etiology

A hormonal etiology has been suggested and is supported by the expression of sex steroid hormone receptors and the association with two conditions (gynaecomastia and pseudoangiomatous stromal hyperplasia) with well-known hormonal etiopathogenesis {1740}.

## Pathogenesis

Myofibroblastoma arises from a precursor cell of the mammary stroma, capable of assuming different sizes and shapes, as well

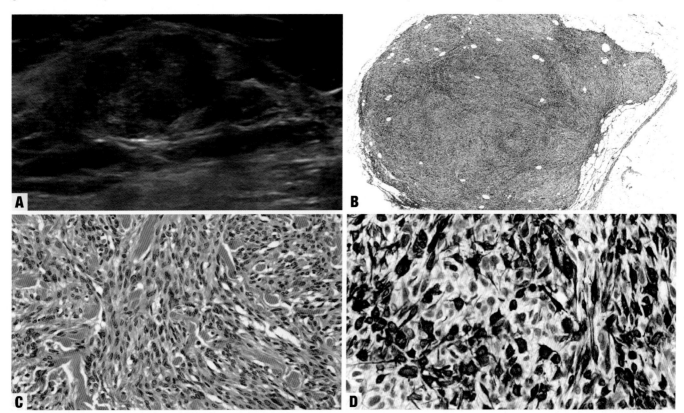

**Fig. 5.15** Myofibroblastoma. **A** Ultrasound shows a well-circumscribed, oval, hypoechoic mass. **B** Low magnification shows a tumour with lobulated, circumscribed borders. **C** Classic type. Bland-looking spindle cell proliferation with interspersed thick eosinophilic collagen fibres. **D** Most neoplastic cells stain strongly with desmin.

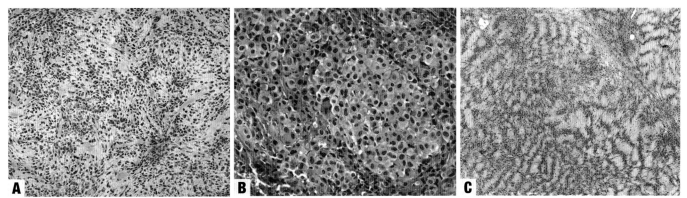

**Fig. 5.16** Myofibroblastoma. **A** Epithelioid cell type. Frozen section diagnosis: epithelioid cells haphazardly arranged in a stroma containing rare collagen fibres. Notice the close resemblance to invasive lobular carcinoma. **B** Deciduoid cell type. Large, deciduoid-like cells with enlarged nuclei are closely packed into solid sheets. **C** Palisaded/schwannoma-like. Spindle cell tumour with Verocay-like bodies, closely reminiscent of schwannoma.

as differentiating along several mesenchymal lineages (especially lipomatous or leiomyomatous tissues) {1272,1271}. Genetically, myofibroblastoma shows monoallelic or biallelic deletions of 13q (13q14), sometimes in combination with monosomy of 16q {1620,1273}. Deletion of 13q results in the loss of RB1 expression by immunohistochemistry {321}. Because spindle cell / pleomorphic lipoma and cellular angiofibroma share with myofibroblastoma not only some morphological and immunohistochemical features but also the same genetic alterations, it has been speculated that these tumours belong to the spectrum of the so-called 13q/Rb family of tumours {1273}.

## Macroscopic appearance
Myofibroblastoma presents as a well-circumscribed, unencapsulated tumour with a rubbery to gelatinous, yellow to whitish/grey cut surface. The tumours range in size from a few millimetres to 15 cm, with most cases not exceeding 3 cm {1268,1269}.

## Histopathology
The tumour has circumscribed margins and usually consists of bland, oval to spindle cells with pale to eosinophilic cytoplasm, arranged haphazardly or in short intersecting fascicles with interspersed variably hyalinized collagen bundles. Areas with storiform or neural-like growth patterns can be seen focally. The nuclei, which are round to oval in shape, may exhibit small

nucleoli, grooves, or pseudoinclusions. Mitoses are absent or rare. Entrapment of breast ducts or lobules is usually not seen. Unusual features include focally infiltrative margins, high cellularity, focal nuclear pleomorphism, multinucleated floret-like cells, intracytoplasmic and extracellular hyaline globules, and extensive myxoedematous stroma with blood vessels containing fibrinoid material, as well as focal smooth muscle and cartilaginous or osseous metaplasia {1268,1269,689,2231}. High mitotic count, necrosis, and extensive infiltrating margins are not features of myofibroblastoma. Five morphological patterns have been described: lipomatous, myxoid, fibrous/collagenized, epithelioid/deciduoid, and palisading/Schwannian-like {1268,1269}.

The tumour cells typically coexpress desmin and CD34, along with ER, PR, and AR {1268,1269}. There is loss of RB1 expression in approximately 90% of cases {321}. α-SMA, calponin, CD10, BCL2, and CD99 are variably expressed. The tumour cells are negative for cytokeratins, EMA, S100, STAT6, ALK, and β-catenin {1270,1267}.

## Cytology
Myofibroblastoma can be suspected on FNA, which shows randomly arranged, single and/or clustered short spindle-shaped cells with finely granular chromatin and small nucleoli {1532}.

## Diagnostic molecular pathology
13q14 deletion can be confirmed by FISH in 70–80% of cases.

## Essential and desirable diagnostic criteria
*Essential:* well-circumscribed margins; a mesenchymal tumour without epimyoepithelial components; none or only mild nuclear atypia or pleomorphism; low mitotic count; short interlacing fascicles.

*Desirable:* positive immunohistochemistry for desmin, CD34, ER/PR/AR; FISH: 13q14 deletion.

See also Box 5.01.

## Staging
Not clinically relevant

## Prognosis and prediction
Myofibroblastoma is cured by excision, with no tendency to recur.

**Box 5.01** Diagnostic criteria for classic-type myofibroblastoma

**Histopathology**
- Purely mesenchymal tumour – epimyoepithelial components absent
- Well-circumscribed margins; rarely focally infiltrative
- Bland-looking, short to elongated spindle cells; minor component: epithelioid to (more rarely) deciduoid-like cells
- No to mild nuclear atypia; nuclear pleomorphism in a minority of cases
- Short, haphazardly intersecting fascicles; focal storiform or neural-like pattern
- Low mitotic count
- Atypical mitoses and necrosis: absent
- Stroma: fibrous to myxoid stroma with interspersed thick collagen bundles
- Intratumoural areas of mature adipose tissue can be seen

**Immunohistochemistry / molecular pathology features**
- Positive markers: vimentin, desmin, CD34, ER/PR/AR
- Variable expression of α-SMA, calponin, CD10, BCL2, CD99
- Negative markers: cytokeratins, EMA, S100, β-catenin, STAT6, RB1, ALK1
- FISH: 13q14 deletion (in 70–80% of cases)

# Desmoid fibromatosis

van de Rijn M
Brogi E
Charville GW
Liegl-Atzwanger B
Shin SJ

## Definition
Desmoid fibromatosis is an infiltrative spindle cell neoplasm characterized by fibroblastic/myofibroblastic differentiation and activation of the WNT/β-catenin pathway.

## ICD-O coding
8821/1 Desmoid-type fibromatosis

## ICD-11 coding
2F75 & XH13Z3 Neoplasms of uncertain behaviour of breast & Aggressive fibromatosis

## Related terminology
*Acceptable:* desmoid tumour; aggressive fibromatosis; musculoaponeurotic fibromatosis.

## Subtype(s)
None

## Localization
Desmoid fibromatosis may arise primarily in the breast parenchyma (primary mammary fibromatosis), but many tumours originate in the pectoral fascia of the chest wall and extend secondarily into the breast {1482,1792}. Localization to the dermis or subcutis is occasionally seen. The tumours are usually solitary, although synchronous and asynchronous bilateralism has been reported {1792,492}.

## Clinical features
The typical presentation is that of a slowly evolving, non-tender, and palpably firm mass with poorly defined boundaries. Rare symptoms include skin retraction or dimpling, nipple discharge, and pain {2230}. Involvement of the axillary soft tissues should not be mistaken for lymphadenopathy. Radiographical findings of an irregularly contoured, spiculated, non-calcified mass often mimic the appearance of malignancy {562}.

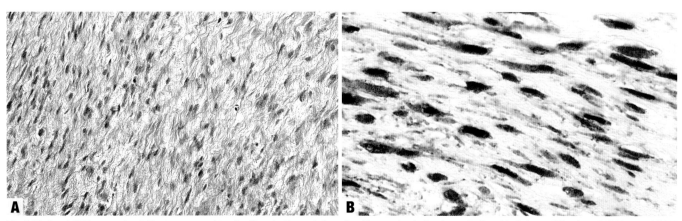

**Fig. 5.17** Desmoid fibromatosis. **A** The tumour consists of uniform-looking spindle cells with occasional pinpoint nucleoli and indistinct cell borders. **B** Evidence of WNT signalling activity may manifest immunohistochemically as nuclear localization of β-catenin.

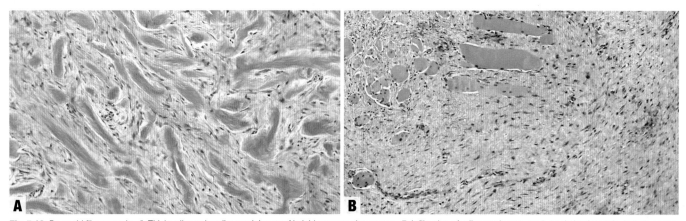

**Fig. 5.18** Desmoid fibromatosis. **A** Thick collagen bundles reminiscent of keloid are sometimes seen. **B** Infiltration of adjacent tissues, such as skeletal muscle, is a characteristic feature.

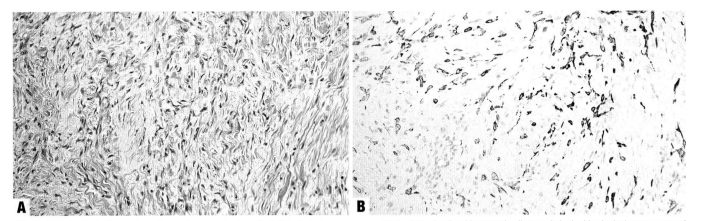

**Fig. 5.19** Fibromatosis-like metaplastic carcinoma of the breast. **A** Relatively homogeneous spindle-shaped cells with stromal collagen mimic the histological appearance of desmoid fibromatosis. **B** Demonstration of cytokeratin expression by immunohistochemistry is critical to the distinction of metaplastic carcinoma from desmoid fibromatosis.

## Epidemiology

Desmoid fibromatosis accounts for < 0.2% of all breast tumours {492}. The median patient age at presentation is in the third to fifth decades of life, but tumours can present at any age {1482, 1792,492}. The overwhelming majority of cases affect females.

## Etiology

More than 90% of desmoid fibromatoses present sporadically, with the remainder arising in the setting of familial adenomatous polyposis. There is a distinct association with prior tissue injury, including surgery, in as many as 44% of cases {1482}.

## Pathogenesis

*CTNNB1* activating mutations have been detected in 83–95% of sporadic desmoid fibromatosis cases {56,1124,533,410}. These mutations have a strong predilection for exon 3 of β-catenin. Activating mutations of *CTNNB1* or inactivating mutations/deletions of *APC* lead to a pathogenic increase in transcriptional signalling through the WNT/β-catenin pathway, which drives cell proliferation. *APC* inactivation via mutation or 5q allelic loss accounts for the majority of remaining sporadic cases, in addition to the bulk of cases associated with familial adenomatous polyposis {5,45,2065}. Application of massively parallel sequencing enables detection of *CTNNB1/APC* mutations with greater sensitivity, along with identification of rare mutations in alternative WNT regulators, such as *BMI1* {410}. Mutations of both *CTNNB1* and *APC* inhibit APC-mediated degradation of β-catenin, which in turn translocates to the nucleus where it regulates gene expression.

## Macroscopic appearance

Desmoid fibromatosis forms a poorly circumscribed mass lesion ranging in size from < 1 cm to > 10 cm in greatest dimension {1482,1792,2230}. The cut surface is tan-white to grey, with a trabeculated or whorled appearance.

## Histopathology

Uniform-looking, slender, spindle-shaped cells form interwoven, arcuate fascicles of varying cellularity that characteristically infiltrate adjacent tissues, such as mammary ducts/lobules, adipose tissue, and skeletal muscle. The relatively small, hypochromatic nuclei may contain a few pinpoint nucleoli. Mitoses are typically absent or rare. The cytoplasm has an eosinophilic hue and a fibrillar texture. Varying degrees of interstitial collagen limit cell–cell contact and nuclear juxtaposition and confer a broad spectrum of morphological manifestations, including those that mimic keloid. Although the stroma of nascent lesions may appear more myxoid, longstanding lesions can develop calcification or chondro-osseous metaplasia. Lymphoid aggregates are commonly seen at the periphery. Morphological features do not always distinguish desmoid fibromatosis from phyllodes tumour or metaplastic carcinoma, which must be excluded with molecular and/or immunohistochemical studies.

By immunohistochemistry, nuclear accumulation of β-catenin is seen in 76–100% of cases {5,163,1409,289,1089}, although patterns of immunoreactivity are sometimes difficult to interpret. Nuclear accumulation of β-catenin does not reliably distinguish desmoid fibromatosis from metaplastic carcinoma or phyllodes tumour {1089,713}. An absence of cytokeratin expression, established using antibodies targeting broad-spectrum, luminal, and basal cytokeratins, is essential to rule out metaplastic carcinoma, especially the fibromatosis-like subtype. Lack of p63 expression also distinguishes desmoid fibromatosis from a subset of metaplastic carcinomas. Unlike in myofibroblastoma and the stroma of phyllodes tumour, there is no expression of CD34 {1068}. ER, PR, and ERBB2 (HER2) are generally not expressed {1144,492}. Most tumours express SMA and calponin {1628}. Desmin immunoreactivity is occasionally seen in a limited fraction of neoplastic cells {1409}.

## Cytology

Classification by FNA is challenging and frequently inconclusive, owing to the indistinct cytomorphological features and low yield of dense fibrous tissue aspirates {1482}; therefore, immunohistochemical and molecular diagnostic assays of WNT/β-catenin pathway activation may be helpful.

## Diagnostic molecular pathology

Given the technical difficulty of interpreting β-catenin immunohistochemistry in some cases, along with the potential benefit of identifying a *CTNNB1* mutation {713}, sequencing may be helpful diagnostically.

## Essential and desirable diagnostic criteria

*Essential:* cytologically bland spindle cell morphology; lack of nuclear pleomorphism and atypical mitoses; lack of circumscription with infiltration of adjacent tissues; exclusion of spindle cell tumours with epithelial, myoepithelial, peripheral nerve sheath, endothelial, and myogenic differentiation by immunohistochemical or molecular assays.

*Desirable:* evidence of WNT/β-catenin activation by nuclear accumulation of β-catenin by immunohistochemistry, or molecular evidence of inactivating *APC* mutation or activating *CTNNB1* mutation.

## Staging

Not clinically relevant

## Prognosis and prediction

Desmoid fibromatosis exhibits infiltrative local growth with no potential for metastasis or evolution to high-grade malignancy. A rare exception is the phenomenon of radiation-induced sarcoma with clonal relationship to the irradiated fibromatosis {2170}. Local recurrence has been reported in 25–29% of breast lesions after local excision {1482,1792,2230}, but the predictive value of surgical margin status is uncertain {152,887, 1668,1353,1644,770}. The serine to phenylalanine substitution at codon 45 of exon 3 (p.Ser45Phe) appears to portend a higher risk of local recurrence in sporadic desmoid-type fibromatosis {1121,392,982,2140}. Growth has generally been regarded as persistent, but renewed interest in non-operative management of desmoid fibromatosis has revealed that growth arrest occurs in a substantial subset of patients who do not undergo surgery {198,640}.

# Inflammatory myofibroblastic tumour

Hornick JL
Liegl-Atzwanger B
Shin SJ

## Definition

Inflammatory myofibroblastic tumour is a fibroblastic/myofibroblastic neoplasm of intermediate biological potential, usually with a prominent inflammatory infiltrate of chiefly lymphocytes and plasma cells.

## ICD-O coding

8825/1 Inflammatory myofibroblastic tumour

## ICD-11 coding

2F30.Y & XH66Z0 Other specified benign neoplasm of breast & Myofibroblastic tumour NOS

## Related terminology

*Not recommended:* inflammatory pseudotumour.

## Subtype(s)

Epithelioid inflammatory myofibroblastic sarcoma

## Localization

The breast is rarely involved, with < 25 reported cases {997, 804,2356,1053}. Most cases occur in the respiratory tract, abdominal cavity, and retroperitoneum {737}.

## Clinical features

Inflammatory myofibroblastic tumour of the breast presents as a painless, circumscribed mass.

## Epidemiology

Tumours of the breast most often affect young to middle-aged females, although the age range is broad {376,1277}.

## Etiology

Unknown

## Pathogenesis

About two thirds of inflammatory myofibroblastic tumours harbour receptor tyrosine kinase gene rearrangements, most often involving the *ALK* locus at 2p23, with diverse fusion partners {1298}. Approximately 5% of inflammatory myofibroblastic tumours harbour *ROS1* gene fusions; other rare gene fusions involve *NTRK3*, *PDGFRB*, and *RET* {1242,73,2311,26,1648}.

## Macroscopic appearance

Most tumours are < 5 cm in size, with white to grey and sometimes yellow cut surfaces.

## Histopathology

Loose fascicles of uniform, plump spindle cells with vesicular chromatin, small nucleoli, and pale eosinophilic to amphophilic cytoplasm are typically observed {376}. The stroma may be myxoid or collagenous, usually containing an inflammatory infiltrate dominated by lymphocytes and plasma cells, with fewer eosinophils and neutrophils. Some tumours exhibit a compact, fascicular architecture with minimal stroma. A subset of tumour cells may resemble ganglion cells. Mitotic activity is low and necrosis is usually absent.

Inflammatory myofibroblastic tumours are nearly always positive for SMA, and more than half of cases are also positive for desmin. Keratin expression is observed in 20–30% of cases. CD34, S100, SOX10, and EMA are negative. About 60% of inflammatory myofibroblastic tumours express ALK (usually with a diffuse cytoplasmic pattern) {397,1648} and approximately 5%

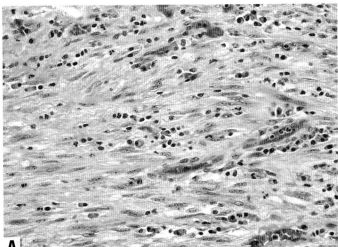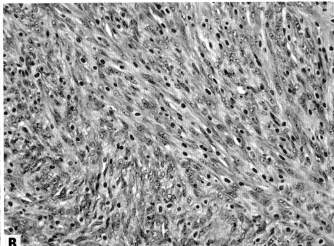

**Fig. 5.20** Inflammatory myofibroblastic tumour. **A** The tumour is composed of loose fascicles of plump spindle cells with vesicular chromatin and scant pale eosinophilic cytoplasm. Note the collagenous stroma and prominent intratumoural plasma cells. **B** This cellular, fascicular example could be mistaken for a sarcoma. Note the prominent intratumoural lymphocytes.

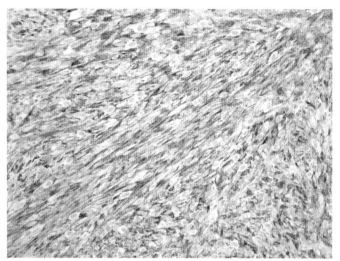

**Fig. 5.21** Inflammatory myofibroblastic tumour. Immunohistochemistry for ALK is positive in the tumour cells, reflecting the presence of an underlying *ALK* gene fusion.

of cases express ROS1, correlating with underlying *ALK* and *ROS1* gene fusions, respectively {875,73}.

## Cytology
Not clinically relevant

## Diagnostic molecular pathology
Confirmation of an appropriate fusion gene supports the diagnosis. However, molecular confirmation is not required if ALK immunohistochemistry is definitively positive.

## Essential and desirable diagnostic criteria
*Essential:* loose fascicles of plump spindle cells without substantial atypia or pleomorphism; inflammatory infiltrate of lymphocytes and plasma cells; consistent SMA expression; frequent ALK expression.

## Staging
Not clinically relevant

## Prognosis and prediction
Inflammatory myofibroblastic tumours of the breast have a low rate of local recurrence (~15%) {202}. Distant metastasis is rare (occurring in < 5% of cases) {2356}; histological features do not reliably predict clinical behaviour {375}.

# Schwannoma

Antonescu CR
Cimino-Mathews A

## Definition
Schwannoma is a benign, typically encapsulated peripheral nerve sheath tumour composed entirely of well-differentiated Schwann cells.

## ICD-O coding
9560/0 Schwannoma NOS

## ICD-11 coding
2F30.Y & XH98Z3 Other specified benign neoplasm of breast & Schwannoma NOS

## Related terminology
*Not recommended:* neurilemmoma.

## Subtype(s)
Cellular schwannoma; epithelioid schwannoma; plexiform schwannoma; melanotic schwannoma

## Localization
Schwannoma can arise within the breast dermis, subcutaneous tissue, breast parenchyma, or axillary soft tissues {2123,139}.

## Clinical features
Schwannomas of the breast can occur in female and male patients {2123,1617}. They most often present as palpable, mobile, non-tender masses {2123}. However, they can also be detected incidentally on routine screening imaging. By ultrasonography and mammography, they are solid, well-circumscribed, oval or round masses that lack calcification {139,346}.

## Epidemiology
Schwannomas of the breast are rare, accounting for < 3% of all schwannomas and < 1% of all primary breast neoplasms {313, 455}.

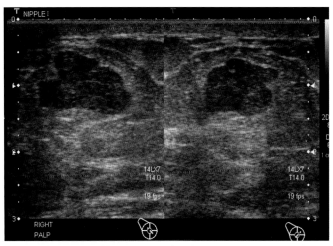

**Fig. 5.22** Schwannoma. Ultrasound scan of a schwannoma in a male breast shows a right retroareolar well-defined, gently lobulated nodule, wider than tall, located 4 mm from the nipple, 7 mm from the skin.

## Etiology
Most schwannomas of the breast are sporadic and non-syndromic {313,2123}. However, the presence of multiple schwannomas should prompt consideration of a syndrome such as neurofibromatosis type 2 or schwannomatosis {634,893}. Melanotic schwannomas in particular are associated with Carney complex {290}.

## Pathogenesis
The *NF2* gene encodes the protein merlin (NF2; also known as schwannomin), which is expressed in Schwann cells. Inactivating mutations of the *NF2* gene have been detected in 60% of all schwannomas {929}. In most cases, such mutations are accompanied by loss of the remaining wildtype allele on 22q. Other cases demonstrate loss of 22q in the absence of detectable

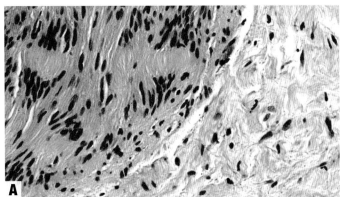
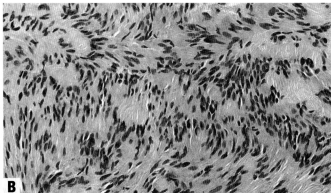

**Fig. 5.23** Schwannoma. **A** Antoni A pattern with nuclear palisading, Verocay bodies, and eosinophilic cell processes on the left, with the less cellular Antoni B pattern on the right. **B** The classic appearance of wavy nuclei with tapering ends stacked in parallel, palisaded alignment (Verocay bodies) is seen in schwannomas of the breast as in other body sites.

*NF2* gene mutations. Nevertheless, loss of merlin (NF2) expression appears to be a universal finding in schwannomas, regardless of their mutation or allelic status {901}. Schwannomas in the setting of neurofibromatosis type 2 show both germline and somatic *NF2* mutations {634}.

The pathogenesis of schwannomas in the setting of familial schwannomatosis occurs in a complex four-hit, three-step model: *SMARCB1* germline mutation (hit 1) is followed by loss of the other chromosome 22 with the wildtype copy of *SMARCB1* and one copy of *NF2* (hits 2 and 3), followed by a somatic mutation in the remaining copy of the *NF2* gene (hit 4) {893,2144}. A second subset of schwannomatosis patients display *LZTR1* germline mutations, following a similar four-hit model and somatically co-inactivating both copies of the *NF2* gene {900}.

Psammomatous melanotic schwannoma is a component of Carney complex, in which patients have loss-of-function germline mutations of the *PRKAR1A* tumour suppressor gene on 17q, which encodes the enzyme PRKAR1A {1023}.

## Macroscopic appearance

Grossly, most breast schwannomas appear as homogeneous, solid, often encapsulated yellowish-tan masses with a circumscribed border and sharp delineation from the adjacent mature adipose tissue or breast parenchyma. They can rarely be infiltrative or exophytic {2123,1131}. Ancient or degenerated schwannomas can display cystic change.

## Histopathology

Conventional schwannomas of the breast display histological features similar to those of their more common soft tissue counterparts {362}. Two architectural patterns are typically present in various proportions: Antoni A areas composed of compact, elongated cells with occasional nuclear palisading (Verocay bodies) and Antoni B areas, which consist of less cellular, loosely textured cells with indistinct processes and variable lipidization. The latter component often contains hyalinized blood vessels and variable lymphoid aggregates. The neoplastic Schwann cells have poorly defined cell borders, a moderate amount of eosinophilic cytoplasm, and euchromatic ovoid nuclei with bipolar tapered ends. Ancient or degenerated schwannomas display nuclear enlargement, pleomorphism, and hyperchromasia (ancient change); however, mitotic figures are scarce and necrosis is absent. By immunohistochemistry, schwannomas label diffusely for S100 and SOX10 {1516,979, 1371}. Schwannomas are negative for ER, actin, and desmin.

The cellular subtype is defined as a hypercellular schwannoma composed exclusively or predominantly of Antoni A tissue and typically lacking Antoni B areas and Verocay bodies. The tumours are composed of densely packed spindled cells arranged in intersecting fascicles, with aggregates of small lymphocytes commonly seen with either perivascular or pericapsular distribution {362}. Mitotic activity can be elevated in this subtype, but the mitotic figures should not be atypical {1224, 2270}.

The epithelioid subtype displays plump cells with dense eosinophilic cytoplasm and round nuclei {1117,1019,826}. Although the majority of schwannomas are negative for epithelial markers, focal keratin labelling has been reported and is particularly seen in the epithelioid subtype {313,614}. Half of the lesions may show loss of SMARCB1 (INI1) nuclear expression {948}.

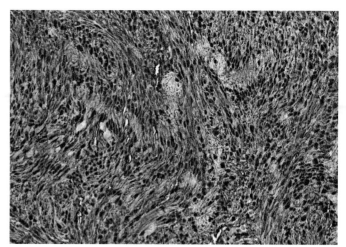

**Fig. 5.24** Schwannoma. Immunostaining for S100 is diffusely positive in the nuclei and cytoplasm of the neoplastic Schwann cells.

Plexiform schwannomas appear as multiple distinct nodules on histological cross-section, owing to their complex, tortuous network-like architecture {143,857}. They are more often dermal-based and can be of either conventional or cellular type.

The melanotic subtype is a rare, circumscribed but unencapsulated, grossly pigmented tumour composed of cells with the ultrastructure and immunophenotype of Schwann cells but containing melanosomes and reactive for melanocytic markers. The tumour is composed of nests and clusters of plump, spindled, and epithelioid cells, with hyperchromatic nuclei and macronucleoli. The cells show abundant intracellular melanin pigment, which is brown and finely granular. Melanotic schwannomas label for melan-A and HMB45 {2094}.

## Cytology

FNA of breast schwannoma reveals clusters of spindled cells indicative of a benign mesenchymal neoplasm {139,147}.

## Diagnostic molecular pathology

Not clinically relevant

## Essential and desirable diagnostic criteria

*Essential:* a mostly encapsulated or well-circumscribed lesion; alternating cellular (Antoni A) and hypocellular (Antoni B) regions; wavy, tapered nuclei with nuclear palisading (Verocay bodies); prominent hyalinized vessels and perivascular/pericapsular lymphoid cuffing; diffuse immunoreactivity for S100 and SOX10.

## Staging

Not clinically relevant

## Prognosis and prediction

Schwannomas are benign neoplasms. Although most schwannomas of the breast are treated with simple wide local excision, conservative expectant management of schwannomas detected on breast core needle biopsy may be a reasonable approach for asymptomatic lesions that lack atypical radiographical features and remain static in size {808}.

# Neurofibroma

Antonescu CR
Cimino-Mathews A

## Definition
Neurofibroma is a benign nerve sheath tumour composed of neoplastic, well-differentiated Schwann cells intermixed with non-neoplastic elements, such as perineurial-like cells, fibroblasts, mast cells, a variably myxoid to collagenous matrix, and residual axons or ganglion cells.

## ICD-O coding
9540/0 Neurofibroma NOS

## ICD-11 coding
2F30.Y & XH87J5 Other specified benign neoplasm of breast & Neurofibroma NOS

## Related terminology
None

## Subtype(s)
Diffuse neurofibroma; atypical neurofibroma; plexiform neurofibroma

## Localization
Neurofibromas involving the breast are most commonly superficial and located in the dermis {313}. However, they can rarely involve the deep breast parenchyma {2079}.

## Clinical features
Neurofibromas of the breast occur in female and male patients {196,1434,945}, typically presenting as palpable and mobile masses. Cutaneous lesions may be pedunculated {196}. They can be detected as incidental masses on routine screening radiography {2079}. On mammography, they are well-circumscribed, round to oval masses; on ultrasonography, they are round, hypoechoic masses with posterior enhancement that can mimic a cyst.

## Epidemiology
Neurofibromas of the breast are rare, accounting for < 1% of all breast neoplasms.

## Etiology
Neurofibromas of the breast are most commonly reported in the nipple–areola complex of patients with neurofibromatosis type 1 (NF1) {196,1434,1330}. Sporadic, solitary neurofibromas of the breast are rare {2079,945}.

## Pathogenesis
Given the mixed cellular composition of neurofibromas, it has been difficult to determine whether they are monoclonal. Notably, allelic loss of the *NF1* gene region of 17q appears to be confined to the S100-positive Schwann cells in neurofibromas {1631}, suggesting that they are the clonal neoplastic element. Mutations in *NF1* lead to loss of function of the neurofibromin (NF1) protein, which regulates cell proliferation via mTOR and via inactivation of p21(ras), a proto-oncogene protein {1330, 634}. The majority of neurofibromas involving the breast occur in patients with NF1, which is due to autosomal dominant mutations in the *NF1* gene, which encodes the protein neurofibromin (NF1) {1330,634}. *CDKN2A/CDKN2B* losses are found in tumours diagnosed as atypical neurofibromas in patients with NF1, suggesting that such tumours may be premalignant lesions {135}.

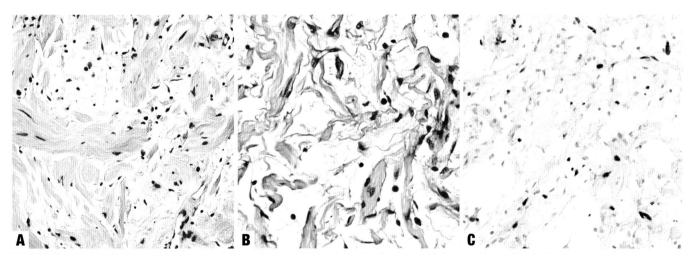

**Fig. 5.25** Neurofibroma. **A** The classic appearance of scattered spindled cells admixed with inflammatory cells in a variably myxoid and collagenous stroma is seen in neurofibromas of the breast as in other body sites. **B** A hypocellular proliferation of bland spindle cells embedded in a collagenous stroma (so-called shredded carrots). **C** Immunostaining for SOX10 shows nuclear positivity in the neoplastic Schwann cells.

## Macroscopic appearance

Grossly, neurofibromas of the breast have a variable appearance; they can be solitary and well circumscribed or multinodular and poorly defined {313}.

## Histopathology

Neurofibromas of the breast display the same histological features as their soft tissue counterparts; however, the diagnosis can be challenging on breast core needle biopsy due to the small sample size and the broad differential diagnosis. Neurofibromas are composed in large part of neoplastic Schwann cells with thin, curved to fusiform nuclei and scant cytoplasm, as well as fibroblasts in a variably collagenous and myxoid matrix. Residual axons are often present within neurofibromas and can be highlighted with neurofilament immunohistochemistry. Stromal collagen varies in abundance and takes the form of dense, refractile bundles (the so-called shredded-carrot appearance) {362}. Solitary neurofibromas are well circumscribed and delineated from the adjacent soft tissue, whereas diffuse neurofibromas lack capsules and infiltrate around adnexal structures or breast ducts and lobules. Intraneural neurofibromas often remain confined to the nerve, encompassed by its thickened perineurium. Diffuse neurofibromas commonly contain highly characteristic tactile-like structures (pseudo-Meissner corpuscles) and occasionally may contain melanotic cells. Ancient neurofibroma is defined by degenerative nuclear atypia alone and should be distinguished from atypical neurofibroma, given the lack of any other features of malignancy.

Atypical neurofibroma is a subtype defined by worrisome features such as high cellularity, scattered mitotic figures, and/or fascicular growth in addition to cytological atypia, and it is notoriously difficult to distinguish from low-grade malignant peripheral nerve sheath tumour {1372}.

Plexiform neurofibroma is a subtype defined by involvement of multiple nerve fascicles, which are expanded by tumour cells and collagen but commonly demonstrate residual nerve fibres at their centres. In contrast to plexiform schwannomas, which are non-syndromic, plexiform neurofibromas are pathognomonic for NF1 {1330,634}.

By immunohistochemistry, a proportion of spindled cells express S100 and SOX10, in contrast to the diffuse labelling seen in schwannomas {1516,979,1371}. This patchy labelling reflects the admixture of the immunoreactive Schwann cells with the other cellular components. Scattered cells, presumably of perineurial origin, show GLUT1 and claudin positivity. EMA typically highlights the residual perineurium. CD34 stains a subset of stromal cells, whereas KIT (CD117) highlights recruited mast cells. Loss of p16 (CDKN2A) expression in cytologically atypical nuclei is an important finding for atypical neurofibroma and distinguishes it from ancient-type change. Neurofibromas are negative for cytokeratins, ER, actin, and desmin.

## Cytology

FNA of breast neurofibroma reveals dispersed spindled cells suggestive of a benign mesenchymal neoplasm {945,863, 1459}.

## Diagnostic molecular pathology

Not clinically relevant

## Essential and desirable diagnostic criteria

*Essential:* bland spindled cells with wavy narrow nuclei; loose shredded-carrot collagen bundles; prominent mast cells; laminated, round, eosinophilic structures (pseudo-Meissner corpuscles); positivity for S100 and CD34 in different cellular subsets.

*Desirable:* loss of p16 expression in atypical nuclei is a hallmark of atypical neurofibroma.

## Staging

Not clinically relevant

## Prognosis and prediction

Neurofibromas are benign neoplasms and are treated with complete conservative (i.e. wide local) excision. However, patients with NF1 should be followed closely, because neurofibromas in these patients are more likely to undergo malignant transformation than sporadic neurofibromas {634}.

# Granular cell tumour

Bui M
Mahar AM
Reis-Filho JS

## Definition
Granular cell tumour is a benign neuroectodermal tumour derived from Schwann cells and composed of epithelioid cells with abundant lysosome-rich granular eosinophilic cytoplasm.

## ICD-O coding
9580/0 Granular cell tumour NOS
9580/3 Granular cell tumour, malignant

## ICD-11 coding
2F30.Y & XH09A9 Other specified benign neoplasm of breast & Granular cell tumour NOS

## Related terminology
*Not recommended:* Abrikossoff tumour; granular cell myoblastoma.

## Subtype(s)
None

## Localization
As many as 8% of all granular cell tumours arise in the breast {1084}. Other common sites include the head and neck (in particular the tongue), proximal extremities, gastrointestinal tract (especially the oesophagus), and respiratory tract. Skin and subcutaneous involvement is most common, although the breast parenchyma can also be involved.

## Clinical features
Representing only 1 in every 1000 breast tumours, granular cell tumours are usually single, but multicentricity has been reported in as many as 18% of patients {15}. These tumours mimic carcinoma clinically (irregular and firm masses) and radiologically (poorly defined or spiculated masses without microcalcifications). Lesions in the skin are firm and flesh-coloured to red, and they can cause skin retraction, nipple inversion, and (more rarely) pectoral fascia involvement. Exceptionally, granular cell tumours can show malignant change (in 1–2% of cases) {615}. Colocalization of granular cell tumour and invasive breast carcinoma has been reported on occasion {25}.

## Epidemiology
Granular cell tumour of the breast usually arises in women, over a wide age range (19–77 years) {1597} and more often in young adult African Americans (mean age: 41 years) than in white Americans (mean age: 54 years) {1597}. Children {1552} and men {1079} are more rarely affected. The tumour can present with coincidental breast carcinoma or be associated with mastectomy scars {1803}. The fact that the driver genes most frequently mutated in granular cell tumours, *ATP6AP1* and *ATP6AP2*, map to the X chromosome may explain the higher prevalence in women {1599,1890}.

## Etiology
There is limited information available on the etiology of granular cell tumour of the breast. Rarely, these tumours have been described in association with other conditions, including Bannayan–Riley–Ruvalcaba syndrome {1292}, neurofibromatosis type 1 {1302}, Noonan syndrome {112}, and LEOPARD syndrome (multiple lentigines, electrocardiographic conduction abnormalities, ocular hypertelorism, pulmonic stenosis, abnormal genitalia, retardation of growth, and sensorineural deafness) {1877}, but most cases, including multifocal presentations, are sporadic.

## Pathogenesis
Granular cell tumours show peripheral nerve sheath (Schwannian) differentiation. Genetic profiling has revealed frequent

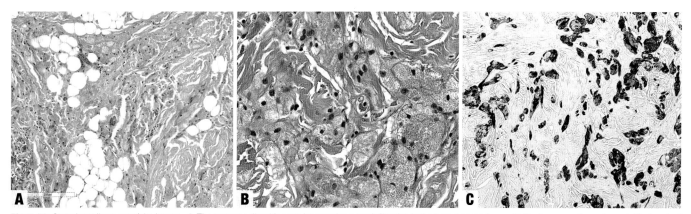

**Fig. 5.26** Granular cell tumour of the breast. **A** The tumour cells with granular cytoplasm are infiltrative in the breast parenchyma. **B** The tumour cells are large, with abundant granular and pale pink cytoplasm, inconspicuous cytoplasmic borders, and bland nuclei. **C** Immunohistochemical staining highlights the infiltrative tumour cells, which show strong and diffuse positivity for S100.

loss-of-function mutations in the *ATP6AP1* and *ATP6AP2* genes, encoding vacuolar H+-ATPase components that regulate endosomal pH. Much less frequently, genes encoding other vacuolar H+-ATPase components are mutated {1599,1890}. These mutations result in impaired vesicular acidification, altered distribution of endosomes, and massive accumulation of intracytoplasmic vesicles, in particular early and recycling endosomes. Although these alterations have been shown to be oncogenic, the mechanistic basis of *ATP6AP1* and *ATP6AP2* loss-of-function mutations remains to be fully elucidated {1599}. These tumours have a low mutation burden.

## Macroscopic appearance
These tumours are homogeneous and white or tan in colour, show regular or infiltrative borders, and can reach up to 5 cm in diameter {15,729}.

## Histopathology
Granular cell tumours have an infiltrative growth pattern, with poorly defined borders. The tumour is composed of sheets, clusters, and trabeculae of large, round to polygonal cells with abundant, eosinophilic, and distinctly granular cytoplasm. The cell borders are indistinct and appear syncytial. The centrally located nuclei are usually small, uniform, and hyperchromatic, more rarely vesicular with prominent nucleoli. The finely granular cytoplasm results from massive accumulation of lysosomes, punctuated by larger intracytoplasmic granules surrounded by clear haloes (pustulo-ovoid bodies of Milian), which are often PAS-positive/diastase-resistant. Perineural and perivascular involvement is frequent {131}. Mitoses are generally scarce {240}. These tumours can elicit exuberant pseudoepitheliomatous hyperplasia when situated in the dermis {1084}. Malignant granular cell tumour (which is exceedingly rare) is recognized by aggressive histological features {615}.

The immunohistochemical profile of granular cell tumours includes strong and diffuse positivity for S100. CD68, CD63 (NKI/C3), and NSE are also positive, most likely due to non-specific reactivity with cytoplasmic lysosomes. Strong nuclear expression of TFE3 and MITF is common, whereas HMB45, melan-A, GFAP, keratins, and NFP are negative {1874,738}. The Ki-67 proliferation index is typically low (< 2%) {250,1122}.

The differential diagnosis includes non-neural granular cell tumours and other diverse tumours with granular cell change, including apocrine neoplasms, naevi, melanomas, fibrous histiocytomas, carcinomas, and alveolar soft part sarcoma.

## Cytology
In FNA samples, the characteristic granular cytoplasm and bland nuclei are useful features {729,566}, but carcinomas (in particular apocrine carcinomas) and histiocytic processes must be considered.

## Diagnostic molecular pathology
Not clinically relevant

## Essential and desirable diagnostic criteria
*Essential:* bland and large cells with granular cytoplasm, often with an infiltrative pattern; S100 strongly and diffusely positive; must exclude other more aggressive neoplasms showing granular cell change (melanoma, breast carcinoma).

## Staging
Not clinically relevant

## Prognosis and prediction
Treatment is local excision {240}. Granular cell tumours of the breast have minimal risk of local recurrence, even when excised with positive margins {1597}. The rare malignant form can give rise to metastasis, including distant dissemination. Features suggestive of malignancy include large tumour size (> 5 cm), cellular and nuclear pleomorphism, prominent nucleoli, increased mitotic activity, tumour necrosis, and local recurrence {1084}.

# Leiomyoma

Creytens D
Flucke U

## Definition
Leiomyoma is a benign tumour of smooth muscle.

## ICD-O coding
8890/0 Leiomyoma NOS

## ICD-11 coding
2F30.Y & XH4CY6 Other specified benign neoplasm of breast & Leiomyoma NOS

## Related terminology
None

## Subtype(s)
*Superficial:* cutaneous (pilar) leiomyoma, leiomyoma of the nipple/areola (muscularis mamillae and areolae).
*Deep:* leiomyoma of the breast parenchyma.

## Localization
Leiomyoma can be localized in the dermis (cutaneous leiomyoma), the nipple/areola, or the breast parenchyma.

## Clinical features
Patients may be asymptomatic or present with pain or a palpable nodule/mass without specific imaging features {1381,27}. Multiple tumours occur rarely.

## Epidemiology
Most patients are women {588}. The age range is broad, from 20 to 70 years, with an average age of 43 years.

## Etiology
A few cases have been reported in association with the syndrome of hereditary leiomyomatosis and renal cell carcinoma, which is attributable to germline mutation of *FH* (encoding fumarate hydratase) {296,2093}.

## Pathogenesis
Unknown

## Macroscopic appearance
In contrast to the poorly defined superficial lesions, deep (parenchymal) lesions are well circumscribed. The neoplasms are firm, rubbery, and grey to tan, with a whorled cut surface. Superficial lesions are commonly smaller than deep-seated ones {588}.

## Histopathology
The histopathology and immunophenotype of these lesions are identical to those of smooth muscle tumours elsewhere in the body {506,1064,1067,1457,1487}. Leiomyoma of the skin or nipple/areolar region shows, in association with the pilar muscle or muscularis mamillae/areolae, a poorly defined disorganized increase in smooth muscle bundles, which can be confluent. The spindle cells have elongated cigar-shaped nuclei and eosinophilic cytoplasm. Focal degenerative cytological atypia may be seen, but mitotic figures are absent. Lesions within the parenchyma are (multi)nodular and well circumscribed. They consist of intersecting fascicles of elongated smooth muscle cells with or without slight degenerative atypia. Mitotic activity is usually absent or low. Oedema and hyalinization may be present. Immunohistochemical markers (SMA and desmin) may be used to confirm a smooth muscle phenotype. Loss of

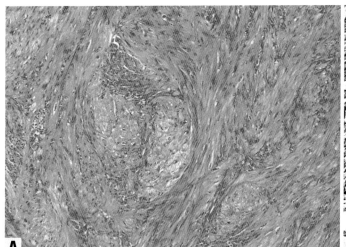
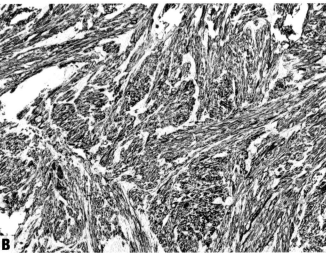

**Fig. 5.27** Leiomyoma. **A** The bland smooth muscle cells proliferate in whorls and fascicles. **B** Immunohistochemistry shows diffuse reactivity for desmin.

expression of fumarate hydratase by immunohistochemistry may suggest the diagnosis of hereditary leiomyomatosis and renal cell carcinoma in the rare familial cases.

## Cytology
Not clinically relevant

## Diagnostic molecular pathology
Not clinically relevant

## Essential and desirable diagnostic criteria
*Essential:* tumour composed of cells with smooth muscle differentiation; absence of atypia and substantial mitotic activity.

## Staging
Not clinically relevant

## Prognosis and prediction
Excision is the treatment of choice. Recurrences are rare {1064, 588,1487}.

# Leiomyosarcoma

Jo VY
Shin SJ

## Definition
Leiomyosarcoma is a malignant tumour with smooth muscle differentiation.

## ICD-O coding
8890/3 Leiomyosarcoma NOS

## ICD-11 coding
2C6Y & XH7ED4 Other specified malignant neoplasms of breast & Leiomyosarcoma NOS

## Related terminology
*Acceptable:* cutaneous leiomyosarcoma; atypical intradermal smooth muscle neoplasm.

## Subtype(s)
None

## Localization
Leiomyosarcoma can be localized in the dermis, the nipple/areola, or the breast parenchyma.

## Clinical features
Leiomyosarcoma of the breast may arise within the deep parenchyma or the nipple. The tumours typically present as a slow-growing palpable mass that may be painful and tender.

## Epidemiology
Primary leiomyosarcomas of the breast are rare, accounting for < 1% of all breast neoplasms. Most patients are affected during adulthood (in the fourth to sixth decades of life). The majority of cases arise superficially in the dermis, especially around the nipple–areola complex, and affect both sexes equally. Leiomyosarcomas arising in deep parenchyma are rare, and most reported cases have been in female patients {899}.

## Etiology
Most reported cases are sporadic, and the etiology is unclear.

## Pathogenesis
Soft tissue leiomyosarcomas usually have highly complex karyotypes, and they show molecular heterogeneity overall. Losses of regions on 16q and 1p have been reported {134}.

## Macroscopic appearance
Cutaneous leiomyosarcomas tend to be small (0.5–1.5 cm in diameter), with indistinct margins. Leiomyosarcomas arising in breast parenchyma are larger (as much as 9.0 cm in greatest dimension) and appear as a well-circumscribed grey, white, or tan fleshy mass; haemorrhage and necrosis are common.

## Histopathology
The histology and immunophenotype of leiomyosarcoma in the breast are similar to those of its counterparts elsewhere in the body {1064}. The lesions typically have irregular infiltrative borders. Leiomyosarcoma is composed of intersecting fascicles of spindle cells with blunt-ended nuclei. The cytoplasm is frequently eosinophilic, although it may occasionally be clear or fibrillary. The cell borders are often well defined. Nuclear atypia, pleomorphism, and mitotic activity are typically prominent {612}. Tumour necrosis may also be observed. Although dermal lesions may appear well circumscribed, they show at least focal infiltration into subcutaneous fat or breast parenchyma. Lesions that are completely confined to the dermis are designated as atypical intradermal smooth muscle neoplasms {1056}.

By immunohistochemistry, most tumours show expression of smooth muscle markers (SMA, desmin, and caldesmon), although staining may be variable. As many as 40% of tumours may be reactive for keratin and/or EMA {241,1370}.

Some fibroadenomas {755} and hamartomas {645,1526} may have stroma showing smooth muscle differentiation; however,

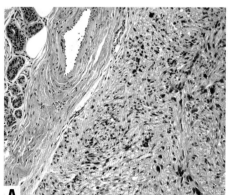
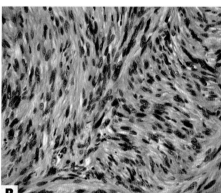
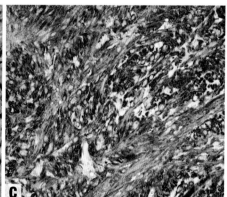

**Fig. 5.28** Leiomyosarcoma. **A** A tumour arising in breast parenchyma. **B** Intersecting fascicles of atypical spindle cells having ovoid nuclei with blunt ends and eosinophilic cytoplasm. **C** Most tumours show expression of SMA (shown here), desmin, and h-caldesmon.

Chapter 5

these lack atypia and mitotic activity. In small biopsies, myofibroblastoma, desmoid fibromatosis, inflammatory myofibroblastic tumour, and schwannoma may resemble leiomyosarcoma. Metaplastic carcinoma must also be distinguished from leiomyosarcoma – p63 and high-molecular weight cytokeratin are most helpful in this {1701}.

## Cytology
Leiomyosarcoma of the breast is only rarely biopsied by FNA, and the aspirate may be indistinguishable from specimens from other spindle cell malignancies, including malignant phyllodes tumour and sarcomatoid carcinoma, without the use of ancillary studies {938}.

## Diagnostic molecular pathology
Not clinically relevant

## Essential and desirable diagnostic criteria
*Essential:* fascicular growth of smooth muscle cells with cytological atypia and increased mitotic activity.
*Desirable:* expression of smooth muscle markers (SMA and desmin or h-caldesmon).

## Staging
See *Mesenchymal tumours of the breast: Introduction* (p. 189).

## Prognosis and prediction
Cutaneous leiomyosarcoma is best treated by complete excision; tumours may recur and rarely metastasize {612}. Tumours confined to the dermis (atypical intradermal smooth muscle neoplasms) show virtually no risk of metastasis {1056}. Mastectomy is appropriate for leiomyosarcoma arising in breast parenchyma. Metastases to distant sites have been reported, although leiomyosarcoma does not metastasize to the lymph nodes. No prognostic parameters have been validated for leiomyosarcomas arising in the breast.

# Lipoma

Nielsen TO
Fletcher CDM
Tay TKY

### Definition
Lipoma is a benign neoplasm of mature fat that displays no cytological atypia.

### ICD-O coding
8850/0 Lipoma NOS

### ICD-11 coding
2F30.Y & XH1PL8 Other specified benign neoplasm of breast & Lipoma NOS

### Related terminology
None

### Subtype(s)
None

### Localization
Not applicable

### Clinical features
Lipomas present as asymptomatic masses. They may feel soft to rubbery on palpation and are mobile over the underlying fascia. MRI can be helpful in identifying lipomas because they are isodense to adjacent fat and typically repress completely when fat-saturation sequences are used. On ultrasonography, lipomas demonstrate echogenicity similar to that of the surrounding fat. Mammography may be less useful in detecting lipomas, especially if they are small or extremely large or if the breast tissue is largely replaced by fat {1114,1186}.

### Epidemiology
Breast lipomas are most commonly brought to clinical attention in middle-aged women and are reported to occur in as many as 4.6% of excision biopsies {1114}.

### Etiology
Unknown

### Pathogenesis
Genetic analyses of lipomas have shown that two thirds of cases involve chromosomal rearrangements; of these, about two thirds harbour gene fusions in which *HMGA2* is the 5′ partner {167,1589}. The 3′ fusion partner is variable and of unclear significance. HMGA2 is normally expressed in replicating cells but is negatively regulated by multiple sequence elements in its 3′ untranslated region. A common feature of documented rearrangements is loss of this repressive 3′ untranslated region. The resulting gene products may also lack some C-terminal HMGA2 sequences but retain its DNA-binding AT-hook domain, which is sufficient to promote tumorigenesis. Similar events are found not only in lipomas but also in several other types of

benign mesenchymal tumours {1871}. Other relatively frequent aberrations that have been described in lipomas involve 13q and 6p {128}.

### Macroscopic appearance
Lipomas are typically well-circumscribed lesions with a homogeneous yellowish-white cut surface. Rarely, lipomas may grow to sizes of > 10 cm {1186}. The clinical concern associated with breast masses means they typically present at a gross size of about 2–3 cm.

### Histopathology
Lipomas are composed of mature adipocytes, which show limited variability in cell size and a small amount of associated fibrous or vascular tissue that is similar to normal subcutaneous fat. A thin capsule may or may not be evident, but the mass is distinct from adjacent breast parenchymal stromal and epithelial elements. Microscopic foci of fat necrosis are quite common, and the presence of histiocytes and giant cells around liquefied adipocytes may raise concern for an atypical lipomatous tumour. Importantly, the adipocytes lack atypical hyperchromatic cells or true lipoblasts, which in conjunction with limited thin stromal collagen helps distinguish conventional lipomas from atypical lipomatous tumours {1806}. Subtypes have been described with increased collagenous or cartilaginous tissues {114}; fibrolipoma and chondrolipoma are considered histological subtypes, but spindle cell lipoma and angiolipoma are distinct diagnostic entities with different molecular biologies. One study suggested that chondrolipoma could be a lipomatous subtype of myofibroblastoma with cartilaginous metaplasia {1929}. The

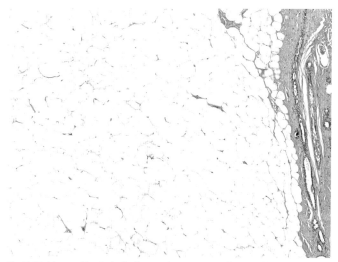

**Fig. 5.29** Lipoma. Histologically, lipoma shows mature adipocytes forming a circumscribed mass distinct from adjacent breast tissues. The adipocytes show neither nuclear atypia nor substantial variation in cell size.

distinction from hamartoma is based on the absence of other epithelial and parenchymal elements.

## Cytology
Not clinically relevant

## Diagnostic molecular pathology
Not clinically relevant

## Essential and desirable diagnostic criteria
*Essential:* mature uniform adipocytes without cytological atypia.

## Staging
Not clinically relevant

## Prognosis and prediction
Lipomas are benign. Due to the clinical concern associated with breast masses, they are often removed surgically. An excisional biopsy procedure is considered adequate treatment.

# Angiolipoma

Nielsen TO
Calhoun BC
Fletcher CDM

## Definition
Angiolipoma is a benign neoplasm of mature fat with clusters of small vessels, some of which contain hyaline microthrombi.

## ICD-O coding
8861/0 Angiolipoma NOS

## ICD-11 coding
2F30.Y & XH3C77 Other specified benign neoplasm of breast & Angiolipoma

## Related terminology
None

## Subtype(s)
None

## Localization
Not applicable

## Clinical features
Unlike their soft tissue counterparts, angiolipomas of the breast generally present as solitary masses, which are not associated with pain {730}. Breast imaging studies may show a homogeneously hyperechoic mass on ultrasonography {944}. The majority are located in subcutis overlying breast, rather than in breast parenchyma.

## Epidemiology
Although more commonly presenting in females, cases can also occur in males {1512}.

## Etiology
Unknown

## Pathogenesis
Although angiolipomas presenting specifically in the breast have yet to be interrogated with modern genomic technologies, a recent next-generation sequencing study including 35 soft tissue angiolipomas found that 80% harboured detectable subclonal mutations in *PRKD2*, the gene encoding the protein kinase PKD2 {866}. PKD2 is a serine/threonine kinase that acts as a major relay node of signal transduction pathways, with a role in transducing proliferative signals in endothelial cells and in activating vascular endothelial growth factor pathways. Within tumour tissue, PKD2 is expressed in both adipocytes and endothelial cells {866}. Activating mutations in the catalytic domain of *PRKD2* are detectable at an allelic frequency of 3–15% (highest in the adipocytic cell fraction), supporting the hypothesis that clonal adipocytic mutant cells secondarily induce the characteristic vessel formation in this tumour. No other chromosomal or consistent RNA-level changes were identified, and this mutation was not seen in other types of fatty tumours.

## Macroscopic appearance
The typical appearance is that of a tan/yellow to brown circumscribed lesion, more commonly located in the subcutaneous fat as opposed to within the breast parenchyma, with a mean size of < 2 cm {1066}.

## Histopathology
In most cases, angiolipomas are predominantly composed of mature fat, but they display obviously increased small vasculature clearly evident even at low magnification. Capillary-sized vessels are often arranged in clusters that are more common towards the periphery of the lesion; fibrin microthrombi are a distinctive histological feature that can be identified in some core biopsies and in the great majority of excision specimens

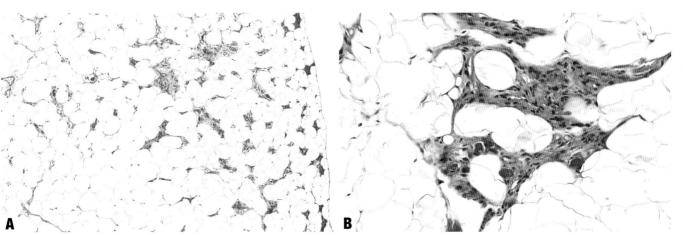

**Fig. 5.30** Angiolipoma. **A** Angiolipomas are characterized by clusters of disorganized small vessels in a background of mature adipocytes. **B** Some vessels display distinctive hyaline microthrombi.

{1066}. Cellular subtypes (with > 50% vascular tissue) occasionally raise concern for angiosarcoma (in particular because they are more likely to present in older patients and with suspicious imaging features), but angiolipomas have monomorphic nuclei generally devoid of substantial cytological atypia or proliferative activity, and they lack infiltrative borders {108,730}.

## Cytology
Not clinically relevant

## Diagnostic molecular pathology
Not clinically relevant

## Essential and desirable diagnostic criteria
*Essential:* a neoplasm composed of benign adipocytes with prominent vessels; microthrombi in small vessels.

## Staging
Not clinically relevant

## Prognosis and prediction
Angiolipomas are benign, with no documented potential for local recurrence or malignant transformation. Definitive diagnosis on core biopsy can obviate the need for excision {1886}.

# Liposarcoma

Folpe AL
Carter JM

### Definition
Liposarcoma is a family of soft tissue neoplasms with lipogenic differentiation and varying biological behaviour, ranging from locally aggressive to metastasizing.

### ICD-O coding
8850/3 Liposarcoma NOS

### ICD-11 coding
2C6Y & XH2J05 Other specified malignant neoplasms of breast & Liposarcoma NOS

### Related terminology
*Acceptable:* atypical lipomatous tumour / well-differentiated liposarcoma; dedifferentiated liposarcoma; myxoid liposarcoma; pleomorphic liposarcoma.

### Subtype(s)
None

### Localization
Liposarcoma arises in mammary parenchyma and adjacent soft tissues.

### Clinical features
Primary liposarcomas of the breast occur across a broad age range in adults, in both women and men. All subtypes have been reported {96}. Patients typically present with palpable, slowly enlarging masses or tumours detected by screening mammography {2138}. By mammography or ultrasonography, the imaging features are nonspecific and may mimic those of other (more common) circumscribed, lobulated lesions of the breast, such as fibroadenoma {311,2138}. "Atypical lipomatous tumour" and "well-differentiated liposarcoma" are related terms for the same (morphologically and genetically identical) tumours. Easily resectable tumours limited to the breast may be labelled atypical lipomatous tumours, whereas more-difficult-to-resect tumours with chest wall involvement are better considered well-differentiated liposarcomas.

### Epidemiology
Primary liposarcomas of the breast are exceptionally rare, with < 50 reported cases. The great majority of liposarcomatous neoplasms in the breast are malignant phyllodes tumours with heterologous liposarcomatous differentiation (see *Phyllodes tumour*, p. 172) {1672,100}. Published series report that primary liposarcomas account for an estimated 1–5% of all sarcomas of the breast, but these data largely predate the advent of diagnostic molecular testing, and the true incidence is unclear {1335,96,232}.

### Etiology
Unknown

### Pathogenesis
Atypical lipomatous tumour / well-differentiated liposarcoma (ALT/WDLPS) and dedifferentiated liposarcoma (DDLPS) almost universally contain supernumerary ring or giant chromosomes containing amplifications of chromosomal region 12q13-q15, including *MDM2*, *CDK4*, and other genes {1986, 977,172}. Overexpression of MDM2 and CDK4 is probably the main genetic driver event in ALT/WDLPS, affecting p53-mediated cell-cycle regulation among other pathways. Myxoid liposarcoma is defined by recurrent *DDIT3* genetic rearrangement: t(12;16)(q13;p11) with *FUS-DDIT3* gene fusion or less commonly t(12;22)(q13;q12) with *EWSR1-DDIT3* gene fusion {413,

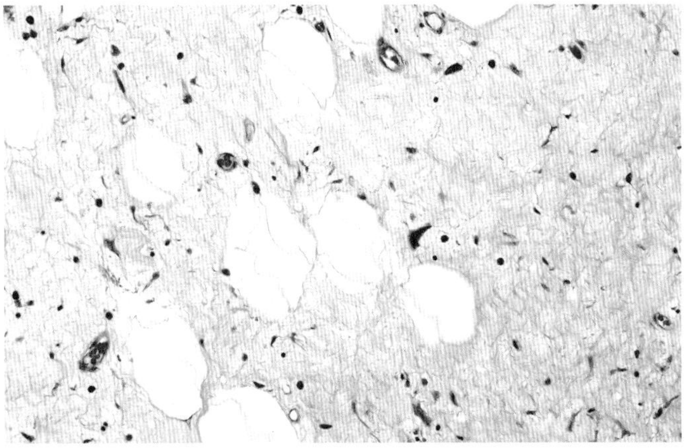

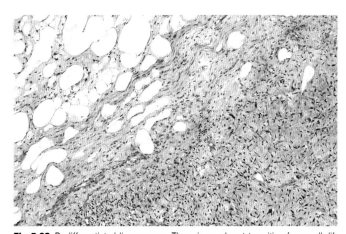

**Fig. 5.31** Well-differentiated liposarcoma. A neoplasm consisting of mature adipose tissue transected by irregular, finely fibrillar septa, containing enlarged, hyperchromatic stromal cells.

**Fig. 5.32** Dedifferentiated liposarcoma. There is an abrupt transition from well-differentiated liposarcoma to an undifferentiated, variably myxoid, spindle cell sarcoma.

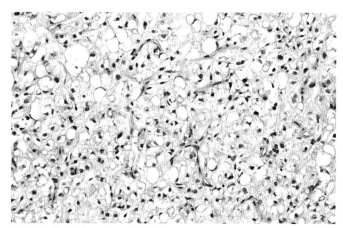

**Fig. 5.33** Myxoid liposarcoma. Abundant myxoid matrix; a well-developed, arborizing capillary vasculature; generally bland, round tumour cells; and scattered lipoblasts.

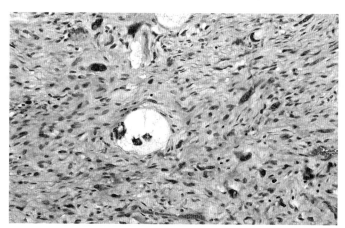

**Fig. 5.34** Pleomorphic liposarcoma. Pleomorphic lipoblasts and undifferentiated-looking spindled cells.

1687,1590}. *DDIT3* encodes a member of the C/EBP family of transcription factors. The DDIT3 fusion proteins probably act as transcriptional dysregulators, and they have been associated with activation of the IGFR/PI3K/AKT signalling axis, but the exact pathogenic mechanisms of myxoid liposarcoma are poorly understood {479}. Pleomorphic liposarcoma has a complex karyotype with numerous chromosomal abnormalities, wherein *TP53* mutations and loss of *RB1* are frequent events, but no recurrent cytogenetic rearrangements have been identified {719}.

### Macroscopic appearance

ALT/WDLPS is a lobulated, typically well-circumscribed, yellow/white mass composed of mature adipose tissue with fibrous strands and variable fat necrosis. DDLPS resembles ALT/WDLPS admixed with firm, fleshy tan/white areas reflecting the high-grade sarcomatous component, and it is often infiltrative. Myxoid liposarcomas are circumscribed, multinodular tumours with a gelatinous cut surface reflecting the myxoid matrix. Fleshy solid areas may be observed and should be well sampled, because they may represent cellular (round cell) change. Grossly, pleomorphic liposarcoma is typically a large, firm, circumscribed tumour, often with necrosis, similar to other high-grade sarcomas.

### Histopathology

ALT/WDLPS is composed of relatively mature adipose tissue transected by irregular fibrous septa containing diagnostic enlarged, hyperchromatic stromal cells. Lipoblasts may be present but are not required for the diagnosis. Some cases of ALT/WDLPS are predominantly composed of fat, whereas others are chiefly fibrous. DDLPS usually shows an abrupt transition from ALT/WDLPS to a higher-grade sarcoma. Most often, the high-grade component of DDLPS resembles undifferentiated pleomorphic sarcoma, but homologous pleomorphic liposarcomatous differentiation {1299}, as well as heterologous mesenchymal differentiation (e.g. myogenic, osteosarcomatous, chondrosarcomatous), can occur.

Myxoid liposarcoma is composed of cytologically bland, small, round to ovoid cells embedded in a myxoid matrix with distinctive small chicken-wire arborizing vasculature. The neoplastic cells tend to cluster around the blood vessels, and the stromal mucin may form large acellular pools. Neither atypia nor mitoses are common. Scattered univacuolated lipoblasts may be present but are not necessary for the diagnosis. Hypercellularity or a round cell component consists of densely packed primitive cells with hyperchromatic nuclei, a high N:C ratio, and no myxoid stroma. When present, the round cell component should be carefully quantified, because myxoid liposarcoma with a > 5% round cell component is associated with aggressive biological behaviour and poor prognosis {439}. Notably, myxoid liposarcoma of the soft tissues has a proclivity for metastasis to unusual sites, including the breast, and metastasis should be carefully excluded before making a diagnosis of primary mammary myxoid liposarcoma {1593,1823,2325}.

Pleomorphic liposarcoma is a high-grade pleomorphic sarcoma with varying numbers of pleomorphic multivacuolated lipoblasts. Myxofibrosarcoma-like areas are a common finding. There is often a high degree of nuclear pleomorphism and the lesional cells are typically spindled, but as many as 25% of cases can be epithelioid and mimic a high-grade carcinoma. By definition, there should be no areas resembling ALT/WDLPS {873}.

Areas indistinguishable from ALT/WDLPS can be found in phyllodes tumours with heterologous liposarcomatous differentiation, but these lack the characteristic 12q13-q15 amplification {1093}. Such tumours are significantly more common in the breast than true ALT/WDLPS, and the presence of an epithelial component should always be carefully searched for with extensive sampling. As noted in the section on breast phyllodes tumours (see *Phyllodes tumour*, p. 172), these low-grade heterotopic adipocytic proliferations with lipoblasts do not represent conventional liposarcoma and thus cannot be used as a criterion for establishing malignancy in phyllodes tumour.

DDLPS can mimic the (much more common) spindle cell subtype of metaplastic breast carcinoma, and other metaplastic breast carcinomas can have pleomorphic liposarcoma–like areas {570}. Careful evaluation for an in situ or conventional carcinoma component and an immunohistochemical panel of broad-spectrum and high-molecular-weight cytokeratin antibodies can help to establish a diagnosis of metaplastic carcinoma.

## Cytology
Not clinically relevant

## Diagnostic molecular pathology
ALT/WDLPS and DDLPS are frequently associated with amplification of *MDM2* and very often of *CDK4* as part of a supernumerary chromosome of 12q13-q15 {1986,977,172}. FISH or immunohistochemistry for MDM2 or CDK4 shows high sensitivity for ALT/WDLPS and DDLPS {2238}. Because myxoid liposarcoma is defined by any one of several recurrent *DDIT3* genetic rearrangements with either *FUS* or *EWSR1*, FISH for *DDIT3* rearrangement or sequencing can be used to confirm the diagnosis {413,1687,1590}. There is typically no role for immunohistochemistry in the diagnosis of myxoid liposarcoma. Although *TP53* mutations are commonly encountered in pleomorphic liposarcoma, molecular diagnostics are not routinely used in this diagnosis. Phyllodes tumour with liposarcomatous differentiation is an important (and more common) entity in the differential diagnosis of both ALT/WDLPS/DDLPS and pleomorphic liposarcoma, in particular on core needle biopsy. Because liposarcomatous phyllodes tumour appears to lack 12q13-q15 (e.g. *MDM2*, *CDK4*) amplification, MDM2/CDK4 testing may be a useful adjunct {1256,923,100}. Extensive sampling to identify a classic malignant phyllodes tumour component should be performed.

## Essential and desirable diagnostic criteria
### ALT/WDLPS and DDLPS
*Essential:* lipogenic tumour with characteristic atypical cells (ALT/WDLPS) and abrupt transition to high-grade sarcoma (DDLPS); exclusion of liposarcomatous phyllodes tumour.
*Desirable:* confirmation of *MDM2/CDK4* amplification or overexpression.

### Myxoid/round cell liposarcoma
*Essential:* characteristic histological features and exclusion of metastasis from other soft tissue site.
*Desirable:* confirmation of *DDIT3* genetic rearrangement, or detection of specific *FUS-DDIT3* or *EWSR1-DDIT3* gene fusion.

### Pleomorphic liposarcoma
*Essential:* high-grade sarcoma with pleomorphic lipoblasts, with exclusion of liposarcomatous malignant phyllodes tumour; exclusion of metaplastic carcinoma with panel of cytokeratin antibodies (as above).
*Desirable:* exclusion of DDLPS with homologous pleomorphic liposarcoma by MDM2/CDK4 testing.

## Staging
Primary liposarcomas of the breast can be staged using the Union for International Cancer Control (UICC) TNM classification system for liposarcomas of soft tissues {229}.

## Prognosis and prediction
The paucity of prognostic and predictive data on liposarcomas of the breast reflects their extreme rarity. Therefore, current prognostication and therapeutic decision-making are largely based on data from their soft tissue counterparts {439}. For ALT/WDLPS, tumour size and surgical resectability are the most important prognostic factors. For DDLPS, anatomical location is also an important prognostic factor. In the breast, surgical resectability and the ability to obtain negative surgical margins predict recurrence likelihood. An estimated 20% of DDLPSs metastasize by haematogenous spread; therefore, there is no indication for lymph node sampling. For myxoid liposarcoma, the presence of a round cell component (the most widely accepted cut-off point is > 5%) is a predictor of aggressive biological behaviour and adverse outcome {439}. As mentioned above, identification of a myxoid liposarcoma within the breast should prompt a thorough clinicoradiological evaluation to exclude metastasis from a distant site {2325,720}. Pooled data on all types of mammary sarcomas (including phyllodes tumours) indicate that tumour size and margin status are the most important prognosticators for recurrence {1335,359}.

# Pseudoangiomatous stromal hyperplasia

Rowe JJ
D'Alfonso TM
Pauwels P
Val-Bernal JF

## Definition

Pseudoangiomatous stromal hyperplasia (PASH) is a stromal myofibroblastic proliferation lining anastomosing slit-like spaces.

## ICD-O coding

None

## ICD-11 coding

GB20.Y Other specified benign breast disease

## Related terminology

None

## Subtype(s)

Fascicular (cellular) pseudoangiomatous stromal hyperplasia; atypical pseudoangiomatous stromal hyperplasia {864}

## Localization

Not applicable

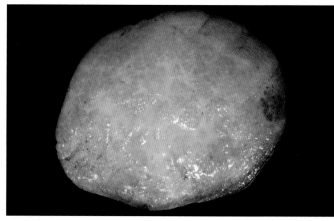

**Fig. 5.35** Pseudoangiomatous stromal hyperplasia. A circumscribed mass with a tan-white cut surface.

## Clinical features

PASH can occur in both sexes and commonly presents as an incidental finding, although it can be associated with other benign or malignant lesions. Palpable mass-forming PASH

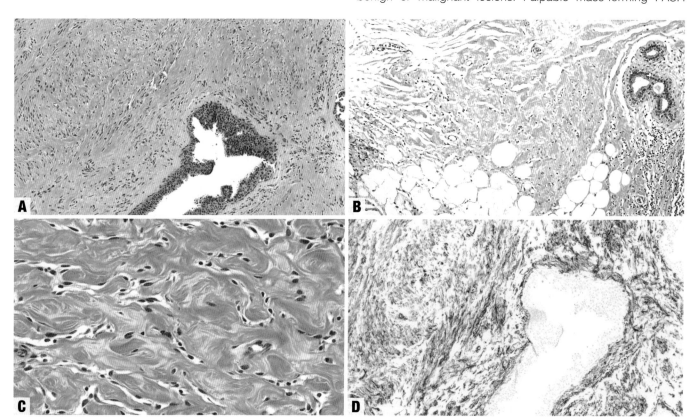

**Fig. 5.36** Pseudoangiomatous stromal hyperplasia. **A** Stromal reaction surrounding a breast duct. The stroma is hypercellular, but without evidence of vascular proliferation. **B** Pseudoangiomatous stromal hyperplasia shows slit-like spaces suggestive of vessels but lined by myofibroblasts with flattened compressed nuclei. **C** Empty anastomosing channels lined by flattened cells resemble a vascular proliferation. **D** CD34 staining highlights the stromal proliferation.

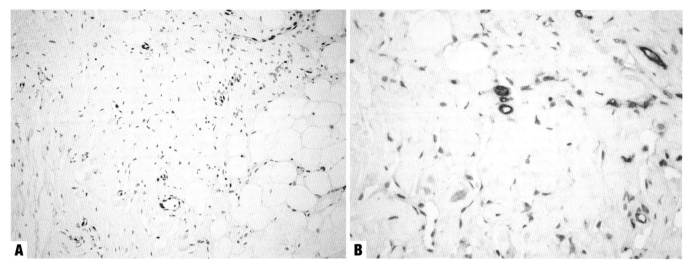

**Fig. 5.37** Pseudoangiomatous stromal hyperplasia (PASH). **A** Immunohistochemistry for ERG, an endothelial marker, is negative along the slit-like spaces of PASH, while staining endothelial nuclei of a few admixed capillaries. **B** Immunohistochemistry for factor VIII, a vascular marker, shows negative staining along the slit-like spaces of PASH, while staining several capillaries in the section.

(so-called nodular PASH or PASH tumour) presents as a painless, unilateral, firm or rubbery mass. In rare instances, PASH can present as rapid diffuse enlargement of both breasts. When visible on mammography, PASH occurs as a mass or focal asymmetry without calcifications; by sonography it appears as a hypoechoic mass and by MRI as either a postcontrast well-delineated mass or an area of non-mass enhancement {1696}. In males, PASH most often occurs as a palpable mass or nodule and is usually associated with gynaecomastia {1373,103}. PASH with stromal giant cells, in the background of gynaecomastia, may be associated with neurofibromatosis type 1 {446}. PASH can occur in accessory breast tissue along the milk line {986}.

### Epidemiology
PASH is most commonly seen in women with a mean age in the fourth to sixth decades of life, but it can also occur in postmenopausal women, in men, and in children {1914,216}.

### Etiology
In premenopausal females and prepubertal boys, PASH is driven by hormonal imbalances. PASH is believed to be an aberrant response of myofibroblasts to endogenous or exogenous hormones – most likely progesterone, because the staining intensity of PR is greater than that of ER {64,2179}.

### Pathogenesis
PASH does not have characteristic molecular features.

### Macroscopic appearance
When mass-forming, PASH occurs as a well-circumscribed, unencapsulated, firm rubbery mass of 1–12 cm in size {1671}, and in some cases it has a multinodular appearance. The cut surface is tan-white and homogeneous.

### Histopathology
PASH is a proliferation of myofibroblasts intermixed with terminal duct lobular units. The stroma is composed of dense collagen with anastomosing, slit-like channels, devoid of red blood cells and lined by spindle cells, which can resemble flattened endothelial cells. The spindle cells most often have bland cytology and lack mitotic activity or atypia. PASH is present as the stromal component of gynaecomastia (in particular florid gynaecomastia), and peri–terminal duct lobular unit oedema and gynaecomastoid-type changes in ductal epithelium are also present. PASH may also be seen in the stroma of fibroadenomas and phyllodes tumours.

The term "fascicular PASH" refers to the formation of cellular bundles of myofibroblasts arranged in a fascicular pattern {1671} lacking slit-like spaces and merging with conventional PASH. Fascicular PASH can mimic myofibroblastoma, but it is differentiated by the presence of typical breast epithelial elements within the borders of the tumour. Rarely, PASH may contain atypical spindle cells with nuclear enlargement and hyperchromasia (atypical PASH), and there is one documented case in the literature in which sarcoma arose from PASH {1464}. Rarely, PASH can show cytoplasmic inclusions similar to those observed in digital fibromas {108}.

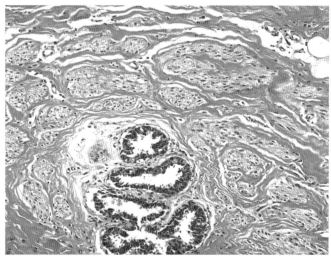

**Fig. 5.38** Fascicular pseudoangiomatous stromal hyperplasia. Short fascicles of spindled myofibroblasts.

The stromal cells of PASH show positive immunohistochemical staining for CD34, actin, desmin, and hormone receptors, with PR staining observed more frequently than ER staining {1671,64}. The stromal cells of PASH are negative for endothelial markers (CD31, ERG, D2-40), cytokeratins, and S100.

PASH must be distinguished from angiosarcoma and other vascular lesions. True blood-filled anastomosing vascular channels lined by malignant endothelial cells are the key feature of angiosarcoma.

## Cytology
FNA of PASH is nonspecific.

## Diagnostic molecular pathology
Not clinically relevant

## Essential and desirable diagnostic criteria
*Essential:* bland spindle cell myofibroblasts; an anastomosing network of slit-like channels; dense acellular collagenous stroma.
*Desirable:* immunohistochemistry negative for endothelial markers if needed; scattered acini and ducts in the background.

## Staging
Not clinically relevant

## Prognosis and prediction
PASH need not be excised when identified in a core biopsy, provided there is histological–imaging concordance. Although local recurrences of PASH have been reported, it is unclear whether excised PASH has truly recurred or whether new PASH foci have arisen in a hormone-rich environment {765}. The clinical implications of atypical PASH are unknown.

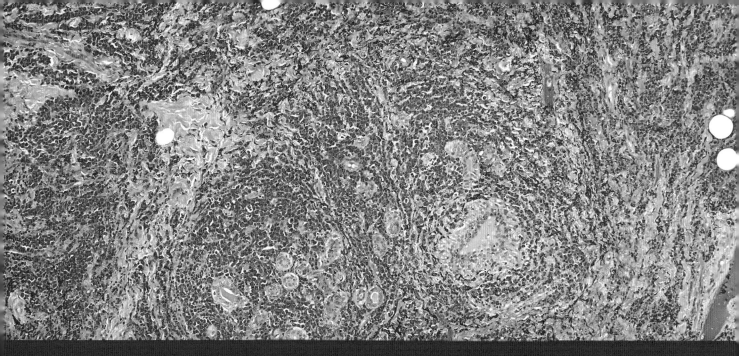

# 6

# Haematolymphoid tumours of the breast

Edited by: Chan JKC

Extranodal marginal zone lymphoma of mucosa-associated lymphoid tissue (MALT lymphoma)
Follicular lymphoma
Diffuse large B-cell lymphoma
Burkitt lymphoma
Breast implant–associated anaplastic large cell lymphoma

# WHO classification of haematolymphoid tumours of the breast

**Lymphoma**
9699/3    Mucosa-associated lymphoid tissue lymphoma
9690/3    Follicular lymphoma NOS
9680/3    Diffuse large B-cell lymphoma NOS
9687/3    Burkitt lymphoma NOS / Acute leukaemia, Burkitt type
        Endemic Burkitt lymphoma
        Sporadic Burkitt lymphoma
        Immunodeficiency-associated Burkitt lymphoma
9715/3    Breast implant–associated anaplastic large cell
    lymphoma

These morphology codes are from the International Classification of Diseases for Oncology, third edition, second revision (ICD-O-3.2) {921}. Behaviour is coded /0 for benign tumours; /1 for unspecified, borderline, or uncertain behaviour; /2 for carcinoma in situ and grade III intraepithelial neoplasia; /3 for malignant tumours, primary site; and /6 for malignant tumours, metastatic site. Behaviour code /6 is not generally used by cancer registries.

This classification is modified from the previous WHO classification, taking into account changes in our understanding of these lesions.

Subtype labels are indented.

# Haematolymphoid tumours of the breast: Introduction

Chan JKC

## Primary lymphoma of the breast

### *Definition*

Primary lymphoma of the breast is often defined as lymphoma confined to one or both breasts and/or regional lymph nodes, in the absence of a prior history of lymphoma {2282,2066,1317, 1814}. However, many studies use criteria less stringent than those for other extranodal lymphomas: presentation with the dominant mass or symptom in the breast in a patient without known lymphoma, even if distant involvement is found on staging {242,891}.

### *Epidemiology*

Primary lymphoma of the breast is uncommon, accounting for < 0.5% of all malignant neoplasms of the breast {1109,2282, 617,891} and approximately 2% of all extranodal lymphomas {680,757}. According to SEER Program data, the incidence of primary breast lymphoma has increased over recent decades, from 0.66 cases per 1 million woman-years in 1975–1977 to 2.96 cases per 1 million woman-years in 2011–2013 {2072}.

### *Clinical features*

Most patients are middle-aged or elderly women, although younger women can also be affected, including pregnant or lactating women presenting with massive bilateral breast masses {2072,2139,2290}. Rarely, men are affected {891,1730, 1814}. Patients usually present with a painless unilateral breast lump, but in some cases the tumour is detected on radiological examination {695}. As many as 11% of cases show bilateral breast involvement {2072,1476,695,2290,1814}.

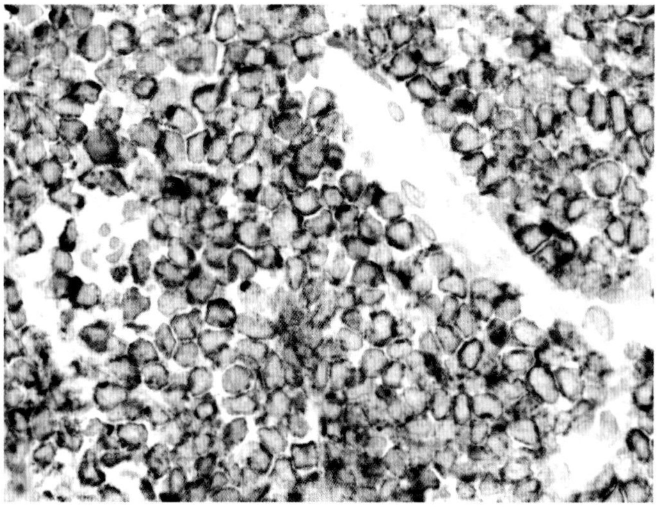

**Fig. 6.02** Myeloid sarcoma of the breast. Positive immunostaining for myeloperoxidase supports a diagnosis of myeloid leukaemia/sarcoma.

Chapter 6

### *Spectrum of primary breast lymphomas*

Although any type of lymphoma can occur as primary breast lymphoma {78,1303}, three histological types account for almost all cases: diffuse large B-cell lymphoma (40–73% of cases), extranodal marginal zone lymphoma of mucosa-associated lymphoid tissue (MALT lymphoma; 9–25%), and follicular lymphoma (13–19%) {2072,695,1304}. Some series report a much higher proportion of diffuse large B-cell lymphoma (84%) or MALT lymphoma (64%) {2139,617}. A site-specific type of

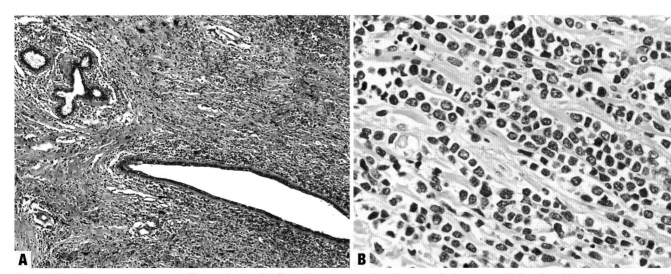

**Fig. 6.01** Myeloid sarcoma of the breast. **A** The neoplastic cells infiltrate the breast parenchyma in a non-cohesive pattern, with formation of single files, mimicking invasive lobular carcinoma. **B** The neoplastic cells are medium-sized and show blastic nuclear features. A single-file pattern of infiltration is present, mimicking invasive lobular carcinoma.

lymphoma is breast implant–associated anaplastic large cell lymphoma, which accounts for 2% of all breast lymphomas {2072}. The breast is also a distinct (though rare) site for the occurrence of Burkitt lymphoma {1476}. Treatment and prognosis depend on the specific type of lymphoma {2290,695,1304}.

## Other haematolymphoid neoplasms of the breast

Plasmacytoma of the breast is uncommon, accounting for 1.5% of all plasmacytomas and 0.2% of malignancies of the breast {2008}. It can occur as solitary extraosseous plasmacytoma or (more commonly {2008}) as a local manifestation of an underlying plasma cell myeloma {464,1024,1354,141}. Occasional cases can show bilateral breast involvement {1481,1557}.

Histiocytic sarcoma, follicular dendritic cell sarcoma, and interdigitating dendritic cell sarcoma have rarely been reported to occur as primary tumours of the breast {1451,1678,644,2128}. Of particular diagnostic interest is a reported case of follicular dendritic cell sarcoma accompanied by abundant myxoid stroma, mimicking mucinous carcinoma {644}.

Myeloid sarcoma can occur in the breast either as a solitary lesion not accompanied by leukaemia or as a local manifestation of acute myeloid leukaemia {1450,1529,2136}. Histologically, it can potentially be mistaken for malignant lymphoma or invasive lobular carcinoma, in particular the latter due to a single-file non-cohesive growth pattern and lack of immunoreactivity for E-cadherin {1304}.

# Extranodal marginal zone lymphoma of mucosa-associated lymphoid tissue (MALT lymphoma)

Ferry JA
Cheng CL

## Definition

Extranodal marginal zone lymphoma of mucosa-associated lymphoid tissue (MALT lymphoma) is a low-grade primary extranodal B-cell lymphoma recapitulating the features of mucosa-associated lymphoid tissue. It is composed mainly of small lymphoid cells, including marginal zone cells.

## ICD-O coding

9699/3 Mucosa-associated lymphoid tissue lymphoma

## ICD-11 coding

2A85.3 Extranodal marginal zone lymphoma, primary site excluding stomach or skin

## Related terminology

None

## Subtype(s)

None

## Localization

Most patients have a single lesion in the breast parenchyma; rare cases are multiple or bilateral {778,1303,2025,751}. Lymphomas are confined to the breast in most cases, occasionally with spread to ipsilateral lymph nodes, and infrequently with more-distant spread {1303,2025,261}.

## Clinical features

Patients typically present with a mass lesion detected on physical examination {1109,2025}. Lesions can also be identified by mammography {1303}. Constitutional symptoms are absent {1303}. Almost all MALT lymphomas involving the breast are primary; rare MALT lymphomas arising in another site can spread to the breast {46}.

## Epidemiology

MALT lymphoma constitutes 7–8% of all B-cell lymphomas {2071}; a small minority of them arise in the breast (2% in one large series) {1006}. In most series, MALT lymphoma is the second most common primary breast lymphoma, after diffuse large B-cell lymphoma (DLBCL) {778,2025,678}. In a few series, follicular lymphomas outnumber MALT lymphomas {46, 1303}. MALT lymphoma mainly affects middle-aged and older adults, almost all women, ranging in age from the fourth to tenth decade of life, with a median age in the sixth or seventh decade {778,1303,1006,1317,551}.

## Etiology

The etiology and risk factors are unknown; rare patients have an autoimmune disease or underlying immunodeficiency {1303, 971,1467,751}.

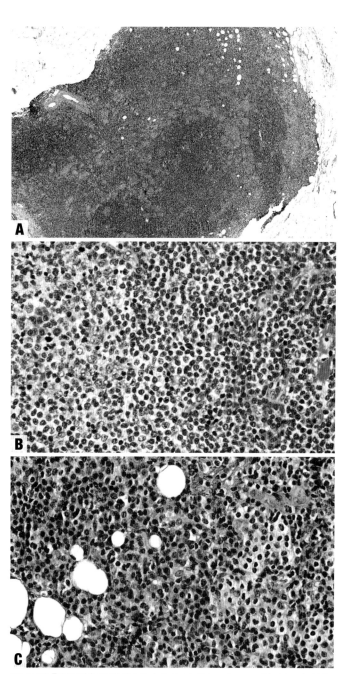

**Fig. 6.03** Extranodal marginal zone lymphoma of mucosa-associated lymphoid tissue (MALT lymphoma) of the breast. **A** Low power shows aggregates of small dark lymphocytes and numerous marginal zone cells with abundant pale cytoplasm. **B** At the left of the image are larger lymphoid cells that represent reactive germinal-centre cells. To the right are smaller, more uniform, neoplastic marginal zone cells, which infiltrate among the germinal-centre cells (follicular colonization). **C** This image shows clusters of marginal zone cells with pale cytoplasm, small lymphocytes, and frequent plasma cells.

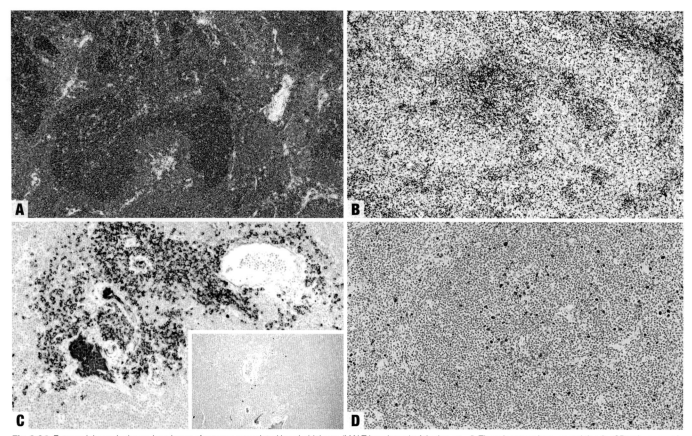

**Fig. 6.04** Extranodal marginal zone lymphoma of mucosa-associated lymphoid tissue (MALT lymphoma) of the breast. **A** There is strong immunostaining for CD20 in a vaguely nodular and diffuse pattern. **B** There are scattered and clustered CD3+ T cells, representing a minority of the lymphoid cells present. **C** Plasma cells are monotypic kappa+ by immunohistochemistry, indicating plasmacytic differentiation. **Inset**: Lambda+ plasma cells are rare by immunohistochemistry. **D** The Ki-67 proliferation index in MALT lymphoma is generally low, as is seen in this case, and some of these proliferating cells may represent remnant germinal-centre cells of colonized follicles.

### Pathogenesis

Recurrent chromosomal translocations that are characteristic of MALT lymphomas in other sites and result in activation of NF-κB {618} are uncommon in MALT lymphoma of the breast {2026,1426,142}. In rare reports, MALT lymphomas of the breast have harboured t(11;18)(q21;q21)/*BIRC3-MALT1* or t(14;18)/ IGH-*MALT1* {1196}. A minority of cases carry trisomy of chromosome 3, 12, or 18 {949,142}.

### Macroscopic appearance

These are solid fleshy lesions ranging from < 1 cm to 20 cm (median: ~3 cm) {1303}.

### Histopathology

Lymphoma should be seen in close proximity to mammary epithelium for a definitive diagnosis of MALT lymphoma of the breast to be established. The histological features of MALT lymphoma of the breast are similar to those of MALT lymphomas in other sites. On low-power examination, the lymphomas have a vaguely nodular to diffuse pattern of growth, often with an infiltrative margin. They are composed of small to medium-sized cells with slightly irregular nuclei and scant to abundant pale cytoplasm (marginal zone cells, previously called centrocyte-like cells). Reactive follicles, sometimes with follicular colonization (infiltration and partial to complete replacement by neoplastic marginal zone cells), and plasmacytic differentiation are found

in some cases. Mitotic activity is low, except in residual reactive follicles. Necrosis and sclerosis are typically absent {2025,142}. Infiltration of epithelial structures by lymphocytes may be seen, but well-formed lymphoepithelial lesions are less commonly found than in MALT lymphomas arising in other sites {2025, 1317,531,142}. Rarely, MALT lymphomas of the breast, usually with plasmacytic differentiation, are associated with localized deposition of amyloid {1109,971,1467}. Rare MALT lymphomas are associated with crystal-storing histiocytosis, wherein there is an accompanying proliferation of histiocytes containing crystalized immunoglobulin {1225,697,142}.

Scattered large cells with the appearance of centroblasts or immunoblasts are usually present but are in the minority. When solid or sheet-like proliferations of large cells are present, the tumour should be diagnosed as DLBCL arising in association with MALT lymphoma. A few cases of DLBCL of the breast have a component of MALT lymphoma, consistent with large cell transformation of a previously undetected MALT lymphoma {1814}.

The neoplastic cells are typically CD20+, CD79a+, CD5–, CD10–, CD23–, CD43+/–, BCL6–, BCL2+, cyclin D1–, and SOX11– B cells, with monotypic cytoplasmic immunoglobulin in the subset of cases with plasmacytic differentiation {551,1196, 617}. The monotypic plasma cells are usually IgM+, although IgG is expressed in some cases. Rare lymphomas expressing monotypic IgG4 are reported, although without associated

IgG4-related disease {142}. If flow cytometry is performed, monotypic surface immunoglobulin may be demonstrated {142}. Proliferation is low. If there are remnants of reactive follicles, the germinal-centre cells are CD10+, BCL6+, and BCL2–, with high proliferation. Markers of follicular dendritic cells (CD21, CD23) typically reveal underlying follicular dendritic meshworks, which may be intact, expanded, or disrupted. Follicular dendritic cell meshworks tend to correlate with areas of vaguely nodular growth. Rare EBV+ MALT lymphomas arising in the breast in solid-organ transplant recipients have been reported {1467,751}.

### Differential diagnosis
The differential diagnosis of MALT lymphoma includes other small B-cell lymphomas and chronic inflammatory processes. Other small B-cell lymphomas are usually associated with more-widespread disease, involving lymph nodes, spleen, and/ or bone marrow. Mantle cell lymphoma is typically composed of a monotonous population of small, dark, irregular lymphoid cells that are CD5+ and cyclin D1+. Follicular lymphoma usually has a predominantly follicular architecture, and it is typically composed of CD10+, BCL6+ B cells that usually coexpress BCL2. Small lymphocytic lymphoma / chronic lymphocytic leukaemia is composed of small round lymphocytes with scattered poorly defined proliferation centres; the neoplastic cells are CD5+, LEF1+ B cells.

Nodal and splenic marginal zone lymphomas {377} and hairy cell leukaemia {619} are B-cell neoplasms that may rarely spread to the breast. Like MALT lymphoma, they are CD5– and CD10–, but information about the distribution of disease can help exclude these entities.

Residual reactive germinal centres can mimic foci of large cell transformation. Germinal centres are CD10+/–, BCL6+, and BCL2–, and they are associated with follicular dendritic cell meshworks. In large cell transformation, neoplastic large cells have a variable immunophenotype, but they are unassociated with follicular dendritic cell meshworks.

Chronic inflammatory processes (including so-called diabetic mastopathy, lymphocytic mastopathy, and lymphocytic lobulitis) do not express monotypic immunoglobulin or show abnormal antigen expression, do not show clonal rearrangement of IGH, and are usually associated with a less dense lymphoid infiltrate; they show fewer but more readily recognizable germinal centres, more marked fibrosis, fewer B cells, and a predominance of IgG+ plasma cells (in contrast to more frequent IgM+ plasma cells in lymphoma) {142}.

### Cytology
FNA can be a useful step in evaluating a lesion {697,2216}, but a larger biopsy or excision is usually required to establish the diagnosis and type of lymphoma.

### Diagnostic molecular pathology
Genetic studies are typically not required for diagnosis, which can be established by histology and immunohistochemistry in most cases. Gene rearrangement studies may be helpful in documenting the presence of a clonal B-cell population, providing evidence against a chronic inflammatory process.

### Essential and desirable diagnostic criteria
*Essential:* involvement of mammary parenchyma; a mass lesion composed of a diffuse or vaguely nodular infiltrate of marginal zone cells and small lymphocytes, often with a few scattered large lymphoid cells; positivity for B-lineage markers; sufficient cytological atypia and immunophenotypic documentation of clonality and/or clonal IGH to exclude a chronic inflammatory process; exclusion of other small B-cell lymphomas.
*Desirable:* the presence of lymphoepithelial lesions; plasmacytic differentiation, with monotypic plasma cells.

### Staging
Lymphoid neoplasms are staged according to the Lugano classification, which has been adopted by the eighth edition of the Union for International Cancer Control (UICC) TNM classification {338}.

### Prognosis and prediction
MALT lymphoma of the breast has a better prognosis than DLBCL {891} and follicular lymphoma {1303} of the breast. Patients often remain well after treatment. A subset of patients develop extranodal relapses involving the ipsilateral or contralateral breast, subcutaneous tissue, larynx, chest wall, orbit, and other sites, or involving lymph nodes, usually without widespread disease {1109,891,779}. Progression to DLBCL may occur {1109,1317}. Although relapses are not uncommon, overall survival is typically excellent {2025}. In one series, the cause-specific survival rates at 3 years, 5 years, and 10 years were 100%, 100%, and 80%, respectively, and the 5-year progression-free survival rate was 56% {1303}. Few patients have died of lymphoma, sometimes after large cell transformation {1317}. Specific prognostic factors are not known.

# Follicular lymphoma

Dogan A
Fend F

## Definition
Follicular lymphoma (FL) is a malignant lymphoid neoplasm of follicle-centre B cells, typically showing follicular architecture.

## ICD-O coding
9690/3 Follicular lymphoma NOS

## ICD-11 coding
2A80.Z Follicular lymphoma, unspecified

## Related terminology
None

## Subtype(s)
None

## Localization
By definition, the tumour presents in the breast parenchyma, with or without local lymph node involvement. Intramammary lymph node involvement without involvement of breast parenchyma should not be considered breast FL.

## Clinical features
FL may present as primary disease in the breast, with or without involvement of axillary lymph nodes, but the proportion of cases with primary versus secondary involvement of the breast varies widely across different series. Although patients may present with a palpable mass, the tumours are more frequently identified by imaging studies performed for breast cancer screening.

## Epidemiology
A variety of low-grade B-cell lymphomas other than extranodal marginal zone lymphoma of mucosa-associated lymphoid tissue (MALT lymphoma) can occur in the breast. Among these,

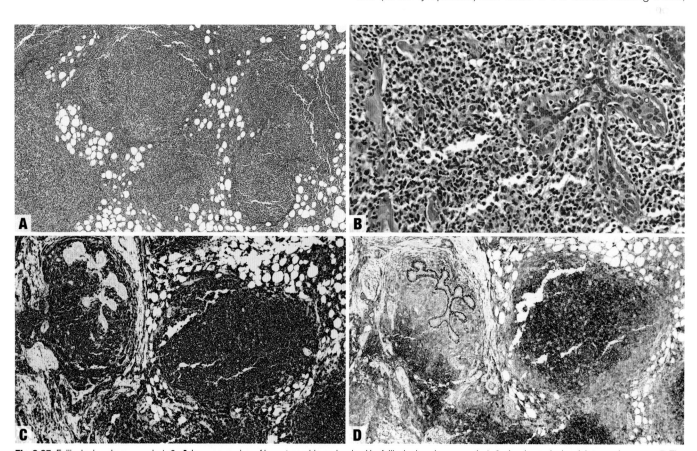

**Fig. 6.05** Follicular lymphoma, grade 1–2. **A** Low-power view of breast core biopsy involved by follicular lymphoma, grade 1–2, showing typical nodular growth pattern. **B** The neoplastic follicles are predominantly composed of centrocytes, with only scattered centroblasts. They are adjacent to the breast ducts, but lymphoepithelial lesions are not present. **C** The neoplastic cells express CD20, consistent with B-cell origin. **D** The neoplastic cells express follicular B-cell marker CD10, both within the follicles and in interfollicular areas.

FL is the most common, accounting for 5–46% of all non-Hodgkin lymphomas in recent series {891,2025,1317,1303,695,1759, 2072}.

## Etiology
Unknown

## Pathogenesis
There have been no systematic studies on the pathogenesis of FLs of the breast. However, limited data suggest that most cases represent secondary involvement by systemic FL {2025}. Therefore, it can be assumed that they share the characteristic phenotypic and molecular features of systemic FL, such as ongoing hypermutation of IGHV genes, and the FL hallmark translocation t(14;18) resulting in fusion of BCL2 and IGH genes. However, it is possible that a subset of cases are of primary breast origin and may represent examples of primary cutaneous follicle-centre cell lymphoma. The morphology, immunophenotype, and molecular genetics of these cases are distinct from those of conventional FL, and they include predominance of large cells, commonly a diffuse growth pattern, lack of expression of BCL2 protein, and usually absence of BCL2 gene rearrangement.

## Macroscopic appearance
Not clinically relevant

## Histopathology
The morphology of breast FL is comparable to that of nodal and other extranodal sites, with both follicular and diffuse growth patterns and a predominance of histological grade 1 or 2 over grade 3A or 3B. The neoplastic follicles show a monotonous pattern and vague borders, and they contain centrocytes with various proportions of centroblasts, depending on grade. The neoplastic follicles can be intimately associated with breast ductules, but lymphoepithelial lesions are usually absent.

The neoplastic follicles show expression of the pan–B-cell markers CD20 and CD79a, as well as CD10, BCL6, and BCL2 in most cases. Follicular dendritic cell networks can be demonstrated by staining for CD21 or CD23, but they may not be as well developed as in nodal cases and often disappear in areas with a diffuse pattern. FL commonly contains a high proportion of reactive T cells.

### Differential diagnosis
The differential diagnosis includes other low-grade B-cell lymphoma subtypes (mainly MALT lymphoma) and chronic mastitis with reactive follicular hyperplasia. The latter may represent so-called cutaneous pseudolymphoma of the skin, especially of the areolar region {209}. Of note, the presence of dense collagenous tissue, especially in core biopsies, may cause a single-file pattern of infiltration and raise the differential diagnosis of lobular carcinoma. These cases can easily be resolved by immunohistochemical analysis.

## Cytology
In some cases, FNA may be the first diagnostic procedure. Smears may show a mixture of centrocytes and centroblasts intermixed with small lymphocytes. The absence of tingible-body macrophages on smears may suggest lymphoid neoplasia, but a definitive diagnosis of B-cell lymphoma cannot be established without immunophenotyping. Even if the immunophenotyping is conclusive of a neoplastic process, a tissue biopsy is required for definitive diagnosis, classification, and grading.

## Diagnostic molecular pathology
The frequency of the characteristic t(14;18)(q32;q21) translocation or other cytogenetic or molecular alterations of FLs has not been assessed systematically for primary FL of the breast.

## Essential and desirable diagnostic criteria
*Essential:* a lymphoid proliferation with cytological features of follicle-centre cells (centrocytes and centroblasts); at least focal atypical follicle formation (crowding, lack of polarization, lack of tingible-body macrophages); expression of B-cell markers (CD20, CD79a, PAX5) and follicle-centre B-cell markers (CD10, BCL6).
*Desirable:* BCL2 positivity.

## Staging
Lymphoid neoplasms are staged according to the Lugano classification, which has been adopted by the eighth edition of the Union for International Cancer Control (UICC) TNM classification {338}.

## Prognosis and prediction
The relapse rates, patterns of spread, and clinical behaviour of primary FL of the breast are believed to be comparable to those of conventional nodal disease. Although a worse prognosis has been reported in a subset of studies {1303}, recent analysis of SEER Program data suggests that patients with low-stage FLs of the breast have a better overall survival than patients with systemic FL {2072}.

# Diffuse large B-cell lymphoma

Medeiros LJ
Piris MA

## Definition

Diffuse large B-cell lymphoma (DLBCL) is a diffuse neoplastic proliferation of large B lymphocytes lacking features of other defined types of large B-cell lymphoma.

## ICD-O coding

9680/3 Diffuse large B-cell lymphoma NOS

## ICD-11 coding

2A81.Z Diffuse large B-cell lymphoma NOS

## Related terminology

*Acceptable:* primary breast DLBCL.

## Subtype(s)

None

## Localization

Primary breast DLBCL is confined to one or both breasts, with or without involvement of regional lymph nodes. Patients with a history of lymphoma or concurrent systemic DLBCL are excluded {2025,946}. The left and right breasts are equally affected. About 2–5% of patients present with bilateral involvement.

## Clinical features

The median patient age is in the seventh decade of life, but there is a wide age range, of 15–90 years in various reports. More than 95% of primary breast DLBCL cases arise in women {1814, 946}. Most patients with primary breast DLBCL present with a painless mass that is growing in size. In about 10% of patients, the lesion may be detected initially by screening mammography {2025,946}. Patients rarely present with skin erythema, oedema, or retraction (features more common in patients with epithelial tumours).

## Epidemiology

The breast may be involved by systemic DLBCL, or the neoplasm may arise in the breast (primary); in one study at a large cancer centre, the ratio was approximately 1:1 {2025}.

DLBCL is the most common type of lymphoma involving the breast. Primary breast DLBCL represents < 1% of all non-Hodgkin lymphomas and about 2% of all extranodal lymphomas {1814,2072,946}. The incidence of primary breast DLBCL has increased over the past 4 decades {2072}. An analysis of SEER Program data showed that in the US population, the incidence is highest in American Indians, Alaskan natives, and Asian/Pacific Islanders and is low in the black population {946}.

## Etiology

There are no known risk factors specific for primary breast DLBCL.

## Pathogenesis

The pathogenesis of primary breast DLBCL is largely unknown. Gene expression profiling can be used to divide DLBCL-NOS into germinal-centre B-cell (GCB), activated B-cell (ABC), and unclassified subtypes, with the ABC subtype associated with a poorer prognosis according to most studies. Primary breast

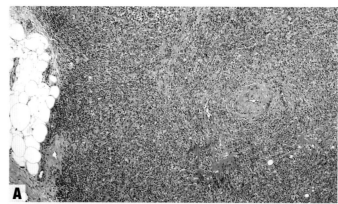
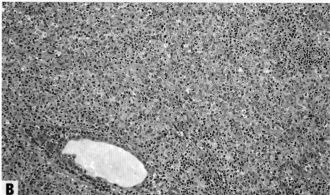
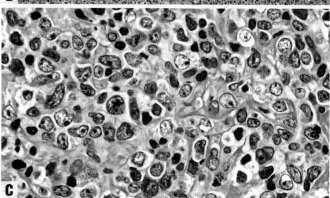

**Fig. 6.06** Primary breast diffuse large B-cell lymphoma. **A** Low power shows the lymphoma surrounding a duct and infiltrating adipose tissue as a mass lesion. **B** Sheets of large lymphoma cells replace breast parenchyma. A residual breast duct is also present in the field (lower left). **C** The lymphoma cells are large, with centroblastic cytological features.

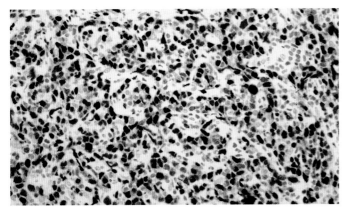

**Fig. 6.07** Primary diffuse large B-cell lymphoma. The lymphoma cells are positive for IRF4 (MUM1) and negative for CD10 (not shown), supporting a non–germinal-centre B-cell immunophenotype.

DLBCL is similarly heterogeneous. In most studies of primary breast DLBCL, 50–90% of cases are of ABC or non-GCB type, with the latter term used for cases characterized by surrogate immunohistochemistry algorithms instead of gene expression profiling {2330,2025}. The remaining cases of primary breast DLBCL are either of GCB type or unclassified. The translocations common in DLBCL-NOS, such as those involving *MYC*, *BCL2*, and *BCL6*, are less frequent in primary breast DLBCL.

The mutation landscape of DLBCL-NOS is fairly well known, but fewer data are available for primary breast DLBCL. *MYD88* and *CD79B* mutations have been reported most often, in approximately 50% and 33% of cases, respectively {2050}. Franco et al. performed targeted sequencing on 18 primary breast DLBCL specimens and showed mutations in *PIM1* (50%); *MYD88* (39%); *CD79B*, *PRDM1*, or *CARD11* (17% each); and *KMT2D*, *TNFAIP3*, or *CREBBP* (11% each) {677}. The available data suggest that *PIM1*, *MYD88*, *CD79B*, and *CARD11* mutations are of gain-of-function type and are predicted to activate the NF-κB pathway. In this study, there was no clear correlation between cell of origin and mutation profile {677}.

## Macroscopic appearance
The median tumour size is 3–4 cm (range: 1–20 cm). Primary breast DLBCL tends to be well circumscribed, unlike systemic DLBCL involving the breast, which tends to be infiltrative and associated with sclerosis {1814,2025}.

## Histopathology
Primary breast DLBCL is composed of large lymphoma cells arranged in a diffuse pattern. The neoplasm replaces breast parenchyma and the lymphoma cells may resemble centroblasts or immunoblasts, or they can uncommonly be anaplastic. The neoplastic cells can preferentially involve breast lobules, imparting a nodular appearance. Lymphoepithelial lesions are uncommon {2025,1176}.

Immunophenotypically, the lymphoma cells are positive for B-cell markers including CD19, CD20, CD22, CD79a, and PAX5. Most cases are positive for surface or cytoplasmic immunoglobulin. Ki-67 staining reveals brisk proliferation, with a median Ki-67 proliferation index of 70–80% {2330,1176}. MYC is often expressed in highly proliferative neoplasms, but usually not uniformly or brightly unless *MYC* is rearranged. ABC/non-GCB–type tumours are usually positive for IRF4 (MUM1) and FOXP1. GCB-type tumours are more often positive for CD10, BCL6 (moderate to strong), GCET1, and LMO2. BCL2 is often positive, but this is usually not associated with *BCL2* translocations. The neoplastic cells are usually negative for CD5 and CD30. There is no evidence of association with EBV.

## Cytology
Smears show large lymphoid cells in a background of small lymphocytes and histiocytes. Necrosis can be present. Obtaining material for immunophenotypic analysis is essential to supplement the interpretation of morphological findings and determine cell lineage.

## Diagnostic molecular pathology
Molecular studies are usually not required to establish the diagnosis. Primary breast DLBCL usually carries monoclonal IGH rearrangements, and TR genes are germline. These tumours are most often of ABC or non-GCB type, with a relatively high frequency of *MYD88* or *CD79B* mutations.

## Essential and desirable diagnostic criteria
*Essential:* restriction to the breast with or without regional lymph node involvement; diffuse proliferation of large atypical lymphoid cells; B-cell lineage.

## Staging
Lymphoid neoplasms are staged according to the Lugano classification, which has been adopted by the eighth edition of the Union for International Cancer Control (UICC) TNM classification {338}. Approximately 60–70% of patients present with localized, stage IE disease, and the remaining patients have regional, usually axillary lymphadenopathy at diagnosis (stage II). Staging of the few patients with bilateral primary breast DLBCL is controversial (stage IE vs IV). The International Prognostic Index (IPI) is useful for prognostication {1814,877}.

## Prognosis and prediction
There is no role for surgical excision; patients are treated with systemic immunochemotherapy, often with involved-field radiotherapy {1814,885}. The 5-year overall survival and event-free survival rates in various studies have been 70–80% and 60–65%, respectively. Cell of origin (GCB vs ABC) is of unproven prognostic value but can guide therapy, particularly at the time of relapse. Relapse occurs in a subset of patients, not uncommonly after 24 months {1248,885}; 10–15% of cases relapse in the same or the contralateral breast, and 15–25% of cases relapse in the CNS {1814,1248,885}.

# Burkitt lymphoma

Leoncini L
Dogan A

## Definition

Burkitt lymphoma (BL) is a highly aggressive B-cell lymphoma characterized by frequent presentation in extranodal sites or as acute leukaemia, with high proliferative activity and usually *MYC* gene translocation to an IG locus.

## ICD-O coding

9687/3 Burkitt lymphoma NOS
9687/3 Acute leukaemia, Burkitt type

## ICD-11 coding

2A85.6 Burkitt lymphoma, including Burkitt leukaemia

## Related terminology

*Acceptable:* Burkitt cell leukaemia.
*Not recommended:* Burkitt tumour; malignant lymphoma, undifferentiated, Burkitt type; malignant lymphoma, small noncleaved, Burkitt type.

## Subtype(s)

Three epidemiological subtypes of BL are recognized: endemic BL, sporadic BL, and immunodeficiency-associated BL.

## Localization

Extranodal sites are most often involved, with some variation according to the epidemiological subtype. Breast involvement (often bilateral and massive) has been associated with onset during puberty, pregnancy, or lactation.

## Clinical features

Patients often present with bulky disease and high tumour burden due to the short doubling time of the tumour. Specific clinical manifestations at presentation vary according to the epidemiological subtype and the site of involvement.

## Epidemiology

Endemic BL occurs in equatorial Africa and in Papua New Guinea, with a distribution that overlaps with regions endemic for malaria. In these areas, BL is the most common childhood malignancy, with an incidence peak among children aged 4–7 years and an M:F ratio of 2:1 {255,2296}.

Sporadic BL is seen throughout the world, mainly in children and young adults {1326}. The incidence is low, with sporadic BL accounting for only 1–2% of all lymphomas in western Europe and the USA. In these parts of the world, BL accounts for approximately 30–50% of all childhood lymphomas. The median age of adult patients is 30 years, but an incidence peak has also been reported in elderly patients {1326}. The M:F ratio is 2:1 to 3:1.

Immunodeficiency-associated BL is more common in the setting of HIV infection than in other forms of inborn or acquired immunodeficiency. In HIV-infected patients, BL appears early in

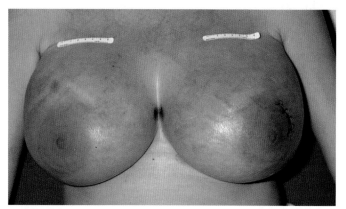

**Fig. 6.08** Burkitt lymphoma of the breast. Bilateral breast involvement may be the presenting manifestation during pregnancy and puberty. Burkitt lymphoma cells have prolactin receptors.

the evolution of the disease, when CD4+ T-cell counts are still high {1725}.

## Etiology

A number of infectious agents (e.g. EBV, *Plasmodium falciparum*, and HIV), environmental factors, and genetic predispositions (e.g. germline mutations in *ATM*, *BLM*, or *SH2D1A*) are known etiological cofactors.

## Pathogenesis

In endemic BL, the EBV genome is present in > 95% of cases. There is also a strong epidemiological link with holoendemic malaria. Therefore, EBV and *P. falciparum* are considered to be associated with endemic BL {491,954}. Recent data have provided new insight into how these two human pathogens interact to cause the disease, supporting the emerging concepts of polymicrobial disease pathogenesis {332,1406,1534,1695, 1771}. The polymicrobial nature of endemic BL is further supported by the status of B-cell receptor, which carries the signs of antigen selection due to chronic antigen stimulation {57,1646}.

In sporadic BL, EBV can be detected in as many as 20–30% of cases {1266}; however, more-sensitive tools are able to identify EBV infection in a higher proportion of cases {1429}. The proportion of EBV+ sporadic BL cases appears to be much higher in adults than in children {1849}.

In immunodeficiency-associated BL, EBV is identified in 25–40% of cases {813,1779}.

The variation in EBV association among the different forms of BL and among different countries makes it difficult to determine the role of the virus in BL pathogenesis. EBV may affect host cell homeostasis in various ways by encoding its own genes and microRNAs and by interfering with cellular microRNA expression {59,989,1158,1647,2165}. However, recent studies have shown that the mutation and viral landscape of BL is more complex than previously reported. In fact, a distinct latency pattern

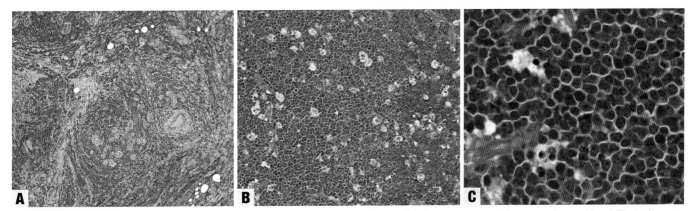

**Fig. 6.09** Burkitt lymphoma of the breast. **A** Low power shows infiltration of the lymphoma cells around the breast structures. **B** Low power shows a diffuse infiltrate of monotonous, intermediate-sized lymphocytes and numerous tingible-body macrophages, giving a starry-sky appearance. **C** On high power, the cells have deeply basophilic cytoplasm and round nuclei with 1–3 nucleoli.

of EBV involving the expression of LMP2A along with that of lytic genes has been demonstrated (non-canonical latency programme) {85,2081}. Nonetheless, expression of the latency pattern in BL is heterogeneous, not only from case to case, but also within a given case from cell to cell, suggesting that the tumour is under selective pressure and needs alternative mechanisms to survive and proliferate. The inverse correlation between the EBV viral load and the number of somatic mutations suggests that these mutations may substitute for the virus in maintaining the neoplastic phenotype {736,1}.

The molecular hallmark of BL is the translocation of *MYC* at band 8q24 to the IGH locus on chromosome 14q32, t(8;14)

(q24;q32), or less commonly to the IGK light chain locus on 2p12 [t(2;8)] or the IGL light chain locus on 22q11 [t(8;22)]. Most breakpoints originate from aberrant somatic hypermutation mediated by activation-induced cytidine deaminase activity. Additional chromosomal abnormalities may also occur in BL, including gains of 1q, 7, and 12 and losses of 6q, 13q32-q34, and 17p. Approximately 10% of classic BL cases lack an identifiable *MYC* rearrangement {821,895,1158}. However, none of the techniques currently used to detect genetic changes can unambiguously rule out all *MYC* translocations. The expression of *MYC* mRNA and MYC protein in these cases suggests that alternative mechanisms deregulating *MYC* also exist {1554,

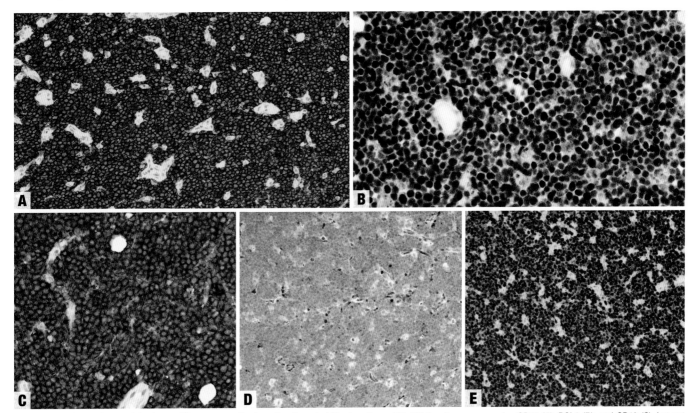

**Fig. 6.10** Burkitt lymphoma of the breast. The tumour cells show the characteristic phenotype of Burkitt lymphoma, expressing CD20 (**A**), BCL6 (**B**), and CD10 (**C**), but not BCL2 (**D**). The Ki-67 proliferation index is 100% (**E**).

1872}. In these cases, strict clinical, morphological, and phenotypic criteria should be used to exclude lymphomas that mimic BL.

Next-generation sequencing analysis has revealed the importance of the B-cell receptor signalling pathway in the pathogenesis of BL. Mutations of the transcription factor *TCF3* (*E2A*) or its negative regulator *ID3* have been reported in about 70% of sporadic BL cases. These mutations activate B-cell receptor signalling, which sustains BL cell survival by engaging the PI3K pathway {1241,1760,1863,1835}. Mutations of *MYC*, *CCND3*, *TP53*, *RHOA*, *SMARCA4*, and *ARID1A* are other recurrent mutations, found in 5–40% of BL cases {736}. The numbers of mutations overall and mutations in *TCF3* or *ID3* are lower in endemic BL than in sporadic BL {1}.

## Macroscopic appearance
Massive bilateral breast involvement may be the presenting manifestation during pregnancy and puberty.

## Histopathology
BL is characterized by a diffuse monotonous infiltrate of medium-sized lymphoid cells. The cells appear to be cohesive but often exhibit squared-off borders of retracted cytoplasm. The nuclei are round with finely clumped chromatin, and they contain multiple basophilic medium-sized paracentrally located nucleoli. The cytoplasm is deeply basophilic and usually contains lipid vacuoles, which are better seen in imprint preparations or FNA specimens. The characteristic lipid vacuoles can also be demonstrated by immunostaining for adipophilin {60}. The tumour has extremely high proliferation, with many mitotic figures, as well as a high rate of spontaneous cell death (apoptosis). A starry-sky pattern is usually present, as a result of the presence of numerous tingible-body macrophages.

The tumour cells typically express moderate to strong membrane IgM with light chain restriction, B-cell antigens (CD19, CD20, CD22, CD79a, and PAX5), and germinal-centre markers (CD10 and BCL6). CD38, CD77, and CD43 are also frequently positive {127,1095,1452}. Almost all BLs show strong expression of MYC protein in the majority of neoplastic cells {58}. Proliferation is very high, with nearly 100% of the cells positive for Ki-67. The neoplastic cells are usually negative for CD5, CD23, CD138, and BCL2. However, BCL2 expression in a variable number of cells may be observed. This immunophenotype may be more variable in sporadic BL in older patients and at extranodal sites {127}. TdT is negative, allowing differential diagnosis from pre-B acute lymphoblastic leukaemia with *MYC* translocation {1452, 516}.

## Cytology
Not clinically relevant

## Diagnostic molecular pathology
Gene and microRNA expression profiling can define molecular signatures that are characteristic of BL and different from those of other lymphomas, such as diffuse large B-cell lymphoma {457,895}. Slight differences in the expression profiles have been identified between the endemic BL and sporadic BL subtypes {1646,1146}.

## Essential and desirable diagnostic criteria
*Classic features*
*Essential:* a diffuse monotonous infiltrate of medium-sized lymphoid cells with squared-off contours, round nuclei with finely clumped chromatin, multiple nucleoli, and basophilic cytoplasm; frequent mitotic figures and apoptotic bodies; immunophenotype: B-lineage marker–positive, CD10+, BCL2–, MYC protein expression in > 80% of neoplastic cells, near 100% Ki-67 proliferation index.

*Cases with deviations from the above-listed features*
*Essential:* when morphology or immunophenotype is atypical and/or MYC protein expression is present in < 80% of neoplastic cells, additional testing is required to confirm a diagnosis of BL: FISH analysis for *MYC*, *BCL2*, and *BCL6* rearrangements and 11q abnormality to exclude high-grade B-cell lymphoma with *MYC* and *BCL2* and/or *BCL6* rearrangements, high-grade B-cell lymphoma NOS, and Burkitt-like lymphoma with 11q abnormality.

## Staging
Paediatric BL is staged according to the system of Murphy et al. {1435}. A revised International Pediatric Non-Hodgkin Lymphoma Staging System (IPNHLSS) has recently been proposed {1799}.

## Prognosis and prediction
BL is a highly aggressive but potentially curable tumour; intensive chemotherapy can result in long-term overall survival in 70–90% of patients, with children doing better than adults. Adverse prognostic factors include advanced-stage disease, bone marrow and CNS involvement, unresected tumour > 10 cm in diameter, and high serum LDH levels {1374,300,245}. The overall survival rate in endemic BL has improved from no more than 10–20% to almost 70% as a result of the introduction of the International Network for Cancer Treatment and Research (INCTR) protocol INCTR 03-06 in African institutions {1493}.

# Breast implant–associated anaplastic large cell lymphoma

Miranda RN
Feldman AL
Soares FA

## Definition

Breast implant–associated anaplastic large cell lymphoma (ALCL) is a T-cell lymphoma, with morphology and immunophenotype similar to those of ALK-negative ALCL, that arises around a breast implant, usually confined by a fibrous capsule.

## ICD-O coding

9715/3 Breast implant–associated anaplastic large cell lymphoma

## ICD-11 coding

2A90.B Anaplastic large cell lymphoma, ALK-negative

## Related terminology

*Acceptable:* seroma-associated ALCL.

## Subtype(s)

None

## Localization

Breast implant–associated ALCL is usually localized to the peri-implant space, but it can progress to involve surrounding soft tissue, breast parenchyma, or regional lymph nodes.

## Clinical features

Most patients had breast implants for cosmetic reasons and one third for reconstruction after breast cancer surgery. The average patient age at diagnosis is 52 years. Patients are women, including (in rare cases) transgender women {1618}. The median time from implant placement to clinical presentation is 8–9 years (range: 2–32 years) {1382}. Most patients present with unilateral effusion around the implant {1774}. Approximately 5% of cases are bilateral. The overlying skin is usually unremarkable but can occasionally be erythematous. B symptoms are typically absent. The volume of effusion can be as high as 700 mL. About one third of patients present with a mass, and about 20% develop regional lymphadenopathy, most commonly in the axilla and supraclavicular fossa. Lymphadenopathy may be the first manifestation of disease. Less commonly, the disease may spread systemically {2368} and even rarely involves bone marrow {1226}. Death from disease, which is uncommon (occurring in < 5% of cases), is usually due to mediastinal extension and bronchial obstruction.

Effusion is best detected with ultrasonography, whereas tumour mass, lymphadenopathy, and follow-up are better assessed by PET {17}. Mammography is suboptimal.

## Epidemiology

Globally, > 10 million women have breast implants. Recent investigations estimate that 1 in 3000–30 000 women with implants develop breast implant–associated ALCL {462,2217}. Cases have been reported in more than 29 countries, with most reported in the USA, Europe, and Australia {1682,1265}. Although most primary lymphomas of the breast are of B-cell lineage {2025}, ALK-negative ALCL is the most common lymphoma type associated with breast implants {1382}.

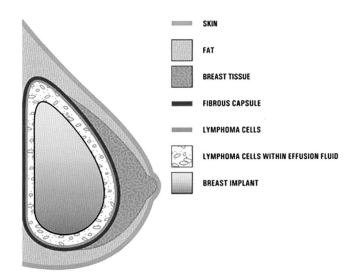

SKIN

FAT

BREAST TISSUE

FIBROUS CAPSULE

LYMPHOMA CELLS

LYMPHOMA CELLS WITHIN EFFUSION FLUID

BREAST IMPLANT

**Fig. 6.11** Schematic diagram of breast implant–associated anaplastic large cell lymphoma. Lymphoma cells are found in the effusion fluid accumulated between the breast implant and the outer fibrous capsule, as well as along the luminal aspect of the fibrous capsule.

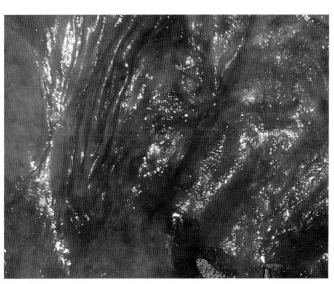

**Fig. 6.12** Breast implant–associated anaplastic large cell lymphoma (ALCL). Gross appearance of a capsule involved by breast implant–associated ALCL. The luminal surface has a fibrinoid appearance, but a distinct lesion is not identified. Microscopic examination reveals tumour cells along the luminal side of the capsule.

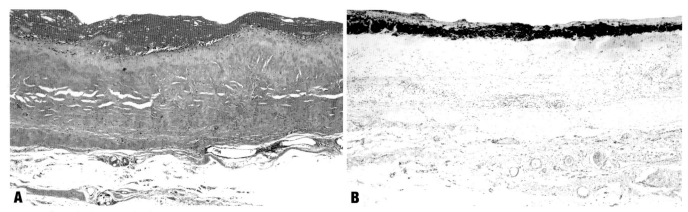

**Fig. 6.13** Breast implant–associated anaplastic large cell lymphoma, pathological stage T1, along the luminal side of the capsule. **A** There is a layer of fibrin and necrotic cells, with only a subset of viable cells. **B** CD30 immunohistochemistry highlights the tumour cells, necrotic cells, and debris along the luminal side of the capsule.

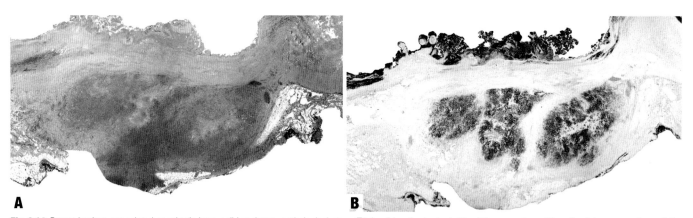

**Fig. 6.14** Breast implant–associated anaplastic large cell lymphoma, pathological stage T4, involving the luminal side of the capsule and invading into surrounding soft tissue. **A** The luminal side appears granular and the tumour mass extends into the surrounding soft tissue. **B** CD30 immunohistochemistry highlights abundant cells and necrotic debris on the luminal side, as well as the tumour cells forming a mass around the capsule.

## Etiology

Most affected patients received implants that had textured as opposed to smooth surfaces {537}. The saline or silicone filling of the implants does not appear to have a pathogenic role {1382}. The suspected pathogenic triggers of lymphoma include a biofilm and the silicone shell that is directly or indirectly immunogenic {1281,920}, and shedding of silicone particles may elicit a host immune response. The bacterial biofilm around textured implants has been suggested as a trigger for immune reaction and lymphoma cell survival {884}. In 2019, the United States Food and Drug Administration (FDA) acknowledged the association, which prompted the world's largest breast implant manufacturer to issue a worldwide recall of textured implants. There are two case reports of breast implant–associated ALCL arising in patients with Li–Fraumeni syndrome, suggesting that germline *TP53* mutations are a predisposing factor {1137,1611}.

## Pathogenesis

Chronic inflammation associated with implants has been proposed as a factor triggering lymphocyte transformation and lymphomagenesis. Biofilm bacteria produce lipopolysaccharide antigens that may stimulate cytokine production resulting in chronic T helper 1 (Th1) cell stimulation {884,968}. Studies in vitro have revealed a genetic and cytokine profile consistent with that of T helper 17 (Th17) cells rather than Th1 or T helper 2 (Th2) subsets {2304,2286}.

The JAK/STAT3 pathway is constitutively activated, which in some cases is associated with recurrent somatic mutations of *JAK1* and/or *STAT3* {1542,1126,496,179}. Other genetic alterations include point mutations in *DNMT3A* and *TP53*. These findings suggest that breast implant–associated ALCL shows more-uniform molecular features than systemic and primary cutaneous ALCLs {1542}. Cytogenetic analysis in a limited number of cases has revealed complex karyotypes without recurrent abnormalities {1542}.

## Macroscopic appearance

The optimal specimen for pathological examination is en bloc resection of the intact capsule containing the implant and effusion. Fluid should be sent for flow cytometry and cytological examination, because some cases involve the effusion only. Fixation on a flat surface allows for optimal orientation. Generous sampling is recommended when a grossly distinct lesion is not identified. Masses appear as necrotic plaque-like lesions. Assessment of the resection margins is essential.

## Histopathology

The physiological reaction to implants is the formation of a fibrous capsule. Silicone material appears as a refringent material that can migrate through surrounding fibrous tissue or to lymph nodes, causing a histiocytic reaction. The capsule is thickened and the luminal side shows necrosis; ghost cells;

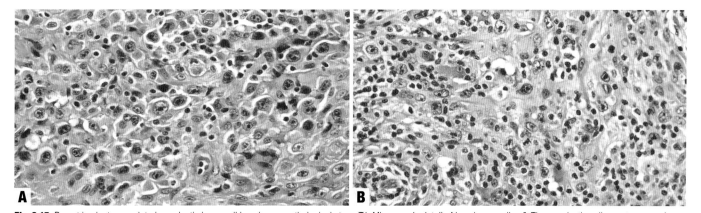

**Fig. 6.15** Breast implant–associated anaplastic large cell lymphoma, pathological stage T4. Microscopic detail of lymphoma cells. **A** The neoplastic cells most commonly appear as sheets of large cells with pleomorphic nuclei and prominent nucleoli. **B** Less frequently, there is a dense inflammatory infiltrate around tumour cells, mimicking Hodgkin lymphoma.

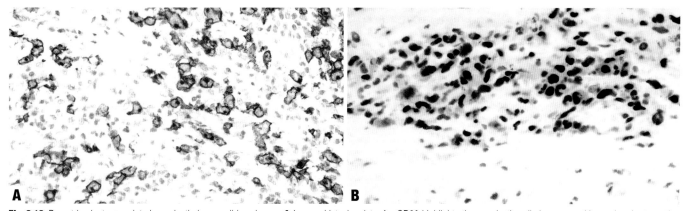

**Fig. 6.16** Breast implant–associated anaplastic large cell lymphoma. **A** Immunohistochemistry for CD30 highlights the neoplastic cells in a case with an abundant reactive infiltrate, mimicking Hodgkin lymphoma. **B** Immunohistochemistry for phosphorylated STAT3 highlights most cells, supporting JAK/STAT pathway activation in most cases.

karyorrhexis; and scattered (< 10%) large, pleomorphic cells, usually arranged as a distinct layer, representing the early pathological stage of disease. In some cases, the only viable lymphoma cells are seen in the effusion/cytological specimen. The neoplastic cells are large, with moderately abundant amphophilic, eosinophilic, or clear cytoplasm and oval to lobated nuclei with small to prominent nucleoli; in about two thirds of cases, hallmark cells are identified. Karyorrhexis is common, and necrosis can be extensive {636}. Upon progression, clusters of cells appear within or beyond the capsule and can infiltrate into surrounding soft tissue or breast parenchyma, usually associated with extensive necrosis {1682}.

Lymph node involvement, when present, is usually sinusoidal and less frequently interfollicular, perifollicular, or diffuse. The infiltrate is best visualized with CD30 immunohistochemistry.

Most or all lymphoma cells are strongly positive for CD30 in a membranous and Golgi pattern. Granular or ghost cell necrosis on the luminal side of the capsule reacts strongly with CD30 and is sometimes the only evidence of disease. Systemic ALCL involvement of the breast does not localize to the capsule, nor are there tumour cells along the luminal side of the capsule {1682}. Similar to ALCL elsewhere, breast implant–associated ALCL is usually negative for CD3, CD5, TRB, and TRG/TRD {24}. The neoplastic cells commonly express CD4, CD43, and CD45RB

and less frequently cytotoxic markers (TIA1, granzyme B, and/ or perforin) {1682}. EBV-encoded small RNA (EBER), LMP1, and ALK are negative. Expression of IL-13 and GATA3, as reported in some series, may suggest an allergic response {969}. Limited studies of the microenvironment show a Th1 and Th17 pattern. Phosphorylated STAT3 is commonly detected, consistent with JAK/STAT pathway activation {1542}. PD1 is negative, whereas PDL1 is expressed in a subset of cases. The immunophenotype can be determined by flow cytometry, and failure is linked with delay in processing, limited volume for testing, and using lymphocyte instead of monocyte gating in the CD45 versus side scatter plot {1682}.

### Cytology
The large lymphoma cells show abundant, often vacuolated, basophilic cytoplasm and cytoplasmic blebs. The nuclei are large, oval, or lobated, with prominent nucleoli. The background commonly shows necrosis and karyorrhexis.

### Diagnostic molecular pathology
Almost 80% of cases have monoclonal rearrangements of the TRG or TRB genes {1542,1682}. Breast implant–associated ALCL is consistently negative for ALCL-related gene rearrangements involving *ALK*, *DUSP22*, and *TP63* {1542}.

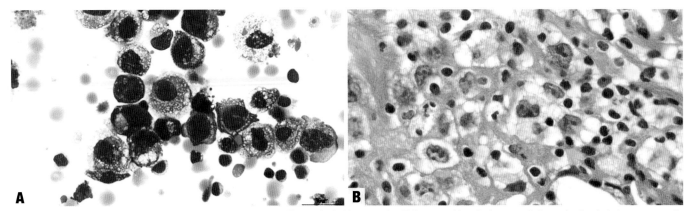

**Fig. 6.17** Breast implant–associated anaplastic large cell lymphoma. **A** The cytological features of an FNA smear of the effusion around a breast implant include numerous cells with abundant vacuolated cytoplasm and large nuclei with prominent nucleoli. Small lymphocytes and histiocytes are noted in the background (Wright–Giemsa stain). **B** A cell block specimen of the effusion around a breast implant shows large cells with vesicular nuclei, prominent nucleoli, and abundant cytoplasm.

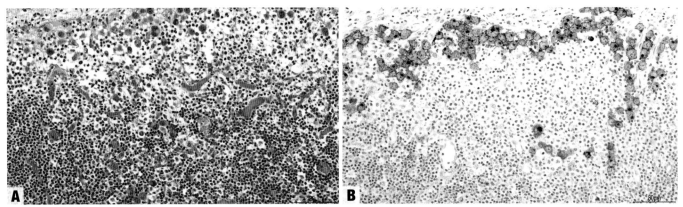

**Fig. 6.18** Breast implant–associated anaplastic large cell lymphoma with axillary lymph node involvement. **A** The lymph node shows hyperplastic changes and sinusoidal distribution of large neoplastic cells. **B** Immunohistochemistry for CD30 highlights the membranes and Golgi bodies of neoplastic cells in the subcapsular sinus.

## Essential and desirable diagnostic criteria

*Essential:* presence of breast implant; CD30+ large lymphoma cells at the luminal side of the capsule; expression of one or more T-lineage–associated markers.

## Staging

A modification of the TNM system has been developed {370}. The pathological T staging is as follows: T1 (tumour confined at the luminal side of the capsule), T2 (superficial infiltration of the capsule), T3 (deep infiltration of the capsule, often accompanied by chronic inflammatory cell infiltration), and T4 (through the capsule) {370,1682}. The proportions of cases showing T1, T2, T3, and T4 stage are 35.6%, 12.6%, 16.1%, and 34.5%, respectively {370,1682}. In addition, lymph node involvement (N1) and distant disease (M1) may occur {370}.

## Prognosis and prediction

The 5-year overall survival rate was 92% in one case series {1382}. Surgery is the cornerstone of therapy, with complete excision of capsule and implant leading to a 5-year overall survival rate of 100% in patients with effusion only {1382,370}. The 5-year overall survival rate is 83.7% for patients with disease beyond the capsule and 75% for patients with lymph node involvement {636}. Incomplete surgery may lead to recurrence or progression of disease {370}. Systemic chemotherapy is recommended for non-resectable disease; brentuximab vedotin is recommended for refractory disease {369}.

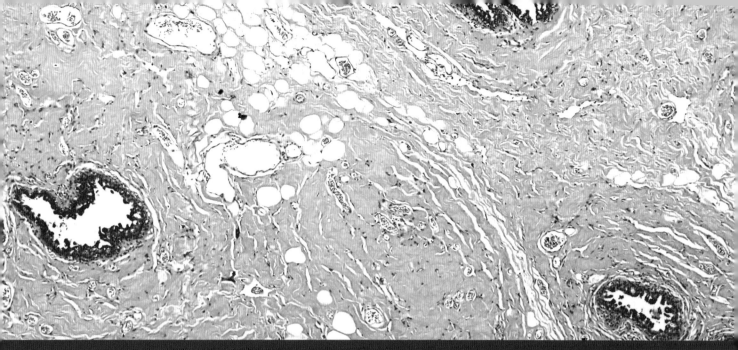

# 7

# Tumours of the male breast

Edited by: van Diest PJ

Epithelial tumours
    Gynaecomastia
    Carcinoma in situ
    Invasive carcinoma

# WHO classification of tumours of the male breast

**Epithelial tumours**

| | |
|---|---|
| | Gynaecomastia |
| |    Florid gynaecomastia |
| |    Fibrous gynaecomastia |
| 8500/2 | Intraductal carcinoma, non-infiltrating, NOS |
| |    Ductal carcinoma in situ |
| |    Lobular carcinoma in situ |
| 8540/3 |    Paget disease of the nipple |
| 8500/3 | Infiltrating duct carcinoma NOS |

---

These morphology codes are from the International Classification of Diseases for Oncology, third edition, second revision (ICD-O-3.2) {921}. Behaviour is coded /0 for benign tumours; /1 for unspecified, borderline, or uncertain behaviour; /2 for carcinoma in situ and grade III intraepithelial neoplasia; /3 for malignant tumours, primary site; and /6 for malignant tumours, metastatic site. Behaviour code /6 is not generally used by cancer registries.

This classification is modified from the previous WHO classification, taking into account changes in our understanding of these lesions.

Subtype labels are indented.

# Tumours of the male breast: Introduction

Foschini MP
Fox SB
Shaaban AM

The male breast is a rudimentary organ, whose glandular composition is limited to ducts located in the retroareolar region. Male breast epithelium shows ER, PR, and AR expression and is exposed to hormonal variation throughout life. In particular, sex chromosome copy-number variations have been demonstrated to be quite frequent in ageing men {928}.

Despite its small size, the male breast can be affected by a variety of benign and malignant diseases, over a wide age range. Clinical and radiological presentation can be similar in benign and malignant nodules {337}, most of which appear as retroareolar lumps. The cytological and histological preoperative diagnoses are similar to those encountered in the female breast. Conversely, the rarity of individual male breast entities makes the acquisition of sufficient knowledge to establish diagnostic, prognostic, and predictive criteria difficult.

Among the male breast lesions, male breast cancer is rare (accounting for ~1% of all breast cancers), and it leads to death in a high proportion of patients. Male breast cancer is treated in a similar manner to female postmenopausal breast cancer. Recurrences are not rare. Over the past decade, studies based on multi-institutional series have shed light on male breast cancer pathogenesis, including differences from female breast carcinoma. Molecular studies have shown a high number of differently expressed genes {272,1660}, among which the *AR* gene seems to play a role as driver in the neoplastic transformation of the male breast epithelial cells.

A potential further challenge might arise from sex reassignment (gender confirmation), either male-to-female or female-to-male. Little evidence is currently available, but published data indicate that hormonal stimulation might induce breast cancer development {827,1996}.

# Gynaecomastia

Foschini MP
Fox SB
Shaaban AM

## Definition

Gynaecomastia is a benign diffuse or focal proliferation of glandular tissue of the male breast.

## ICD-O coding

None

## ICD-11 coding

GB22 Gynaecomastia

## Related terminology

None

## Subtype(s)

Florid gynaecomastia; fibrous gynaecomastia

## Localization

Most cases are retroareolar and bilateral.

## Clinical features

Gynaecomastia commonly presents as bilateral diffuse or discrete masses in the retroareolar area. It can be painful or painless, and it may be an incidental finding. Physiological gynaecomastia during puberty or in the neonatal period is a temporary, often self-limited, enlargement. It is important to identify patients with an underlying pathological cause through clinical history, physical examination, and laboratory and imaging tests. Lipomastia (pseudogynaecomastia) may be confused with true gynaecomastia.

## Epidemiology

Gynaecomastia in infants, children, and adolescents is common and frequently physiological. In a minority of males, more commonly aged > 26 years, it is pathological and related to underrecognized conditions causing hormonal imbalance {1159,1483}.

## Etiology

The majority of cases result from an abnormal androgen-to-estrogen ratio and AR absence or alterations. Gynaecomastia can result from exposure to exogenous estrogens (e.g. dietary phytoestrogens), drugs (including anabolic steroids), an increase in endogenous estrogen production (due to testicular or adrenal tumours or increased aromatization of androgens),

**Table 7.01** Summary of causes and mechanisms of production of gynaecomastia

| Etiology | Age group | Mechanism of production of gynaecomastia |
|---|---|---|
| Physiological | Children and adolescents | Estrogens and androgens hormonal imbalance {793} |
| Physiological senile | Elderly adults | Relative increase in estrogen levels {996} |
| Familial increased aromatization of androgens | Children | Increased aromatization of androgens {2084} |
| X-linked disorders | All ages | Full or partial androgen insensitivity syndromes {1032,2009} |
| Klinefelter syndrome | All ages | AR gene with higher number of CAG repeats leading to a reduction in its activity {1777} |
| Carney complex | Children | Development of Sertoli cell tumours {556} |
| Peutz–Jeghers syndrome | Children | Loss of heterozygosity of STK11 leading to increased aromatase expression in testicular Sertoli cells and in breast tissue {2350} |
| Exogenous estrogens | Adults | Estrogens and androgens hormonal imbalance {402} |
| Androgen deprivation therapy for prostate cancer | Adults | Unopposed estrogen activity {1615} |
| Testicular or adrenal tumours | Mainly adults | Increased estrogen production {33} |
| Aromatase excess syndrome | All ages | Alterations in the aromatase gene {687} |
| Drugs | Mainly adults | Several mechanisms, depending on the type of drug; reviewed by Nuttall et al. {1523} and Costanzo et al. {402} |
| Obesity | All ages | Dependent on cause of obesity {1075} |
| Alcohol-induced cirrhosis | Adults | Several mechanisms proposed, such as reduced activity of cytochrome P450 and abnormal testosterone-to-estrogen ratio {514} |
| Spinobulbar muscular atrophy | All ages | Similar to in Klinefelter syndrome – an increased number of CAG repeats in the AR gene {1798} |
| Unknown | Mainly adults | Reviewed by Costanzo et al. {402} |

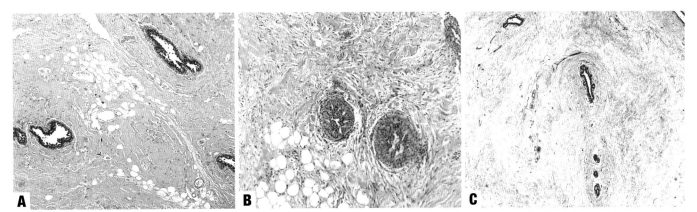

**Fig. 7.01** Gynaecomastia. **A** Florid pattern: breast ducts surrounded by pseudoangiomatous hyperplasia. **B** Florid pattern: ducts are lined by florid epithelium and surrounded by stromal hyperplasia. **C** Fibrous pattern: characterized by fibrous stroma and flat epithelium lining the ducts.

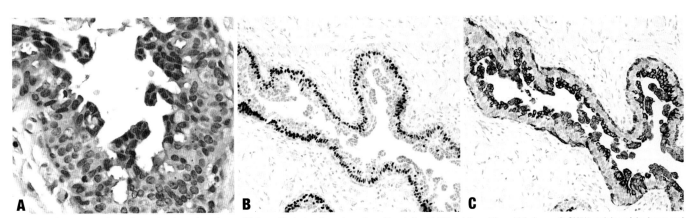

**Fig. 7.02** Gynaecomastia. **A** Ducts showing a three-layered lining, with dark cells and small papillary tufts. **B** ER staining of the middle layer. **C** CK5/6 staining of the inner and outer layers.

obesity, alcohol-induced cirrhosis, renal failure, ageing, and hyperthyroidism. Androgen deficiencies (hypogonadism, either primary or secondary) can result primarily from Klinefelter syndrome, chemotherapy, radiotherapy, or drugs that affect enzymes related to androgen synthesis (spironolactone, metronidazole). Drugs for the treatment of prostate cancer or a range of AR defects (e.g. AR insensitivity syndromes resulting in end-organ resistance) can also cause gynaecomastia. In > 40% of cases, no cause is identified {402}.

## Pathogenesis

Estrogen, progesterone, and androgens are thought to play a role in the pathogenesis of gynaecomastia. Additional pathways mediated through receptors for prolactin, IGF1, IGF2, LH, and/or hCG have also been implicated {1455}. Leptin and polymorphisms in its receptor might contribute to gynaecomastia by altering expression of adipocyte aromatase or via a paracrine effect through the epithelial component {591}.

Table 7.01 summarizes the causes and mechanisms of production of gynaecomastia. Patients with Klinefelter syndrome (47,XXY) show gynaecomastia in 50–70% of cases. In this syndrome, there is an increase in the number of CAG repeats in the *AR* gene, leading to a reduction in its activity {1777}. More repeats have been associated with clinically more-prominent gynaecomastia. Klinefelter syndrome patients can develop hCG-secreting germ cell tumours as a further cause

of gynaecomastia {2272}. Other genetic syndromes associated with gynaecomastia are spinobulbar muscular atrophy (through a similar mechanism of expanded CAG repeats in exon 1 of *AR*) {1798}, full or partial androgen insensitivity syndrome {1032,2009}, androgen excess syndrome (from alterations in the aromatase gene or adjacent enhancer) {687}, and Peutz–Jeghers syndrome {2350} and Carney complex {556} (causing increased aromatase expression in testicular Sertoli cells and in breast tissue).

## Macroscopic appearance

Gynaecomastia manifests as a discrete, soft, rubbery to firm, grey or white mass or a poorly defined area of induration under the nipple.

## Histopathology

The histopathological appearance is dependent on the relative proportion of ducts and stroma. The ducts are increased in number and lined by a characteristic bilayer of epithelial cells {1048} and an outer layer of myoepithelial cells. The inner epithelial cell layer and the outer myoepithelial cells may be demonstrated by CK5/6 and CK14, and the middle epithelial layer is positive for ER, PR, and AR {1048}. The ducts are surrounded by stroma admixed with adipose tissue. There are two main histological patterns that may coexist. The florid pattern is characterized by irregular branching ducts lined by mildly to moderately proliferative cells with small tufts, pyramid-shaped micropapillae, occasional true papillae, or cribriform structures. Concomitant myoepithelial hyperplasia may be present. The surrounding stroma, often appearing as concentric cuffs around the ducts, can be loose, myxoid, or cellular (fibroblastic). Pseudoangiomatous stromal hyperplasia is often present. The fibrous pattern is characterized by hyalinized, hypocellular periductal stroma, often in a confluent pattern due to expansion of concentric cuffs. An intermediate phase including a mixture of florid and fibrous patterns can also be seen. Rarely, apocrine or squamous metaplasia may be observed. Multinucleated stromal cells as seen in the female breast have also been described and have been reported in patients with neurofibromatosis type 1 {446}. In Klinefelter syndrome, dense hyalinized stroma with few ducts may be seen {1503}.

Gynaecomastoid hyperplasia should be distinguished from atypical ductal hyperplasia and ductal carcinoma in situ. Staining for basal cytokeratins and ER may be helpful.

## Cytology

Cytology reveals a biphasic population of epithelial and stromal fragments with small to medium-sized flat sheets of ductal cells surrounded by scattered single bipolar nuclei. Spindle cells, apocrine cells, and foamy macrophages may also be present. Some dyscohesion of ductal cells and nuclear enlargement with hyperchromasia may occur {1581}. Core needle biopsy is recommended for diagnosis.

## Diagnostic molecular pathology
Not clinically relevant

## Essential and desirable diagnostic criteria
*Essential:* benign ductular and stromal proliferation with characteristic stromal cuffing.
*Desirable:* typical three-layered ductal lining (two basal layers and one luminal layer); pseudoangiomatous stromal hyperplasia.

## Staging
Not clinically relevant

## Prognosis and prediction
Gynaecomastia is not associated with risk of developing breast carcinoma. Because most cases of gynaecomastia regress within 2 years, treatment is not usually indicated, except in the specific clinical context of sudden or symptomatic gynaecomastia. Medical treatment includes aromatase inhibitor, anti-estrogen, and/or androgen therapy. Hormonal treatment is most effective for florid {1694} and pubertal {1115} gynaecomastia.

# Carcinoma in situ

Foschini MP
Fox SB
Shaaban AM

## Definition

Carcinoma in situ of the male breast is a neoplastic proliferation of epithelial cells confined to the mammary ducts encompassing the entire spectrum of carcinoma in situ observed in the female breast.

## ICD-O coding

8500/2 Intraductal carcinoma, non-infiltrating, NOS

## ICD-11 coding

2E65.2 & XH4V32 Ductal carcinoma in situ of breast & Ductal carcinoma in situ NOS
2E65.0 & XH6EH0 Lobular carcinoma in situ of breast & Lobular carcinoma in situ NOS

## Related terminology

None

## Subtype(s)

Ductal carcinoma in situ; lobular carcinoma in situ; Paget disease of the nipple

## Localization

Carcinoma of the male breast is almost exclusively localized in the retroareolar region.

## Clinical features

Carcinoma in situ of the male breast presents in three different clinical settings: as an occasional finding in gynaecomastia, in association with invasive carcinoma, or as pure carcinoma in situ with variable symptoms and clinical features. Symptom duration ranges from a few months to 8 years {425,859,1739}. Pure carcinoma in situ most often presents as a retroareolar mass affecting elderly men, with a mean age range of 58–65 years {425,859}, and it can be bilateral {1930}. Rarely, carcinoma in situ can affect young men and adolescents {425}. Large duct involvement is associated with bloody nipple discharge {226, 1739,425}. In Paget disease, there is an enlarging eczematous lesion of the nipple–areola complex {11,1235}. Diagnosis by mammography alone can be difficult, and MRI can be helpful in reaching the correct diagnosis {226,1739}.

## Epidemiology

Male carcinoma in situ, which is almost exclusively ductal carcinoma in situ (DCIS), is associated with invasive carcinoma in as many as 46.2% of cases {525}. Pure carcinoma in situ is rarer, with recent data indicating it constitutes 10% of all male breast cancers {576} and 18% of breast cancers occurring in young and adolescent boys {651}. The incidence of carcinoma in situ in gynaecomastia has been reported to be 6.76%, but this is based on a small series {1930}. Paget disease accounts for 1.45% of all male breast cancers {11}.

## Etiology

The etiological factors are similar to those of invasive carcinoma of the female breast and are discussed in that section (p. 82).

## Pathogenesis

The pathogenesis is similar to that of invasive male breast carcinoma (see *Invasive carcinoma*, p. 257). Data on the molecular profile of male carcinoma in situ, which are scant and concern DCIS, point towards a close relationship between in situ and associated invasive carcinoma, with similar mutations in *PIK3CA*, *TP53*, and *GATA3* {525} and copy-number aberrations for common oncogenes {2168}. In rare cases, columnar cell–like changes present adjacent to DCIS, and invasive carcinoma showed the same mutation profile {525}. X chromosome aneusomy associated with *AR* copy-number gain has been identified in DCIS {497}.

## Macroscopic appearance

Pure carcinoma in situ presents as an irregular, sometimes cystic mass {425}.

## Histopathology

Although the entire spectrum of carcinoma in situ observed in the female breast can also be found in the male breast {2183}, the vast majority (97.9%) of male carcinoma in situ is DCIS, whereas lobular carcinoma in situ is rare {525}. Most pure DCIS is of low or intermediate nuclear grade {859} and of papillary or micropapillary architecture, whereas high-grade DCIS with comedonecrosis is usually associated with high-grade invasive carcinoma. The nuclear grade, histotype, and immunophenotype of DCIS usually correlate with the grade and type of associated invasive carcinoma. DCIS seems to be associated

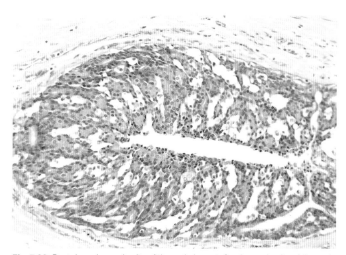

**Fig. 7.03** Ductal carcinoma in situ of the male breast. Carcinoma in situ of the male breast is most frequently of ductal type, as in this example with papillary and cribriform features.

Chapter 7

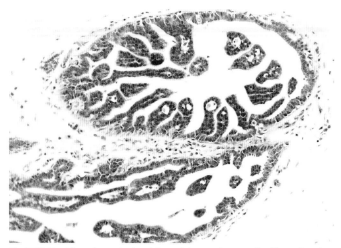

**Fig. 7.04** Ductal carcinoma in situ of the male breast. An example with papillary features.

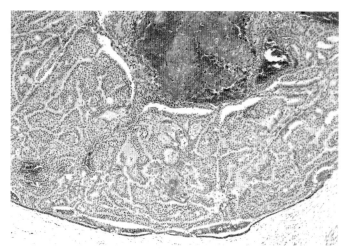

**Fig. 7.05** Ductal carcinoma in situ of the male breast. Encapsulated papillary carcinoma.

with invasive carcinoma of no special type (NST), whereas the rare cases of lobular carcinoma in situ were associated with invasive lobular carcinoma, invasive carcinoma NST, or invasive carcinoma of mixed type {525}. The ER, PR, and ERBB2 (HER2) status in the in situ component mirrors that of the invasive component {525}.

On rare occasions, carcinoma in situ has the features of encapsulated papillary carcinoma and can lack a myoepithelial layer {953}. Paget disease is similar to that in the female breast {11, 2166}. Columnar cell–like changes can be associated with DCIS {2172,525}. These cases are characterized by dilated ducts, lined by monomorphic mildly atypical cells with apical snouts. Rarely, microcalcifications and secretions are present {2172,1739}.

## Cytology

There is no FNA literature focused on pure male carcinoma in situ. Core needle biopsy is preferred for diagnosis.

## Diagnostic molecular pathology

Not clinically relevant

## Essential and desirable diagnostic criteria

The diagnostic criteria are similar to those of invasive carcinoma of the female breast and are discussed in that section (p. 82).

## Staging

The staging is similar to that of invasive carcinoma of the female breast and is discussed in that section (p. 82).

## Prognosis and prediction

Carcinoma in situ associated with invasive carcinoma is treated similarly to invasive disease. For pure DCIS, the prognosis is good. In one series, 4 of 31 cases recurred: 1 case as DCIS and 3 cases as invasive carcinoma {425}. It has been suggested that the presence of DCIS next to invasive carcinoma is associated with longer overall survival in the luminal A and luminal B HER2-enriched groups {525}.

# Invasive carcinoma

Foschini MP
Fox SB
Shaaban AM

## Definition

Invasive carcinoma of the male breast is a rare malignant epithelial tumour that is histologically similar to its counterpart in the female breast.

## ICD-O coding

8500/3 Infiltrating duct carcinoma NOS

## ICD-11 coding

2C61.0 & XH7KH3 Invasive carcinoma of breast NOS & Infiltrating duct carcinoma NOS

## Related terminology

Similar to that of invasive carcinoma of the female breast

## Subtype(s)

Same as those observed in the female breast

## Localization

Male breast cancer is usually localized in the retroareolar region.

## Clinical features

Male breast cancer usually presents as a unilateral painless mass in the subareolar region, often slightly eccentric to the nipple. Bloody or serous discharge may be the presenting symptom. Due to the usually small amount of mammary tissue in men, tumours can easily infiltrate the overlying skin or underlying fascia/muscle.

## Epidemiology

Male breast cancer accounts for < 1% of all breast cancers {1218} and for < 0.5% of all cancer deaths in men in the USA {1939}. Over the past few decades, the incidence of male breast cancer has risen in the United Kingdom, USA, Canada, and Australia {1983,1939}. The highest incidence has been reported in Israel (1.24 cases per 100 000 man-years) and the lowest in Thailand (0.16 cases per 100 000 man-years) {1255}. Male breast cancer is more common in black men, in whom breast cancer also occurs at a younger age, presents at a more advanced stage, and is associated with higher breast cancer–specific mortality {2006}. Whereas female breast cancer shows two age peaks, male breast cancer occurs at a slightly older age (median: 68.4 years) than breast cancer in postmenopausal women. However, it can also affect young and adolescent boys {1181}. Klinefelter syndrome confers a relative risk of male breast cancer of 30–50 (as a result of increased circulating estrogen); it accounts for as many as 5% of male breast cancers {894} and a 57.8-fold increase in mortality {1181}. The risk of developing breast cancer might also be influenced by hormonal changes associated with sex reassignment (gender confirmation), both male-to-female and female-to-male {827,1996,976,756}.

## Etiology

Hormonal imbalance leading to a relative excess of estrogen (as seen in liver cirrhosis or Klinefelter syndrome) has been most commonly implicated in male breast cancer development. As is seen with other cancers, age increases the risk of developing breast cancer in men. Obesity has also been linked to the disease, with a recent increase in body mass index having a significant effect {231,896}. Cryptorchidism, mumps, orchitis, testicular trauma, and prostate cancer also increase the risk of male breast cancer {1810}.

Approximately 20% of male breast cancer patients have a first-degree family member with breast cancer {130}. Men with a family history of female or male breast cancer have a 2–3 times increased risk of developing breast carcinoma. One third of familial male breast cancers seem to arise in *BRCA1/2* mutation carriers, with the remainder associated with other genes (e.g. *CHEK2* and *PALB2*), whereas other cases have unknown underlying genetic mechanisms {1946}. Mutations and rearrangements of *BRCA2* are more frequent than those of *BRCA1* in male breast cancer. About 5–10% of male *BRCA2* carriers develop breast cancer in their lifetime {1810}, compared with 1–2% of *BRCA1* carriers. *BRCA1/2* male breast

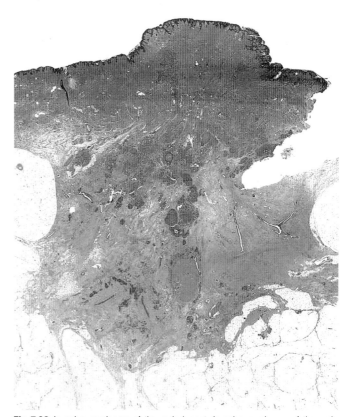

**Fig. 7.06** Invasive carcinoma of the male breast. Invasive carcinoma of the male breast is most frequently located in the retroareolar area.

cancers display pathological characteristics distinct from those of *BRCA1/2* female breast cancers, and they show a more aggressive phenotype {1946}.

Environmental factors such as ionizing radiation and electromagnetic exposure, alcohol consumption, smoking, and red meat consumption have been linked to increased male breast cancer incidence {637}. Most studies have found no convincing causative link between gynaecomastia and male breast cancer.

## Pathogenesis

The precise pathogenesis is not fully understood, but genetic, hormonal, and environmental factors are thought to lead to hormonal imbalance, with a relative excess of estrogen-to-androgen ratio, causing enhanced proliferation of mammary epithelial cells. Several recently published molecular studies {1660,272} show differences between male and female breast cancer, with proportionately more luminal cancers in males than in females and almost half the proportion of ERBB2 (HER2), basal, and triple-negative subtypes among male breast cancers compared with female breast cancers {470,1047}.

The pattern of chromosomal gains and losses in ER-positive male breast cancer is similar to that of ER-positive female breast cancer, except for gains on the X chromosome in male breast cancer. A substantial proportion of male breast cancers have a *BRCA2*-like profile {169}. Male breast cancer shows more frequent *CCND1* amplification, fewer copy-number changes on chromosome 17 {1086}, and less frequent copy-number loss on 16q {1085,1042}. The role of *AR* as a driver gene in male breast cancer {272} has been well established. AR is highly expressed in male breast cancer {1044,498}, with X chromosome aneusomy and consequent *AR* gene polysomy described in about 74% of cases {497}. These data are consistent with the recent observation of the value of anti-androgen therapy in male breast cancer {1903}.

mRNA expression profiling in male breast cancer shows differences compared with female breast cancer, with minimal overlap {950,272,951}. Losses of 16q and mutations found in ER-positive, HER2-negative tumours (e.g. mutations in *PIK3CA* and *TP53* {469}) are less frequent in male breast cancer, which is enriched for mutations in the DNA repair–related genes {1660}. There is frequent activation of the PI3K/AKT/mTOR {469} and FGFR2 pathways in male breast cancers, a finding which may provide promising future targets for therapy. There are similarities and differences in methylated genes in male breast cancer compared with female breast cancer, with lower methylation rates in male breast cancer overall {725,1043} but relatively frequent *ESR1* and *GSTP1* methylation in high-grade male breast cancer {1043}. There are only limited data on a limited number of microRNAs in male breast cancer, but again these differ from those in female breast cancer {1141,624}.

## Macroscopic appearance

Male breast cancer usually forms a large stellate or nodular mass, which may also involve the nipple.

## Histopathology

The most common type of invasive male breast cancer is invasive ductal carcinoma of no special type (NST). Unlike among female breast cancers, the second most common tumour is papillary carcinoma. Invasive lobular carcinoma is extremely rare. Other special types, such as mucinous, tubular, and metaplastic carcinomas, are also extremely rare. Most tumours are grade 2 {897,470}. In high-grade male breast cancer, a fibrotic focus may be found {1045,471}.

Male breast cancer is usually ER-positive and/or PR-positive (> 90% of cases) {897,1046}, with frequent AR expression {1088}. HER2-positive, triple-negative, and basal-like tumours are rare {1905,470,1046}. Typical markers of breast epithelium, such as GATA3, cyclin D1, mammaglobin, BCL2, and GCDFP-15 (BRST-2), are expressed in most male breast cancers and maintained in metastases {175,1046}.

Sentinel node and axillary clearance specimens are reported using the same guidelines as for female breast cancer. Primary male breast cancer should be differentiated from metastases to the breast, including metastatic prostate cancer, which is positive for PSA, PSMA, and NKX3-1.

## Cytology

FNA, when performed by an experienced cytopathologist, can lead to accurate diagnosis {1782}. The cytological features are similar to those of female breast cancer. Core needle biopsy is the gold standard for diagnosis of male breast cancer.

## Diagnostic molecular pathology

Not clinically relevant

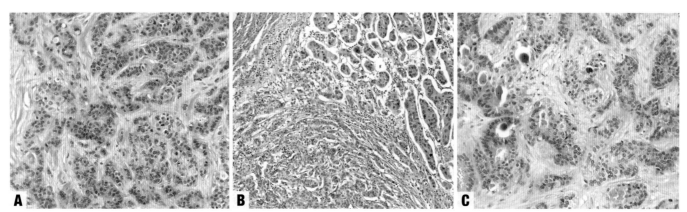

**Fig. 7.07** Invasive carcinoma of the male breast. **A** Most invasive carcinomas are of no special type (NST). **B** Invasive carcinoma NST shows micropapillary features. **C** Microcalcifications can occur.

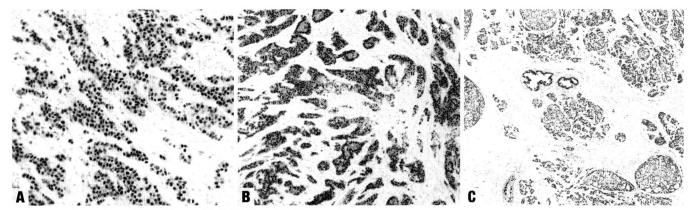

**Fig. 7.08** Invasive carcinoma of the male breast. ER (**A**), PR (**B**), and AR (**C**) are usually strongly positive.

## Essential and desirable diagnostic criteria

*Essential:* the diagnostic criteria are identical to those of female breast cancer; invasive malignant process of breast epithelium lacking a peripheral myoepithelial cell layer (immunohistochemistry may be required), with or without carcinoma in situ; ER, PR, and HER2 immunohistochemistry to guide classification, treatment, and prognosis.

## Staging

The eighth edition of the Union for International Cancer Control (UICC) TNM classification {229} should be used as for female breast cancer.

## Prognosis and prediction

Data from the EORTC 10085/TBCRC/BIG/NABCG International Male Breast Cancer Program demonstrate that most patients with male breast cancer present with T1 (48.7%) or T2 (38.3%) disease. There is axillary lymph node metastasis in 40.6% of cases, with low-volume nodal involvement (N1: 32.2%, N2: 5.3%, and N3: 3%) {2169}. Distant metastases at presentation have been reported in a small proportion of cases (5.1%) {284}.

Disease outcome is influenced by stage, hormone receptor status, mitotic count, grade, molecular subtype, and nodal status {1045,1047,1042,1043,1046,1087,2169}. Nodal positivity has an adverse effect on disease-free survival and overall survival {897}. Despite contradictory data, the general understanding is that male breast cancer has a prognosis similar to that of female breast cancer with equivalent stage and patient age {2337, 2006,1218,316}. It has been suggested that married patients have a significantly better 5-year survival rate, indicating the importance of spousal support {1217}.

There are few if any prognostic markers, owing to the low numbers of male breast cancers reported. Nevertheless, as with female breast cancer, hormone receptor expression and HER2 status are used as predictors of therapy response. Prognostic models applied in female breast cancer, such as the Morphometric Prognostic Index (MPI), the Nottingham Prognostic Index (NPI), and Predict, can also be of practical management value in male breast cancer {2145}. The role of grading performed according to the criteria followed in female breast cancer has been challenged {2169}, because thresholds for mitotic count may differ. A *BRCA2*-like profile may indicate benefit from targeted therapy, as seen in female breast cancer {169}.

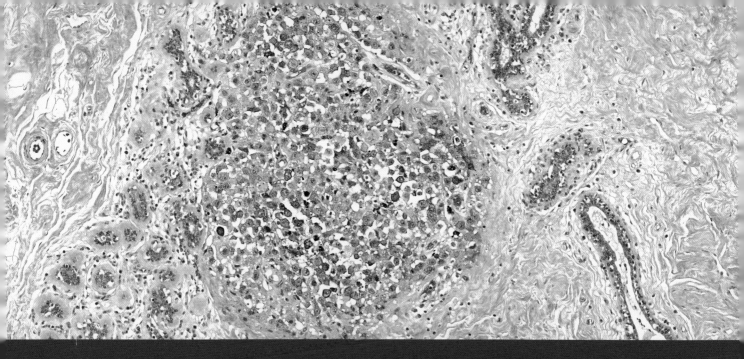

# 8

# Metastases to the breast

Edited by: van Diest PJ

# Metastases to the breast

Kulka J
Varga Z

## Definition
Metastases to the breast are malignant tumours in the breast originating from an extramammary organ or site.

## ICD-O coding
Code as original tumour

## ICD-11 coding
2E0Y & XA12C1 Malignant neoplasm metastasis in other specified sites & Breast

## Related terminology
None

## Subtype(s)
None

## Localization
The upper-outer quadrant is the most common site {805}.

## Clinical features
The clinical findings in patients with primary breast cancer and those with metastasis to the breast overlap. Metastases to the breast occur more often in advanced-stage cancer in patients in their fifth to sixth decade of life {191}, but they may also be the first sign of an extramammary primary tumour {249}. In about one third of patients presenting with metastasis, this is the first indication of malignancy {1128}. Females are more frequently affected than males {191,1128,476,249,2274}. In children and adolescents, rhabdomyosarcoma metastases have been described {987}. The tumours are typically a rapidly growing, painless, firm, palpable mass (or masses), and bilateral involvement may also occur {191}. Occasionally, oedematous thickening of the skin, mimicking inflammatory breast cancer, is seen {54}.

On mammography and ultrasonography, breast metastases appear as relatively small, superficial, poorly defined, irregular nodules. Stellate configuration, which is common in primary breast cancer, is not a typical mammographic feature. Microcalcifications may accompany serous carcinoma metastases {1136,2274}.

## Epidemiology
Metastatic solid tumours in the breast account for 0.2–1.1% of all breast malignancies, and 0.02–0.4% are due to systemic involvement by haematological malignancies {191}. In autopsy studies, breast involvement occurs in 3.9% of haematological malignancies and in 1.4% of extramammary solid tumours {1839,6}. The most common source of breast metastases is contralateral breast cancer. However, the majority of bilateral

**Table 8.01** Useful antibodies and their specificity in the differential diagnosis of breast metastases

| Immunohistochemistry | Specificity in primary breast cancer | Specificity in non-breast primaries | References |
|---|---|---|---|
| GATA3 | High | Intermediate in urothelial neoplasms | {1499,879,758,1840} |
| NY-BR-1 | High | High in salivary gland tumours | {175,2292,2157} |
| AR | High | High in prostate cancers | {205} |
| ER | High (in luminal-type cases) | Intermediate-high in ovarian and gastric cancers | {879} |
| SOX10 | High (in triple-negative cases) | High in melanomas, Schwannian tumours, and myoepithelial carcinomas | {1479,1371} |
| GCDFP-15 | Intermediate-high | High in salivary gland tumours and apocrine tumours; low in lung cancers | {1499,879,758,1840} |
| Mammaglobin | Intermediate-high | Intermediate in salivary gland tumours | {1499,879,758,1840,2292} |
| CK7 | Intermediate-high | High in tubo-ovarian cancers | {879} |
| CK20 | Absent | High in gastrointestinal cancers | {1128} |
| PAX8 | Low-absent | High in serous tubo-ovarian and endometrial cancers | {2292,596,1517} |
| p53 | Low-absent | High in serous tubo-ovarian, endometrial, and gastrointestinal cancers | {1128} |
| CA125 | Low-absent | High in serous ovarian, biliary, and pancreatic cancers | {1128} |
| Melan-A (MART1) | Absent | High in melanomas | {99} |
| TTF1 | Low-absent | High in lung adenocarcinomas | {1128} |
| S100 | Low-intermediate | Low-intermediate in melanomas and peripheral nerve sheath tumours | {99} |

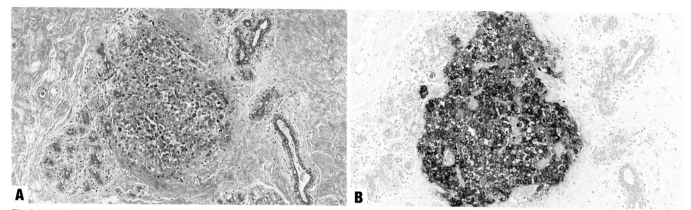

**Fig. 8.01** Melanoma metastatic to the breast. **A** Metastatic melanoma with prominent pigment. **B** Pigmented tumour cells are diffusely positive for HMB45.

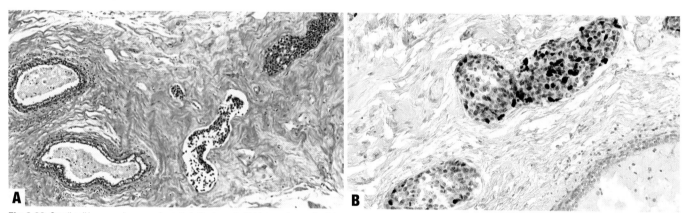

**Fig. 8.02** Small cell lung carcinoma metastatic to the breast. **A** Metastatic small cell lung carcinoma is seen within lymphovascular spaces. **B** Tumour cells are positive for TTF1.

breast cancers seem to be independent primaries: a molecular genetic relationship has recently been found in < 10% of cases {135A}.

## Etiology
The etiology varies according to the primary tumour.

## Pathogenesis
Although breast cancer may spread to the contralateral breast via lymphatics or blood vessels, metastases from extramammary malignant tumours mainly reach the breast via blood circulation. However, given that in lung cancer metastatic to the breast the secondary tumour is often ipsilateral and accompanied by ipsilateral axillary metastases, it has been suggested that tumour cells preferentially spread through a retrograde axillary lymphatic drainage {886}. The available reviews and several case reports list the following primary tumours as the most common sources of breast metastases: lymphoma/leukaemia, melanoma, pulmonary carcinoma, ovarian carcinoma, gastric carcinoma, prostatic carcinoma, renal cell carcinoma, colorectal carcinoma, sarcomas (rhabdomyosarcoma metastases have been described in children and adolescents {987}), malignant mesothelioma, neuroendocrine tumours (NETs), and squamous cell carcinoma of the uterine cervix.

## Macroscopic appearance
Solitary or multiple nodules may be present. Although there are no specific macroscopic features, in some cases the gross appearance may suggest the primary tumour, as in a metastasis from a heavily pigmented melanoma.

## Histopathology
Key morphological clues for the recognition of metastatic tumours are unusual histological patterns, lack of an in situ component, predominant periductal and/or perilobular distribution, and (in some) extensive lymphovascular involvement. Clinical history is often helpful. Some tumours metastatic to the breast show characteristic features (and do not cause diagnostic problems): typical nuclear features and pigment in melanoma, nuclear features in lymphomas, chromatin pattern in NETs, typical appearance of colorectal adenocarcinomas, and papillary architecture and psammoma bodies in serous carcinomas. However, at least one third of epithelial tumours metastatic to the breast lack any specific histological features and are high-grade, making the diagnosis difficult. Comparison of the mammary and extramammary malignant tumours is essential in this situation.

If metastasis to the breast is suspected and there is no known extramammary malignant tumour, a broad panel of organ- or tumour-specific immunohistochemical markers can be applied to delineate the likely primary site. If there is known previous or synchronous malignancy, a smaller panel of immunohistochemical markers is sufficient (see Table 8.01 and Fig. 8.03).

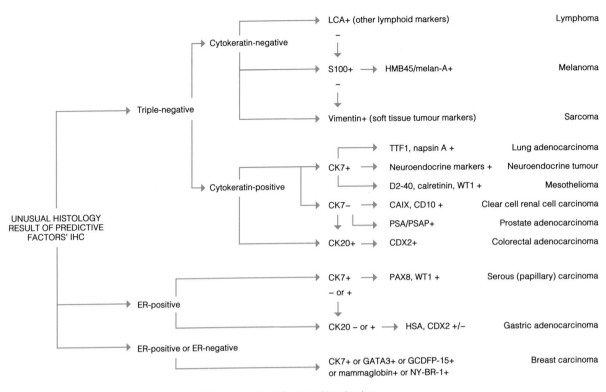

Fig. 8.03 Suggested algorithm for breast tumours suspected to be metastatic. IHC, immunohistochemistry.

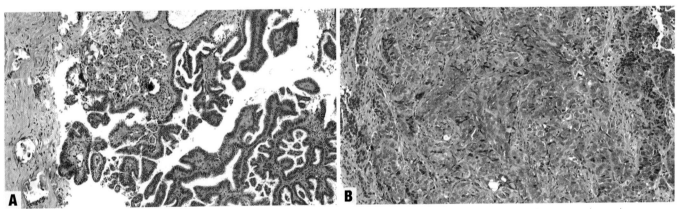

Fig. 8.04 Metastases to the breast. **A** Histological appearance of metastatic low-grade serous ovarian carcinoma. **B** Metastatic high-grade serous ovarian carcinoma.

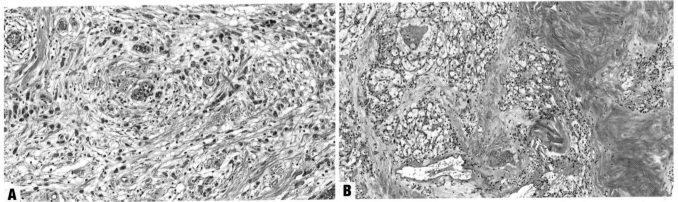

Fig. 8.05 Metastases to the breast. **A** Metastatic poorly cohesive gastric carcinoma may mimic invasive lobular carcinoma. **B** Clear cell renal cell carcinoma metastatic to the breast.

Breast metastases may spread via small lymphatics in such a manner that the distended lymphatics mimic carcinoma in situ and thus mislead the pathologist. In case of doubt, the use of lymphatic endothelial immunohistochemical markers may be helpful. With a triple-negative immunophenotype, especially without a known history of extramammary malignancy, the following primaries must be considered: melanoma (both skin and ocular), lymphoma (most often diffuse large B-cell lymphoma), lung cancer (mainly adenocarcinomas {32}), gastrointestinal adenocarcinomas, NETs, renal cell carcinomas, and soft tissue sarcomas. In men, prostatic carcinoma may metastasize to the breast. Lung adenocarcinomas may express ER, and breast carcinomas can (rarely) express TTF1 {1772}. SOX10 is considered the most specific antibody for the distinction of TTF1-negative lung adenocarcinoma from triple-negative breast carcinoma {1118A}, and it may be combined with GATA3 {2099A}. Gastric adenocarcinomas with intestinal and signet-ring cell histology are ER-negative {891A} and frequently HNF4A-positive {2145A}.

In ER-positive tumours, high-grade serous ovarian / fallopian tube / peritoneal carcinoma should be considered in the differential diagnosis. If there is any uncertainty, a panel of breast-related immunohistochemical markers (CK7, GATA3, GCDFP-15, mammaglobin, NY-BR-1) is helpful to rule out a metastasis. Carcinoma in situ and stromal elastosis are characteristic of primary breast cancer {1128}.

## Cytology
The cytological features depend on the type of metastatic tumour.

## Diagnostic molecular pathology
The diagnostic molecular pathology is related to the primary tumour.

## Essential and desirable diagnostic criteria
The essential and desirable diagnostic criteria vary according to the primary tumour.

## Staging
The primary tumour should be staged according to the eighth edition of the Union for International Cancer Control (UICC) TNM classification {229}.

## Prognosis and prediction
Most metastases to the breast occur as part of disseminated disease, and the prognosis is therefore very poor. Survival for > 1 year has been reported in patients with lymphoma and NETs {2274}. One study suggested that patients who underwent surgery for breast metastases had better overall survival {2274}.

# 9

# Genetic tumour syndromes of the breast

Edited by: Lakhani SR, Lazar AJ

*BRCA1/2*-associated hereditary breast and ovarian cancer syndrome
Cowden syndrome
Ataxia–telangiectasia
Li–Fraumeni syndrome, *TP53*-associated
Li–Fraumeni syndrome, *CHEK2*-associated
*CDH1*-associated breast cancer
*PALB2*-associated cancers
Peutz–Jeghers syndrome
Neurofibromatosis type 1
The polygenic component of breast cancer susceptibility

# Genetic tumour syndromes of the breast: Introduction

Lazar AJ
Salgado R

In this section, we discuss the genetics of familial predisposition to breast cancer and some of the established and emerging genes that are a source of discussion within genetic clinics. *BRCA1* and *BRCA2* have now been well established, and *PALB2* is increasingly also considered an important predisposition gene; all three would be considered for testing in patients suspected to have a familial predisposition. However, many other genes (*ATM*, *CHEK2*, etc.) have limited evidence for their use in routine testing – mostly due to limited data on penetrance and frequency in the population and a lack of data on ethnic variations. In part because of these limitations, variants of unknown significance are commonly encountered in these genes, making patient management a challenge. There is now increasing interest in multigene breast cancer susceptibility and the use of polygenic risk scores; these topics are covered in the multigene section at the end of this chapter (see *The polygenic component of breast cancer susceptibility*, p. 292). Table 9.01 lists details of the familial syndromes covered in this chapter, as well as details of some additional syndromes of relevance to breast cancer that are not covered in this volume because breast cancer is not the major feature of the syndrome; most of these syndromes are covered in detail in other volumes of this series.

**Table 9.01** Genetic syndromes associated with an increased susceptibility to breast cancer {405,1405,1403,1404,1449}

| Disease/phenotype | MIM number | Inheritance | Locus | Gene | Gene/locus MIM number | Protein | Normal protein function |
|---|---|---|---|---|---|---|---|
| Familial breast-ovarian cancer 1 (BROVCA1) | 604370 | Mu, AD | 17q21.31 | *BRCA1* | 113705 | BRCA1 | DNA repair |
| Familial breast-ovarian cancer 2 (BROVCA2) | 612555 | AD | 13q13.1 | *BRCA2* | 600185 | BRCA2 | DNA repair |
| Familial breast-ovarian cancer 3 (BROVCA3) | 613399 | Unknown | 17q22 | *RAD51C* | 602774 | RAD51C | DNA repair |
| Familial breast-ovarian cancer 4 (BROVCA4) | 614291 | Unknown | 17q12 | *RAD51D* | 602954 | RAD51D | DNA repair |
| Cowden syndrome / Lhermitte–Duclos disease | 158350 | AD | 10q23.31 | *PTEN* | 601728 | PTEN | A phosphatase; regulation of cell division (tumour suppressor) |
| Ataxia–telangiectasia | 208900 | SMu, AD | 11q22.3 | *ATM* | 607585 | ATM | DNA damage response (DNA repair, apoptosis, cell cycle, stress response) |
| Li–Fraumeni syndrome, *TP53*-associated | 151623 | SMu, AD | 17p13.1 | *TP53* | 191170 | p53 | Regulation of cell division (tumour suppressor) |
| Li–Fraumeni syndrome, *CHEK2*-associated | 609265 | SMu, AD | 22q12.1 | *CHEK2* | 604373 | CHK2 | Induction of cell-cycle arrest and apoptosis after DNA damage |
| *CDH1*-associated breast cancer | 137215 | SMu, AD | 16q22.1 | *CDH1* | 192090 | E-cadherin (cadherin 1) | Calcium-dependent cell–cell adhesion |
| *PALB2*-associated breast cancer | 114480 | SMu, AD | 16p12.1 | *PALB2* | 610355 | PALB2 | DNA repair in collaboration with BRCA1 |
| Peutz–Jeghers syndrome | 175200 | AD | 19p13.3 | *STK11* | 602216 | STK11 | Suppression of cell division |
| Neurofibromatosis type 1 | 162200 | AD | 17q11.2 | *NF1* | 613113 | Neurofibromin (NF1) | Negative regulation of RAS |
| Lynch syndrome[a] | Various | AD | Various | Various | Various | Various | DNA mismatch repair |

AD, autosomal dominant; Mu, multifocal; SMu, somatic mutation.
[a]There is no conclusive evidence that susceptibility to breast carcinoma is increased in Lynch syndrome.

Screening for familial predisposition can also impact the pathologist. Clinical, morphological, and immunohistochemical features of tumours can be identified by pathologists as being potentially related to some hereditary syndromes. For example, hereditary syndromes associated with BRCA1 and BRCA2 mutations tend to be related to bilateral tumours arising mostly at a young age, and in the case of BRCA1-associated syndromes, to well-demarcated tumours composed of solid nests and a lymphoplasmacytic infiltrate, prominent nuclear atypia, high grade, and high mitotic activity. A panel of immunohistochemical markers has been proven to be useful in discriminating between BRCA1/2-related and sporadic cancers {2193}. Cowden syndrome preferentially gives rise to PTEN-negative apocrine cancers. Recent technological advances in high-throughput and large-scale sequencing testing, which is increasingly including both tumour and normal sequencing, have enabled the identification of germline variants that may identify underlying hereditary syndromes that otherwise would not have been recognized. This has been exemplified in patients with advanced renal cancer {1286} and across a large variety of heterogeneous tumours when universal tumour–normal sequencing is performed on a large institutional patient population. This development is reminiscent of an evolving population-based screening concept using cancer-focused panels that include relevant cancer predisposition genes {672}. In addition, whole-exome or whole-genome sequencing on formalin-fixed, paraffin-embedded specimens has been shown to be feasible and potentially applicable in a routine clinical environment {1770}, suggesting a path forwards beyond targeted sequencing in daily clinical practice sequencing. There is growing awareness of the ethical considerations of tumour sequencing {2195}.

Specific breast cancer subtypes like triple-negative breast cancer are an additional indicator of underlying germline mutations associated with homologous recombination deficiency, demonstrating, for example, deleterious mutations in BRCA1 in 14.8% of patients with triple-negative breast cancer {883}, whereas none of the carriers of ATM, RAD51D, CHEK2, or PALB2 mutations had a family history. This concept of testing triple-negative breast cancer patients irrespective of family history or patient age therefore emphasizes the importance to the pathologist of adequate and reliable identification of those patients with specific breast cancer subtypes, in this case triple-negative breast cancer. The importance of the pathologist lies in the potential identification of those patients based on detailed morphological and immunohistochemical analysis. It has been clearly shown that attempting to identify patients with high-risk mutations in cancer susceptibility genes by merely focusing on family history is not only laborious but can also result in a substantial proportion of patients being missed.

Patients with homologous recombination deficiency, which is most commonly associated with germline and/or somatic mutations in BRCA1 and/or BRCA2, show sensitivity to poly (ADP-ribose) polymerase (PARP) inhibitors {1257}. The emerging use of immunohistochemistry for markers like RAD51 to evaluate prediction for PARP inhibition in breast cancer is therefore intrinsically linked with the further merging of the disciplines of pathology and genetics {301}. Pathologists can assist in the identification of these patients by knowing the situations in which these biomarkers are best applied and the context of their interpretation.

# BRCA1/2-associated hereditary breast and ovarian cancer syndrome

Shaaban AM
Cheung AN
Fox SB
Jones JL
Khoo US

## Definition
BRCA1/2-associated hereditary breast and ovarian cancer syndrome is an autosomal dominant inherited disorder with germline mutations in BRCA1 and BRCA2 and in which the risk of breast cancer (especially before the age of 50 years) and ovarian cancer is higher than normal. There is also an increased risk of other cancer types.

## MIM numbering
604370 Familial breast-ovarian cancer 1 (BROVCA1)
612555 Familial breast-ovarian cancer 2 (BROVCA2)

## ICD-11 coding
2C65 Hereditary breast and ovarian cancer syndrome

## Related terminology
*Acceptable:* hereditary breast-ovarian cancer syndrome.

## Subtype(s)
None

## Localization
BRCA1/2-associated hereditary breast and ovarian cancer syndrome is associated with cancers of the breast, ovary, pancreas, prostate, and potentially other sites.

## Clinical features
The clinical features are dependent on the presentation of the tumour; there is no specific phenotype.

## Epidemiology
In a meta-analysis of 60 studies involving 105 220 breast cancer patients, 3588 patients (3.4%) were BRCA1/2 mutation carriers. Germline mutations in BRCA1 and BRCA2 are known to confer a high lifetime risk of breast and ovarian cancers {327}, as well as contralateral breast cancer {1320}. In the USA, the number of women who carry actionable BRCA1 and BRCA2 mutations is estimated to be 1 in 300–500 {1020}. More-recent large international studies have refined risk estimates. The Consortium of Investigators of Modifiers of BRCA1/2 (CIMBA) assembled data on 29 700 families with BRCA1 or BRCA2 mutations on six continents and found that breast and ovarian cancer risks varied by type and location of BRCA1/2 mutations {1985}. The incidence rates of breast cancer were 46% (BRCA1) and 52% (BRCA2), and of ovarian cancer 12% (BRCA1) and 6% (BRCA2). The incidence rates of breast and ovarian cancers together were 5% (BRCA1) and 2% (BRCA2); 37% of BRCA1 and 40% of BRCA2 mutation carriers were without cancer {1985}. The consortium also observed substantial variation in mutation type and frequency by geographical region and race/ethnicity. Besides the known founder mutations, other mutations of relatively high frequency were also identified in specific

**Table 9.02** Risk of cancers other than breast and ovarian cancers in BRCA1 and BRCA2 mutation carriers

| Cancer | Risk in mutation carriers | |
|---|---|---|
| | BRCA1 | BRCA2 |
| Prostate | Possible | Definite |
| Pancreas | Possible | Definite |
| Fallopian tube | Definite | Definite |
| Endometrium | Possible | No evidence |
| Cervix | No evidence | Possible |
| Hepatobiliary | Possible | Possible |
| Stomach | Possible | Possible |
| Colorectal | Possible | No evidence |
| Head and neck | No evidence | Possible |
| Melanoma | No evidence | Possible |
| Risk to male carriers | Little/none | Definite |

racial/ethnic or geographical groups. A recent meta-analysis of breast and ovarian cancers in India revealed 18 novel BRCA1 and 16 BRCA2 variants that were not previously reported or included in the Breast Cancer Information Core (BIC) or ClinVar databases {1912}. Three founder mutations of BRCA1 and BRCA2 are found in approximately 2.5% of the Ashkenazi Jewish population {1162}. Knowledge of the population-specific BRCA1 and BRCA2 mutation spectrum could inform efficient strategies for genetic testing and may justify more broad-based oncogenetic testing in some populations {1732}.

BRCA1 and BRCA2 mutations also increase the risk of male breast cancer, with a higher frequency of BRCA2 mutations found in such cases. In high-risk families, BRCA2 mutations account for 60–76% of male breast cancers and BRCA1 mutations for 10–16% {1768}.

### Other cancers in carriers of BRCA1/2 mutations
BRCA1 or BRCA2 mutation carriers, besides being subject to increased lifetime risks of breast and ovarian cancers, have also been reported to have increased susceptibility to prostate, pancreas, stomach, and colon carcinomas (see Table 9.02) {1355,223,2077}. A trend of increased incidence of melanoma in BRCA1 mutation carriers and cervical cancer in BRCA2 mutation carriers has been observed {1355}. A recent subgroup meta-analysis reporting evaluations adjusted for sex and age demonstrated an increased risk of colorectal cancer associated with BRCA1 but not BRCA2 mutations {1535}.

### Risk modifiers in carriers of BRCA1/2 mutations
The penetrance of BRCA1 and BRCA2 mutations is likely to be modified by genetic, lifestyle, and reproductive factors, as well

as genetic variants {1453,1378,682}. Such information is important for predicting the risk of breast and other cancers among carriers of *BRCA1* and *BRCA2* mutations to improve prevention of cancer development.

### Lifestyle factors

Reproductive and lifestyle factors have been reported as risk modifiers of breast cancers among individuals with *BRCA1* and *BRCA2* mutations. A higher number of term pregnancies is associated with reduced risk of breast cancer among *BRCA1* and *BRCA2* mutation carriers {1011,1605,2096,1606}. Breastfeeding has been reported to be a protective factor in *BRCA1* mutation carriers {942,772,1051,2096}. However, no significant association can be found between breastfeeding and breast cancer risk in *BRCA2* mutation carriers {1051}. Earlier menarche has been found to be associated with increased risk of breast cancer in *BRCA2* but not *BRCA1* mutation carriers {1011,1605}. In contrast, late age at menopause shows a protective effect against breast cancer in BRCA mutation carriers {2096}. There is no significant association between the use of oral contraceptives {1605,2096} and breast cancer among BRCA mutation carriers.

Interestingly, a recent study using consortia data from *BRCA1* and *BRCA2* mutation carriers showed that height and height genetic score are positively associated with risk of breast cancer, although the association with height genetic score was not statistically significant {869}. Observed body mass index and body mass index genetic score are inversely associated with breast cancer risk. Body mass index was found to be associated with premenopausal breast cancer. These environmental and lifestyle factors are particularly important in women with a strong family history {1681}.

### Etiology

The BRCA genes are tumour suppressor genes coding for proteins engaged in the highly conserved homologous recombination repair pathway to accurately repair DNA breaks using the sister chromatid as a template. If not repaired, such breaks promote genomic instability and lead to the development of cancer. A recent study using whole-genome sequencing of tumours from patients with germline *BRCA1/2* mutations and non-carriers showed that some patients have unreported, dual pathogenic germline variants in cancer risk genes (*BRCA1/BRCA2*; *BRCA1/MUTYH*). It also showed that 100% of tumours from *BRCA1* carriers and 91% of tumours from *BRCA2* carriers exhibited biallelic inactivation of the respective gene, together with somatic mutation signatures suggestive of a functional deficiency in homologous recombination {1518}. Although BRCA mutations are spread widely over these large genes, there is an association between mutations in the central part of *BRCA2* (the ovarian cluster region) and an increase in the likelihood of ovarian carcinoma. *BRCA1* is localized to chromosome 17q21 and contains 23 coding exons. It encodes a nuclear protein of 1863 amino acids. A RING finger domain at the N-terminus mediates interactions with other proteins. *BRCA1* is often mutated in three domains: the RING domain, exons 11–13, and the BRCA1 C-terminal domain {365}. *BRCA2* maps to chromosome 13q13.1 and consists of 27 coding exons. The BRCA2 protein includes 3418 amino acids. The BRCA1 and BRCA2 proteins share no structural homology with any other protein

{2154}. Fig. 9.01 illustrates the functional domains in the BRCA1 and BRCA2 proteins.

### Pathogenesis

DNA repair is essential for cell survival, and cells have developed a number of mechanisms to ensure genomic integrity. During replication, double-strand breaks at replication forks lead to the loss of genome segments with rearrangements. Loss of the tumour suppressor function of BRCA1 and BRCA2 is probably central to the development of cancer, but it is still unclear why BRCA-associated cancers are mostly restricted to the breast and/or ovary. It has been suggested that, at least for *BRCA1*, homologous recombination–independent functions in transcription may account for the development of breast cancers {2352}.

BRCA gene mutations and promoter methylation have been linked to risk of breast cancer and have been reported to be mutually exclusive. BRCA methylation has been reported to be more common in sporadic breast cancer {2194} and linked to increased breast cancer risk {1508}. A recent systematic review concluded that BRCA methylation is found in 1.3% and 1.1% of breast and ovarian carcinomas, respectively, in BRCA mutation carriers {2196}. The frequency of BRCA mutation varies considerably between CpG sites in *BRCA1* and *BRCA2* promotors.

Numerous genetic events, as identified by population-based genome-wide association and multiconsortial studies, have

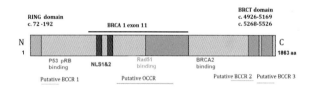

**A**

**B**

**Fig. 9.01** Functional domains in the BRCA proteins. **A** The BRCA1 protein. The RING domain contains a C3HC4 motif that interacts with other proteins. **B** The BRCA2 protein. There are eight BRC repeats, in the central domain of the protein, that interact with RAD51. The oligonucleotide/oligosaccharide-binding (OB) domains have a strong affinity for single-stranded DNA. aa, amino acids; BCCR, breast cancer cluster region; BRCT, BRCA1 C-terminal; C, C-terminus; N, N-terminus; NLS, nuclear localization signal; OCCR, ovarian cancer cluster region.

been reported to affect the real risk of breast cancers among *BRCA1* and *BRCA2* mutation carriers {406,1733}. The spectrum of *BRCA1* and *BRCA2* mutations with indels, missense, nonsense, and splice site mutations has been found to be similar and constitutes 67% of *BRCA1* and 56% of *BRCA2* mutations, as well as about 33% and 45%, respectively, of variants of unknown significance {1239}. In contrast, these mutations were reported to constitute only about 8% of variants of unknown significance in earlier studies on *BRCA1* mutation {407}. This observation is thought to reflect the fact that advances in mutation detection have far exceeded those in mutation interpretation {1239}. Indeed, a variety of technical approaches have been adopted to evaluate the pathogenicity of variants of unknown significance, which need to be further clarified.

Breast and ovarian cancer risks vary with the type and location of *BRCA1/2* mutations. Three breast cancer cluster regions and an ovarian cancer cluster region, found in exon 11, have been identified in *BRCA1* {1733}. Mutations in the BRCA1 C-terminal domain region are associated with a higher susceptibility to breast cancers than other *BRCA1* mutations {1606}. This may be because BRCA1 C-terminal phosphoprotein recognition is crucial for *BRCA1* tumour suppression effect {1909}. In *BRCA2*, multiple breast cancer cluster regions have been found, together with three ovarian cancer cluster regions. Mutations conferring nonsense-mediated decay have been associated with differential breast or ovarian cancer risks and an earlier age of breast cancer diagnosis in both *BRCA1* and *BRCA2* mutation carriers {1733}.

Mutations at specific regions such as those on 11q22.3 {809} and 19p13 {1120} have been found to be significantly associated with breast cancer risk among *BRCA1* mutation carriers. Although data regarding *BRCA2* are less available, a susceptibility allele at 6p24 that is specifically and inversely associated with breast cancer risk in *BRCA2* mutation carriers has been reported. This variant was found to be associated with risk of breast cancer in neither *BRCA1* mutation carriers nor the general population {705}. The signal interaction network of BRCA variants, particularly genes involved in DNA damage repair and cell-cycle regulation (e.g. *ATM*, *ATR*, *TP53*, *RB1*, and *RAD51*), is another factor that may also affect penetrance {353,1029,1239}.

Large-scale studies using whole-genome sequencing have identified distinct patterns of genomic alterations (called mutation signatures) across different tumour types {30}. An algorithm integrating six of these mutation signatures, including those reflecting homologous recombination deficiency, could identify *BRCA1/2* sporadic and germline mutation–associated tumours with as high as 98.7% sensitivity {458}, suggesting that this approach could be useful in identifying patients who may benefit from poly (ADP-ribose) polymerase (PARP) inhibitors.

Gene expression analysis has revealed that *BRCA1* tumours are characterized by alterations in genes involved in proliferation, adhesion, angiogenesis, motility, transcription, and DNA repair, whereas *BRCA2* tumours are characterized by alterations in genes involved in proliferation, adhesion, signal transduction, and extracellular matrix production.

BRCA-positive breast cancers have significantly higher numbers of tumour-infiltrating lymphocytes {1974}, and recent studies in mouse models suggest a possible role for combined immune-checkpoint blockade {1515}; however, the data are still preliminary.

## Macroscopic appearance

These tumours demonstrate features similar to those of breast cancers that are not BRCA-associated, although with higher proportions of smooth circumscribed boundaries and an internal lobulated cut surface with areas of haemorrhage and necrosis.

## Histopathology

Tumours arising in *BRCA1* and *BRCA2* mutation carries are more likely than sporadic breast cancers to have certain histological and molecular characteristics (see Table 9.03). In addition, breast cancers in *BRCA1* mutation carriers are associated with more-aggressive tumour characteristics than in *BRCA2* mutation carriers {323,799}. Tumours in *BRCA1* (vs *BRCA2*) mutation carriers have been found to exhibit significantly higher nuclear and histological grades, with prominent lymphocytic infiltrate. They were more often of the triple-negative type, whereas *BRCA2* tumours were more frequently of the ER-positive phenotype. Invasive breast carcinomas of no special type (NST), invasive breast carcinomas with medullary pattern (formerly designated medullary carcinomas), and metaplastic carcinomas have been reported in *BRCA1* mutation carriers {227,2354}. *BRCA2* tumours more frequently present with

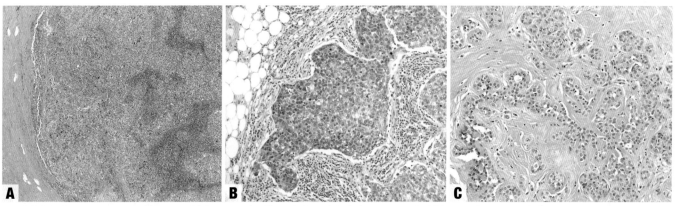

**Fig. 9.02** Histological features of *BRCA1/2*-associated tumours. **A,B** The typical morphological appearance of a *BRCA1* mutation–associated breast cancer: a well-circumscribed tumour with a pushing margin, syncytial growth, and an associated prominent lymphocytic infiltrate (**A**). Note the ample mitoses and adjacent lymphocytic infiltrate (**B**). **C** Lobular carcinoma in situ in a prophylactic mastectomy specimen from a *BRCA2* mutation carrier. There is a proliferation of atypical dyscohesive cells involving terminal duct lobular units.

**Table 9.03** Histological characteristics and molecular phenotype of breast cancer in *BRCA1* and *BRCA2* mutation carriers compared with sporadic breast cancer

| Characteristic(s) | Typical findings in mutation carriers | |
|---|---|---|
| | **BRCA1** | **BRCA2** |
| Clinical | More lung and brain metastases | More bone and soft tissue metastases |
| Margin | Well demarcated, solid nests, no tubule formation | More often pushing borders |
| Lymphocytic infiltrate | Prominent lymphoplasmacytic infiltrate | Less lymphoplasmacytic infiltrate than in *BRCA1* carriers, but more than in sporadic cancer |
| Necrosis | Often necrosis, fibrotic focus | May be present |
| Lymphovascular invasion | Often present | Less common |
| Grade | High histological grade | Variable histological grade (mainly grade 2 or 3) |
| Histological types | IBC, IBC with medullary pattern, metaplastic | IBC-NST, tubular, cribriform, mucinous, classic/pleomorphic lobular |
| In situ cancer | Little DCIS | More frequently present with DCIS alone |
| | Little LCIS | LCIS may be present |
| Immunophenotype | ER/PR− | ER/PR+ |
| | ERBB2 (HER2)− | ERBB2 (HER2)− |
| | High MIB1 | Variable MIB1 |
| Molecular type | Triple-negative: ER−, PR−, ERBB2 (HER2)− | Luminal A: ER+, PR+, ERBB2 (HER2)− |
| | Basal-like: CK5/6+, CK14+ or EGFR (HER1)+ | CK5/6−/CK14− |
| Gene expression | Genes involved in proliferation, adhesion, angiogenesis, motility, transcription, DNA repair | Genes involved in proliferation, adhesion, signal transduction, extracellular matrix production |
| | CK8/18− | CK8/18+ |
| | EGFR (HER1)+ | EGFR (HER1)+ |
| | p53+, very often *TP53* mutations | p53+/−, ~50% *TP53* mutations |
| | Cyclin D1−, cyclin A and cyclin E high | Cyclin D1+, cyclin A and cyclin E variable |
| | BCL2 low | BCL2 high |
| | HIF1α+ | FGF1+, FGFR1+, FGFR2+ |
| | p63+, P-cadherin+, caveolin-1+, vimentin+, laminin+ | |

DCIS, ductal carcinoma in situ; IBC, invasive breast carcinoma; LCIS, lobular carcinoma in situ; NST, of no special type.

ductal carcinoma in situ alone, and they more frequently exhibit calcifications that are more easily detectable by mammography {1057}. Lobular carcinoma in situ has been reported in *BRCA2* carriers mostly as an incidental finding in prophylactic mastectomy specimens. Limited data suggest that younger patients with inflammatory breast cancer may be more likely to harbour a BRCA mutation {795}.

Because the histopathological features of cancers in BRCA mutation carriers differ from those of cancers with no known mutation, these features have been considered useful for mutation prediction, risk prediction algorithms, and statistical modelling to assess the pathogenicity of BRCA variants of uncertain clinical significance, as well as for informing clinical strategies for screening and prophylaxis. The proportions of ER-negative breast tumours and triple-negative tumours decrease with increasing patient age at diagnosis among *BRCA1* mutation carriers, but they increase with age at diagnosis among *BRCA2* carriers. In both *BRCA1* and *BRCA2* carriers, ER-negative tumours have been found to be of higher histological grade than ER-positive tumours {1319}. Interestingly, in addition to many cases being of basal-like phenotype (see below), a substantial portion of BRCA carriers have recently been found to have the

luminal A subtype. These cases were mainly in *BRCA2* carriers (35%) rather than *BRCA1* carriers (9%). The luminal B subtype was more frequent than the luminal A subtype and was also found in a higher proportion of *BRCA2* carriers (40% in *BRCA2* carriers vs 21% in *BRCA1* carriers) {1975}.

The distribution of histological types of *BRCA1*-associated breast cancers differs from that of sporadic breast cancers {456}, with the majority being invasive breast carcinoma NST; approximately 15% are classified as invasive breast carcinoma with medullary pattern (formerly designated medullary carcinoma), histological grade 3, with heavy lymphocytic infiltration and pushing margins {1099}. Triple-negative breast cancers expressing epithelial keratins (CK5/6), referred to as the basal phenotype, are overrepresented among *BRCA1* tumours {673}. Although basal cytokeratin and/or EGFR (HER1) expression can be used to identify triple-negative breast cancers with basal-like phenotype, the expression of these markers alone is not sufficient to determine which women with triple-negative breast cancers are likely to harbour *BRCA1* germline mutations {390}. *BRCA2*-associated breast cancers do not appear to exhibit a specific pathological phenotype, although lobular tumours have been found to be more likely to be *BRCA2*-related {1319}.

Analysis of large pathology datasets accrued by CIMBA and the Breast Cancer Association Consortium (BCAC) showed that ER-positive phenotype negatively predicted *BRCA1* mutation status, irrespective of grade. Patient age at diagnosis is an important variable, with ER-negative grade 3 histopathology being more predictive of positive *BRCA1* mutation status in women aged 50 years or older (likelihood ratio: 4.13; range: 3.70–4.62) than in women younger than 50 years (likelihood ratio: 3.16; range: 2.96–3.37), likewise for triple-negative tumour status in women aged 50 years or older (likelihood ratio: 4.41; range: 3.86–5.04) versus women younger than 50 years (likelihood ratio: 3.73; range: 3.43–4.05). These features were only modestly predictive for *BRCA2* mutation cases, with grade being more informative than ER status {1985}.

*BRCA2* male breast cancers are of significantly higher stage and grade than *BRCA2* female breast cancers. In SEER Program data, the grade was also higher than that of sporadic male breast cancers {1946}.

## Cytology
The cytology of BRCA-associated breast cancers is the same as that of non–BRCA-associated breast cancers, apart from the individual features associated with the relative frequency of *BRCA1*-associated cases with medullary pattern.

## Diagnostic molecular pathology
*BRCA1/2*-associated hereditary breast and ovarian cancer syndrome is an autosomal dominant inherited disorder with germline mutations in *BRCA1* and *BRCA2*.

## Essential and desirable diagnostic criteria
*Essential:* identification of germline *BRCA1* and *BRCA2* pathogenic mutations; the eligibility of patients for germline *BRCA1/2* testing is determined using tools including the BRCAPRO model, the Breast and Ovarian Analysis of Disease Incidence and Carrier Estimation Algorithm (BOADICEA), and the Manchester scoring system {1402,51,123,868,1997,1211}.

## Staging
The staging of cancers in the setting of *BRCA1/2*-associated hereditary breast and ovarian cancer syndrome is similar to that of non-BRCA cancers.

## Prognosis and prediction
In one study, cases with *BRCA1/2* germline mutations were associated with worse overall survival and disease-specific survival than were *BRCA1/2*-wildtype cases {123}. Several meta-analyses have supported these findings {2362,1211}, whereas other meta-analyses have found the results to be inconclusive {2142, 2367}. A prospective cohort study of outcome in 2733 women who developed breast cancer at or before the age of 40 years, of whom 12% were found to be *BRCA1/2* mutation carriers, showed no significant difference in survival between *BRCA1/2* carriers and non-carriers over about 10 years of follow-up (median: 8.2 years). Among patients with triple-negative breast cancer, BRCA mutation carriers had a better overall survival than non-carriers after 2 years of follow-up but not after 5 or 10 years {399}.

The difference in overall survival between *BRCA1* and *BRCA2* breast cancer patients could be ascribed to tumour biology. Although breast cancer patients with *BRCA1* mutation may have a lower 10-year disease-free survival rate than *BRCA2* breast cancer patients, chemotherapy and risk-reducing contralateral mastectomy can reduce mortality for both *BRCA1* and *BRCA2* mutation carriers {1968}. Cisplatin and oophorectomy have been demonstrated to be effective therapies for women with breast cancer and a *BRCA1* mutation {1454}.

The term "synthetic lethality" refers to the scenario in which an individual mutation in either of two genes has no effect on cell viability but mutations in both of the genes lead to cell death {1997}. One of the most well known examples of synthetic lethality relates to *BRCA1/2* and PARP inhibitors. The *BRCA1/2* genes are responsible for repairing double-strand DNA breaks, and PARP is responsible for repairing single-strand DNA breaks through base excision repair. PARP inhibitors have been found to be effective in patients with ovarian cancer associated with either germline or somatic *BRCA1/2* mutations {2015}, with greater clinical benefit seen in patients with platinum-sensitive disease {660}. Similar promising results have also been found for BRCA1/2-deficient breast carcinomas {527}, with a response rate of 41% among patients with advanced-stage *BRCA1/2*-mutated breast carcinoma {93}. The application of mutation signatures, as described above, may be useful in identifying these patients.

Besides the possibility of surveillance strategies and chemoprevention, in the USA, the National Comprehensive Cancer Network (NCCN) and the Society of Gynecologic Oncology (SGO) guidelines recommend risk-reducing salpingo-oophorectomy for germline *BRCA1/2* mutation carriers at the age of 35–40 years or once childbearing is complete, together with prophylactic mastectomy {1468,530}. This has been found to reduce the risk of breast cancer by as much as 90%.

# Cowden syndrome

Brosens LAA
Jansen M

## Definition
Cowden syndrome (CS), also known as *PTEN* hamartoma tumour syndrome (PHTS), is a heterogeneous group of disorders with autosomal dominant inheritance caused by germline mutation of the *PTEN* gene, characterized by multiple hamartomas and a predisposition to cancer.

## MIM numbering
158350 Cowden syndrome

## ICD-11 coding
LD2D.Y Other specified phakomatoses or hamartoneoplastic syndromes – Cowden syndrome

## Related terminology
*Acceptable:* multiple hamartoma syndrome; *PTEN* hamartoma tumour syndrome.

## Subtype(s)
Bannayan–Riley–Ruvalcaba syndrome; Proteus syndrome

## Localization
CS involves organs derived from any of the three germ layers.

## Clinical features
CS is characterized by mucocutaneous lesions (multiple facial trichilemmomas, acral keratoses, papillomatous papules, and mucosal lesions are considered pathognomonic), an increased cancer risk, benign hamartomatous overgrowth of tissues (including hamartomatous / juvenile gastrointestinal polyposis), and macrocephaly {1650,1492}. Diffuse oesophageal glycogenic acanthosis in combination with colonic polyposis may be diagnostic of CS {400,1160}. Cancer risk is relatively widespread, including risk for breast, thyroid, endometrial, renal cell, and colon cancers, as well as melanoma {589,1492}.

PHTS also includes Bannayan–Riley–Ruvalcaba syndrome and Proteus syndrome. However, most PHTS cases correspond to CS, and these terms are often used interchangeably {861}.

## Epidemiology
The prevalence has been estimated at about 1 case per 200 000–250 000 individuals in a European population. This may be an underestimate given the difficulty in diagnosing this syndrome {1477}. Female CS patients have a cumulative lifetime breast cancer risk (to the age of 70 years) as high as 85% and a relative risk of 25 {2035,1761}. Multifocal and bilateral breast cancer has been reported in 34% of CS patients with breast cancer {1761,1492}. Male CS patients are also at increased risk of breast cancer, although the exact magnitude of risk is unclear {609,1492}. Benign breast lesions can be found in the majority of female CS patients {1878}.

**Box 9.01** The International Cowden Consortium (ICC) operational diagnostic criteria {2034}

**Pathognomonic criteria**
- Adult Lhermitte–Duclos disease (cerebellar tumours)
- Mucocutaneous lesions
  - Facial trichilemmomas, any number[a] (≥ 2 biopsy-proven trichilemmomas[b])
  - Acral keratoses
  - Papillomatous papules
- Mucosal lesions
- Autism spectrum disorder

**Major criteria**
- Breast cancer
- Non-medullary thyroid cancer
- Megalocephaly
- Endometrial carcinoma
- Mucocutaneous lesions[b]
  - 1 biopsy-proven trichilemmoma
  - Multiple palmoplantar keratoses
  - Multifocal cutaneous facial papules
  - Macular pigmentation of the glans penis
- Multiple gastrointestinal hamartomas or ganglioneuromas[b]

**Minor criteria**
- Other thyroid lesions (follicular adenomas, multinodular goitre)
- Mental retardation (i.e. IQ of ≤ 75)
- Gastrointestinal hamartomas[a] (single gastrointestinal hamartoma or ganglioneuroma[b])
- Fibrocystic breast disease
- Lipomas
- Fibromas
- Genitourinary tumours (especially renal cell carcinoma)
- Genitourinary malformations[a]
- Uterine fibroids
- Autism spectrum disorder[b]

**Relaxed ICC operational diagnostic criteria for Cowden syndrome**
≥ 1 pathognomonic criterion
*or*
≥ 2 major or minor criteria

[a]Present in this section as defined by ICC criteria only. [b]Present in this section as defined by National Comprehensive Cancer Network (NCCN) 2010 criteria only.

## Etiology
CS is an autosomal dominant disorder with age-related penetrance and variable expression. Germline mutation in *PTEN* (10q23.3) is found in about 85% of CS cases, as well as in subsets of other PHTS disorders (65% in Bannayan–Riley–Ruvalcaba syndrome, 20% in Proteus syndrome, and 50% in Proteus-like syndrome) {861,1558,1191,1478}. Individualized risk calculation may aid in the assessment of a patient's risk of carrying a germline *PTEN* mutation on the basis of clinical features {2034}.

Germline SDH mutations have been found in about 5% of patients with *PTEN* mutation–negative CS/CS-like phenotypes, and they are associated with increased frequencies of breast,

Chapter 9

**Table 9.04** Lifetime cancer risks and general screening recommendations in *PTEN* hamartoma tumour syndrome {2035,1356,1650}

| Cancer | Lifetime risk | Patient age at cancer diagnosis | Predominant histology | Recommended screening |
|--------|--------------|--------------------------------|----------------------|----------------------|
| Breast (female) | 25–85% | 38–50 years | Ductal adenocarcinoma | Starting at age 30 years: annual mammogram; consider MRI for patients with dense breasts |
| Thyroid | 35% | Unknown | Follicular carcinoma | Annual ultrasound |
| Endometrial | 19–28% | < 50 years | Endometrioid adenocarcinoma | Starting at age 30 years: annual endometrial biopsy or transvaginal ultrasound |
| Renal cell | 34% | Unknown | Unknown | Starting at age 40 years: renal imaging every 2 years |
| Colon | 9% | < 50 years | n/a | Starting at age 40 years: colonoscopy every 2 years |
| Melanoma | 6% | Unknown | n/a | Annual dermatological examination |

n/a, not applicable.

thyroid, and renal cancers beyond those conferred by germline *PTEN* mutation {1498}.

## Pathogenesis

PTEN, which is a virtually ubiquitously expressed tumour suppressor, is a dual-specificity lipid and protein phosphatase that regulates cell proliferation, cell migration, and apoptosis through inhibition of AKT via the PI3K/AKT pathway {1356}. Inactivation of the second copy of the gene allows deregulation of the AKT pathway.

## Macroscopic appearance

Not clinically relevant

## Histopathology

Benign breast pathologies occur in about 75% of female CS patients and include ductal hyperplasia, intraductal papillomatosis, adenosis, lobular atrophy, fibroadenomas, and fibrocystic change. Many patients show features suggestive of a breast hamartoma. Malignant breast lesions are mostly invasive carcinoma of no special type (NST), often associated with ductal carcinoma in situ {1878}. A recent report suggests that apocrine differentiation is common in breast cancers from patients with germline *PTEN* mutations, and expression profiling puts these cancers in the molecular apocrine category {115}.

## Cytology

Not clinically relevant

## Diagnostic molecular pathology

CS is caused by germline *PTEN* mutations.

## Essential and desirable diagnostic criteria

The International Cowden Consortium (ICC) operational diagnostic criteria are listed in Box 9.01 (p. 275).

## Staging

Not clinically relevant

## Prognosis and prediction

Patients with PHTS are at increased risk of several types of cancer, and interval screening is recommended (see Table 9.04) {2035,1356,243}.

# Ataxia–telangiectasia

Chenevix-Trench G
Mills AM
Vincent-Salomon A
Weigelt B

## Definition

Ataxia–telangiectasia (AT) is an autosomal recessive syndrome characterized by progressive cerebellar ataxia, oculomotor apraxia, choreoathetosis, sinopulmonary infections, oculocutaneous telangiectasia, variable immune deficiency, sterility, a high risk of malignancy, and sensitivity to ionizing radiation, caused by germline mutations in the *ATM* gene.

## MIM numbering

208900 Ataxia–telangiectasia

## ICD-11 coding

4A01.31 DNA repair defects other than combined T-cell or B-cell immunodeficiencies – Ataxia–telangiectasia

## Related terminology

*Acceptable:* immunodeficiency with ataxia–telangiectasia; Louis–Bar syndrome; cerebello-oculocutaneous telangiectasia.

## Subtype(s)

None

## Localization

AT patients show a high incidence of malignancy, in particular of leukaemias and lymphomas {785}. Heterozygotes have an elevated risk of breast cancer. There is also some evidence for an increased risk of ovarian cancer {1245} and digestive tract cancers {762,1773}.

## Clinical features

Heterozygous germline mutations in *ATM* have been associated with young age at breast cancer onset {1992,234,2076,333, 149,2060,744,1179,1980}. Heterozygous carriers of *ATM* variants do not show the severe toxic effects of radiation therapy that can occur in AT patients {2002}, but there is an elevated risk of contralateral breast cancer in heterozygous carriers of deleterious *ATM* mutations treated with radiotherapy {148,150}.

The major characteristics of AT are generally consistent, but there is variability in the age of onset, progression, and severity of symptoms, as well as in the occurrence of cancer. In particular, it has been observed that *ATM* missense mutations resulting in some protein expression and residual kinase activity may result in an attenuated phenotype {2167}. In this regard, the c.7271T>G missense mutation has been of interest, because rare homozygotes for this mutation showed a less severe form of AT and normal levels of ATM protein {1992}. In addition, elevated rates of breast cancer have been observed in homozygote and heterozygote carriers {333,149}.

## Epidemiology

AT is a rare condition, with an estimated prevalence of 1 case per 40 000–100 000 live births {1805}.

## Etiology

Classic AT is a monogenic disease caused by germline mutations in the *ATM* gene. Most AT patients are compound heterozygotes for mutations in *ATM* {394,1337,1161,1805}.

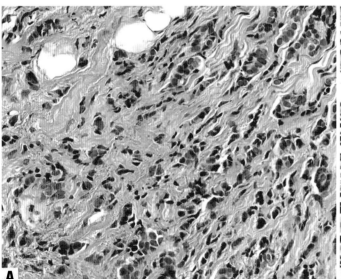 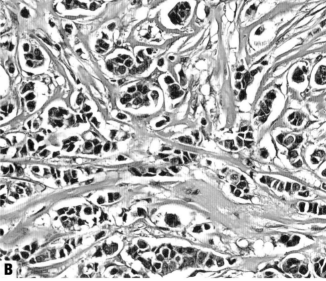

**Fig. 9.03** *ATM*-associated breast cancer. **A,B** Two examples of breast carcinoma from patients with germline *ATM* mutations. Both demonstrate ductal morphology with lobular features including cells infiltrating singly and in strands. Both tumours were ER/PR-positive; the tumour shown in panel A was ERBB2 (HER2)-negative, whereas the tumour in panel B was HER2-amplified. Neither tumour demonstrates the high nuclear grade or brisk immune response often associated with BRCA-mutated tumours.

Chapter 9

## Pathogenesis

The *ATM* gene extends over 150 kb of DNA and has 66 exons. The *ATM* transcript is 13 kb, encoding a 3056 amino acid protein of 350 kDa. The initiating codon is within exon 4 {2133}. ATM, which is expressed in all normal tissues {1851}, is a serine/threonine kinase that belongs to the PI3K-related kinase family, with conserved kinase and regulatory domains in the C-terminal region {1145}. ATM has a large number of phosphorylation targets, including major human tumour suppressors such as p53 and BRCA1. In response to DNA damage, in particular double-strand DNA breaks, ATM is activated by autophosphorylation. Many of its known functions relate to the activation of cell-cycle checkpoints that impede progression of the cell cycle in cells with damaged DNA. ATM functions to slow S-phase progression via phosphorylation of components of the MRN complex and direct phosphorylation of BRCA1, FANCD2, and SMC1. Phosphorylation of CHK2, BRCA1, and RAD17 contributes to the G2/M checkpoint {998,1918}. ATM is also known to contribute to DNA repair through CHK2-mediated phosphorylation of BRCA1 and regulation of chromatin dynamics, and it has been implicated in the maintenance of telomere length {998,1918}.

More than 500 unique germline mutations in *ATM* have been reported, distributed throughout the gene, with no mutation hotspots {394}. *ATM* mutations can be broadly categorized as (1) protein-truncating, non-expressing mutations; (2) in-frame deletions encoding mutant protein without kinase activity; or (3) missense mutations encoding mutant protein with reduced kinase activity {2167,2064}. Most AT patients carry protein-truncating, non-expressing mutations. Approximately 90% of AT patients have no detectable ATM protein, 10% have trace amounts, and 1% express a normal amount of protein without kinase activity. Detection of ATM protein and in vitro assays for radiosensitivity and ATM kinase activity may form part of diagnostic testing for AT {1629}.

The current estimate of relative risk of breast cancer in *ATM* mutation carriers is 2.8 (95% CI: 2.2–3.7) for truncating mutations {560}, with a higher risk (11.0; 95% CI: 1.42–85.7) for the c.7271T>G (p.Val2424Gly) mutation {1980,149,333,744}. This finding led to the hypothesis that carriers of *ATM* mutations were at increased risk of breast cancer and that the risk might be higher for carriers of missense mutations because of a dominant-negative effect on protein function {703}. However, the rarity of individual variants of *ATM* poses an ongoing challenge to researchers seeking to elucidate precise genotype–phenotype correlates of breast cancer incidence, features, and outcome.

There is evidence that inhibition of PARP1 is synthetically lethal with mutation or loss of *ATM* and that the effect is mediated through mitotic catastrophe independently of apoptosis {2267}. It was therefore thought that *ATM* mutation carriers with breast cancer might be candidates for treatment with poly (ADP-ribose) polymerase (PARP) inhibitors, similar to carriers of mutations in *BRCA1* and *BRCA2* {348}. However, recent analyses have shown that breast tumours from *ATM* mutation carriers often harbour biallelic inactivation of *ATM* but lack mutation signatures of homologous recombination deficiency {2244} and large-scale genomic instability {1750}, suggesting that they might not be susceptible to PARP inhibitors.

## Macroscopic appearance

Not clinically relevant

## Histopathology

There is limited information on the histopathology of breast cancers occurring in carriers of *ATM* variants, and no distinctive tumour phenotype has been reproducibly identified {744}. One series revealed no significant morphological differences between *ATM*-mutated cancers and controls {111}. Others have reported that *ATM*-mutated cancers are usually luminal B {1750} and hormone receptor–positive {2244}, with double positivity for ER and PR. Notably, although ATM plays a similar role in DNA damage repair as BRCA1/2, no series has identified a predominance of the high-grade, lymphocyte-rich morphology typical of *BRCA1/2* mutation–associated cancers among breast tumours with *ATM* abnormalities {111,1342,2244}. Instead, most reported cases are invasive carcinoma of no special type (NST; > 80%) {1750} or with mixed ductal and lobular-like morphology associated with a tumour-infiltrating lymphocyte–poor stroma. Breast tumours in *ATM* heterozygotes are usually hormone receptor–positive, display minimal immune infiltrate, and are wildtype for *TP53* {2244}.

## Cytology

Not clinically relevant

## Diagnostic molecular pathology

AT is caused by pathogenic germline mutation in *ATM*.

## Essential and desirable diagnostic criteria

*Essential:* characteristic clinical scenario.

## Staging

Not clinically relevant

## Prognosis and prediction

Not clinically relevant

# Li–Fraumeni syndrome, *TP53*-associated

Lax SF
Soares FA

## Definition
*TP53*-associated Li–Fraumeni syndrome (LFS) is an autosomal dominant cancer predisposition syndrome caused by germline mutations of the *TP53* gene.

## MIM numbering
151623 Li–Fraumeni syndrome

## ICD-11 coding
None

## Related terminology
*Not recommended:* sarcoma family syndrome of Li and Fraumeni.

## Subtype(s)
None

## Localization
*TP53*-associated LFS is associated with cancers of the breast, soft tissue, bone, brain, and adrenal glands.

## Clinical features
LFS is characterized by the early onset of a broad spectrum of cancers and a high lifetime cancer risk. Breast and adrenocortical carcinoma, brain tumours (particularly choroid plexus carcinoma), leukaemia, and soft tissue and bone sarcomas are considered to be the main cancer types or component or core tumours, which constitute about 70% of LFS-related neoplasms {55}. In addition, a broad range of other tumours, including lymphomas, gastrointestinal malignancies (gastric and colorectal cancers), melanoma, and lung cancer has been described in

**Box 9.02** The Chompret criteria for *TP53* germline testing, amended in line with 2019 WHO Classification of Tumours terminology {210}

**Familial presentation:** Proband with a tumour belonging to the Li–Fraumeni syndrome tumour spectrum (cancers of the breast, soft tissue, bone, brain, or adrenal glands) before the age of 46 years; AND at least one first- or second-degree relative with a Li–Fraumeni syndrome tumour (with the exception of breast cancer if the proband has breast cancer) before the age of 56 years, or with multiple tumours

**Multiple primary tumours:** Proband with multiple tumours (with the exception of multiple breast tumours), two of which belong to the Li–Fraumeni syndrome tumour spectrum – the first of which occurred before the age of 46 years

**Rare tumours:** Patient with embryonal rhabdomyosarcoma, choroid plexus tumour, or adrenocortical carcinoma, irrespective of family history

**Early-onset breast cancer:** Breast cancer occurring before 31 years of age

LFS families, occurring at younger ages than usual {752,972, 1500}. More-recent studies have also reported cancers of the female reproductive organs (ovarian and endometrial carcinomas), the urogenital tract (carcinomas of the kidney and the prostate), and the eyes {1547,1563}.

The classic definition of LFS required sarcoma in a patient aged < 45 years, a first-degree relative with any cancer before the age of 45 years, and a first- or second-degree relative with any cancer before the age of 45 years or sarcoma at any age {1873}. This clinical definition has since been expanded to allow a broader recognition of individuals and families with LFS (see Box 9.02).

Patients and families without the full spectrum of classic criteria have been designated as having Li–Fraumeni–like syndrome (LFL), which has been further defined clinically by two sets of criteria, proposed by Birch and Eeles, respectively {1873}. The Birch criteria are close to those of classic LFS but do not require

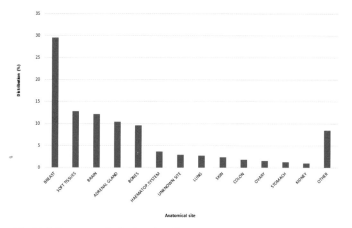

**Fig. 9.04** Percentage distribution of 2095 tumours associated with *TP53* germline mutations, by anatomical site (adapted from the IARC *TP53* Database).

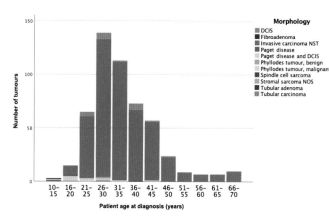

**Fig. 9.05** Frequency distribution of 522 breast tumours in 324 families with *TP53* germline mutations, by 5-year age group and histological type: 491 invasive carcinomas of no special type (NST); 10 ductal carcinomas in situ (DCIS); 10 malignant phyllodes tumours; and 1 each of benign phyllodes tumour, fibroadenoma, tubular adenoma, and tubular carcinoma (modified according to the IARC *TP53* Database).

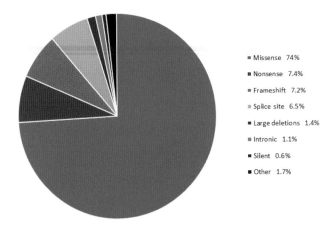

**Fig. 9.06** Percentage distribution of 1219 *TP53* germline mutations by mutation type.

Legend:
- Missense 74%
- Nonsense 7.4%
- Frameshift 7.2%
- Splice site 6.5%
- Large deletions 1.4%
- Intronic 1.1%
- Silent 0.6%
- Other 1.7%

a sarcoma, whereas the Eeles definition of LFL includes two first- or second-degree relatives with LFS component tumours at any age, rather than the three required by the classic criteria {1873}. The investigation of other family genes and non-coding regions of the *TP53* gene may explain the occurrence of LFL {1624}.

About one third of breast cancers associated with LFS or LFL seem to occur before the age of 30 years, whereas they are less common after the age of 50 years. Approximately 3–8% of breast cancer patients aged < 30 years are estimated to carry *TP53* germline mutation, regardless of family history {972}. In a cohort of 70 breast cancer patients who were carriers of the *TP53* p.Arg337His mutation, 49 were aged < 45 years and 21 were aged > 55 years {726}. Therefore, early onset of breast cancer in the absence of other malignancies points towards LFS, whereas later onset of cancers has been encountered in LFL {983}. Soft tissue sarcomas are the second most frequent type of cancer, with a wide range of tumour onset age (6 months to 70 years), whereas osteosarcomas mainly occur in children {210}.

### Epidemiology

More than 1200 germline mutations associated with LFS, LFL, and probands with a family history or fulfilling the Chompret criteria are included in version R19 (August 2018) of the International Agency for Research on Cancer (IARC) *TP53* Database from 1990 onwards {907,208}. The incidence of *TP53* germline mutation in Europe and North America seems to be 1 case per 5000–20 000 person-years {752,1102A}. In southern Brazil, a specific germline mutation at codon 337 (p.Arg337His) occurs with an incidence of 1 case per 650 person-years and is found in 0.3% of the general population {8,726}. There is recent evidence of the occurrence of de novo *TP53* mutations in about 10–20% of individuals with LFS; about 20% of these mutations seem to occur during embryogenesis {1751}. The highest pickup rate of *TP53* germline variants seems to be in patients with early-onset breast cancer {663}.

### Etiology

The genetic basis of LFS is a germline mutation of the *TP53* gene {1283,1987}. A broad spectrum of *TP53* germline mutations involving the coding regions of the gene has been found in LFS families, but 20–40% of LFS individuals and the majority

of LFL families may lack detectable mutations {1547,2160}. The lack of 100% concordance between *TP53* mutations and the classic LFS phenotype may be explained in several ways, including posttranslational alterations, complete deletion, the effects of modifier genes, and alterations of other genes influencing the phenotype generated by the presence of specific germline alterations {1282}. Mutations may occur at specific hotspot codons that either interfere with DNA binding or disrupt the structure of the binding surface, thus interfering with its ability to modulate the transcription of target genes {1548}. Missense mutations lead to a codon change, posing challenges to the functional interpretation of new variants {1149}. Further mutations may occur outside of the DNA-binding domain and include rearrangements and deletions {2137}. In the IARC *TP53* Database, more than 1500 different germline mutations are listed, with only four patterns accounting for about 80% of the mutations: G:C>A:T at CpG islands in almost 50%, followed by A:T>G:C, G:C>A:T, and deletions (in ~10% each), predominantly involving 11 codons within the coding regions of exons 5–8, most commonly codons 175, 245, 248, 273, and 282 {907,208}. Lesions within introns or the regulatory regions of the gene have been identified, although their functional significance is unclear and there are open questions about the significance of some *TP53* variants occurring in cancer {1148}. There is some evidence that genes of the Fanconi pathway, RECQ family genes, and other genes found in breast cancer are associated with LFL cancers {1624}. Future studies with novel sequencing technologies such as next-generation sequencing may be able to uncover a higher number of mutations in *TP53*, as well as in other genes in LFS and LFL {1563}.

### Pathogenesis

*TP53* is one of the most prominent tumour suppressors, whose activation as a transcription factor stimulates downstream pathways leading to protective cellular processes including cell-cycle arrest, apoptosis, and senescence to prevent the propagation of genetically altered cells {2188}. The importance of these cellular responses has recently been challenged by findings in mouse models {862}. Under normal conditions, the p53 protein is maintained at low levels as a result of rapid turnover mediated by MDM2, its main negative regulator {1148}. Recent evidence has linked *TP53* function to regulation of metabolism and the redox balance to maintain intracellular homeostasis. Cells from LFS individuals exhibit genomic instability, telomere dysfunction, and spontaneous immortalization {1594}.

### Macroscopic appearance

Not clinically relevant

### Histopathology

Breast cancer is by far the most frequent malignancy associated with LFS, accounting for 29.5% of cases (618 of 2095 included tumours) in version R19 (August 2018) of the IARC *TP53* Database {907,208}. There is limited evidence on the histopathological and molecular types of LFS-associated breast cancer. The largest published series (of 43 tumours from 39 women) consisted of 32 invasive carcinomas of no special type (NST; invasive ductal carcinomas) and 11 cases of ductal carcinoma in situ; no other histological types were observed {1308}. The median patient age at diagnosis was 32 years (range: 22–46 years). Interestingly, the ERBB2 (HER2)-amplified molecular subtype (both classic and variant) predominated. Of the invasive carcinomas, 84% were positive for ER and/or PR, 81% were high-grade, 63% were positive for HER2 (immunohistochemistry 3+ or FISH amplified), and 53% were positive for both ER and HER2. Of the ductal carcinoma in situ cases, 73% were positive for HER2 and 27% for ER and HER2. The high frequency of HER2 positivity has been confirmed by others {1345, 2278}. Malignant phyllodes tumours of the breast may also be associated with LFS {174}, whereas male breast cancer seems to be uncommon.

Other cancers may involve many other organs aside from the breast, but soft tissue and bone sarcomas, brain tumours, and adrenocortical carcinomas are the most frequent {210}. The most frequent types of soft tissue sarcomas were found to be leiomyosarcomas, rhabdomyosarcomas, liposarcomas, and undifferentiated sarcomas that can be challenging to classify. Osteosarcoma is the most frequent bone tumour. Among the brain tumours, glioblastomas and other types of gliomas, choroid plexus carcinomas, medulloblastomas, and ependymomas were found.

## Cytology
Not clinically relevant

## Diagnostic molecular pathology
Candidates for *TP53* germline testing are identified on the basis of the 2015 Chompret criteria (see Box 9.02, p. 279) {210} and the recommendations of the National Comprehensive Cancer Network (NCCN; see Box 9.03) {2187}. In the era of testing by next-generation sequencing, it may be necessary to further broaden the criteria to find a greater number of *TP53* germline mutations {1563}. *TP53* should be considered in addition to *BRCA1*, *BRCA2*, and other genes for germline panel testing of young breast cancer patients {1624}.

## Essential and desirable diagnostic criteria
*Essential:* pathogenic germline mutation in *TP53*; appropriate family history.

**Box 9.03** Testing criteria for Li–Fraumeni syndrome as recommended by the National Comprehensive Cancer Network (NCCN) {2187}

Person diagnosed with sarcoma at < 45 years of age AND a first-degree relative diagnosed with cancer at < 45 years of age AND an additional first- or second-degree relative with cancer diagnosed at < 45 years of age or sarcoma diagnosed at any age[a]

Person with a tumour associated with Li–Fraumeni syndrome diagnosed before the age of 46 years AND at least one first- or second-degree relative with a tumour associated with Li–Fraumeni syndrome[b] (other than breast cancer if the proband has breast cancer) before the age of 56 years or with multiple primaries at any age[c]

Person with multiple primaries (except multiple breast primaries), with at least two primaries associated with Li–Fraumeni syndrome[b], before the age of 46 years[c]

Person with adrenocortical carcinoma, choroid plexus carcinoma, or rhabdomyosarcoma of embryonal anaplastic subtype diagnosed at any age, regardless of family history[c]

Person with breast cancer before the age of 31 years[c]

Person from a family with known *TP53* mutation

[a]Classic Li–Fraumeni syndrome criteria. [b]Cancers associated with Li–Fraumeni syndrome: soft tissue sarcoma, osteosarcoma, CNS tumour, breast cancer, and adrenocortical carcinoma. [c]Chompret criteria.

## Staging
Not clinically relevant

## Prognosis and prediction
In males, the specific cancer risks at ≤ 15 years, 16–45 years, and > 45 years are 19%, 27%, and 54%, respectively. In females, the respective risks in these same age groups are 12%, 82%, and 100%, with breast cancer incidence responsible for the observed sex difference {2297}. Mutated *TP53* as seen in LFS confers an elevated risk of radiation-induced secondary malignancies and possibly increased sensitivity to low-dose radiation exposure by diagnostic methods such as mammography {1979}.

# Li–Fraumeni syndrome, CHEK2-associated

van Diest PJ
Hahnen E
Schoolmeester JK

## Definition
CHEK2-associated Li–Fraumeni syndrome (also called Li–Fraumeni syndrome 2) is a hereditary cancer susceptibility syndrome resulting from germline mutations in the CHEK2 gene.

## MIM numbering
609265 Li–Fraumeni syndrome 2

## ICD-11 coding
None

## Related terminology
Acceptable: CHK2.

## Subtype(s)
None

## Localization
In addition to breast cancer, germline CHEK2 c.1100delC heterozygosity has also been associated with an increased risk of gastric, colon, thyroid, kidney, and prostate cancers, as well as sarcoma {1458} and non-Hodgkin lymphoma {77,2221}.

## Clinical features
CHEK2 is a moderately penetrant breast cancer predisposition gene, with an estimated lifetime risk of 20–30% for women {1860,560,2320,1344,2252}. The estimated cumulative risks for development of ER-positive and ER-negative tumours by the age of 80 years in female CHEK2 c.1100delC carriers were 20% and 3%, respectively {1860}. CHEK2 c.1100delC–associated breast cancer seems to be associated with a higher contralateral breast cancer rate for women {1060,2253,655,1861,1361}.

## Epidemiology
Breast cancers resulting from an underlying CHEK2 germline mutation account for 1–3% of all breast cancer cases in females {405,835} and 4–9% in males {1676,1341,318}. The c.1100delC variant is the most prevalent, with an overall odds ratio of 2.89 that stratifies to 2.88 for female breast cancer and 3.13 for male breast cancer {1188}. The frequency of c.1100delC varies among regional breast cancer populations, from 0% (in Malaysia) to 2.7% (in the Russian Federation). In population-based studies of asymptomatic carriers, the frequency ranges from 0% (in Spain) to 0.7% (in Sweden) {77}.

## Etiology
CHEK2 is a 54.6 kb gene located at chromosome 22q12.1. CHEK2 mutations produce malfunctioning proteins, resulting in a disruption of DNA repair and consequent accumulation of genetic events that contribute to carcinogenesis. No external factors are known to influence carcinogenesis in patients with CHEK2 germline mutations.

## Pathogenesis
CHEK2 is a tumour suppressor gene that encodes the serine/threonine cell-cycle checkpoint kinase CHK2 {1341}. The CHK2 protein is activated by double-strand DNA breaks and in turn activates downstream repair proteins including BRCA1 and p53, playing an important role in DNA damage response by regulating cell-cycle checkpoints and triggering DNA repair by homologous recombination {1998,317}. The most common genetic alteration is the c.1100delC truncating loss-of-function mutation that yields an unstable CHK2 protein incapable of kinase activity {1431,1485}. For female CHEK2 c.1100delC mutation carriers, there is currently no evidence that risk varies by PR or ERBB2 (HER2) status after adjustment for ER status, nor any evidence for variation in relative risk by grade or morphology {1861}.

Array comparative genomic hybridization of c.1100delC cases showed recurrent losses at 1p13.3-p31.3, 8p21.1-p21.2, 8p23.1-p23.2, and 17p12-p13.1, as well as gains of 12q13.11-q13.13, 16p13.3, and 19p13.3 {1433}. In gene expression analysis, 26 CHEK2 c.1100delC–mutant tumours clustered with hormone receptor–positive breast cancers as luminal A (n = 8) or luminal B (n = 18) intrinsic subtype breast cancers {1442}. Another study pointed to CLCA1 on 1p22 and CALCOCO1, MUCL1 (SBEM), and LRP1 on 12q13 as candidates for CHEK2 c.1100delC–associated tumour-progression drivers {1433}.

Most of the data on CHEK2 relate to the c.1100delC variant, which is found frequently in northern European populations {1341,1860}. The risk of breast cancer is probably higher in homozygous c.1100delC carriers than in heterozygous females {892,12}. CHEK2 missense variants such as c.470T>C (p.Ile157Thr) may confer a lower risk of female breast cancer than the CHEK2 c.1100delC truncating variant {560,1007}. The p.Ile157Thr variant corrupts proper dimerization of the CHK2 protein, resulting in a dysfunctional protein that affects interactions at the interface of forkhead-associated and kinase domains {265}. The p.Ile157Thr variant was found to be associated with a luminal A phenotype and lower E-cadherin (CDH1) expression {902,1431}, and CHEK2 truncating mutations appear to be associated with a luminal B phenotype {902}. More than 200 pathogenic or likely pathogenic CHEK2 germline alterations have been reported (according to the ClinVar database as of November 2018), of which the c.1100delC and c.470T>C (p.Ile157Thr) missense variants appear to be most prevalent.

## Macroscopic appearance
The macroscopic appearance is not known to be at variance with that of sporadic breast cancer.

## Histopathology

Collective reports of the morphological and biomarker immunophenotypic features of *CHEK2*-associated breast carcinoma are conflicting. Some studies have identified a propensity for high-grade tumours, whereas others have described an increased frequency of low-grade carcinomas {428,461,528, 1431,1485,1875}. All combinations of ER, PR, and HER2 expression have also been identified, but c.1100delC carriers tend to develop hormone receptor–positive tumours {428,528,461,1431, 1875}. A strong link to lobular phenotype has been reported in carriers of the p.Ile157Thr variant {902,1431}. When parsed by mutation, the c.1100delC variant is associated with a luminal B phenotype, whereas the p.Ile157Thr variant is associated with a luminal A phenotype {1431,528}. Differences in tumour pathology may be related to the type of *CHEK2* mutation.

## Cytology

The cytology is not known to be at variance with that of sporadic breast cancer.

## Diagnostic molecular pathology

Not clinically relevant

## Essential and desirable diagnostic criteria

*Essential:* pathogenic germline mutation in *CHEK2*.

## Staging

The staging is not at variance with that of sporadic breast cancer.

## Prognosis and prediction

Patients with c.1100delC-associated breast cancer experience decreased survival {1060,461,1431}. Furthermore, no significant difference in response to adjuvant chemotherapy has been reported in these patients {1060}. *CHEK2* p.Ile157Thr carriers have survival comparable to that of non-carriers {1431,903}.

# CDH1-associated breast cancer

van Deurzen CHM
Carneiro F
Hornick JL
Provenzano E

## Definition

*CDH1*-associated breast cancer is a cancer susceptibility syndrome characterized by lobular carcinoma of the breast, caused by inactivating germline mutations in *CDH1*, the gene encoding E-cadherin. Invasive lobular breast cancer can also occur in the setting of hereditary diffuse gastric cancer (HDGC), which is also caused by germline mutations in *CDH1*.

## MIM numbering

192090 Cadherin 1; *CDH1*

## ICD-11 coding

None

## Related terminology

*Acceptable:* hereditary lobular breast cancer; hereditary diffuse gastric cancer (HDGC).

## Subtype(s)

None

## Localization

There is no specific localization of *CDH1*-associated breast cancer. HDGC can affect all topographical regions of the stomach.

## Clinical features

Female *CDH1* mutation carriers have a 40% lifetime risk of developing lobular breast carcinoma {820}. The clinical presentation of invasive lobular carcinoma (ILC) is described in detail in the section *Invasive lobular carcinoma* (p. 114). There are no widely used clinical criteria for *CDH1* genetic screening with respect to lobular carcinoma predisposition not associated with gastric cancer. However, an international expert panel on hereditary lobular breast carcinoma suggested criteria for *CDH1* testing (see *Essential and desirable diagnostic criteria*, below).

## Epidemiology

The frequency of a germline *CDH1* mutation is very low (~1%) in women with early-onset or familial lobular breast carcinoma without a family history of gastric carcinoma {1876}. Pathogenic germline *CDH1* mutations have been identified in 4 of 50 patients with bilateral lobular carcinoma in situ or ILC {1639}.

## Etiology

*CDH1* is located at 16q22.1, comprises 16 exons, and encodes E-cadherin. E-cadherin is a transmembrane protein that is predominantly expressed at the basolateral membrane of epithelial cells and is involved in homophilic cell–cell adhesion and transduction of mechanical force {228,1127}. Its cytoplasmic domain interacts with numerous structural and regulatory proteins, including the catenin family {228}. These interactions influence cell survival signalling, the microtubule network, and the organization of the cortical actin cytoskeleton {228}, with a profound impact on cell shape, polarity, and motility {1127}.

## Pathogenesis

Several *CDH1* germline alterations have been reported to be associated with an increased risk of lobular breast carcinoma. Classically, lobular breast carcinomas in patients with *CDH1* germline mutations are also associated with a predisposition for HDGC {820}. However, recent studies have identified *CDH1*

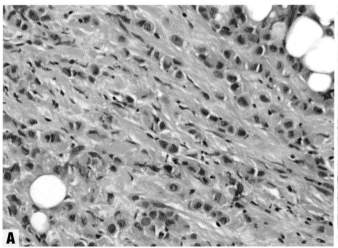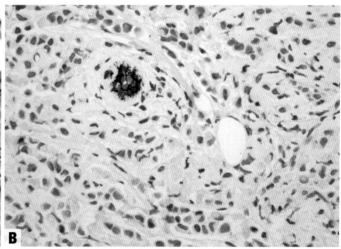

**Fig. 9.07** Invasive lobular carcinoma of breast. **A** The cells are present without glands, singly and in single files. The nuclei are minimally pleomorphic with occasional nucleoli and intracytoplasmic inclusions (see *Invasive lobular carcinoma*, p. 114, for additional images of invasive lobular carcinoma). **B** Typical loss of E-cadherin expression. Note the immunoreactivity in normal epithelium.

variants with a potential pathogenic role in hereditary lobular breast cancer in the absence of a family history of gastric carcinoma {140,1639,2000}. The loss of E-cadherin expression identified in breast tumours occurs via various somatic mechanisms: somatic *CDH1* mutations, loss of heterozygosity, *CDH1* promoter hypermethylation, and allelic imbalance {334,761,118, 1546}.

## Macroscopic appearance

There is no specific information on macroscopic findings in *CDH1* mutation carriers; however, ILCs often present as poorly defined masses that can be difficult to delineate macroscopically. There may be a vague area of increased firmness rather than a discrete mass, and the final tumour diameter often exceeds the macroscopic size estimate.

## Histopathology

*CDH1* germline mutations have specifically been associated with ILCs. Most published series do not provide more-detailed histological information such as grade or size in *CDH1* mutation carriers.

ILC is described in detail in the section *Invasive lobular carcinoma* (p. 114), but in summary, it is characterized by diffuse infiltration by small round cells with monomorphic nuclei that invade individually or as single files and cords. There is minimal disruption of background breast architecture, and the tumour cells often surround existing structures, forming a targetoid arrangement. On occasion, the cells may have prominent intracytoplasmic mucin vacuoles or pale foamy cytoplasm imparting a histiocytoid appearance. There are subtypes with solid, alveolar, or tubulolobular growth patterns, as well as a pleomorphic subtype with marked nuclear pleomorphism that often has apocrine morphology with abundant eosinophilic cytoplasm. Classic ILCs are almost always ER-positive and ERBB2 (HER2)-negative, although the pleomorphic subtype may be ER-negative and is HER2-positive in approximately 15–40% of cases. Loss of E-cadherin membrane staining occurs in ILC irrespective of germline mutation {2303}.

## Cytology

Cytologically, aspirates of ILC contain small monomorphic cells with mild atypia, often with intracytoplasmic mucin vacuoles. The cells are present singly, as loose clusters, or forming cords. Some series have shown an increased false negative rate by FNA, with ILC largely related to low tumour cellularity, although the cells are sometimes so bland that they may be mistaken for lymphocytes {1348}. A more detailed description is provided in the section *Invasive lobular carcinoma* (p. 114).

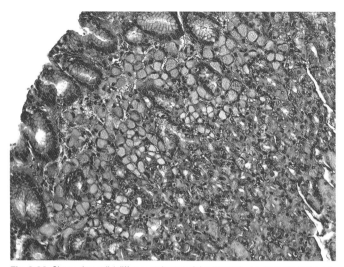

**Fig. 9.08** Signet-ring cell / diffuse carcinoma of the stomach. An example in the setting of hereditary diffuse gastric cancer (HDGC), in which invasive lobular carcinoma can also develop.

## Diagnostic molecular pathology

Genetic testing for *CDH1* germline mutations should be considered in two settings. In the absence of a family history of gastric cancer, the two criteria for genetic testing are (1) bilateral ILC with or without a family history of ILC, with patient age at onset of < 50 years, and (2) unilateral ILC with a family history of ILC and patient age at onset of < 45 years {401}. In the setting of HDGC, the criterion for genetic testing is a personal or family (first- or second-degree relative) history of diffuse gastric cancer and ILC, with one diagnosed at an age < 50 years {2145B}.

## Essential and desirable diagnostic criteria

*Essential:* pathogenic germline mutation in *CDH1*.

## Staging

The staging is the same as for other breast carcinomas.

## Prognosis and prediction

The estimated cumulative risk of gastric cancer is 70% for male and 56% for female *CDH1* mutation carriers {820,2145B}. Female carriers have a 40% lifetime risk of developing ILC {820}. In the setting of HDGC, diffuse gastric cancer is the main cause of mortality in both sexes.

# PALB2-associated cancers

Mills AM
Furukawa T

## Definition

PALB2-associated cancers occur due to germline mutations in the PALB2 gene, which is a partner of BRCA2 {2302,2347, 2016}.

## MIM numbering

610355 Partner and localizer of BRCA2; PALB2

## ICD-11 coding

None

## Related terminology

Acceptable: DNA double-strand break repair; homologous recombination repair; pancreatic cancer 3; Fanconi anaemia, complementation group N.

## Subtype(s)

Germline monoallelic mutations are associated with increased cancer risk. Germline biallelic mutations are associated with the genetic syndrome Fanconi anaemia, complementation group 2.

## Localization

PALB2 mutations are associated with cancers of the breast and the pancreas.

## Clinical features

Patients with monoallelic germline PALB2 mutations have increased susceptibility to breast and pancreatic cancers {75, 299,2358,1693,962}. PALB2 was originally considered to be a moderate-risk gene for breast cancer; however, subsequent work has led to its reclassification as high-risk: PALB2 mutations are associated with a breast cancer risk as much as 9-fold higher than average, with an average lifetime risk of about 14% {75}. The risk imparted by the loss-of-function gene mutation appears to synergize with uncharacterized additional genetic factors, because the mean risk for carriers varies with family history {75}. For example, a 70-year-old carrier with no immediate family history of breast cancer bears only a 33% risk, but that risk nearly doubles, to 58%, when two first-degree relatives have a history of breast cancer {75}.

Biallelic mutations in PALB2 lead to the autosomal recessive genetic syndrome Fanconi anaemia, complementation group 2 {2302,2083}. Patients with Fanconi anaemia demonstrate hypersensitivity to DNA crosslinking agents, short stature, microcephaly, hypertelorism, bone marrow failure, and developmental abnormalities in major organ systems. Furthermore, Fanconi anaemia is associated with early onset of a variety of childhood malignancies, including acute leukaemias, neuroblastoma, Wilms tumour, and medulloblastoma {2083}. Somatic mutations of PALB2 in breast cancer tissues are infrequently observed. In a whole-genome analysis of breast cancer tissues, somatic mutations of PALB2 were found in 8 of 560 samples (1.4%) {1507}. According to the Catalogue Of Somatic Mutations In Cancer (COSMIC), somatic mutations of PALB2 were found in 52 of 4060 breast cancer samples (~1.3%) {2258}.

## Epidemiology

Although rare in the general population (< 1%), monoallelic germline PALB2 mutations are identified in 1–5% of familial breast cancer patients {299,933}. Unlike BRCA mutations, PALB2 mutations do not appear to be strongly associated with either Ashkenazi Jewish heritage or ethnically diverse Jewish ancestry {299,304}. Fanconi anaemia has a prevalence of about 1 case per 130 000 live births in the USA, and only a subset of these cases are attributable to biallelic PALB2 mutations {1738, 2301}.

## Etiology

Patients with PALB2-associated familial breast cancers inherit a monoallelic germline mutation in the gene. The acquisition of a second hit, whether through somatic point mutations or loss of heterozygosity, causes biallelic inactivation in the majority of cancers, leading to PALB2 loss of function {1133}.

## Pathogenesis

PALB2 is a 38 kb gene located on chromosome 16p12.2 that spans 13 exons and encodes the tumour suppressor protein PALB2, which is involved in DNA double-strand break repair by homologous recombination. One of its critical roles is the binding to and stabilization of BRCA2, permitting nuclear BRCA2 accumulation {2302,2347,2016}. PALB2 also promotes the incorporation of the tumour suppressor protein RAD51 into the processed single-stranded DNA end for strand exchange in homologous recombination repair {2302,2347,2016}. Impairments in PALB2 function therefore lead to defective double-strand break repair, which facilitates non-homologous end joining of DNA breaks and accumulation of mutations.

## Macroscopic appearance

The macroscopic appearance is not known to be at variance with that of sporadic breast cancer.

## Histopathology

There has been limited morphological study of breast cancers associated with PALB2 mutations. One study of a series of 28 cases compared cancers from patients with PALB2 mutations to BRCA-associated and non-familial cancers, and found that the only morphological feature characteristic of the PALB2 group was minimal stromal sclerosis. Despite the functional relationship between the PALB2 and BRCA2 proteins, features more typically associated with BRCA-affiliated cancers, such as high-grade histology and robust lymphoid infiltration, were not predictive of PALB2 mutations in this small series {2068}.

## Cytology

The cytology is not known to be at variance with that of sporadic breast cancer.

## Diagnostic molecular pathology

*PALB2* mutations are most often identified by next-generation sequencing performed on patient blood samples. Increasingly, these tests use multigene panels that assess for a large number of genes affiliated with familial breast cancer risk.

## Essential and desirable diagnostic criteria

*Essential:* pathogenic germline mutation in *PALB2*.

## Staging

The staging is the same as for sporadic breast cancer.

## Prognosis and prediction

Breast cancer patients with *PALB2* mutations are at an increased risk not only for secondary breast cancers, but also for pancreatic cancers. Increased screening may therefore be warranted in this population {75,299,2358}. Recent studies suggest that *PALB2* pathogenic germline variants are associated with functional BRCA deficiency, raising the possibility of therapeutic intervention with poly (ADP-ribose) polymerase (PARP) inhibitors {458,1518}.

# Peutz–Jeghers syndrome

Jansen M
Brosens LAA

## Definition

Peutz–Jeghers syndrome (PJS) is an autosomal dominant polyp and cancer predisposition syndrome characterized by mucocutaneous melanin pigmentation and gastrointestinal polyposis associated with *STK11* mutation.

## MIM numbering

175200 Peutz–Jeghers syndrome

## ICD-11 coding

LD2D.0 Peutz–Jeghers syndrome

## Related terminology

None

## Subtype(s)

None

## Localization

Polyps in PJS typically occur in the small intestine (in 95% of PJS patients). About 25% of patients have polyps in the colon and stomach {239}. The second most common organ site for malignancy in women is the breast.

## Clinical features

Presenting symptoms include abdominal pain, intestinal bleeding, anaemia, and intussusception, which typically manifest in the first two decades of life {238}. If present, the characteristic mucocutaneous pigmentation allows diagnosis of asymptomatic patients in familial cases, but the characteristic Peutz–Jeghers polyps constitute the main clinical hallmark.

PJS is associated with a moderate or high risk of a range of malignancies, with an overall risk of any cancer by the age of 70 years of 81% (see Table 9.05) {838,727,728}. Well-documented extraintestinal tumours include carcinomas of the breast and pancreas, as well as otherwise rare gonadal lesions, including sex cord tumour with annular tubules of the ovary and Sertoli cell tumour of the testis.

## Epidemiology

The incidence of PJS is roughly one tenth that of familial adenomatous polyposis, with an estimated incidence of 1 case per 50 000–200 000 births.

## Etiology

A germline mutation in the tumour suppressor gene *STK11* (formerly *LKB1*) encoding a serine/threonine kinase can be found in > 90% of PJS patients. Most germline defects are point mutations and small intragenic deletions, but larger deletions of one or more exons have also been described {467}.

## Pathogenesis

The direct precursor to gastrointestinal cancer in PJS patients remains unknown {934}. Peutz–Jeghers polyps are probably an epiphenomenon to the cancer-prone condition and not obligate malignant precursors {934,1112}. There are no data on the pathogenesis of breast cancer.

## Macroscopic appearance

The macroscopic appearance is not known to be at variance with that of sporadic breast cancer.

## Histopathology

There are few data on breast cancer phenotypes in PJS, but the very limited data suggest that akin to cancers in *BRCA2* carriers, breast cancers in PJS are likely to be of intermediate-high grade, ER-positive and PR-positive, and ERBB2 (HER2)-negative {1210}. Gastrointestinal Peutz–Jeghers polyps have been described in detail in the *Digestive system tumours* volume of this series {2270A}.

## Cytology

The cytology is not known to be at variance with that of sporadic breast cancer.

## Diagnostic molecular pathology

Not clinically relevant

**Table 9.05** Peutz–Jeghers syndrome cancer risks for specific anatomical localizations at 65–70 years of age

| Site | Cancer risk |
|------|-------------|
| Colorectum | 39% |
| Small intestine | 13% |
| Stomach | 29% |
| Pancreas | 11–36% |
| Breast | 32–54% |
| Uterus | 9% |
| Ovary | 21% |
| Cervix | 10% |
| Testis | 9% |
| Lung | 7–17% |

### Essential and desirable diagnostic criteria

The diagnostic criteria for PJS are presented in Box 9.04.

### Staging

The staging is the same as for sporadic breast cancer.

### Prognosis and prediction

The prognosis for patients with PJS is now mainly determined by the risk of malignancy, and an increased cancer mortality has been shown in PJS {2150}. PJS patients should be surveilled to prevent gastrointestinal complications and cancer {2018}. Specific data for breast cancer are not available.

**Box 9.04** Diagnostic criteria for Peutz–Jeghers syndrome (PJS)

1. ≥ 3 histologically confirmed Peutz–Jeghers polyps
2. Any number of Peutz–Jeghers polyps with a family history of PJS
3. Characteristic, prominent[a] mucocutaneous pigmentation with a family history of PJS
4. Any number of Peutz–Jeghers polyps and characteristic, prominent mucocutaneous pigmentation

[a]Some melanin pigmentation is also regularly seen in unaffected individuals, hence the emphasis on the prominence of the pigmentation; moreover, the pigmentation in patients with PJS may disappear with time and can in rare cases be absent altogether.

# Neurofibromatosis type 1

Frayling IM
Arends MJ

## Definition
Neurofibromatosis type 1 (NF1) is an inherited, multisystem, neurocutaneous disorder that predisposes individuals to the development of both benign and malignant tumours.

## MIM numbering
162200 Neurofibromatosis, type 1

## ICD-11 coding
LD2D.10 Neurofibromatosis type 1

## Related terminology
*Acceptable:* von Recklinghausen disease.

## Subtype(s)
None

## Localization
Tumours associated with NF1 are localized in the brain, central and peripheral nerves, and breast.

## Clinical features
There are no specific clinical features of NF1-associated breast cancer (NF1-BC), although patients with deletions of the whole *NF1* gene (so-called microdeletions), who tend to experience more-severe NF1-related disease, including a higher incidence of malignant tumours such as malignant peripheral nerve sheath tumours, paradoxically appear to be at low risk of NF1-BC {679}. However, although NF1-BC can occur at any age, it tends to occur at younger ages and is more malignant {606,2132}.

## Epidemiology
NF1 has a prevalence of 1 case per 2000–3500 individuals, consistent across all populations tested {796}. NF1-BC occurs in both males and females, sometimes bilaterally, consistent with predisposition {2209,2277,2132}. Both the absolute and relative risks of NF1-BC in females up to the age of 50 years are increased: 7.8–8.4% versus 2% in the general population, with standardized incidence ratios of 4.0–8.8 (see Table 9.06).

## Etiology
NF1 is an autosomal dominant tumour predisposition syndrome due to heritable pathogenic variants in the *NF1* gene (17q11.2) {2129}. A high proportion of cases are due to de novo mutations. The expressivity and age-related penetrance are variable. There is evidence that NF1-BC is more likely in patients with pathogenic variants of *NF1* that confer a gain of function {679}. This is consistent with a study of somatic *NF1* mutations observed in sporadic cancers, in which breast cancer stands out as being the only type of malignancy in which amplification of *NF1* is common (and, importantly, is independent of *ERBB2* amplification) {1645,679}.

## Pathogenesis
Neurofibromin (NF1) is a large (2485 amino acid) cytoplasmic protein predominantly expressed in neurons, Schwann cells, and oligodendrocytes. It has a number of domains and is a major regulator of several intracellular pathways (e.g. RAS/cAMP), the MAPK/ERK cascade, adenylyl cyclase, and cytoskeletal assembly {1857}. A potential direct functional link to ER signalling has recently been demonstrated in a rat model {518}.

## Macroscopic appearance
There are no specific macroscopic features associated with NF1-BC.

## Histopathology
Breast cancers occurring in NF1 are mostly adenocarcinomas of no special type (NST), but lobular neoplasms also occur. Recent data have also shown an association with sporadic metaplastic carcinoma in which overrepresentation of somatic *NF1* mutations was noted {1328}.

## Cytology
Not clinically relevant

**Table 9.06** Neurofibromatosis type 1–associated breast cancer risk estimates

| Reference(s) | Standardized incidence ratio (95% CI) | | |
| --- | --- | --- | --- |
| | Overall | At < 50 years | At ≥ 50 years |
| Sharif et al., 2007 {1911} | 3.5 (1.9–5.9) | 4.9 (2.4–8.8) | |
| Wang et al., 2012 {2220} | 5.2 (2.4–9.8) | 8.8 (3.2–19.2) | 2.8 (0.6–8.2) |
| Madanikia et al., 2012 {1264} | 2.7 (0.7–7.3)[a] | 4.41 (1.1–12.0)[a] | 0.94 (0.05–4.6)[a] |
| Seminog and Goldacre, 2013 {1895} | 2.3 (1.7–2.9) | | |
| Uusitalo et al., 2017 {2132}, Frayling et al., 2018 {679} | 2.8 (1.92–4.0) | 5.1 (2.9–8.1)[b] | 2.0 (1.2–3.1)[b] |

[a]Adjusted for race, neurofibromatosis type 1 prevalence, and date of diagnosis. [b]Calculated, using Poisson regression, from the published observed and expected values.

## Diagnostic molecular pathology

No consistent features, such as positivity for ER, PR, or ERBB2 (HER2), have been noted for NF1-BC, but there is a lack of definitive evidence to exclude a relationship.

## Essential and desirable diagnostic criteria

Two of the following criteria are required to diagnose NF1: ≥ 6 café-au-lait patches, neurofibromas (i.e. peripheral nerve sheath tumours manifesting as cutaneous, subcutaneous, or plexiform lesions), skin-fold freckling, ≥ 2 iris Lisch nodules, an optic pathway glioma, a specific bony dysplasia (thinning of the long bone cortex, sphenoid wing dysplasia), an affected first-degree relative {2129}.

## Staging

The staging of breast cancer in NF1 is the same as for sporadic breast cancer.

## Prognosis and prediction

Given the increased risk of breast cancer in NF1, screening for breast cancer in women with NF1 may be advised. However, recent work showing that the risk of breast cancer may be higher in relation to specific *NF1* variants, and that patients with whole gene deletions may be at reduced risk, indicates that generalizing the risk in individuals may be of limited utility; in the future, more-personalized mutation-specific advice may be possible {679}.

NF1-BC tends to have a poorer prognosis, and this may be related to presentation at later stages, which is likely to be due in part to patients with NF1 often having learning difficulties, a well-recognized risk factor in late diagnosis {1336,2005}. Three human studies have reported increased mortality and unfavourable prognostic factors with NF1-BC {606,2132,2317}.

# The polygenic component of breast cancer susceptibility

Hollestelle A
Southey MC

Pathogenic variants in known breast cancer susceptibility genes account for only a small proportion of the familial risk of breast cancer. Several breast cancer susceptibility genes have been identified that, when mutated in the germ line, substantially increase the risk of developing breast cancer (i.e. by 2-fold to 20-fold). These are *BRCA1*, *BRCA2*, *TP53*, *PTEN*, *STK11*, *CDH1*, *PALB2*, *CHEK2*, *ATM*, and *NBN* (*NBS1*); together they explain about 20–25% of the familial breast cancer risk {560}.

Over the past decade, another 18% of the familial breast cancer risk has been explained by the identification of more than 170 common genetic variants that are most often located outside of coding regions and are each associated with an increase in breast cancer risk as high as 1.3-fold {1365,1380}. Unlike pathogenic variants associated with high penetrance, these variants are common in the population and are often referred to as low-penetrance alleles. These so-called low-penetrance breast cancer susceptibility alleles are commonly identified through genome-wide association studies in which SNPs tagging genomic loci are compared between women affected by breast cancer (cases) and women unaffected by breast cancer (controls), thereby taking advantage of the linkage disequilibrium structure in the human genome. Because the breast cancer risk associated with each of these variants is so small, large numbers of subjects are required for genome-wide association studies; consequently, the establishment of large research consortia has been pivotal to the continued identification of these variants. The most recent and largest breast cancer genome-wide association study, from the Breast Cancer Association Consortium (BCAC), measured 11.8 million SNPs for 137 045 cases and 119 078 controls. The study led to the identification of 65 new breast cancer risk loci and replicated low-penetrance alleles from 49 previously identified loci {1365}. In total, 172 low-penetrance breast cancer susceptibility alleles have been identified to date (see Table 9.07, p. 294). However, it is estimated that these represent only 44% of the familial breast cancer risk that can be explained by the polygenic component of breast cancer susceptibility {1365}.

## Breast cancer subtypes

The majority of the low-penetrance breast cancer susceptibility alleles are associated with higher risks for ER-positive rather than ER-negative breast cancer {1365,1380}. In fact, most common genetic variants associated with overall breast cancer risk also show an association with ER-positive breast cancer. Only 20 low-penetrance breast cancer susceptibility alleles are associated with ER-negative breast cancer alone. This demonstrates that ER-positive and ER-negative breast cancers share a common genetic etiology, with subtype-specific genetic features.

Low-penetrance breast cancer susceptibility alleles associated with ER-negative breast cancer are also associated with breast cancer risk in *BRCA1* pathogenic variant carriers – a finding consistent with the observation that the majority of *BRCA1*

pathogenic variant carriers develop ER-negative disease {1319, 1070}. In addition, 24 of the low-penetrance breast cancer susceptibility alleles associated with overall breast cancer risk are also associated with breast cancer risk for *BRCA1* pathogenic variant carriers {1380}. Similarly, *BRCA2* pathogenic variant carriers commonly develop ER-positive disease, and the low-penetrance breast cancer susceptibility alleles that are associated with overall breast cancer (predominantly ER-positive disease) risk are also associated with breast cancer risk in *BRCA2* pathogenic variant carriers {1319,1070}.

Although most breast cancers are of ductal histology, there have also been efforts to identify low-penetrance breast cancer susceptibility alleles that specifically predispose individuals to other histological subtypes. One low-penetrance breast cancer susceptibility allele at 7q34 is specifically associated with lobular breast cancer. Seven alleles show significant differences between ER-positive breast cancers with invasive ductal carcinoma histology and those with invasive lobular carcinoma histology. Three of these alleles showed stronger associations with invasive lobular carcinoma than invasive ductal carcinoma, and the other four were specifically associated with invasive ductal carcinoma {1853}. No low-penetrance breast cancer susceptibility alleles were identified that were specifically associated with ductal carcinoma in situ, suggesting that ductal carcinoma in situ and invasive ductal carcinoma have a common genetic etiology {1638}.

Few of the low-penetrance breast cancer susceptibility alleles have been definitively associated with other cancer types. A rare exception is the low-penetrance breast cancer susceptibility allele at 19p13, which is also associated with ovarian cancer {1120}. Interestingly, common genetic variants in the 9p21.3 region are associated with multiple disease phenotypes, including stroke, coronary artery disease {1834}, diabetes {2345}, and several types of cancer (including breast cancer {2121}, oesophageal squamous cell carcinoma {1206}, oral cancer {1153}, and multiple myeloma {1386}). Common genetic variation in this region has also been associated with a global DNA methylation pattern in glioma {436}. Additionally, a large germline deletion of this region (involving nine genes) has been reported in a family that presented with familial melanoma, astrocytoma, and breast cancer {2162}.

Most low-penetrance breast cancer susceptibility alleles have been identified in populations of European descent. Because there are differences in linkage disequilibrium structure between populations of European and non-European descent, this may influence the breast cancer risks for some loci in some populations {1642}. African women have an increased incidence of ER-negative breast cancer, which may also be partially explained by genetic risk factors {354}. This highlights the need for larger genome-wide association studies in non-European populations, in particular African populations.

## Breast cancer–specific survival

The potential for germline genetic information to add to the routinely collected tumour-derived prognostic factors has been investigated in numerous settings. The possible association between common genetic variation and breast cancer–specific survival has been examined in candidate gene studies {1758} and pooled analyses {787,1653}. These studies have identified and further evaluated numerous common genetic variants nominally associated with outcome, but few have been replicated and/or reached genome-wide significance. Breast cancer subtype–specific survival analyses conducted as part of a large meta-analysis of European genome-wide association studies identified an (imputed) common genetic variant associated with ER-negative disease with genome-wide significance {787}. However, larger studies with the necessary design and data are needed to provide enough statistical power to definitively identify common genetic variants associated with survival and to support breast cancer subtype analyses.

## Assigning causation to genetic variation

Genome-wide association studies take advantage of the linkage disequilibrium structure of the human genome and identify common variants that are likely to tag a genomic region associated with the disease. These region-tagging common genetic variants are associated with breast cancer risk, but they are seldom the cause of the genetic susceptibility. Considerable work has therefore been invested into further fine-scale mapping of these regions of interest, combined with in silico analysis and molecular experiments, in order to identify the so-called causal variants and their mechanisms of action. Such post–genome-wide association study analyses have been performed for 22 of the 172 risk loci and have provided several new insights into how low-penetrance breast cancer susceptibility alleles might increase breast cancer risk {1767}. For example, a single breast cancer risk locus is likely to harbour multiple causal variants. Breast cancer risk loci at 1p11.2, 2q33, 4q24, 5p12, 5p15.33, 5q11.2, 6q25.1, 8q24, 9q31.2, 10q21, 10q26, 11q13, and 12p11 are likely to each contain two to five distinct causal variants. Furthermore, each causal variant has been predicted to regulate two to three different target genes. Deregulating target genes or non-coding RNAs at the transcriptional level is a common theme among these low-penetrance breast cancer susceptibility alleles. Consequently, these alleles are usually located in regulatory regions that are associated with sites of open chromatin, transcription factor binding sites, and sites of chromatin interaction and histone modification {1767}. In contrast to the high- and moderate-penetrance breast cancer susceptibility genes, the genes that are deregulated by these low-penetrance alleles are not necessarily involved in the DNA damage response pathways, but rather affect known somatic breast cancer driver genes. Pathway analysis for 689 predicted target genes from 128 breast cancer risk loci revealed the FGF, PDGF, and WNT signalling pathways to be involved, as well as the ERK1/2 cascade, immune response, and cell-cycle pathways {1365}. However, the expression of breast cancer driver genes is not necessarily deregulated in the same direction by the germline variants as by somatic mutations {189,681,739}. For example, expression of MAP3K1 is upregulated in the germ line by low-penetrance variants at the 5q11.2 locus {739}. In contrast, somatic driver mutations in MAP3K1 are inactivating and thus associated with downregulation of expression {1993}.

## Polygenic risk score

The magnitude of risk associated with each individual low-penetrance breast cancer susceptibility allele is very low, but these risks appear to combine multiplicatively, so that the breast cancer risk associated with carrying a large proportion of these alleles can be substantial. A polygenic risk score (PRS), which is calculated as the sum of the log odds ratios for each common risk-associated variant, can now be used to identify whether risk-reducing interventions should be explored for every woman, even in the absence of a high-risk pathogenic variant {1856}. The most recent estimates, based on 77 risk-associated alleles, place women who are in the highest 1% of the PRS distribution at a 3.4-fold increased risk of breast cancer compared with women in the middle quintile of the PRS {1321}. The addition of further risk-associated alleles into the PRS is anticipated and likely to further stratify breast cancer risk in the general population, providing additional support for the utility of the PRS in the preventive setting {1365,1380}.

The PRS has also been shown to be useful for further stratifying breast cancer risk within carriers of BRCA1, BRCA2, and CHEK2 germline pathogenic variants {1069,1432}. Particularly for BRCA1 and BRCA2 pathogenic variant carriers, who (on average) have a high risk of developing breast cancer during their lifetime, information about the PRS could modify their risk sufficiently to support a change to their clinical risk management. PRSs that can stratify breast cancer risk for PALB2 and ATM pathogenic variant carriers are likely to be developed in the future.

Several breast cancer risk prediction models that make use of various clinical variables such as family history, reproductive history, and breast density are currently applied in the clinical setting, such as the Breast and Ovarian Analysis of Disease Incidence and Carrier Estimation Algorithm (BOADICEA), the BRCAPRO model, the Breast Cancer Risk Assessment Tool (BCRAT), and the International Breast Cancer Intervention Studies (IBIS) risk assessment tool. Remarkably, combining the 77-risk-allele PRS with these clinical models improved breast cancer risk prediction by > 20% in women aged < 50 years {519}. However, some of the clinical variables incorporated into these risk models are also hereditary traits; therefore, there is likely some overlap in the risk-associated genetic variants associated with these traits and breast cancer. For example, 18% of the known low-penetrance breast cancer susceptibility alleles are also associated with mammographic breast density, an important breast cancer risk factor {1207,1995}. Therefore, understanding how much of these heritable risk factors the breast cancer PRS already encompasses is an important area of future research.

**Table 9.07** 172 low-risk loci associated with breast cancer

| Locus | Strongest associated SNP | Candidate causal gene | MAF | Breast cancer subtype | OR | 95% CI | P value from meta-analysis | Reference(s) |
|---|---|---|---|---|---|---|---|---|
| 1p11.2 | rs11249433 | EMBP1 | 0.41 | Overall | 1.11 | (1.09–1.13) | $1.8 \times 10^{-52}$ | {2073} |
| 1p12 | rs7529522 | | 0.23 | Overall | 1.06 | (1.04–1.08) | $1.7 \times 10^{-10}$ | {1365} |
| 1p13.2 | rs11552449 | DCLRE1B | 0.17 | Overall | 1.04 | (1.01–1.06) | $4.6 \times 10^{-11}$ | {1364} |
| 1p22.3 | rs17426269 | | 0.15 | Overall | 1.05 | (1.02–1.07) | $1.7 \times 10^{-8}$ | {1365} |
| 1p32.3 | rs140850326 | | 0.49 | Overall | 0.97 | (0.95–0.99) | $3.9 \times 10^{-8}$ | {1365} |
| 1p34.1 | rs1707302 | PIK3R3, LOC101929626 | 0.34 | Overall | 0.96 | (0.95–0.98) | $3.0 \times 10^{-8}$ | {1365} |
| 1p34.2 | rs4233486 | | 0.36 | Overall | 0.97 | (0.95–0.98) | $9.1 \times 10^{-9}$ | {1365} |
| 1p34.2 | rs79724016 | HIVEP3 | 0.03 | Overall | 0.93 | (0.88–0.97) | $3.5 \times 10^{-8}$ | {1365} |
| 1p36.13 | rs2992756 | KLHDC7A | 0.49 | Overall | 1.06 | (1.04–1.08) | $1.6 \times 10^{-15}$ | {1365} |
| 1p36.22 | rs616488 | PEX14 | 0.33 | Overall | 0.94 | (0.93–0.96) | $5 \times 10^{-20}$ | {1364} |
| 1q21.1 | rs12405132 | RNF115 | 0.37 | Overall | 0.97 | (0.95–0.99) | $6.3 \times 10^{-10}$ | {1363} |
| 1q21.2 | rs12048493 | OTUD7B | 0.38 | Overall | 1.04 | (1.02–1.06) | $8.6 \times 10^{-14}$ | {1363} |
| 1q22 | rs4971059 | TRIM46 | 0.35 | Overall | 1.05 | (1.03–1.07) | $4.8 \times 10^{-11}$ | {1365} |
| 1q32.1 | rs6678914 | LGR6 | 0.41 | Overall | 1.00 | (0.99–1.02) | $3 \times 10^{-1}$ | {699} |
| 1q32.1 | rs4245739 | MDM4 | 0.26 | Overall | 1.02 | (1.00–1.04) | $1.3 \times 10^{-4}$ | {699} |
| 1q32.1 | rs4951011 | ZC3H11A | 0.16 | Overall | 1.04 | (1.02–1.07) | $1.3 \times 10^{-5}$ | {263} |
| 1q32.1 | rs35383942 | PHLDA3 | 0.06 | Overall | 1.12 | (1.08–1.17) | $3.8 \times 10^{-13}$ | {1365} |
| 1q41 | rs11117758 | ESRRG | 0.21 | Overall | 0.95 | (0.93–0.97) | $3.9 \times 10^{-9}$ | {1365} |
| 1q43 | rs72755295 | EXO1 | 0.03 | Overall | 1.15 | (1.09–1.20) | $1.7 \times 10^{-14}$ | {1363} |
| 2p23.2 | rs4577244 | WDR43 | 0.23 | ER–/BRCA1 | 1.01 | (0.99–1.03) | $4.3 \times 10^{-1}$ | {404} |
| 2p23.3 | rs6725517 | ADCY3 | 0.41 | Overall | 0.96 | (0.94–0.98) | $2.9 \times 10^{-12}$ | {1365} |
| 2p24.1 | rs12710696 | | 0.37 | Overall | 1.03 | (1.01–1.04) | $1.3 \times 10^{-8}$ | {699} |
| 2p25.1 | rs113577745 | GRHL1 | 0.10 | Overall | 1.08 | (1.05–1.11) | $3.9 \times 10^{-10}$ | {1365} |
| 2q13 | rs71801447 | BCL2L11 | 0.06 | Overall | 1.09 | (1.05–1.13) | $3.7 \times 10^{-8}$ | {1365} |
| 2q14.1 | rs4849887 | | 0.10 | Overall | 0.91 | (0.88–0.94) | $6.9 \times 10^{-20}$ | {1364} |
| 2q31.1 | rs2016394 | DLX2-DT (DLX2-AS1) | 0.47 | Overall | 0.95 | (0.94–0.97) | $6.2 \times 10^{-12}$ | {1364} |
| 2q31.1 | rs1550623 | CDCA7 | 0.15 | Overall | 0.95 | (0.93–0.98) | $5.4 \times 10^{-10}$ | {1364} |
| 2q33.1 | rs1830298 | CASP8, FLACC1 (ALS2CR12) | 0.28 | Overall | 1.06 | (1.04–1.08) | $1.9 \times 10^{-16}$ | {1263,1205} |
| 2q35 | rs4442975 | IGFBP5 | 0.50 | ER+ | 0.89 | (0.87–0.90) | $1.1 \times 10^{-95}$ | {1989,723} |
| 2q35 | rs34005590 | IGFBP5 | 0.05 | Overall | 0.82 | (0.79–0.86) | $3.2 \times 10^{-41}$ | {1989,2300} |
| 2q35 | rs16857609 | DIRC3 | 0.26 | Overall | 1.06 | (1.04–1.09) | $1.8 \times 10^{-25}$ | {1364} |
| 2q36.3 | rs12479355 | | 0.21 | Overall | 0.96 | (0.94–0.98) | $2.4 \times 10^{-8}$ | {1365} |
| 3p12.1 | rs13066793 | VGLL3 | 0.09 | Overall | 0.94 | (0.91–0.97) | $1.0 \times 10^{-9}$ | {1365} |
| 3p12.1 | rs9833888 | CMSS1, FILIP1L | 0.22 | Overall | 1.06 | (1.04–1.08) | $5.2 \times 10^{-10}$ | {1365} |
| 3p13 | rs6805189 | FOXP1 | 0.48 | Overall | 0.97 | (0.95–0.99) | $4.6 \times 10^{-8}$ | {1365} |
| 3p14.1 | rs1053338 | ATXN7 | 0.14 | Overall | 1.05 | (1.02–1.07) | $5.3 \times 10^{-11}$ | {1379} |
| 3p21.31 | rs6796502 | | 0.10 | Overall | 0.92 | (0.89–0.95) | $5.5 \times 10^{-15}$ | {1363} |
| 3p24.1 | rs4973768 | SLC4A7 | 0.47 | Overall | 1.11 | (1.09–1.13) | $4.8 \times 10^{-57}$ | {19} |
| 3p24.1 | rs12493607 | TGFBR2 | 0.34 | Overall | 1.05 | (1.03–1.07) | $6.9 \times 10^{-14}$ | {1364} |

CI, confidence interval; MAF, minor allele frequency; OR, odds ratio; SNP, single nucleotide polymorphism.

**Table 9.07** 172 low-risk loci associated with breast cancer (continued)

| Locus | Strongest associated SNP | Candidate causal gene | MAF | Breast cancer subtype | OR | 95% CI | P value from meta-analysis | Reference(s) |
|---|---|---|---|---|---|---|---|---|
| 3p26.1 | rs6762644 | EGOT, ITPR1 | 0.38 | Overall | 1.05 | (1.03–1.07) | $4 \times 10^{-18}$ | {1364} |
| 3q23 | rs34207738 | ZBTB38 | 0.41 | Overall | 1.06 | (1.04–1.08) | $3.2 \times 10^{-15}$ | {1365} |
| 3q26.31 | rs58058861 | | 0.21 | Overall | 1.06 | (1.04–1.09) | $1.9 \times 10^{-10}$ | {1365} |
| 4p14 | rs6815814 | | 0.26 | Overall | 1.06 | (1.04–1.08) | $6.1 \times 10^{-13}$ | {1365} |
| 4q21.23 | 4:84370124 | HELQ | 0.47 | Overall | 1.04 | (1.02–1.05) | $2.2 \times 10^{-9}$ | {1365} |
| 4q22.1 | rs10022462 | LOC105369192 | 0.44 | Overall | 1.04 | (1.02–1.06) | $1.6 \times 10^{-9}$ | {1365} |
| 4q24 | rs9790517 | TET2 | 0.23 | Overall | 1.04 | (1.01–1.06) | $5 \times 10^{-11}$ | {1364} |
| 4q28.1 | rs77528541 | | 0.13 | Overall | 0.95 | (0.92–0.97) | $1.4 \times 10^{-9}$ | {1365} |
| 4q34.1 | rs6828523 | ADAM29 | 0.12 | Overall | 0.91 | (0.88–0.93) | $1.8 \times 10^{-25}$ | {1364} |
| 5p12 | rs10941679 | FGF10, MRPS30 | 0.25 | ER+ | 1.15 | (1.13–1.18) | $5.6 \times 10^{-73}$ | {1988} |
| 5p13.3 | rs2012709 | | 0.48 | Overall | 1.02 | (1.00–1.04) | $1.2 \times 10^{-8}$ | {1363} |
| 5p15.1 | rs13162653 | | 0.45 | Overall | 0.99 | (0.97–1.01) | $5.4 \times 10^{-7}$ | {1363} |
| 5p15.33 | rs10069690 | TERT | 0.26 | ER− | 1.06 | (1.04–1.08) | $7.8 \times 10^{-17}$ | {803} |
| 5p15.33 | rs3215401 | TERT | 0.31 | Overall | 0.93 | (0.91–0.95) | $1.1 \times 10^{-20}$ | {189} |
| 5p15.33 | rs116095464 | AHRR | 0.05 | Overall | 1.06 | (1.02–1.10) | $3.8 \times 10^{-9}$ | {1365} |
| 5q11.1 | rs72749841 | | 0.16 | Overall | 0.93 | (0.91–0.96) | $7.2 \times 10^{-10}$ | {1365} |
| 5q11.1 | rs35951924 | | 0.32 | Overall | 0.95 | (0.93–0.97) | $1.3 \times 10^{-11}$ | {1365} |
| 5q11.2 | rs62355902 | MAP3K1 | 0.16 | Overall | 1.18 | (1.15–1.21) | $6.8 \times 10^{-98}$ | {561} |
| 5q11.2 | rs10472076 | RAB3C | 0.38 | Overall | 1.03 | (1.01–1.04) | $9.6 \times 10^{-9}$ | {1364} |
| 5q11.2 | rs1353747 | PDE4D | 0.09 | Overall | 0.96 | (0.93–0.99) | $4.1 \times 10^{-9}$ | {1364} |
| 5q14.2 | rs7707921 | ATG10 | 0.25 | Overall | 0.96 | (0.94–0.98) | $1.7 \times 10^{-12}$ | {1363} |
| 5q14.3 | rs10474352 | ARRDC3 | 0.16 | Overall | 0.94 | (0.92–0.97) | $4.5 \times 10^{-11}$ | {263} |
| 5q22.1 | rs6882649 | NREP | 0.34 | Overall | 0.97 | (0.95–0.99) | $3.7 \times 10^{-9}$ | {1365} |
| 5q31.1 | rs6596100 | HSPA4 | 0.25 | Overall | 0.94 | (0.92–0.96) | $7.7 \times 10^{-9}$ | {1365} |
| 5q33.3 | rs1432679 | EBF1 | 0.43 | Overall | 1.08 | (1.06–1.10) | $6.6 \times 10^{-31}$ | {1364} |
| 5q35.1 | rs4562056 | | 0.33 | Overall | 1.05 | (1.03–1.07) | $4.7 \times 10^{-10}$ | {1365} |
| 6p22.1 | rs9257408 | | 0.41 | Overall | 1.02 | (1.00–1.04) | $6.9 \times 10^{-8}$ | {1363} |
| 6p22.2 | rs71557345 | | 0.07 | Overall | 0.92 | (0.88–0.96) | $3.9 \times 10^{-10}$ | {1365} |
| 6p22.3 | rs3819405 | ATXN1 | 0.33 | Overall | 0.96 | (0.94–0.97) | $1.7 \times 10^{-8}$ | {1365} |
| 6p22.3 | rs2223621 | CDKAL1 | 0.38 | Overall | 1.04 | (1.02–1.06) | $3.0 \times 10^{-10}$ | {1365} |
| 6p23 | rs204247 | RANBP9 | 0.44 | Overall | 1.04 | (1.02–1.06) | $7.9 \times 10^{-13}$ | {1364} |
| 6p24.3 | rs9348512 | TFAP2A | 0.33 | BRCA2 | 1.00 | (0.99–1.02) | $8 \times 10^{-1}$ | {705} |
| 6p25.3 | rs11242675 | FOXQ1 | 0.37 | Overall | 1.00 | (0.98–1.02) | $1 \times 10^{-4}$ | {1364} |
| 6q14.1 | rs17529111 | | 0.22 | ER− | 1.02 | (1.00–1.04) | $1.3 \times 10^{-9}$ | {1937} |
| 6q14.1 | rs12207986 | | 0.47 | Overall | 0.97 | (0.95–0.98) | $1.5 \times 10^{-9}$ | {1365} |
| 6q23.1 | rs6569648 | L3MBTL3 | 0.24 | Overall | 0.94 | (0.92–0.96) | $3.0 \times 10^{-12}$ | {1365} |
| 6q25 | rs3757322 | ESR1 | 0.32 | ER− | 1.08 | (1.06–1.10) | $3.3 \times 10^{-41}$ | {2121,552} |
| 6q25 | rs9397437 | ESR1 | 0.07 | ER− | 1.17 | (1.14–1.21) | $4.8 \times 10^{-54}$ | {2121,552} |
| 6q25 | rs2747652 | ESR1 | 0.48 | ER− | 0.94 | (0.92–0.96) | $1.3 \times 10^{-26}$ | {2121,552} |
| 6q25.1 | rs9485372 | TAB2 | 0.19 | Overall | 0.96 | (0.93–0.98) | $3.5 \times 10^{-6}$ | {1232} |
| 7p15.1 | rs17156577 | CREB5 | 0.11 | Overall | 1.05 | (1.02–1.08) | $4.3 \times 10^{-9}$ | {1365} |

CI, confidence interval; MAF, minor allele frequency; OR, odds ratio; SNP, single nucleotide polymorphism.

Chapter 9

**Table 9.07** 172 low-risk loci associated with breast cancer (continued)

| Locus | Strongest associated SNP | Candidate causal gene | MAF | Breast cancer subtype | OR | 95% CI | *P* value from meta-analysis | Reference(s) |
|---|---|---|---|---|---|---|---|---|
| 7p15.3 | rs7971 | DNAH11, CDCA7L | 0.35 | Overall | 0.96 | (0.94–0.98) | $1.9 \times 10^{-8}$ | {1365} |
| 7q21.2 | rs6964587 | AKAP9 | 0.39 | Overall | 1.03 | (1.02–1.05) | $9 \times 10^{-11}$ | {1379} |
| 7q21.3 | rs17268829 | | 0.28 | Overall | 1.05 | (1.03–1.07) | $4.5 \times 10^{-13}$ | {1365} |
| 7q22.1 | rs71559437 | CUX1 | 0.12 | Overall | 0.93 | (0.91–0.96) | $5.1 \times 10^{-12}$ | {1365} |
| 7q32.3 | rs4593472 | LINC-PINT (FLJ43663) | 0.35 | Overall | 0.97 | (0.95–0.99) | $1.8 \times 10^{-11}$ | {1363} |
| 7q34 | rs11977670 | | 0.43 | Lobular | 1.06 | (1.04–1.08) | $1 \times 10^{-16}$ | {1853} |
| 7q35 | rs720475 | NOBOX, ARHGEF6 | 0.25 | Overall | 0.96 | (0.94–0.98) | $1.2 \times 10^{-11}$ | {1364} |
| 8p11.23 | rs13365225 | | 0.18 | Overall | 0.91 | (0.89–0.93) | $1.4 \times 10^{-20}$ | {1363} |
| 8p12 | rs9693444 | | 0.32 | Overall | 1.06 | (1.04–1.08) | $1.6 \times 10^{-21}$ | {1364} |
| 8q21.11 | rs6472903 | | 0.17 | Overall | 0.94 | (0.92–0.96) | $4.4 \times 10^{-21}$ | {1364} |
| 8q21.11 | rs2943559 | HNF4G | 0.08 | Overall | 1.10 | (1.07–1.14) | $4 \times 10^{-24}$ | {1364} |
| 8q22.3 | rs514192 | | 0.32 | Overall | 1.05 | (1.03–1.07) | $5.6 \times 10^{-9}$ | {1365} |
| 8q23.1 | rs12546444 | ZFPM2 | 0.10 | Overall | 0.93 | (0.91–0.96) | $7.5 \times 10^{-11}$ | {1365} |
| 8q23.3 | rs13267382 | LINC00536 | 0.36 | Overall | 1.03 | (1.01–1.05) | $1.6 \times 10^{-11}$ | {1363} |
| 8q24.13 | rs58847541 | | 0.15 | Overall | 1.08 | (1.05–1.10) | $5.5 \times 10^{-13}$ | {1365} |
| 8q24.21 | rs13281615 | | 0.41 | Overall | 1.11 | (1.09–1.13) | $1.9 \times 10^{-57}$ | {561} |
| 8q24.21 | rs11780156 | MYC | 0.17 | Overall | 1.05 | (1.03–1.08) | $1.1 \times 10^{-13}$ | {1364} |
| 9p21.3 | rs1011970 | CDKN2A, CDKN2B | 0.16 | Overall | 1.07 | (1.04–1.09) | $1 \times 10^{-15}$ | {2121} |
| 9q31.2 | rs10816625 | | 0.06 | Overall | 1.11 | (1.07–1.15) | $5 \times 10^{-18}$ | {656,1559} |
| 9q31.2 | rs13294895 | | 0.18 | Overall | 1.06 | (1.03–1.08) | $6.5 \times 10^{-17}$ | {656,1559} |
| 9q31.2 | rs676256 | | 0.38 | Overall | 0.91 | (0.90–0.93) | $3.5 \times 10^{-53}$ | {656,1559} |
| 9q31.2 | rs10759243 | | 0.29 | Overall | 1.06 | (1.04–1.08) | $2.2 \times 10^{-18}$ | {1364} |
| 9q33.1 | rs1895062 | ASTN2 | 0.41 | Overall | 0.94 | (0.92–0.95) | $1.1 \times 10^{-14}$ | {1365} |
| 9q33.3 | rs10760444 | LMX1B | 0.43 | Overall | 1.03 | (1.02–1.05) | $9.1 \times 10^{-9}$ | {1365} |
| 9q34.2 | rs8176636 | ABO | 0.20 | Overall | 1.03 | (1.01–1.06) | $1.4 \times 10^{-8}$ | {1365} |
| 10p12.31 | rs7072776 | DNAJC1 | 0.29 | Overall | 1.05 | (1.03–1.07) | $1.8 \times 10^{-19}$ | {1364} |
| 10p12.31 | rs11814448 | DNAJC1 | 0.02 | Overall | 1.12 | (1.06–1.19) | $6.1 \times 10^{-18}$ | {1364} |
| 10p14 | rs67958007 | | 0.12 | Overall | 1.09 | (1.06–1.12) | $1.7 \times 10^{-10}$ | {1365} |
| 10p15.1 | rs2380205 | ANKRD16 | 0.44 | Overall | 0.98 | (0.96–0.99) | $1.7 \times 10^{-4}$ | {2121} |
| 10q21.2 | rs10995201 | ZNF365 | 0.16 | Overall | 0.90 | (0.88–0.92) | $1.6 \times 10^{-51}$ | {262,453} |
| 10q22.3 | rs704010 | ZMIZ1 | 0.38 | Overall | 1.07 | (1.05–1.09) | $1.7 \times 10^{-35}$ | {2121} |
| 10q23.33 | rs140936696 | | 0.18 | Overall | 1.04 | (1.02–1.07) | $4.2 \times 10^{-8}$ | {1365} |
| 10q25.2 | rs7904519 | TCF7L2 | 0.46 | Overall | 1.03 | (1.01–1.05) | $1.5 \times 10^{-13}$ | {1364} |
| 10q26.12 | rs11199914 | | 0.32 | Overall | 0.96 | (0.94–0.98) | $6.5 \times 10^{-12}$ | {1364} |
| 10q26.13 | rs2981578 | FGFR2 | 0.47 | Overall | 1.23 | (1.21–1.25) | $1.3 \times 10^{-245}$ | {561,1362} |
| 10q26.13 | rs35054928 | FGFR2 | 0.40 | Overall | 1.27 | (1.25–1.30) | $2.3 \times 10^{-322}$ | {561,1362} |
| 10q26.13 | rs45631563 | FGFR2 | 0.05 | Overall | 0.81 | (0.78–0.85) | $7.3 \times 10^{-37}$ | {561,1362} |
| 11p15 | rs6597981 | PIDD1 | 0.48 | Overall | 0.96 | (0.94–0.97) | $1.4 \times 10^{-12}$ | {1365} |
| 11p15.5 | rs3817198 | LSP1 | 0.32 | Overall | 1.05 | (1.03–1.07) | $9.9 \times 10^{-19}$ | {561} |
| 11q13.1 | rs3903072 | | 0.47 | Overall | 0.97 | (0.95–0.97) | $2.3 \times 10^{-12}$ | {1364} |
| 11q13.3 | rs554219 | CCND1 | 0.13 | ER+ | 1.21 | (1.18–1.24) | $5.8 \times 10^{-47}$ | {2121,681} |

CI, confidence interval; MAF, minor allele frequency; OR, odds ratio; SNP, single nucleotide polymorphism.

**Table 9.07** 172 low-risk loci associated with breast cancer (continued)

| Locus | Strongest associated SNP | Candidate causal gene | MAF | Breast cancer subtype | OR | 95% CI | P value from meta-analysis | Reference(s) |
|---|---|---|---|---|---|---|---|---|
| 11q13.3 | rs75915166 | CCND1 | 0.06 | ER+ | 1.28 | (1.24–1.33) | $4.1 \times 10^{-95}$ | {2121,681} |
| 11q24.3 | rs11820646 | | 0.40 | Overall | 0.96 | (0.94–0.98) | $2.1 \times 10^{-14}$ | {1364} |
| 12p11.22 | rs7297051 | | 0.24 | ER−/BRCA1 | 0.89 | (0.87–0.91) | $3 \times 10^{-60}$ | {404} |
| 12p13.1 | rs12422552 | | 0.26 | Overall | 1.06 | (1.04–1.08) | $3.6 \times 10^{-15}$ | {1364} |
| 12q21.31 | rs202049448 | | 0.34 | Overall | 0.95 | (0.93–0.97) | $2.7 \times 10^{-8}$ | {1365} |
| 12q22 | rs17356907 | NTN4 | 0.30 | Overall | 0.91 | (0.90–0.93) | $1 \times 10^{-39}$ | {1364} |
| 12q24.21 | rs1292011 | TBX3 | 0.42 | Overall | 0.92 | (0.90–0.94) | $4.4 \times 10^{-39}$ | {724} |
| 12q24.31 | rs206966 | | 0.16 | Overall | 1.05 | (1.02–1.07) | $3.8 \times 10^{-8}$ | {1365} |
| 13q13.1 | rs11571833 | BRCA2 | 0.01 | Overall | 1.35 | (1.23–1.48) | $3.1 \times 10^{-15}$ | {1364} |
| 13q22.1 | rs6562760 | | 0.24 | ER−/BRCA1 | 0.95 | (0.93–0.97) | $1.5 \times 10^{-9}$ | {404} |
| 14q13.3 | rs2236007 | PAX9 | 0.21 | Overall | 0.93 | (0.91–0.95) | $4.2 \times 10^{-21}$ | {1364} |
| 14q24.1 | rs999737 | RAD51B | 0.23 | Overall | 0.91 | (0.89–0.93) | $6.5 \times 10^{-39}$ | {2073} |
| 14q24.1 | rs2588809 | RAD51B | 0.17 | Overall | 1.06 | (1.03–1.08) | $6.3 \times 10^{-14}$ | {1364} |
| 14q32.11 | rs941764 | CCDC88C | 0.35 | Overall | 1.03 | (1.02–1.05) | $8.2 \times 10^{-13}$ | {1364} |
| 14q32.12 | rs11627032 | RIN3 | 0.25 | Overall | 0.96 | (0.94–0.98) | $4.1 \times 10^{-11}$ | {1363} |
| 14q32.33 | rs10623258 | ADSSL1 | 0.45 | Overall | 1.04 | (1.02–1.06) | $2.3 \times 10^{-8}$ | {1365} |
| 15q26.1 | rs2290203 | PRC1 | 0.21 | Overall | 0.94 | (0.92–0.96) | $8.07 \times 10^{-10}$ | {263} |
| 16q12.1 | rs4784227 | TOX3 | 0.24 | Overall | 1.23 | (1.20–1.25) | $6.8 \times 10^{-201}$ | {561,2125} |
| 16q12.2 | rs11075995 | FTO | 0.24 | Overall | 1.03 | (1.01–1.06) | $8.7 \times 10^{-9}$ | {699} |
| 16q12.2 | rs17817449 | FTO | 0.41 | Overall | 0.95 | (0.93–0.96) | $2.5 \times 10^{-21}$ | {1364} |
| 16q12.2 | rs28539243 | | 0.49 | Overall | 1.05 | (1.03–1.07) | $9.1 \times 10^{-15}$ | {1365} |
| 16q13 | rs2432539 | AMFR | 0.40 | Overall | 1.03 | (1.02–1.05) | $4.0 \times 10^{-8}$ | {1365} |
| 16q23.2 | rs13329835 | CDYL2 | 0.23 | Overall | 1.07 | (1.05–1.09) | $8.8 \times 10^{-27}$ | {1364} |
| 16q24.2 | rs4496150 | | 0.25 | Overall | 0.96 | (0.94–0.98) | $8.1 \times 10^{-9}$ | {1365} |
| 17q11.2 | rs146699004 | ATAD5 | 0.27 | Overall | 0.97 | (0.95–0.99) | $2 \times 10^{-9}$ | {1363} |
| 17q21.2 | rs72826962 | CNTNAP1 | 0.01 | Overall | 1.20 | (1.11–1.30) | $4.6 \times 10^{-9}$ | {1365} |
| 17q21.31 | rs2532263 | KANSL1 | 0.19 | Overall | 0.95 | (0.93–0.97) | $6.9 \times 10^{-13}$ | {1365} |
| 17q22 | rs2787486 | | 0.30 | Overall | 0.93 | (0.91–0.94) | $5.6 \times 10^{-29}$ | {19,452} |
| 17q25.3 | rs745570 | | 0.50 | Overall | 1.03 | (1.01–1.05) | $3.9 \times 10^{-10}$ | {1363} |
| 18q11.2 | rs527616 | | 0.38 | Overall | 0.97 | (0.95–0.98) | $6.7 \times 10^{-15}$ | {1364} |
| 18q11.2 | rs1436904 | CHST9 | 0.40 | Overall | 0.95 | (0.94–0.97) | $9.9 \times 10^{-15}$ | {1364} |
| 18q12.1 | rs117618124 | GAREM1 | 0.05 | Overall | 0.89 | (0.85–0.92) | $5.5 \times 10^{-12}$ | {1365} |
| 18q12.3 | rs6507583 | SETBP1 | 0.07 | Overall | 0.92 | (0.89–0.96) | $2.2 \times 10^{-12}$ | {1363} |
| 19p13.11 | rs67397200 | | 0.30 | BRCA1 | 1.03 | (1.01–1.05) | $1.6 \times 10^{-8}$ | {76,1120} |
| 19p13.11 | rs4808801 | ELL | 0.34 | Overall | 0.93 | (0.91–0.95) | $4.7 \times 10^{-28}$ | {1364} |
| 19p13.11 | rs2965183 | GATAD2A, MIR640 | 0.35 | Overall | 1.04 | (1.02–1.06) | $6.3 \times 10^{-12}$ | {1365} |
| 19p13.12 | rs2594714 | | 0.23 | Overall | 0.97 | (0.95–0.99) | $1.1 \times 10^{-8}$ | {1365} |
| 19p13.13 | rs78269692 | NFIX | 0.05 | Overall | 1.09 | (1.04–1.13) | $1.9 \times 10^{-9}$ | {1365} |
| 19q13.22 | rs71338792 | GIPR | 0.23 | Overall | 1.05 | (1.03–1.07) | $3.5 \times 10^{-9}$ | {1365} |
| 19q13.31 | rs3760982 | KCNN4/LYPD5 | 0.46 | Overall | 1.05 | (1.03–1.07) | $1.4 \times 10^{-16}$ | {1364} |
| 20p12.3 | rs16991615 | MCM8 | 0.06 | Overall | 1.10 | (1.06–1.14) | $1.9 \times 10^{-9}$ | {1365} |

CI, confidence interval; MAF, minor allele frequency; OR, odds ratio; SNP, single nucleotide polymorphism.

**Table 9.07** 172 low-risk loci associated with breast cancer (continued)

| Locus | Strongest associated SNP | Candidate causal gene | MAF | Breast cancer subtype | OR | 95% CI | *P* value from meta-analysis | Reference(s) |
|---|---|---|---|---|---|---|---|---|
| 20q11.22 | rs2284378 | *RALY* | 0.32 | Overall | 1.00 | (0.98–1.02) | $3.2 \times 10^{-2}$ | {1937} |
| 20q13.13 | rs6122906 | | 0.18 | Overall | 1.05 | (1.03–1.07) | $2.5 \times 10^{-10}$ | {1365} |
| 21q21.1 | rs2823093 | *NRIP1* | 0.27 | Overall | 0.94 | (0.92–0.96) | $1.5 \times 10^{-20}$ | {724} |
| 22q12.1 | rs17879961 | *CHEK2* | 0.01 | Overall | 1.26 | (1.11–1.42) | $9.7 \times 10^{-9}$ | {806,1364} |
| 22q12.2 | rs132390 | *EMID1* | 0.04 | Overall | 1.04 | (0.99–1.09) | $1.2 \times 10^{-8}$ | {1364} |
| 22q13.1 | chr22:39359355 | *APOBEC3A, APOBEC3B* | 0.10 | Overall | 1.10 | (1.07–1.14) | $4.9 \times 10^{-12}$ | {1233} |
| 22q13.1 | rs6001930 | *MRTFA (MKL1)* | 0.10 | Overall | 1.12 | (1.09–1.16) | $4.4 \times 10^{-34}$ | {1364} |
| 22q13.1 | rs738321 | *PLA2G6* | 0.38 | Overall | 0.95 | (0.93–0.97) | $1.0 \times 10^{-13}$ | {1365} |
| 22q13.2 | rs73161324 | *XRCC6* | 0.06 | Overall | 1.06 | (1.02–1.09) | $2.0 \times 10^{-9}$ | {1365} |
| 22q13.31 | rs28512361 | | 0.11 | Overall | 1.05 | (1.02–1.08) | $2.3 \times 10^{-8}$ | {1365} |

CI, confidence interval; MAF, minor allele frequency; OR, odds ratio; SNP, single nucleotide polymorphism.

# Contributors

**ALBARRACIN, Constance T.**
University of Texas
MD Anderson Cancer Center
1515 Holcombe Boulevard
Houston TX 77030
USA

**ALLISON, Kimberly H.**
Stanford University School of Medicine
300 Pasteur Drive
Stanford CA 94305-5324
USA

**ANTONESCU, Cristina R.**
Memorial Sloan Kettering Cancer Center
1275 York Avenue
New York NY 10065
USA

**ARENDS, Mark J.**
Cancer Research UK Edinburgh Centre
MRC Institute of Genetics & Molecular
Medicine
University of Edinburgh
Crewe Road South
Edinburgh EH4 2XR
UNITED KINGDOM

**BALDEWIJNS, Marcella**
University Hospital Leuven
Herestraat 49
3000 Leuven
BELGIUM

**BILLINGS, Steven D.**
Cleveland Clinic
9500 Euclid Avenue, L25
Cleveland OH 44195
USA

**BOULOS, Fouad**
American University of Beirut Medical Center
Cairo Street, 3rd Floor
Beirut 1107 2020
LEBANON

**BRENN, Thomas**
Cumming School of Medicine
University of Calgary
9-3535 Research Road North-West
Calgary AB T2L 2K8
CANADA

**BROGI, Edi***
Memorial Sloan Kettering Cancer Center
1275 York Avenue
New York NY 10065
USA

**BROSENS, Lodewijk A.A.**
University Medical Center Utrecht
Heidelberglaan 100
3584 CX Utrecht
NETHERLANDS

**BU, Hong**
West China Hospital, Sichuan University
Chengdu, Sichuan
Chengdu 610041
CHINA

**BUI, Marilyn**
Moffitt Cancer Center
12902 Magnolia Drive
Tampa FL 33612
USA

**CALHOUN, Benjamin C.**
University of North Carolina at Chapel Hill
160 North Medical Drive, Campus Box 7525
Chapel Hill NC 27599
USA

**CALONJE, Jaime E.**
St John's Institute of Dermatology
St Thomas' Hospital
Westminster Bridge Road
London SE1 7EH
UNITED KINGDOM

**CARNEIRO, Fátima**
Ipatimup/i3S
Rua Júlio Amaral de Carvalho 45
4200-135 Porto
PORTUGAL

**CARTER, Jodi M.**
Mayo Clinic
200 First Street South-West
Rochester MN 55905
USA

**CHAN, John K.C.**
Queen Elizabeth Hospital
30 Gascoigne Road
Kowloon, Hong Kong SAR
CHINA

**CHARVILLE, Gregory W.**
Stanford University School of Medicine
300 Pasteur Drive, Room L235
Stanford CA 94305
USA

**CHEN, Yunn-Yi**
University of California, San Francisco
1825 Fourth Street, M-2358
San Francisco CA 94143
USA

**CHENEVIX-TRENCH, Georgia**
QIMR Berghofer
300 Herston Road
Brisbane QLD 4006
AUSTRALIA

**CHENG, Chee Leong**
Singapore General Hospital
Pathology Department
Academia, Level 10, Diagnostics Tower
20 College Road
Singapore 169856
SINGAPORE

**CHEUNG, Annie Nga-Yin**
University of Hong Kong
Queen Mary Hospital
Pok Fu Lam Road
Hong Kong SAR
CHINA

**CIMINO-MATHEWS, Ashley**
Johns Hopkins University School of Medicine
401 North Broadway
Baltimore MD 21287
USA

**COLLINS, Laura C.**
Beth Israel Deaconess Medical Center
330 Brookline Avenue
Boston MA 02215
USA

**CREE, Ian A.**
International Agency for Research on Cancer
150 Cours Albert Thomas
69372 Lyon
FRANCE

**CREYTENS, David**
Department of Pathology
Ghent University Hospital, Ghent University
Corneel Heymanslaan 10
9000 Ghent
BELGIUM

**CSERNI, Gábor**
Bács-Kiskun County Teaching Hospital /
University of Szeged
Nyíri út 38
Kecskemét 6000
HUNGARY

* Indicates disclosure of interests (see p. 305).

D'ALFONSO, Timothy M.*
Memorial Sloan Kettering Cancer Center
1275 York Avenue
New York NY 10065
USA

DECKER, Thomas
Dietrich Bonhoeffer Medical Centre
Salvador-Allende-Straße 30
17036 Neubrandenburg
GERMANY

DENKERT, Carsten*
Institute of Pathology
Philipps-University Marburg
University Hospital Marburg (UKGM)
Baldingerstraße 1
35042 Marburg
GERMANY

DESMEDT, Christine
KU Leuven
Herestraat 49
3000 Leuven
BELGIUM

DOGAN, Ahmet
Memorial Sloan Kettering Cancer Center
1275 York Avenue
New York NY 10065
USA

ELLIS, Ian O.
University of Nottingham
Department of Histopathology
Nottingham City Hospital Campus
Nottingham University Hospitals
Hucknall Road
Nottingham NG7 1DD
UNITED KINGDOM

FELDMAN, Andrew L.*
Mayo Clinic College of Medicine and Science
200 First Street South-West
Rochester MN 55905
USA

FEND, Falko
Institute of Pathology
Tübingen University Hospital
Liebermeisterstraße 8
72076 Tübingen
GERMANY

FERRY, Judith A.
Massachusetts General Hospital
55 Fruit Street
Boston MA 02114
USA

FITZGIBBONS, Patrick L.
St. Jude Medical Center
101 East Valencia Mesa Drive
Fullerton CA 92835
USA

FLETCHER, Christopher D.M.
Brigham and Women's Hospital
75 Francis Street
Boston MA 02115
USA

FLUCKE, Uta
Radboudumc
Geert Grooteplein Zuid 10
6500 HB Nijmegen
NETHERLANDS

FOLPE, Andrew L.*
Mayo Clinic
200 First Street South-West
Rochester MN 55905
USA

FOSCHINI, Maria Pia*
Department of Biomedical and Neuromotor
Sciences
University of Bologna
Anatomic Pathology Bellaria Hospital
Via Altura 3
40139 Bologna BO
ITALY

FOX, Stephen B.*
Peter MacCallum Cancer Centre and
University of Melbourne
305 Grattan Street
Melbourne VIC 3000
AUSTRALIA

FRAYLING, Ian M.
Institute of Medical Genetics
University Hospital of Wales
Cardiff CF14 4XW
UNITED KINGDOM

FURUKAWA, Toru*
Tohoku University Graduate School of
Medicine
2-1 Seiryomachi, Aoba-ku
Sendai 980-8575
JAPAN

GATALICA, Zoran*
Caris Life Sciences
4610 South 44th Place
Phoenix AZ 85040
USA

GEYER, Felipe C.
Novartis Institutes for BioMedical Research
250 Massachusetts Avenue
Cambridge MA 02139
USA

GILL, Anthony J.
Royal North Shore Hospital
Pacific Highway
St Leonards NSW 2065
AUSTRALIA

GOBBI, Helenice
Institute of Health Sciences
Federal University of Triângulo Mineiro
Avenida Getúlio Guaritá 130
Uberaba MG 38025-440
BRAZIL

GOLDBLUM, John R.
Cleveland Clinic
9500 Euclid Avenue L25
Cleveland OH 44195
USA

HAHNEN, Eric*
University Hospital Cologne
Kerpener Straße 34
50931 Cologne
GERMANY

HARADA, Oi*
Showa University
1-5-8 Hatanodai, Shinagawa-ku
Tokyo 142-8666
JAPAN

HAYES, Malcolm M.
British Columbia Cancer Agency
600 West 10th Avenue
Vancouver BC V5Z 4E6
CANADA

HOLLESTELLE, Antoinette
Erasmus MC Cancer Institute
Doctor Molewaterplein 40
3015 CN Rotterdam
NETHERLANDS

HORII, Rie*
Cancer Institute Hospital
Japanese Foundation for Cancer Research
3-8-31 Ariake, Koto-ku
Tokyo 135-8550
JAPAN

HORLINGS, Hugo M.
Netherlands Cancer Institute
Plesmanlaan 121
1066 CX Amsterdam
NETHERLANDS

HORNICK, Jason L.*
Brigham and Women's Hospital
Harvard Medical School
75 Francis Street
Boston MA 02115
USA

---

* Indicates disclosure of interests (see p. 305).

HUNT, Kelly K.*
University of Texas
MD Anderson Cancer Center
1400 Pressler Street, Unit 1434
Houston TX 77030
USA

JAFFER, Shabnam M.
Mount Sinai
1 Gustave L. Levy Place
Department of Pathology, PO Box 1194
New York NY 10029
USA

JANSEN, Marnix*
University College London
21 University Street, Rockefeller Building
Room 410, Histopathology Department
London WC1E 6DE
UNITED KINGDOM

JO, Vickie Y.*
Brigham and Women's Hospital
Harvard Medical School
75 Francis Street
Boston MA 02115
USA

JONES, J. Louise
Barts Cancer Institute
Charterhouse Square
London EC1M 6BQ
UNITED KINGDOM

KARIM, Rooshdiya Z.
Royal Prince Alfred Hospital
Missenden Road, Camperdown
Sydney NSW 2050
AUSTRALIA

KHOO, Ui-Soon
University of Hong Kong
Queen Mary Hospital
Pok Fu Lam Road
Hong Kong SAR
CHINA

KING, Tari A.*
Brigham and Women's Hospital /
Dana-Farber Cancer Institute
450 Brookline Avenue
Boston MA 02215
USA

KOO, Ja Seung
Yonsei University College of Medicine
50 Yonsei-ro, Seodaemun-gu
Seoul 03722
REPUBLIC OF KOREA

KRINGS, Gregor
University of California, San Francisco
1825 Fourth Street, M-2355
San Francisco CA 94143
USA

KRISTIANSEN, Glen
Institute of Pathology
Sigmund-Freud-Straße 25
53127 Bonn
GERMANY

KULKA, Janina
Semmelweis University Budapest
Üllői út 93
Budapest 1091
HUNGARY

LAKHANI, Sunil R.*
University of Queensland and
Pathology Queensland
Royal Brisbane and Women's Hospital
Campus
Herston QLD 4029
AUSTRALIA

LAX, Sigurd F.*
General Hospital Graz II
Medical University of Graz
Göstinger Straße 22
8020 Graz
AUSTRIA

LAZAR, Alexander J.
University of Texas
MD Anderson Cancer Center
1515 Holcombe Boulevard, Unit 85
Houston TX 77030
USA

LEE, Andrew H.S.
Nottingham University Hospitals
City Hospital Campus
Hucknall Road
Nottingham NG5 1PB
UNITED KINGDOM

LEONCINI, Lorenzo
University of Siena
Department of Medical Biotechnology
Pathological Anatomy Division
Via dele Scotte
53100 Siena SI
ITALY

LERWILL, Melinda*
Massachusetts General Hospital
55 Fruit Street
Boston MA 02114
USA

LESTER, Susan C.
Brigham and Women's Hospital
Dana-Farber Cancer Institute
Harvard Medical School
75 Francis Street
Boston MA 02115
USA

LIEGL-ATZWANGER, Bernadette
Medical University of Graz
Neue Stiftingtalstraße 6
8010 Graz
AUSTRIA

LOKUHETTY, Dilani
International Agency for Research on Cancer
150 Cours Albert Thomas
69372 Lyon
FRANCE

MAC GROGAN, Gaëtan
Institut Bergonié
229 Cours de l'Argonne
33076 Bordeaux
FRANCE

MAGRO, Gaetano
University of Catania
Via Santa Sofia 87
95123 Catania CT
ITALY

MAHAR, Annabelle M.
Royal Prince Alfred Hospital
Missenden Road
Sydney NSW 2050
AUSTRALIA

MARCHIÒ, Caterina
Department of Medical Sciences
University of Turin /
Candiolo Cancer Institute - FPO, IRCCS
Strada Provinciale 142, km 3.95
10060 Candiolo TO
ITALY

MASUDA, Shinobu*
Nihon University School of Medicine
30-1 Ohyaguchikami-cho, Itabashi-ku
Tokyo 173-8610
JAPAN

McCART REED, Amy E.
University of Queensland
Building 71/918
Brisbane QLD 4029
AUSTRALIA

McHUGH, Jonathan B.
Michigan Medicine – University of Michigan
2800 Plymouth Road
Ann Arbor MI 48109
USA

* Indicates disclosure of interests (see p. 305).

MEDEIROS, L. Jeffrey
MD Anderson Cancer Center
1515 Holcombe Boulevard
Houston TX 77030
USA

MILLS, Anne M.
University of Virginia
1215 Lee Street, HEP 3rd Floor, Room 3001
Charlottesville VA 22908
USA

MIRANDA, Roberto N.*
University of Texas
MD Anderson Cancer Center
1515 Holcombe Boulevard
Houston TX 77030
USA

MOCH, Holger
University of Zurich and
University Hospital Zurich
12 Schmelzbergstrasse
8091 Zurich
SWITZERLAND

MORITANI, Suzuko
Shiga University of Medical Science
Setatsukinowa-cho
Otsu 520-2192
JAPAN

MORIYA, Takuya
Kawasaki Medical School
577 Matsushima
Kurashiki 701-0192
JAPAN

MORRIS, Elizabeth A.
Memorial Sloan Kettering Cancer Center
300 East 66th Street, Suite 723
New York NY 10065
USA

NIELSEN, Torsten O.*
University of British Columbia
Anatomical Pathology JPN 1401
Vancouver Hospital, 855 West 12th Avenue
Vancouver BC V5Z 1M9
CANADA

NISHIMURA, Rieko
National Hospital Organization
Nagoya Medical Center
4-1-1 Sannomaru, Naka-ku
Nagoya 460-0001
JAPAN

OCHIAI, Atsushi
National Cancer Center
6-5-1 Kashiwanoha
Kashiwa 277-8577
JAPAN

OLIVA, Esther
Massachusetts General Hospital
55 Fruit Street
Boston MA 02114
USA

OYAMA, Tetsunari
Gunma University Graduate School of
Medicine
3-39-22 Showa
Maebashi 371-8511
JAPAN

PALACIOS, José
Hospital Universitario Ramón y Cajal,
IRYCIS, CIBERONC
Carretera de Colmenar Viejo, km 9, 100
28034 Madrid
SPAIN

PAUWELS, Patrick
Universitair Ziekenhuis Antwerpen
Wilrijkstraat 10
2650 Edegem
BELGIUM

PENAULT-LLORCA, Frédérique*
Centre Jean Perrin
58 Rue Montalembert
63011 Clermont-Ferrand
FRANCE

PINDER, Sarah E.
King's College London
Innovation Hub, Guy's Cancer Centre
London SE1 9RT
UNITED KINGDOM

PIRIS, Miguel A.*
Fundación Jiménez Díaz
Avenida de los Reyes Católicos 4
28040 Madrid
SPAIN

PROVENZANO, Elena
Addenbrooke's Hospital
Hills Road
Cambridge CB2 0QQ
UNITED KINGDOM

PURDIE, Colin A.
NHS Tayside
Ninewells Hospital & Medical School
Dundee DD1 9SY
UNITED KINGDOM

RAKHA, Emad A.
University of Nottingham
80 Russell Drive
Nottingham NG8 2BE
UNITED KINGDOM

REIS-FILHO, Jorge S.*
Memorial Sloan Kettering Cancer Center
1275 York Avenue
New York NY 10065
USA

ROUS, Brian
Public Health England
Victoria House, Capital Park
Fulbourn, Cambridge CB21 XB
UNITED KINGDOM

ROWE, J. Jordi
Cleveland Clinic
9500 Euclid Avenue
Cleveland OH 44195
USA

SAHIN, Aysegul
University of Texas
MD Anderson Cancer Center
1515 Holcombe Boulevard
Houston TX 77005
USA

SALGADO, Roberto*
GZA-ZNA Hospitals
Lindendreef 1
2020 Antwerp
BELGIUM

SANDERS, Melinda E.
Vanderbilt University Medical Center
1301 Medical Center Drive, 4918A-TVC
Nashville TN 37232
USA

SAPINO, Anna
Candiolo Cancer Institute, FPO-IRCCS
Candiolo TO, ITALY, and
Department of Medical Sciences
University of Turin
ITALY

SASANO, Hironobu*
Tohoku University School of Medicine
2-1 Seiryou-machi, Aoba-ku
Sendai 980-8575
JAPAN

SCHMITT, Fernando
IPATIMUP and
Medical Faculty of Porto University
Rua Júlio Amaral de Carvalho 45
4200-135 Porto
PORTUGAL

SCHNITT, Stuart J.
Brigham and Women's Hospital /
Dana-Farber Cancer Institute
75 Francis Street
Boston MA 02115
USA

---

* Indicates disclosure of interests (see p. 305).

SCHOOLMEESTER, J. Kenneth
Mayo Clinic
200 First Street South-West
Rochester MN 55905
USA

SHAABAN, Abeer M.
Queen Elizabeth Hospital Birmingham and
University of Birmingham
Birmingham B15 2GW
UNITED KINGDOM

SHIN, Sandra J.
Albany Medical College
47 New Scotland Avenue
Albany NY 12208
USA

SILVA, Leonard
Grupo Oncoclínicas
Avenida Juscelino Kubitschek 510, 2° andar
Vila Nova Conceição
São Paulo SP 04532-002
BRAZIL

SIMPSON, Peter T.
University of Queensland
Royal Brisbane and Women's Hospital
Building 71/918
Brisbane QLD 4029
AUSTRALIA

SINGH, Rajendra
Icahn School of Medicine at Mount Sinai
1 Gustave L. Levy Place
New York NY 10029
USA

SOARES, Fernando Augusto
Rede D'Or Hospitals
Rua das Perobas 266
São Paulo SP 04120-080
BRAZIL

SORENSEN, Poul H.B.
University of British Columbia
675 West 10th Avenue, Room 4112
Vancouver BC V5Z 1L3
CANADA

SOTIRIOU, Christos
Institut Jules Bordet (Université Libre de
Bruxelles)
Rue Héger-Bordet 1
1000 Brussels
BELGIUM

SOUTHEY, Melissa C.
Monash University
246 Clayton Road, Clayton
Melbourne VIC 3168
AUSTRALIA

SRIGLEY, John R.
Trillium Health Partners
Credit Valley Hospital Site
2200 Eglinton Avenue West
Mississauga ON L5M 2N1
CANADA

TAN, Benjamin Yongcheng
Department of Anatomical Pathology
Singapore General Hospital
Academia, Level 10, Diagnostics Tower
Singapore 169856
SINGAPORE

TAN, Puay Hoon*
Singapore General Hospital
20 College Road
Academia, Level 7, Diagnostics Tower
Singapore 169856
SINGAPORE

TAY, Timothy Kwang Yong
Singapore General Hospital
20 College Road
Academia, Level 10, Diagnostics Tower
Department of Anatomical Pathology
Singapore 169856
SINGAPORE

THIKE, Aye Aye
Singapore General Hospital
20 College Road
Academia, Diagnostics Tower
Singapore 169856
SINGAPORE

THOMPSON, Lester D.R.
Woodland Hills Medical Center
5601 De Soto Avenue
Woodland Hills CA 91365
USA

THWAY, Khin
Royal Marsden Hospital /
Institute of Cancer Research
203 Fulham Road
London SW3 6JJ
UNITED KINGDOM

TROXELL, Megan L.*
Stanford University School of Medicine
300 Pasteur Drive, L235
Stanford CA 94305
USA

TSAO, Ming S.*
University Health Network
200 Elizabeth Street, 11th Floor
Toronto ON M5G 2C4
CANADA

TSE, Gary
Prince of Wales Hospital
Ngan Shing Street
Hong Kong SAR
CHINA

TSUDA, Hitoshi*
National Defense Medical College Japan
3-2 Namiki
Tokorozawa 359-8513
JAPAN

TSUZUKI, Toyonori
Aichi Medical University Hospital
1-1 Yazakokarimata
Nagakute 480-1195
JAPAN

VAL-BERNAL, José Fernando
Pathology Unit
Department of Medical and Surgical Sciences
University of Cantabria
Avenida Cardenal Herrera Oria s/n
39011 Santander
SPAIN

VAN DE RIJN, Matt
Stanford University Medical Center
1291 Welch Road
Stanford CA 94305-5324
USA

VAN DEURZEN, Carolien H.M.
Erasmus MC Cancer Institute
PO Box 2040
3000 CA Rotterdam
NETHERLANDS

VAN DIEST, Paul J.
University Medical Center Utrecht
PO Box 85500
3508 GA Utrecht
NETHERLANDS

VARGA, Zsuzsanna
University Hospital Zurich
Institute of Pathology and Molecular
Pathology
12 Schmelzbergstrasse
8091 Zurich
SWITZERLAND

VINCENT-SALOMON, Anne
Institut Curie
25 Rue d'Ulm
75005 Paris
FRANCE

VISSCHER, Daniel W.
Mayo Clinic
200 First Street South-West
Rochester MN 55905
USA

---

* Indicates disclosure of interests (see p. 305).

**VRANIC, Semir**
Qatar University
Al Jamiaa Street, PO Box 2713
Doha
QATAR

**WAITZBERG, Angela Flávia Logullo**
EPM-UNIFESP - Federal University of São
Paulo
Rua Itajubá 64, Pacaembu
São Paulo SP 01249-020
BRAZIL

**WASHINGTON, Mary K.**
Vanderbilt University Medical Center
C-3321 MCN
Nashville TN 37232
USA

**WEAVER, Donald L.**
University of Vermont
89 Beaumont Avenue
Burlington VT 05405-0068
USA

**WEIGELT, Britta***
Memorial Sloan Kettering Cancer Center
1275 York Avenue
New York NY 10065
USA

**WEN, Hannah Y.**
Memorial Sloan Kettering Cancer Center
1275 York Avenue
New York NY 10065
USA

**WESSELING, Jelle**
Netherlands Cancer Institute
Plesmanlaan 121
1066 CX Amsterdam
NETHERLANDS

**WU, Yun**
University of Texas
MD Anderson Cancer Center
1515 Holcombe Boulevard
Houston TX 77030
USA

**YAMAGUCHI, Rin***
Kurume University Medical Center
155-1 Kokubu
Kurume 839-0863
JAPAN

**YANG, Wen-Tao**
Fudan University Shanghai Cancer Center
270 Dong An Road
Shanghai 200032
CHINA

---

\* Indicates disclosure of interests (see p. 305).

# Declaration of interests

Dr **Brogi** reports holding intellectual property rights to *Rosen's Breast Pathology* (2014) and *Rosen's Diagnosis of Breast Pathology by Needle Core Biopsy* (2016) in her capacity as associate editor at Wolters Kluwer Lippincott.

Dr **D'Alfonso** reports receiving personal consultancy fees from Paige.AI.

Dr **Denkert** reports receiving personal consultancy fees from Daiichi and Roche, that his unit at Charité University Hospital benefits from research funding from Cepheid, being a cofounder and shareholder of EndoPredict Assay from Sividon Diagnostics, holding patent PCT/EP2015/052081 together with Sividon Diagnostics, and holding intellectual property rights to software for image analysis together with VMScope.

Dr **Feldman** reports that Mayo Clinic holds patents U.S. 8.679.743 and U.S. 9.677.137, on which he is a named inventor.

Dr **Folpe** reports receiving personal consultancy fees from Ultragenyx.

Dr **Foschini** reports having received personal consultancy fees from Biocartis and benefiting from research funding from Roche and Devicor Mammotome.

Dr **Fox** reports having received research funding and/or in-kind support from MSD, Bristol-Myers Squibb, AstraZeneca, Amgen, Biocartis, and Roche and that the Peter MacCallum Cancer Centre has received his consultancy fees from Roche, Pfizer, Novartis, AstraZeneca, Bristol-Myers Squibb, and MSD.

Dr **Furukawa** reports having benefited from research funding from AstraZeneca.

Dr **Gatalica** reports holding stocks and several patents in his capacity as executive medical director at Caris Life Sciences.

Dr **Hahnen** reports having received personal consultancy fees and benefiting from research funding from AstraZeneca.

Dr **Harada** reports being an external advisory consultant for Philips Digital Pathology Solutions Japan.

Dr **Horii** reports that his unit at the Cancer Institute Hospital benefits from research funding from Ventana Medical Systems.

Dr **Hornick** reports receiving personal consultancy fees from Epizyme and Eli Lilly.

Dr **Hunt** reports receiving personal consultancy fees from ArmadaHealth and that her unit at MD Anderson Cancer Center benefits from research funding from Endomag.

Dr **Jansen** reports benefiting from research funding from Rosetrees Trust and the Engineering and Physical Sciences Research Council (EPSRC).

Dr **Jo** reports that her spouse is an employee of Merck & Co., for which he receives a salary and stock options.

Dr **King** reports receiving speaker fees from Genomic Health.

Dr **Lakhani** reports receiving personal consultancy fees from Sullivan Nicolaides Pathology and educational funding from Roche and Ventana Medical Systems.

Dr **Lax** reports having received personal consultancy fees from Roche, AstraZeneca, Novartis, and Biomedica in his role as a scientific advisory board member.

Dr **Lerwill** reports having provided expert opinion in a medical malpractice case concerning a breast cancer diagnosis.

Dr **Masuda** reports that her unit at Nihon University School of Medicine benefited from research funding from Chugai Pharmaceutical Co.

Dr **Miranda** reports having received personal consultancy fees from Allergan in his capacity as a scientific advisory board member.

Dr **Nielsen** reports receiving personal consultancy fees and having benefited from research support from NanoString Technologics, benefiting from research support from Novartis and Epizyme, and holding a patent licensed to NanoString Technologies developed in collaboration with Bioclassifier LLC.

Dr **Penault-Llorca** reports that she and her unit at Centre Jean Perrin receive consultancy fees from Roche and that her unit benefits from research funding from Roche, AstraZeneca, Bristol-Myers Squibb, and MSD.

Dr **Piris** reports receiving personal consultancy fees from Celgene, Gilead Sciences, Janssen, Kyowa Kirin, NanoString Technologies, and Takeda in his capacity as a scientific advisory board member. He also reports receiving other personal consultancy fees from Janssen and Takeda, as well as research funding from Gilead Sciences, Kura Oncology, and Millennium/Takeda.

Dr **Reis-Filho** reports receiving personal consultancy fees from Goldman Sachs, as well as from VolitionRx and Paige.AI in his capacity as a scientific advisory board member.

Dr **Salgado** reports receiving research funding from Roche/Genentech, Merck, and Puma; receiving personal consultancy fees from Roche/Genentech; and benefiting from support for travel and congress registration from Roche/Genentech, AstraZeneca, and Merck.

Dr **Sasano** reports receiving honoraria from Pfizer Oncology, Novartis Oncology, and Teijin Medical.

Dr **P.H. Tan** reports holding patents on "breast fibroadenoma susceptibility mutations and use thereof" and "method and kit for pathologic grading of breast neoplasm".

Dr **Troxell** reports having received support from Ventana Roche in the capacity of invited speaker.

Dr **Tsao** reports that his institute receives research funding from Pfizer, Merck, and AstraZeneca. He also reports receiving personal consultancy fees from Merck, AstraZeneca, Bristol-Myers Squibb, Pfizer, Takeda, Bayer, and Hoffmann-La Roche.

Dr **Tsuda** reports that his unit at National Defense Medical College Japan benefits from research funding from Chugai Pharmaceutical Co. and Taiho Pharmaceutical Co.

Dr **Weigelt** reports that her spouse receives personal consultancy fees from Goldman Sachs, as well as from VolitionRx and Paige.AI in his capacity as a scientific advisory board member. She also reports having received research funding from Basser Center, Kaleidoscope of Hope Ovarian Cancer Foundation, and Cycle for Survival.

Dr **Yamaguchi** reports that Kurume University receives research support from Chugai Pharmaceutical Co.

# IARC/WHO Committee for the International Classification of Diseases for Oncology (ICD-O)

CREE, Ian A.
International Agency for Research on Cancer
150 Cours Albert Thomas
69372 Lyon
FRANCE

FERLAY, Jacques
International Agency for Research on Cancer
150 Cours Albert Thomas
69372 Lyon
FRANCE

JAKOB, Robert
Data Standards and Informatics
World Health Organization (WHO)
20 Avenue Appia
1211 Geneva
SWITZERLAND

ROUS, Brian
Public Health England
Victoria House, Capital Park
Fulbourn, Cambridge CB21 XB
UNITED KINGDOM

WATANABE, Reiko
National Cancer Center Hospital East
6-5-1 Kashiwanoha, Kashiwa-shi
Chiba 277-8577
JAPAN

WHITE, Valerie A.
International Agency for Research on Cancer
150 Cours Albert Thomas
69372 Lyon
FRANCE

ZNAOR, Ariana
International Agency for Research on Cancer
150 Cours Albert Thomas
69372 Lyon
FRANCE

# Sources

### TNM staging tables

## Figures

| | | | | | |
|---|---|---|---|---|---|
| 2.01A,B | Schnitt SJ | 2.24A,B | Moritani S | 2.56 | Mac Grogan G |
| 2.02A,B | Schnitt SJ | 2.25A,B | Tan PH | 2.57A,B | Mac Grogan G |
| 2.03A,B | Tan PH | 2.26 | Moritani S | 2.58A–D | Chen YY |
| 2.04A,B | Tan PH | 2.27A,B | Moritani S | 2.59 | Chen YY |
| 2.05A,B | Allison KH | 2.28A,B | Hayes MM | 2.60A,B | Chen YY |
| 2.06 | Allison KH | 2.29A,B | Foschini MP | 2.61A,B | Chen YY |
| 2.07A,B | Allison KH | 2.30A | Hayes MM | 2.62A,B | Chen YY |
| 2.08 | Allison KH | 2.30B | Nishimura R | 2.63A,B | Pinder SE |
| 2.09A,B | Allison KH | 2.31 | Foschini MP | 2.64 | Pinder SE |
| 2.10A–C | Allison KH | 2.32A,B | Tan PH | 2.65A,B | Pinder SE |
| 2.11A–D | Allison KH | 2.33A–C | Hayes MM | 2.66A,B | Pinder SE |
| 2.12A–C | Sahin A | 2.34A–C | Hayes MM | 2.67 | Pinder SE |
| 2.13A,B | Sahin A | 2.35A,B | Horii R | 2.68A,B | Pinder SE |
| 2.14A,B | Sahin A | 2.36 | Troxell ML | 2.69 | Pinder SE |
| 2.15A,B | Sahin A | 2.37A–C | Troxell ML | 2.70A–C | Pinder SE |
| 2.16A | Moritani S | 2.38A–C | Yamaguchi R | 2.71 | Pinder SE |
| 2.16B | Waitzberg AFL | 2.39A,B | © Ichihara S Lakhani SR, Ellis IO, Schnitt SJ, et al., editors. WHO classification of tumours of the breast. Lyon (France): International Agency for Research on Cancer; 2012. (WHO classification of tumours series, 4th ed.; vol. 4). http://publications.iarc.fr/14. | 2.72 | Ferlay J, Ervik M, Lam F, et al. Global Cancer Observatory: Cancer Today [Internet]. Lyon (France): International Agency for Research on Cancer; 2018 [accessed 2019 Feb]. Available from: https://gco.iarc.fr/today. |
| 2.16C | © Drijkoningen M Lakhani SR, Ellis IO, Schnitt SJ, et al., editors. WHO classification of tumours of the breast. Lyon (France): International Agency for Research on Cancer; 2012. (WHO classification of tumours series, 4th ed.; vol. 4). http://publications.iarc.fr/14. | | | 2.73 | Thompson LDR |
| | | 2.40A–D | Troxell ML | 2.74 | © Wilson R Lakhani SR, Ellis IO, Schnitt SJ, et al., editors. WHO classification of tumours of the breast. Lyon (France): International Agency for Research on Cancer; 2012. (WHO classification of tumours series, 4th ed.; vol. 4). http://publications.iarc.fr/14. |
| | | 2.41A,B | Brogi E | | |
| | | 2.42 | Brogi E | | |
| | | 2.43A–C | Brogi E | | |
| | | 2.44A–C | Brogi E | | |
| 2.16D | Schnitt SJ | 2.45A,B | Troxell ML | | |
| 2.17A,B | Moritani S | 2.46A,B | Troxell ML | | |
| 2.17C | van Diest PJ | 2.47 | Brogi E | | |
| 2.18A–D | Sahin A | 2.48A,B | Mac Grogan G | | |
| 2.19A,B | Sahin A | 2.49A–C | Mac Grogan G | | |
| 2.20 | Chan JKC | 2.50A,B | Mac Grogan G | | |
| 2.21A,B | Gary J. Whitman, Breast Imaging and Radiation Oncology, University of Texas MD Anderson Cancer Center, Houston TX, USA | 2.51A,B | Mac Grogan G | 2.75 | Tsuda H |
| | | 2.52A,B | Mac Grogan G | 2.76A | Rakha EA |
| | | 2.53 | Mac Grogan G | 2.76B | Tsuda H |
| | | 2.54A,B | Mac Grogan G | 2.77 | Allison KH |
| 2.22A–C | Sahin A | 2.55 | Mac Grogan G | 2.78 | Allison KH |
| 2.23A–C | Sahin A | | | 2.79 | Allison KH |
| | | | | 2.80 | Allison KH |

| | |
|---|---|
| 2.81 | Allison KH |
| 2.82 | Allison KH |
| 2.83 | Allison KH |
| 2.84 | Allison KH |
| 2.85A,B | Rakha EA |
| 2.86A–D | © Dabbs D<br>Lakhani SR, Ellis IO, Schnitt SJ, et al., editors. WHO classification of tumours of the breast. Lyon (France): International Agency for Research on Cancer; 2012. (WHO classification of tumours series, 4th ed.; vol. 4). http://publications.iarc.fr/14. |
| 2.87A,B | Tan PH |
| 2.88 | Sotiriou C |
| 2.89A–D | Horii R |
| 2.90A–D | Horii R |
| 2.91A–C | Rakha EA |
| 2.92A,B | Vincent-Salomon A |
| 2.93 | Rakha EA |
| 2.94A–C | Allison KH |
| 2.95A,B | Allison KH |
| 2.96A,B | Allison KH |
| 2.97 | Allison KH |
| 2.98 | Allison KH |
| 2.99A,B | Tan PH |
| 2.100A–C | Foschini MP |
| 2.101A–C | Yang WT |
| 2.102A–C | Yang WT |
| 2.103A,B | Huaye Ding, Seventh Medical Center of the Chinese PLA General Hospital, Beijing, China |
| 2.104 | Rakha EA |
| 2.105 | Cserni G |
| 2.106A,B | Koo JS |
| 2.107 | Koo JS |
| 2.108A–C | Cserni G |
| 2.109 | Koo JS |
| 2.110 | Koo JS |
| 2.111A,B | © Tabár L<br>Lakhani SR, Ellis IO, Schnitt SJ, et al., editors. WHO classification of tumours of the breast. Lyon (France): International Agency for Research on Cancer; 2012. (WHO classification of tumours series, 4th ed.; vol. 4). http://publications.iarc.fr/14. |
| 2.112 | © Sastre-Garau X<br>Lakhani SR, Ellis IO, Schnitt SJ, et al., editors. WHO classification of tumours of the breast. Lyon (France): International Agency for Research on Cancer; 2012. (WHO classification of tumours series, 4th ed.; vol. 4). http://publications.iarc.fr/14. |
| 2.113 | D'Alfonso TM |
| 2.114 | Chen YY |
| 2.115A,B | Chan JKC |
| 2.116A,B | Chen YY |
| 2.117 | Shin SJ |
| 2.118A–C | Shin SJ |
| 2.119 | © Tabár L<br>Lakhani SR, Ellis IO, Schnitt SJ, et al., editors. WHO classification of tumours of the breast. Lyon (France): International Agency for Research on Cancer; 2012. (WHO classification of tumours series, 4th ed.; vol. 4). http://publications.iarc.fr/14. |
| 2.120A,B | van Deurzen CHM |
| 2.121A–C | Purdie CA |
| 2.122 | Wen HY |
| 2.123 | Wen HY |
| 2.124A,B | Wen HY |
| 2.125A,B | Wen HY |
| 2.126A–C | Brogi E |
| 2.127A,B | Wen HY |
| 2.128 | Brogi E |
| 2.129 | Brogi E |
| 2.130A,B | Vincent-Salomon A |
| 2.131A | Marchiò C |
| 2.131B,C | Dara S. Ross, Department of Pathology, Memorial Sloan Kettering Cancer Center, New York NY, USA |
| 2.132A | Vranic S |
| 2.132B | Provenzano E |
| 2.133A,B | Rakha EA |
| 2.134 | Rakha EA |
| 2.135A–D | Rakha EA |
| 2.136A,B | Foschini MP |
| 2.137 | Nishimura R |
| 2.138A,B | Foschini MP |
| 2.139A–C | Foschini MP |
| 2.140A–D | Foschini MP |
| 2.141 | Nishimura R |
| 2.142A–C | Hayes MM |
| 2.143 | Adapted, with permission, from: Triche TJ, Hicks MJ, Sorensen PH. Diagnostic pathology of pediatric malignancies. In: Pizzo PA, Poplack DG, editors. Principles and practice of pediatric oncology. 7th ed. Alphen aan den Rijn (Netherlands): Wolters Kluwer Health; 2016. pp. 131–84. Copyright Wolters Kluwer Health. |
| 2.144A–D | Krings G |
| 2.145 | Krings G |
| 2.146 | Krings G |
| 2.147A–D | Foschini MP |
| 2.148A–C | Foschini MP |
| 2.149A,B | Guido Ficarra, Clinical Pathology, Policlinico di Modena, Modena, Italy |
| 2.150 | Foschini MP |
| 2.151A,B | Yang WT |
| 2.152A,B | Yang WT |
| 2.152C | Foschini MP |
| 2.153A,B | Wu Y |
| 2.154A,B | Sapino A |
| 2.155A–C | Wu Y |
| 2.156A,B | Brogi E |
| 2.157 | Brogi E |
| 3.01 | Koo JS |
| 3.02A,B | Tan PH |
| 3.03 | Tse G |
| 3.04A | Thike AA |
| 3.04B | Tan PH |
| 3.05A,B | Tse G |
| 3.06 | Tan PH |
| 3.07A,B | Tse G |
| 3.08A–C | Thike AA |
| 3.08D | Tan PH |
| 3.09 | Mihir Gudi, Department of Pathology and Laboratory Medicine, KK Women's and Children's Hospital, Singapore |
| 3.10 | Thompson LDR |
| 3.11A,C | Tse G |
| 3.11B | Tan PH |
| 3.12 | Tse G |
| 3.13 | Tan PH |
| 3.14 | Tan PH |
| 3.15 | Tan PH |
| 3.16 | Tse G |
| 3.17 | Thike AA |
| 3.18 | Tan PH |
| 4.02A,B | Lester SC |
| 4.03 | Lester SC |
| 4.04 | Lester SC |
| 4.05 | Albarracin CT |
| 4.06A–C | Albarracin CT |
| 4.07 | Albarracin CT |
| 5.01A | Alfonso Vega, Santander, Spain |
| 5.01B | Val-Bernal JF |
| 5.02 | Val-Bernal JF |
| 5.03A,B | Val-Bernal JF |
| 5.04A,B | Schnitt SJ |
| 5.05A,B | Schnitt SJ |
| 5.06A,B | Brenn T |
| 5.07A,B | Brenn T |
| 5.08 | Antonescu CR |
| 5.09A,C,D | Billings SD |
| 5.09B | Antonescu CR |
| 5.10 | Billings SD |
| 5.11 | Antonescu CR |
| 5.12A–D | Antonescu CR |
| 5.13 | Karim RZ |
| 5.14A–D | Karim RZ |
| 5.15A–D | Magro G |
| 5.16A–C | Magro G |
| 5.17A,B | Charville GW |
| 5.18A,B | Charville GW |
| 5.19A,B | Charville GW |
| 5.20A,B | Hornick JL |
| 5.21 | Hornick JL |
| 5.22 | Lester Leong, Department of Diagnostic Radiology, Singapore General Hospital, Singapore |
| 5.23A,B | Cimino-Mathews A |
| 5.24 | Cimino-Mathews A |
| 5.25A–C | Cimino-Mathews A |
| 5.26A–C | Bui M |
| 5.27A,B | Creytens D |
| 5.28A–C | Jo VY |
| 5.29 | Nielsen TO |
| 5.30A,B | Nielsen TO |
| 5.31 | Folpe AL |
| 5.32 | Folpe AL |
| 5.33 | Folpe AL |
| 5.34 | Folpe AL |
| 5.35 | D'Alfonso TM |
| 5.36A,D | Rowe JJ |
| 5.36B | Tan PH |
| 5.36C | D'Alfonso TM |

| | |
|---|---|
| 5.37A,B | Tan PH |
| 5.38 | D'Alfonso TM |
| | |
| 6.01A,B | Chan JKC |
| 6.02 | Chan JKC |
| 6.03A–C | Ferry JA |
| 6.04A–C | Ferry JA |
| 6.04D | Cheng CL |
| 6.05A–D | Dogan A |
| 6.06A–C | Medeiros LJ |
| 6.07 | Medeiros LJ |
| 6.08 | © Jaffe ES<br>Lakhani SR, Ellis IO, Schnitt SJ, et al., editors. WHO classification of tumours of the breast. Lyon (France): International Agency for Research on Cancer; 2012. (WHO classification of tumours series, 4th ed., vol. 4). http://publications.iarc.fr/14. |
| 6.09A | Chan JKC |
| 6.09B,C | Dogan A |
| 6.10A–E | Dogan A |
| 6.11 | Adapted, with kind permission, from: Thompson PA, Lade S, Webster H, et al. Effusion-associated anaplastic large cell lymphoma of the breast: time for it to be defined as a distinct clinico-pathological entity. Haematologica. 2010 Nov;95(11):1977–9. PMID:20801901.<br>and<br>FDA. U.S. Food & Drug Administration [Internet]. Silver Spring (MD): FDA; 2011. Anaplastic large cell lymphoma (ALCL) in |

| | |
|---|---|
| | women with breast implants: preliminary FDA findings and analyses; updated 2017 Mar 21. Available from: http://wayback.archive-it.org/7993/20171115053750/https://www.fda.gov/MedicalDevices/ProductsandMedicalProcedures/ImplantsandProsthetics/BreastImplants/ucm239996.htm |
| 6.12 | Miranda RN |
| 6.13A,B | Miranda RN |
| 6.14A,B | Miranda RN |
| 6.15A,B | Miranda RN |
| 6.16A | Miranda RN |
| 6.16B | Feldman AL |
| 6.17A,B | Miranda RN |
| 6.18A,B | Miranda RN |
| | |
| 7.01A | Chan JKC |
| 7.01B,C | Shaaban AM |
| 7.02A–C | Chan JKC |
| 7.03 | Shaaban AM |
| 7.04 | Shaaban AM |
| 7.05 | Shaaban AM |
| 7.06 | Foschini MP |
| 7.07A–C | Shaaban AM |
| 7.08A,B | Shaaban AM |
| 7.08C | Foschini MP |
| | |
| 8.01A,B | Kulka J |
| 8.02A,B | Kulka J |
| 8.03 | Kulka J |
| 8.04A,B | Kulka J |
| 8.05A,B | Kulka J |

| | |
|---|---|
| 9.01 | Adapted, with permission from Springer Nature, from: van der Groep P, van der Wall E, van Diest PJ. Pathology of hereditary breast cancer. Cell Oncol (Dordr). 2011 Apr;34(2):71–88. PMID:21336636. Copyright 2011. |
| 9.02A–C | Shaaban AM |
| 9.03A,B | Mills AM |
| 9.04 | Adapted from: IARC TP53 Database [Internet]. Lyon (France): International Agency for Research on Cancer; 2018. Version R19, August 2018. Available from: http://p53.iarc.fr/. |
| 9.05 | Adapted from: IARC TP53 Database [Internet]. Lyon (France): International Agency for Research on Cancer; 2018. Version R19, August 2018. Available from: http://p53.iarc.fr/. |
| 9.06 | Adapted from: IARC TP53 Database [Internet]. Lyon (France): International Agency for Research on Cancer; 2018. Version R19, August 2018. Available from: http://p53.iarc.fr/. |
| 9.07A,B | Provenzano E |
| 9.08 | Carneiro F |

## Tables

| | |
|---|---|
| 1.01 | Adapted, with permission, from: Lakhani SR, Ellis IO, Schnitt SJ, et al., editors. WHO classification of tumours of the breast. Lyon (France): International Agency for Research on Cancer; 2012. (WHO classification of tumours series, 4th ed.; vol. 4). http://publications.iarc.fr/14. |
| 2.01 | Tan PH |
| 2.02 | Brogi E |
| 2.03 | Adapted from: Lakhani SR, Ellis IO, Schnitt SJ, et al., editors. WHO classification of tumours of the breast. Lyon (France): International Agency for Research on Cancer; 2012. (WHO classification of tumours series, 4th ed.; vol. 4). http://publications.iarc.fr/14. |
| 2.04 | Adapted from: Lakhani SR, Ellis IO, Schnitt SJ, et al., editors. WHO classification of tumours of the breast. Lyon (France): International Agency for Research on Cancer; 2012. (WHO classification of tumours series, 4th ed.; vol. 4). http://publications.iarc.fr/14. |
| 2.06 | Lakhani SR, Ellis IO, Schnitt SJ, et al., editors. WHO classification of tumours of the breast. Lyon (France): International Agency for Research on Cancer; 2012. (WHO classification of tumours series, 4th ed.; vol. 4). http://publications.iarc.fr/14. Adapted, with permission, from Elston CW, Ellis IO. Pathological prognostic factors in breast cancer. I. The value of histological grade in breast cancer: experience from a large study with long-term follow-up. Histopathology. 1991 Nov;19(5):403–10. PMID:1757079. |
| 2.07 | Allison KH |
| 2.08 | Adapted, with permission, from: Brandão M, Pondé N, Piccart-Gebhart M. Mammaprint™: a comprehensive review. Future Oncol. 2019 Jan;15(2):207–24. PMID:30156427. |
| 2.09 | Lokuhetty D |
| 3.01 | Adapted from: Lakhani SR, Ellis IO, Schnitt SJ, et al., editors. WHO classification of tumours of the breast. Lyon |

(France): International Agency for Research on Cancer; 2012. (WHO classification of tumours series, 4th ed.; vol. 4). http://publications.iarc.fr/14.

| | |
|---|---|
| 7.01 | Foschini MP |
| 8.01 | Varga Z |
| 9.02 | Adapted from: a presentation by van Diest PJ |
| 9.03 | Adapted from: a presentation by van Diest PJ |
| 9.05 | WHO Classification of Tumours Editorial Board. Digestive system tumours. Lyon (France): International Agency for Research on Cancer; 2019. (WHO classification of tumours series, 5th ed.; vol. 1). http://publications.iarc.fr/579. |
| 9.06 | Frayling IM |
| 9.07 | Adapted from: Lilyquist J, Ruddy KJ, Vachon CM, et al. Common genetic variation and breast cancer risk-past, present, and future. Cancer Epidemiol Biomarkers Prev. 2018 Apr;27(4):380–94. PMID:29382703. |

## Boxes

| | |
|---|---|
| 2.01 | Adapted, with permission, from: Goldhirsch A, Winer EP, Coates AS, et al. Personalizing the treatment of women with early breast cancer: highlights of the St Gallen International Expert Consensus on the Primary Therapy of Early Breast Cancer 2013. Ann Oncol. 2013 Sep;24(9):2206–23. PMID:23917950. |
| 5.01 | Magro G |
| 9.01 | Reprinted, with permission from Elsevier, from: Tan MH, Mester J, Peterson C, et al. A clinical scoring system for selection of patients for PTEN mutation testing is proposed on the basis of a prospective study of 3042 probands. Am J Hum Genet. 2011 Jan 7;88(1):42–56. PMID:21194675. Copyright 2011. |
| 9.03 | Reprinted, with permission, from: Vogel WH. Li-Fraumeni syndrome. J Adv Pract Oncol. 2017 Nov-Dec;8(7):742–6. PMID:30333936. |
| 9.04 | WHO Classification of Tumours Editorial Board. Digestive system tumours. |

Lyon (France): International Agency for Research on Cancer; 2019. (WHO classification of tumours series, 5th ed.; vol. 1). http://publications.iarc.fr/579.

## Images on the cover

| | |
|---|---|
| Top left | Fig. 2.21A: Gary J. Whitman, Breast Imaging and Radiation Oncology, University of Texas MD Anderson Cancer Center, Houston TX, USA |
| Top centre | Fig. 2.47: Brogi E |
| Top right | Fig. 6.11: Adapted, with kind permission, from: Thompson PA, Lade S, Webster H, et al. Effusion-associated anaplastic large cell lymphoma of the breast: time for it to be defined as a distinct clinico-pathological entity. Haematologica. 2010 Nov;95(11):1977–9. PMID:20801901. and FDA. U.S. Food & Drug Administration [Internet]. Silver Spring (MD): FDA; 2011. Anaplastic large cell lymphoma (ALCL) in women with breast implants: preliminary FDA findings and analyses; updated 2017 Mar 21. Available from: http://wayback.archive-it.org/7993/20171115053750/https://www.fda.gov/MedicalDevices/ProductsandMedicalProcedures/ImplantsandProsthetics/BreastImplants/ucm239996.htm |
| Middle left | Fig. 2.22B: Sahin A |
| Middle centre | Fig. 2.150: Foschini MP |
| Middle right | Fig. 6.17A: Miranda RN |
| Bottom left | Fig. 2.49C: Mac Grogan G |
| Bottom centre | Fig. 5.11: Antonescu CR |
| Bottom right | Fig. 6.16A: Miranda RN |

## Images on the chapter title pages

| | |
|---|---|
| Chapter 1 | Fig. 2.91A: Rakha EA |
| Chapter 2 | Fig. 2.113: D'Alfonso TM |
| Chapter 3 | Fig. 3.11C: Tse G |
| Chapter 4 | Fig. 4.06B: Albarracin CT |
| Chapter 5 | Fig. 5.12B: Antonescu CR |
| Chapter 6 | Fig. 6.09A: Chan JKC |
| Chapter 7 | Fig. 7.01A: Chan JKC |
| Chapter 8 | Fig. 8.01A: Kulka J |
| Chapter 9 | Fig. 9.02A: Shaaban AM |

# References

**1.** Abate F, Ambrosio MR, Mundo L, et al. Distinct viral and mutational spectrum of endemic Burkitt lymphoma. PLoS Pathog. 2015 Oct 15;11(10):e1005158. PMID:26468873

**2.** Abdalla HM, Sakr MA. Predictive factors of local recurrence and survival following primary surgical treatment of phyllodes tumors of the breast. J Egypt Natl Canc Inst. 2006 Jun;18(2):125–33. PMID:17496937

**3.** Abdel-Fatah TM, Powe DG, Hodi Z, et al. High frequency of coexistence of columnar cell lesions, lobular neoplasia, and low grade ductal carcinoma in situ with invasive tubular carcinoma and invasive lobular carcinoma. Am J Surg Pathol. 2007 Mar;31(3):417–26. PMID:17325484

**4.** Abdel-Fatah TM, Powe DG, Hodi Z, et al. Morphologic and molecular evolutionary pathways of low nuclear grade invasive breast cancers and their putative precursor lesions: further evidence to support the concept of low nuclear grade breast neoplasia family. Am J Surg Pathol. 2008 Apr;32(4):513–23. PMID:18223478

**5.** Abraham SC, Reynolds C, Lee JH, et al. Fibromatosis of the breast and mutations involving the APC/beta-catenin pathway. Hum Pathol. 2002 Jan;33(1):39–46. PMID:11823972

**6.** Abrams HL, Spiro R, Goldstein N. Metastases in carcinoma; analysis of 1000 autopsied cases. Cancer. 1950 Jan;3(1):74–85. PMID:15405683

**7.** Acevedo F, Armengol VD, Deng Z, et al. Pathologic findings in reduction mammoplasty specimens: a surrogate for the population prevalence of breast cancer and high-risk lesions. Breast Cancer Res Treat. 2019 Jan;173(1):201–7. PMID:30238276

**8.** Achatz MI, Olivier M, Le Calvez F, et al. The TP53 mutation, R337H, is associated with Li-Fraumeni and Li-Fraumeni-like syndromes in Brazilian families. Cancer Lett. 2007 Jan 8;245(1-2):96–102. PMID:16494995

**9.** Acs G, Lawton TJ, Rebbeck TR, et al. Differential expression of E-cadherin in lobular and ductal neoplasms of the breast and its biologic and diagnostic implications. Am J Clin Pathol. 2001 Jan;115(1):85–98. PMID:11190811

**10.** Acs G, Simpson JF, Bleiweiss IJ, et al. Microglandular adenosis with transition into adenoid cystic carcinoma of the breast. Am J Surg Pathol. 2003 Aug;27(8):1052–60. PMID:12883237

**11.** Adams SJ, Kanthan R. Paget's disease of the male breast in the 21st century: a systematic review. Breast. 2016 Oct;29:14–23. PMID:27394005

**12.** Adank MA, Jonker MA, Kluijt I, et al. CHEK2*1100delC homozygosity is associated with a high breast cancer risk in women. J Med Genet. 2011 Dec;48(12):860–3. PMID:22058428

**13.** Adegbola T, Connolly CE, Mortimer G. Small cell neuroendocrine carcinoma of the breast: a report of three cases and review of the literature. J Clin Pathol. 2005 Jul;58(7):775–8. PMID:15976350

**14.** Adem C, Reynolds C, Ingle JN, et al. Primary breast sarcoma: clinicopathologic series from the Mayo Clinic and review of the literature. Br J Cancer. 2004 Jul 19;91(2):237–41.

PMID:15187996

**15.** Adeniran A, Al-Ahmadie H, Mahoney MC, et al. Granular cell tumor of the breast: a series of 17 cases and review of the literature. Breast J. 2004 Nov-Dec;10(6):528–31. PMID:15569210

**16.** Adrada B, Arribas E, Gilcrease M, et al. Invasive micropapillary carcinoma of the breast: mammographic, sonographic, and MRI features. AJR Am J Roentgenol. 2009 Jul;193(1):W58-63. PMID:19542384

**17.** Adrada BE, Miranda RN, Rauch GM, et al. Breast implant-associated anaplastic large cell lymphoma: sensitivity, specificity, and findings of imaging studies in 44 patients. Breast Cancer Res Treat. 2014 Aug;147(1):1–14. PMID:25073777

**18.** Ahmed AA, Heller DS. Malignant adenomyoepithelioma of the breast with malignant proliferation of epithelial and myoepithelial elements: a case report and review of the literature. Arch Pathol Lab Med. 2000 Apr;124(4):632–6. PMID:10747327

**19.** Ahmed S, Thomas G, Ghoussaini M, et al. Newly discovered breast cancer susceptibility loci on 3p24 and 17q23.2. Nat Genet. 2009 May;41(5):585–90. PMID:19330027

**20.** Aida Y, Takeuchi E, Shinagawa T, et al. Fine needle aspiration cytology of lipid-secreting carcinoma of the breast. A case report. Acta Cytol. 1993 Jul-Aug;37(4):547–51. PMID:8328251

**21.** Akbulut M, Zekioglu O, Ozdemir N, et al. Fine needle aspiration cytology of mammary carcinoma with choriocarcinomatous features: a report of 2 cases. Acta Cytol. 2008 Jan-Feb;52(1):99–104. PMID:18323284

**22.** Al Sarakbi W, Worku D, Escobar PF, et al. Breast papillomas: current management with a focus on a new diagnostic and therapeutic modality. Int Semin Surg Oncol. 2006 Jan 17;3:1. PMID:16417642

**23.** Al-Abbadi MA, Almasri NM, Al-Quran S, et al. Cytokeratin and epithelial membrane antigen expression in angiosarcomas: an immunohistochemical study of 33 cases. Arch Pathol Lab Med. 2007 Feb;131(2):288–92. PMID:17284115

**24.** Aladily TN, Medeiros LJ, Amin MB, et al. Anaplastic large cell lymphoma associated with breast implants: a report of 13 cases. Am J Surg Pathol. 2012 Jul;36(7):1000–8. PMID:22613996

**25.** Al-Ahmadie H, Hasselgren PO, Yassin R, et al. Colocalized granular cell tumor and infiltrating ductal carcinoma of the breast. Arch Pathol Lab Med. 2002 Jun;126(6):731–3. PMID:12033967

**26.** Alassiri AH, Ali RH, Shen Y, et al. ETV6-NTRK3 is expressed in a subset of ALK-negative inflammatory myofibroblastic tumors. Am J Surg Pathol. 2016 Aug;40(8):1051–61. PMID:27259007

**27.** Alawad AA. Multiple parenchymal leiomyomas of the breast in a Sudanese female. Breast Dis. 2014 Jan 1;34(4):165–7. PMID:24898199

**28.** Albonico G, Querzoli P, Ferretti S, et al. Biological profile of in situ breast cancer investigated by immunohistochemical technique. Cancer Detect Prev. 1998;22(4):313–8. PMID:9674874

**29.** Alenda C, Aranda FI, Seguí FJ, et al.

Secretory carcinoma of the male breast: correlation of aspiration cytology and pathology. Diagn Cytopathol. 2005 Jan;32(1):47–50. PMID:15584046

**30.** Alexandrov LB, Nik-Zainal S, Wedge DC, et al. Signatures of mutational processes in human cancer. Nature. 2013 Aug 22;500(7463):415–21. PMID:23945592

**31.** Ali RH, Hayes MM. Combined epithelial-myoepithelial lesions of the breast. Surg Pathol Clin. 2012 Sep;5(3):661–99. PMID:26838284

**32.** Ali RH, Taraboanta C, Mohammad T, et al. Metastatic non-small cell lung carcinoma a mimic of primary breast carcinoma-case series and literature review. Virchows Arch. 2018 May;472(5):771–7. PMID:29105026

**33.** Ali SN, Jayasena CN, Sam AH. Which patients with gynaecomastia require more detailed investigation? Clin Endocrinol (Oxf). 2018 Mar;88(3):360–3. PMID:29193251

**34.** Ali-Fehmi R, Carolin K, Wallis T, et al. Clinicopathologic analysis of breast lesions associated with multiple papillomas. Hum Pathol. 2003 Mar;34(3):234–9. PMID:12673557

**35.** Alkaied H, Harris K, Brenner A, et al. Does hormonal therapy have a therapeutic role in metastatic primary small cell neuroendocrine breast carcinoma? Case report and literature review. Clin Breast Cancer. 2012 Jun;12(3):226–30. PMID:22424945

**36.** Allen S, Levine EA, Lesko N, et al. Is excisional biopsy and chemoprevention warranted in patients with atypical lobular hyperplasia on core biopsy? Am Surg. 2015 Sep;81(9):876–8. PMID:26350664

**37.** Allison KH. Ancillary prognostic and predictive testing in breast cancer: focus on discordant, unusual, and borderline results. Surg Pathol Clin. 2018 Mar;11(1):147–76. PMID:29413654

**38.** Allison KH, Abraham LA, Weaver DL, et al. Trends in breast biopsy pathology diagnoses among women undergoing mammography in the United States: a report from the Breast Cancer Surveillance Consortium. Cancer. 2015 May 1;121(9):1369–78. PMID:25603785

**39.** Allison KH, Eby PR, Kohr J, et al. Atypical ductal hyperplasia on vacuum-assisted breast biopsy: suspicion for ductal carcinoma in situ can stratify patients at high risk for upgrade. Hum Pathol. 2011 Jan;42(1):41–50. PMID:20970167

**40.** Allison KH, Mohsin SK, Dabbs DJ. Gross examination of breast specimens. In: Dabbs DJ, editor. Breast pathology. 2nd ed. Philadelphia (PA): Elsevier; 2017. pp. 76–102.

**41.** Allison KH, Reisch LM, Carney PA, et al. Understanding diagnostic variability in breast pathology: lessons learned from an expert consensus review panel. Histopathology. 2014 Aug;65(2):240–51. PMID:24511905

**42.** Allison KH, Rendi MH, Peacock S, et al. Histological features associated with diagnostic agreement in atypical ductal hyperplasia of the breast: illustrative cases from the B-Path study. Histopathology. 2016 Dec;69(6):1028–46. PMID:27398812

**43.** Allred DC, Anderson SJ, Paik S, et al. Adjuvant tamoxifen reduces subsequent breast cancer in women with estrogen receptor-positive ductal carcinoma in situ: a study based on NSABP protocol B-24. J Clin Oncol. 2012

Apr 20;30(12):1268–73. PMID:22393101

**44.** Allred DC, Wu Y, Mao S, et al. Ductal carcinoma in situ and the emergence of diversity during breast cancer evolution. Clin Cancer Res. 2008 Jan 15;14(2):370–8. PMID:18223211

**45.** Alman BA, Li C, Pajerski ME, et al. Increased beta-catenin protein and somatic APC mutations in sporadic aggressive fibromatoses (desmoid tumors). Am J Pathol. 1997 Aug;151(2):329–34. PMID:9250146

**46.** Alsadi A, Lin D, Alnajar H, et al. Hematologic malignancies discovered on investigation of breast abnormalities. South Med J. 2017 Oct;110(10):614–20. PMID:28973700

**47.** Alsadoun N, MacGrogan G, Truntzer C, et al. Solid papillary carcinoma with reverse polarity of the breast harbors specific morphologic, immunohistochemical and molecular profile in comparison with other benign or malignant papillary lesions of the breast: a comparative study of 9 additional cases. Mod Pathol. 2018 Sep;31(9):1367–80. PMID:29785016

**48.** Alsaedi M, Shoimer I, Kurwa HA. Basal cell carcinoma of the nipple-areola complex. Dermatol Surg. 2017 Jan;43(1):142–6. PMID:27571043

**49.** Alsharif S, Daghistani R, Kamberoğlu EA, et al. Mammographic, sonographic and MR imaging features of invasive micropapillary breast cancer. Eur J Radiol. 2014 Aug;83(8):1375–80. PMID:24913934

**50.** AlSharif S, Tremblay F, Omeroglu A, et al. Infiltrating syringomatous adenoma of the nipple: sonographic and mammographic features with pathologic correlation. J Clin Ultrasound. 2014 Sep;42(7):427–9. PMID:24648330

**51.** Alsop K, Fereday S, Meldrum C, et al. BRCA mutation frequency and patterns of treatment response in BRCA mutation-positive women with ovarian cancer: a report from the Australian Ovarian Cancer Study Group. J Clin Oncol. 2012 Jul 20;30(21):2654–63. PMID:22711857

**52.** Alvarado-Cabrero I, Picón Coronel G, Valencia Cedillo R, et al. Florid lobular intraepithelial neoplasia with signet ring cells, central necrosis and calcifications: a clinicopathological and immunohistochemical analysis of ten cases associated with invasive lobular carcinoma. Arch Med Res. 2010 Aug;41(6):436–41. PMID:21044747

**53.** Alvarenga CA, Paravidino PI, Alvarenga M, et al. Reappraisal of immunohistochemical profiling of special histological types of breast carcinomas: a study of 121 cases of eight different subtypes. J Clin Pathol. 2012 Dec;65(12):1066–71. PMID:22944625

**54.** Alvarez RH, Gong Y, Ueno NT, et al. Metastasis in the breast mimicking inflammatory breast cancer. J Clin Oncol. 2012 Aug 1;30(22):e202–6. PMID:22734030

**55.** Amadou A, Waddington Achatz MI, Hainaut P. Revisiting tumor patterns and penetrance in germline TP53 mutation carriers: temporal phases of Li-Fraumeni syndrome. Curr Opin Oncol. 2018 Jan;30(1):23–9. PMID:29076966

**56.** Amary MF, Pauwels P, Meulemans E, et al. Detection of beta-catenin mutations in paraffin-embedded sporadic desmoid-type fibromatosis by mutation-specific restriction enzyme

digestion (MSRED): an ancillary diagnostic tool. Am J Surg Pathol. 2007 Sep;31(9):1299–309. PMID:17721184
**57.** Amato T, Abate F, Piccaluga P, et al. Clonality analysis of immunoglobulin gene rearrangement by next-generation sequencing in endemic Burkitt lymphoma suggests antigen drive activation of BCR as opposed to sporadic Burkitt lymphoma. Am J Clin Pathol. 2016 Jan;145(1):116–27. PMID:26712879
**58.** Ambrosio MR, Lazzi S, Bello GL, et al. MYC protein expression scoring and its impact on the prognosis of aggressive B-cell lymphoma patients. Haematologica. 2019 Jan;104(1):e25–8. PMID:29954940
**59.** Ambrosio MR, Navari M, Di Lisio L, et al. The Epstein Barr-encoded BART-6-3p microRNA affects regulation of cell growth and immuno response in Burkitt lymphoma. Infect Agent Cancer. 2014 Apr 14;9:12. PMID:24731550
**60.** Ambrosio MR, Piccaluga PP, Ponzoni M, et al. The alteration of lipid metabolism in Burkitt lymphoma identifies a novel marker: adipophilin. PLoS One. 2012;7(8):e44315. PMID:22952953
**60A.** American Society of Clinical Oncology, College of American Pathologists. Estrogen and progesterone receptor testing in breast cancer: American Society of Clinical Oncology / College of American Pathologists Clinical Practice Guideline Update. Forthcoming 2019. Available from: https://www.cap.org/protocols-and-guidelines/cap-guidelines/current-cap-guidelines/guideline-recommendations-for-immunohistochemical-testing-of-estrogen-and-progesterone-receptors-in-breast-cancer.
**61.** Amin MB, Edge S, Greene F, et al., editors. AJCC cancer staging manual. 8th ed. New York (NY): Springer; 2017.
**62.** Amin MB, Greene FL, Edge SB, et al. The Eighth Edition AJCC Cancer Staging Manual: continuing to build a bridge from a population-based to a more "personalized" approach to cancer staging. CA Cancer J Clin. 2017 Mar;67(2):93–9. PMID:28094848
**63.** Andersen JA. Lobular carcinoma in situ of the breast. An approach to rational treatment. Cancer. 1977 Jun;39(6):2597–602. PMID:872058
**64.** Anderson C, Ricci A Jr, Pedersen CA, et al. Immunocytochemical analysis of estrogen and progesterone receptors in benign stromal lesions of the breast. Evidence for hormonal etiology in pseudoangiomatous hyperplasia of mammary stroma. Am J Surg Pathol. 1991 Feb;15(2):145–9. PMID:1989462
**65.** Anderson JM, Ariga R, Govil H, et al. Assessment of Her-2/Neu status by immunohistochemistry and fluorescence in situ hybridization in mammary Paget disease and underlying carcinoma. Appl Immunohistochem Mol Morphol. 2003 Jun;11(2):120–4. PMID:12777994
**66.** Anderson KN, Schwab RB, Martinez ME. Reproductive risk factors and breast cancer subtypes: a review of the literature. Breast Cancer Res Treat. 2014 Feb;144(1):1–10. PMID:24477977
**67.** Anderson WF, Chu KC, Chang S, et al. Comparison of age-specific incidence rate patterns for different histopathologic types of breast carcinoma. Cancer Epidemiol Biomarkers Prev. 2004 Jul;13(7):1128–35. PMID:15247123
**68.** Anderson WF, Rosenberg PS, Prat A, et al. How many etiological subtypes of breast cancer: two, three, four, or more? J Natl Cancer Inst. 2014 Aug 12;106(8):dju165. PMID:25118203
**69.** Andrade VP, Morrogh M, Qin LX, et al. Gene expression profiling of lobular carcinoma in situ reveals candidate precursor genes for invasion. Mol Oncol. 2015 Apr;9(4):772–82. PMID:25601220
**69A.** André F, Ciruelos E, Rubovszky G, et al. Alpelisib for PIK3CA-mutated, hormone receptor-positive advanced breast cancer. N Engl J Med. 2019 May 16;380(20):1929–40. PMID:31091374
**70.** Andreasen S, Tan Q, Agander TK, et al. Adenoid cystic carcinomas of the salivary gland, lacrimal gland, and breast are morphologically and genetically similar but have distinct microRNA expression profiles. Mod Pathol. 2018 Aug;31(8):1211–25. PMID:29467480
**71.** Ansquer Y, Delaney S, Santulli P, et al. Risk of invasive breast cancer after lobular intra-epithelial neoplasia: review of the literature. Eur J Surg Oncol. 2010 Jul;36(7):604–9. PMID:20541352
**72.** Antonescu C. Malignant vascular tumors–an update. Mod Pathol. 2014 Jan;27 Suppl 1:S30–8. PMID:24384851
**73.** Antonescu CR, Suurmeijer AJ, Zhang L, et al. Molecular characterization of inflammatory myofibroblastic tumors with frequent ALK and ROS1 gene fusions and rare novel RET rearrangement. Am J Surg Pathol. 2015 Jul;39(7):957–67. PMID:25723109
**74.** Antonescu CR, Yoshida A, Guo T, et al. KDR activating mutations in human angiosarcomas are sensitive to specific kinase inhibitors. Cancer Res. 2009 Sep 15;69(18):7175–9. PMID:19723655
**75.** Antoniou AC, Casadei S, Heikkinen T, et al. Breast-cancer risk in families with mutations in PALB2. N Engl J Med. 2014 Aug 7;371(6):497–506. PMID:25099575
**76.** Antoniou AC, Wang X, Fredericksen ZS, et al. A locus on 19p13 modifies risk of breast cancer in BRCA1 mutation carriers and is associated with hormone receptor-negative breast cancer in the general population. Nat Genet. 2010 Oct;42(10):885–92. PMID:20852631
**77.** Apostolou P, Papasotiriou I. Current perspectives on CHEK2 mutations in breast cancer. Breast Cancer (Dove Med Press). 2017 May 12;9:331–5. PMID:28553140
**78.** Arber DA, Simpson JF, Weiss LM, et al. Non-Hodgkin's lymphoma involving the breast. Am J Surg Pathol. 1994 Mar;18(3):288–95. PMID:8116797
**79.** Arce C, Cortes-Padilla D, Huntsman DG, et al. Secretory carcinoma of the breast containing the ETV6-NTRK3 fusion gene in a male: case report and review of the literature. World J Surg Oncol. 2005 Jun 17;3:35. PMID:15963235
**80.** Aroner SA, Collins LC, Schnitt SJ, et al. Columnar cell lesions and subsequent breast cancer risk: a nested case-control study. Breast Cancer Res. 2010;12(4):R61. PMID:20691043
**81.** Arpino G, Allred DC, Mohsin SK, et al. Lobular neoplasia on core-needle biopsy–clinical significance. Cancer. 2004 Jul 15;101(2):242–50. PMID:15241819
**82.** Arpino G, Bardou VJ, Clark GM, et al. Infiltrating lobular carcinoma of the breast: tumor characteristics and clinical outcome. Breast Cancer Res. 2004;6(3):R149–56. PMID:15084238
**83.** Arpino G, Clark GM, Mohsin S, et al. Adenoid cystic carcinoma of the breast: molecular markers, treatment, and clinical outcome. Cancer. 2002 Apr 15;94(8):2119–27. PMID:12001107
**84.** Arslan A, Güldoğan N, Kapucuoğlu N, et al. A rare case of pleomorphic adenoma of the breast: ultrasonography and pathology findings. Breast J. 2018 Nov;24(6):1069–70. PMID:30240069
**85.** Arvey A, Ojesina AI, Pedamallu CS, et al. The tumor virus landscape of AIDS-related lymphomas. Blood. 2015 May 14;125(20):e14–22. PMID:25827832
**86.** Ashikari R, Huvos AG, Urban JA, et al. Infiltrating lobular carcinoma of the breast. Cancer. 1973 Jan;31(1):110–6. PMID:4345605
**87.** Ashikari R, Park K, Huvos AG, et al. Paget's disease of the breast. Cancer. 1970 Sep;26(3):680–5. PMID:4318756
**88.** Asioli S, Marucci G, Ficarra G, et al. Polymorphous adenocarcinoma of the breast. Report of three cases. Virchows Arch. 2006 Jan;448(1):29–34. PMID:16220292
**89.** Asirvatham JR, Falcone MM, Kleer CG. Atypical apocrine adenosis: diagnostic challenges and pitfalls. Arch Pathol Lab Med. 2016 Oct;140(10):1045–51. PMID:27684975
**90.** Astvatsaturyan K, Yue Y, Walts AE, et al. Androgen receptor positive triple negative breast cancer: clinicopathologic, prognostic, and predictive features. PLoS One. 2018 Jun 8;13(6):e0197827. PMID:29883487
**91.** Atkins KA, Cohen MA, Nicholson B, et al. Atypical lobular hyperplasia and lobular carcinoma in situ at core breast biopsy: use of careful radiologic-pathologic correlation to recommend excision or observation. Radiology. 2013 Nov;269(2):340–7. PMID:23901123
**92.** Aubele MM, Cummings MC, Mattis AE, et al. Accumulation of chromosomal imbalances from intraductal proliferative lesions to adjacent in situ and invasive ductal breast cancer. Diagn Mol Pathol. 2000 Mar;9(1):14–9. PMID:10718208
**93.** Audeh MW, Carmichael J, Penson RT, et al. Oral poly(ADP-ribose) polymerase inhibitor olaparib in patients with BRCA1 or BRCA2 mutations and recurrent ovarian cancer: a proof-of-concept trial. Lancet. 2010 Jul 24;376(9737):245–51. PMID:20609468
**94.** Auger M, Hüttner I. Fine-needle aspiration cytology of pleomorphic lobular carcinoma of the breast. Comparison with the classic type. Cancer. 1997 Feb 25;81(1):29–32. PMID:9100538
**95.** Aulmann S, Elsawaf Z, Penzel R, et al. Invasive tubular carcinoma of the breast frequently is clonally related to flat epithelial atypia and low-grade ductal carcinoma in situ. Am J Surg Pathol. 2009 Nov;33(11):1646–53. PMID:19675453
**96.** Austin RM, Dupree WB. Liposarcoma of the breast: a clinicopathologic study of 20 cases. Hum Pathol. 1986 Sep;17(9):906–13. PMID:3019868
**96A.** Avigdor BE, Beierl K, Gocke CD, et al. Whole-exome sequencing of metaplastic breast carcinoma indicates monoclonality with associated ductal carcinoma component. Clin Cancer Res. 2017 Aug 15;23(16):4875–884. PMID:28424200
**97.** Azzopardi JG, Eusebi V. Melanocyte colonization and pigmentation of breast carcinoma. Histopathology. 1977 Jan;1(1):21–30. PMID:615831
**98.** Azzopardi JG, Muretto P, Goddeeris P, et al. 'Carcinoid' tumours of the breast: the morphological spectrum of argyrophil carcinomas. Histopathology. 1982 Sep;6(5):549–69. PMID:6183185
**99.** Bacchi CE, Wludarski SC, Ambaye AB, et al. Metastatic melanoma presenting as an isolated breast tumor: a study of 20 cases with emphasis on several primary mimickers. Arch Pathol Lab Med. 2013 Jan;137(1):41–9. PMID:23276173
**100.** Bacchi CE, Wludarski SC, Lamovec J, et al. Lipophyllodes of the breast. A reappraisal of fat-rich tumors of the breast based on 22 cases integrated by immunohistochemical study, molecular pathology insights, and clinical follow-up. Ann Diagn Pathol. 2016 Apr;21:1–6. PMID:27040923
**101.** Bachmeier BE, Nerlich AG, Mirisola V, et al. Lineage infidelity and expression of melanocytic markers in human breast cancer. Int J Oncol. 2008 Nov;33(5):1011–5. PMID:18949364
**102.** Baddoura FK, Judd RL. Apocrine adenoma of the breast: report of a case with investigation of lectin binding patterns in apocrine breast lesions. Mod Pathol. 1990 May;3(3):373–6. PMID:2362943
**103.** Badve S, Sloane JP. Pseudoangiomatous hyperplasia of male breast. Histopathology. 1995 May;26(5):463–6. PMID:7544764
**104.** Badyal RK, Bal A, Das A, et al. Invasive micropapillary carcinoma of the breast: immunophenotypic analysis and role of cell adhesion molecules (CD44 and E-cadherin) in nodal metastasis. Appl Immunohistochem Mol Morphol. 2016 Mar;24(3):151–8. PMID:26200840
**105.** Bagaria SP, Shamonki J, Kinnaird M, et al. The florid subtype of lobular carcinoma in situ: marker or precursor for invasive lobular carcinoma? Ann Surg Oncol. 2011 Jul;18(7):1845–51. PMID:21287281
**106.** Bailar JC 3rd. Diagnostic drift in the reporting of cancer incidence. J Natl Cancer Inst. 1998 Jun 3;90(11):863–4. PMID:9625178
**107.** Baildam AD, Higgins RM, Hurley E, et al. Cyclosporin A and multiple fibroadenomas of the breast. Br J Surg. 1996 Dec;83(12):1755–7. PMID:9038560
**108.** Baker GM, Schnitt SJ. Vascular lesions of the breast. Semin Diagn Pathol. 2017 Sep;34(5):410–9. PMID:28676174
**109.** Bal A, Joshi K, Sharma SC, et al. Prognostic significance of micropapillary pattern in pure mucinous carcinoma of the breast. Int J Surg Pathol. 2008 Jul;16(3):251–6. PMID:18387988
**110.** Balasubramanian I, Fleming CA, Corrigan MA, et al. Meta-analysis of the diagnostic accuracy of ultrasound-guided fine-needle aspiration and core needle biopsy in diagnosing axillary lymph node metastasis. Br J Surg. 2018 Sep;105(10):1244–53. PMID:29972239
**111.** Balleine RL, Murali R, Bilous AM, et al. Histopathological features of breast cancer in carriers of ATM gene variants. Histopathology. 2006 Nov;49(5):523–32. PMID:17064299
**112.** Bamps S, Oyen T, Legius E, et al. Multiple granular cell tumors in a child with Noonan syndrome. Eur J Pediatr Surg. 2013 Jun;23(3):257–9. PMID:22915371
**113.** Bane AL, Tjan S, Parkes RK, et al. Invasive lobular carcinoma: to grade or not to grade. Mod Pathol. 2005 May;18(5):621–8. PMID:15605082
**114.** Banev SG, Filipovski VA. Chondrolipoma of the breast–case report and a review of literature. Breast. 2006 Jun;15(3):425–6. PMID:16131470
**115.** Banneau G, Guedj M, MacGrogan G, et al. Molecular apocrine differentiation is a common feature of breast cancer in patients with germline PTEN mutations. Breast Cancer Res. 2010;12(4):R63. PMID:20712882
**116.** Baraban E, Zhang PJ, Jaffer S, et al. MYB rearrangement and immunohistochemical expression in adenomyoepithelioma of the breast: a comparison with adenoid cystic carcinoma. Histopathology. 2018 Dec;73(6):897–903. PMID:30003572
**117.** Barbashina V, Corben AD, Akram M, et al. Mucinous micropapillary carcinoma of the breast: an aggressive counterpart to conventional pure mucinous tumors. Hum Pathol. 2013 Aug;44(8):1577–85. PMID:23517923
**118.** Barber M, Murrell A, Ito Y, et al. Mechanisms and sequelae of E-cadherin silencing in hereditary diffuse gastric cancer. J Pathol. 2008 Nov;216(3):295–306.

PMID:18788075

**119.** Barbosa ML, Ribeiro EM, Silva GF, et al. Cytogenetic findings in phyllodes tumor and fibroadenomas of the breast. Cancer Genet Cytogenet. 2004 Oct 15;154(2):156–9. PMID:15474152

**120.** Barco I, Vidal M, Fraile M, et al. MOHS micrographic surgery for treating erosive adenoma of the nipple: a case report and review of the literature. Int J Dermatol. 2017 Dec;56(12):1451–4. PMID:28960299

**121.** Barco Nebreda I, Vidal MC, Fraile M, et al. Lactating adenoma of the breast. J Hum Lact. 2016 Aug;32(3):559–62. PMID:27197575

**122.** Bareche Y, Venet D, Ignatiadis M, et al. Unravelling triple-negative breast cancer molecular heterogeneity using an integrative multiomic analysis. Ann Oncol. 2018 Apr 1;29(4):895–902. PMID:29365031

**123.** Baretta Z, Mocellin S, Goldin E, et al. Effect of BRCA germline mutations on breast cancer prognosis: a systematic review and meta-analysis. Medicine (Baltimore). 2016 Oct;95(40):e4975. PMID:27749552

**124.** Bari VB, Bholay SU, Sane KC. Invasive lobular carcinoma of the breast with extracellular mucin - a new rare variant. J Clin Diagn Res. 2015 Apr;9(4):ED05–06. PMID:26023557

**125.** Barkley CR, Ligibel JA, Wong JS, et al. Mucinous breast carcinoma: a large contemporary series. Am J Surg. 2008 Oct;196(4):549–51. PMID:18809061

**126.** Barnard ME, Boeke CE, Tamimi RM. Established breast cancer risk factors and risk of intrinsic tumor subtypes. Biochim Biophys Acta. 2015 Aug;1856(1):73–85. PMID:26071880

**127.** Barth TF, Müller S, Pawlita M, et al. Homogeneous immunophenotype and paucity of secondary genomic aberrations are distinctive features of endemic but not of sporadic Burkitt's lymphoma and diffuse large B-cell lymphoma with MYC rearrangement. J Pathol. 2004 Aug;203(4):940–5. PMID:15258997

**128.** Bartuma H, Hallor KH, Panagopoulos I, et al. Assessment of the clinical and molecular impact of different cytogenetic subgroups in a series of 272 lipomas with abnormal karyotype. Genes Chromosomes Cancer. 2007 Jun;46(6):594–606. PMID:17370328

**129.** Basbug M, Akbulut S, Arikanoglu Z, et al. Mucoepidermoid carcinoma in a breast affected by burn scars: comprehensive literature review and case report. Breast Care (Basel). 2011 Aug;6(4):293–7. PMID:22135628

**130.** Basham VM, Lipscombe JM, Ward JM, et al. BRCA1 and BRCA2 mutations in a population-based study of male breast cancer. Breast Cancer Res. 2002;4(1):R2. PMID:11879560

**130A.** Bataillon G, Fuhrmann L, Girard E, et al. High rate of PIK3CA mutations but no TP53 mutations in low-grade adenosquamous carcinoma of the breast. Histopathology. 2018 Aug;73(2):273–83. PMID:29537649

**131.** Battistella M, Cribier B, Feugeas JP, et al. Vascular invasion and other invasive features in granular cell tumours of the skin: a multicentre study of 119 cases. J Clin Pathol. 2014 Jan;67(1):19–25. PMID:23908453

**132.** Bauermeister DE, Hall MH. Specimen radiography–a mandatory adjunct to mammography. Am J Clin Pathol. 1973 Jun;59(6):782–9. PMID:4709078

**133.** Bean GR, Krings G, Otis CN, et al. CRTC1-MAML2 fusion in mucoepidermoid carcinoma of the breast. Histopathology. 2019 Feb;74(3):463–73. PMID:30380176

**134.** Beck AH, Lee CH, Witten DM, et al. Discovery of molecular subtypes in leiomyosarcoma through integrative molecular profiling. Oncogene. 2010 Feb

11;29(6):845–54. PMID:19901961

**135.** Beert E, Brems H, Daniëls B, et al. Atypical neurofibromas in neurofibromatosis type 1 are premalignant tumors. Genes Chromosomes Cancer. 2011 Dec;50(12):1021–32. PMID:21987445

**135A.** Begg CB, Ostrovnaya I, Geyer FC, et al. Contralateral breast cancers: independent cancers or metastases? Int J Cancer. 2018 Jan 15;142(2):347–56. PMID:28921573

**136.** Beguinot M, Dauplat MM, Kwiatkowski F, et al. Analysis of tumour-infiltrating lymphocytes reveals two new biologically different subgroups of breast ductal carcinoma in situ. BMC Cancer. 2018 Feb 3;18(1):129. PMID:29394917

**137.** Begum SM, Jara-Lazaro AR, Thike AA, et al. Mucin extravasation in breast core biopsies– clinical significance and outcome correlation. Histopathology. 2009 Nov;55(5):609–17. PMID:19912367

**138.** Behjati S, Tarpey PS, Sheldon H, et al. Recurrent PTPRB and PLCG1 mutations in angiosarcoma. Nat Genet. 2014 Apr;46(4):376–9. PMID:24633157

**139.** Bellezza G, Lombardi T, Panzarola P, et al. Schwannoma of the breast: a case report and review of the literature. Tumori. 2007 May-Jun;93(3):308–11. PMID:17679472

**140.** Benusiglio PR, Malka D, Rouleau E, et al. CDH1 germline mutations and the hereditary diffuse gastric and lobular breast cancer syndrome: a multicentre study. J Med Genet. 2013 Jul;50(7):486–9. PMID:23709761

**141.** Ben-Yehuda A, Steiner-Saltz D, Libson E, et al. Plasmacytoma of the breast. Unusual initial presentation of myeloma: report of two cases and review of the literature. Blut. 1989 Mar;58(3):169–70. PMID:2649190

**142.** Berg AN, Soma L, Clark BZ, et al. Evaluating breast lymphoplasmacytic infiltrates: a multiparameter immunohistochemical study, including assessment of IgG4. Hum Pathol. 2015 Aug;46(8):1162–70. PMID:26026200

**143.** Berg JC, Scheithauer BW, Spinner RJ, et al. Plexiform schwannoma: a clinicopathologic overview with emphasis on the head and neck region. Hum Pathol. 2008 May;39(5):633–40. PMID:18439936

**144.** Berg JW, Hutter RV. Breast cancer. Cancer. 1995 Jan 1;75(1) Suppl:257–69. PMID:8001000

**145.** Berg WA, Mrose HE, Ioffe OB. Atypical lobular hyperplasia or lobular carcinoma in situ at core-needle breast biopsy. Radiology. 2001 Feb;218(2):503–9. PMID:11161169

**146.** Berna JD, Arcas I, Ballester A, et al. Adenomyoepithelioma of the breast in a male. AJR Am J Roentgenol. 1997 Sep;169(3):917–8. PMID:9275934

**147.** Bernardello F, Caneva A, Bresaola E, et al. Breast solitary schwannoma: fine-needle aspiration biopsy and immunocytochemical analysis. Diagn Cytopathol. 1994;10(3):221–3. PMID:8050328

**148.** Bernstein JL, Haile RW, Stovall M, et al. Radiation exposure, the ATM gene, and contralateral breast cancer in the women's environmental cancer and radiation epidemiology study. J Natl Cancer Inst. 2010 Apr 7;102(7):475–83. PMID:20305132

**149.** Bernstein JL, Teraoka S, Southey MC, et al. Population-based estimates of breast cancer risks associated with ATM gene variants c.7271T>G and c.1066-6T>G (IVS10-6T>G) from the Breast Cancer Family Registry. Hum Mutat. 2006 Nov;27(11):1122–8. PMID:16958054

**150.** Bernstein JL, WECARE Study Collaborative Group, Concannon P. ATM, radiation, and the risk of second primary breast cancer. Int J Radiat Biol. 2017 Oct;93(10):1121–7. PMID:28627265

**151.** Bernstein L, Deapen D, Ross RK. The descriptive epidemiology of malignant cystosarcoma phyllodes tumors of the breast. Cancer. 1993 May 15;71(10):3020–4. PMID:8387873

**152.** Bertani E, Testori A, Chiappa A, et al. Recurrence and prognostic factors in patients with aggressive fibromatosis. The role of radical surgery and its limitations. World J Surg Oncol. 2012 Sep 10;10:184. PMID:22963172

**153.** Berx G, Van Roy F. The E-cadherin/catenin complex: an important gatekeeper in breast cancer tumorigenesis and malignant progression. Breast Cancer Res. 2001;3(5):289–93. PMID:11597316

**154.** Beumer IJ, Persoon M, Witteveen A, et al. Prognostic value of MammaPrint® in invasive lobular breast cancer. Biomark Insights. 2016 Dec 11;11:139–46. PMID:27980389

**155.** Beute BJ, Kalisher L, Hutter RV. Lobular carcinoma in situ of the breast: clinical, pathologic, and mammographic features. AJR Am J Roentgenol. 1991 Aug;157(2):257–65. PMID:1853802

**156.** Bezić J, Forempoher G, Poljicanin A, et al. Apocrine adenoma of the breast coexistent with invasive carcinoma. Pathol Res Pract. 2007;203(11):809–12. PMID:17936522

**157.** Bezić J, Karaman I, Šundov D. Combined fibroadenoma and tubular adenoma of the breast: rare presentation that confirms common histogenesis. Breast J. 2015 May-Jun;21(3):309–11. PMID:25775939

**158.** Bhagavan BS, Patchefsky A, Koss LG. Florid subareolar duct papillomatosis (nipple adenoma) and mammary carcinoma: report of three cases. Hum Pathol. 1973 Jun;4(2):289–95. PMID:4350340

**159.** Bhargava R, Dabbs DJ. Use of immunohistochemistry in diagnosis of breast epithelial lesions. Adv Anat Pathol. 2007 Mar;14(2):93–107. PMID:17471116

**160.** Bhargava R, Esposito NN, Dabbs DJ. Intracystic papillary carcinomas of the breast are more similar to in situ carcinomas than to invasive carcinoma. Am J Surg Pathol. 2011 May;35(5):778–9, author reply 779–81. PMID:21451361

**161.** Bhargava R, Florea AV, Pelmus M, et al. Breast tumor resembling tall cell variant of papillary thyroid carcinoma: a solid papillary neoplasm with characteristic immunohistochemical profile and few recurrent mutations. Am J Clin Pathol. 2017 Apr 1;147(4):399–410. PMID:28375433

**162.** Bhasin SD, Vyas JJ. Angiomatosis of the breast–a case report with review of literature. Indian J Pathol Microbiol. 1991 Oct;34(4):296–8. PMID:1818036

**163.** Bhattacharya B, Dilworth HP, Iacobuzio-Donahue C, et al. Nuclear beta-catenin expression distinguishes deep fibromatosis from other benign and malignant fibroblastic and myofibroblastic lesions. Am J Surg Pathol. 2005 May;29(5):653–9. PMID:15832090

**164.** Bhattarai S, Kapila K, Verma K. Phyllodes tumor of the breast. A cytohistologic study of 80 cases. Acta Cytol. 2000 Sep-Oct;44(5):790–6. PMID:11015981

**165.** Bhutani N, Kajal P, Singla S. Adenoid cystic carcinoma of the breast: experience at a tertiary care centre of Northern India. Int J Surg Case Rep. 2018;51:204–9. PMID:30189404

**166.** Bianchi S, Vezzosi V. Microinvasive carcinoma of the breast. Pathol Oncol Res. 2008 Jun;14(2):105–11. PMID:18493870

**167.** Bianchini L, Birtwisle L, Saâda E, et al. Identification of PPAP2B as a novel recurrent translocation partner gene of HMGA2 in lipomas. Genes Chromosomes Cancer. 2013 Jun;52(6):580–90. PMID:23508853

**168.** Bibbo M, Hanau C. Cytopathology of the

breast. In: Tavassoli FA, editor. Pathology of the breast. 2nd ed. Stamford (CT): Appleton & Lange; 1999. pp. 82–3.

**169.** Biesma HD, Schouten PC, Lacle MM, et al. Copy number profiling by array comparative genomic hybridization identifies frequently occurring BRCA2-like male breast cancer. Genes Chromosomes Cancer. 2015 Dec;54(12):734–44. PMID:26355282

**170.** Bijker N, Peterse JL, Duchateau L, et al. Risk factors for recurrence and metastasis after breast-conserving therapy for ductal carcinoma-in-situ: analysis of European Organization for Research and Treatment of Cancer Trial 10853. J Clin Oncol. 2001 Apr 15;19(8):2263–71. PMID:11304780

**171.** Billings SD, McKenney JK, Folpe AL, et al. Cutaneous angiosarcoma following breast-conserving surgery and radiation: an analysis of 27 cases. Am J Surg Pathol. 2004 Jun;28(6):781–8. PMID:15166670

**172.** Binh MB, Sastre-Garau X, Guillou L, et al. MDM2 and CDK4 immunostainings are useful adjuncts in diagnosing well-differentiated and dedifferentiated liposarcoma subtypes: a comparative analysis of 559 soft tissue neoplasms with genetic data. Am J Surg Pathol. 2005 Oct;29(10):1340–7. PMID:16160477

**173.** Binokay F, Balal M, Demir E, et al. Risk of developing fibroadenoma with the use of cyclosporine A in renal transplant recipients. Ren Fail. 2005;27(6):721–5. PMID:16350824

**174.** Birch JM, Alston RD, McNally RJ, et al. Relative frequency and morphology of cancers in carriers of germline TP53 mutations. Oncogene. 2001 Aug 2;20(34):4621–8. PMID:11498785

**175.** Biserni GB, Di Oto E, Moskovszky LE, et al. Preferential expression of NY-BR-1 and GATA-3 in male breast cancer. J Cancer Res Clin Oncol. 2018 Feb;144(2):199–204. PMID:29116378

**176.** Bishop JA, Taube JM, Su A, et al. Secretory carcinoma of the skin harboring ETV6 gene fusions: a cutaneous analogue to secretory carcinomas of the breast and salivary glands. Am J Surg Pathol. 2017 Jan;41(1):62–6. PMID:27631515

**177.** Black J, Metcalf C, Wylie EJ. Ultrasonography of breast hamartomas. Australas Radiol. 1996 Nov;40(4):412–5. PMID:8996902

**178.** Blair SL, Emerson DK, Kulkarni S, et al. Breast surgeon's survey: no consensus for surgical treatment of pleomorphic lobular carcinoma in situ. Breast J. 2013 Jan-Feb;19(1):116–8. PMID:23231019

**179.** Blombery P, Thompson ER, Jones K, et al. Whole exome sequencing reveals activating JAK1 and STAT3 mutations in breast implant-associated anaplastic large cell lymphoma anaplastic large cell lymphoma. Haematologica. 2016 Sep;101(9):e387–90. PMID:27198716

**180.** Bodian CA, Perzin KH, Lattes R. Lobular neoplasia. Long term risk of breast cancer and relation to other factors. Cancer. 1996 Sep 1;78(5):1024–34. PMID:8780540

**181.** Bodian CA, Perzin KH, Lattes R, et al. Reproducibility and validity of pathologic classifications of benign breast disease and implications for clinical applications. Cancer. 1993 Jun 15;71(12):3908–13. PMID:8508356

**182.** Boecker W, Buerger H, Schmitz K, et al. Ductal epithelial proliferations of the breast: a biological continuum? Comparative genomic hybridization and high-molecular-weight cytokeratin expression patterns. J Pathol. 2001 Nov;195(4):415–21. PMID:11745672

**183.** Boecker W, Buerger H. Usual and atypical ductal hyperplasia—members of the same family? Diagn Histopathol (Oxf). 2004 Jun;10(3):175–82. doi:10.1016/j.

cdip.2004.03.010.

**184.** Boecker W, Junkers T, Reusch M, et al. Origin and differentiation of breast nipple syringoma. Sci Rep. 2012;2:226. PMID:22355740

**185.** Boecker W, Moll R, Dervan P, et al. Usual ductal hyperplasia of the breast is a committed stem (progenitor) cell lesion distinct from atypical ductal hyperplasia and ductal carcinoma in situ. J Pathol. 2002 Dec;198(4):458–67. PMID:12434415

**186.** Boecker W, Stenman G, Loening T, et al. Differentiation and histogenesis of syringomatous tumour of the nipple and low-grade adenosquamous carcinoma: evidence for a common origin. Histopathology. 2014 Jul;65(1):9–23. PMID:24382117

**187.** Boelens MC, Nethe M, Klarenbeek S, et al. PTEN loss in E-cadherin-deficient mouse mammary epithelial cells rescues apoptosis and results in development of classical invasive lobular carcinoma. Cell Rep. 2016 Aug 23;16(8):2087–101. PMID:27524621

**188.** Bogina G, Munari E, Brunelli M, et al. Neuroendocrine differentiation in breast carcinoma: clinicopathological features and outcome. Histopathology. 2016 Feb;68(3):422–32. PMID:26114478

**189.** Bojesen SE, Pooley KA, Johnatty SE, et al. Multiple independent variants at the TERT locus are associated with telomere length and risks of breast and ovarian cancer. Nat Genet. 2013 Apr;45(4):371–84, e1–2. PMID:23535731

**190.** Boldt V, Stacher E, Halbwedl I, et al. Positioning of necrotic lobular intraepithelial neoplasias (LIN, grade 3) within the sequence of breast carcinoma progression. Genes Chromosomes Cancer. 2010 May;49(5):463–70. PMID:20155841

**191.** Bombonati A, Lerwill MF. Metastases to and from the breast. Surg Pathol Clin. 2012 Sep;5(3):719–47. PMID:26838286

**192.** Bombonati A, Sgroi DC. The molecular pathology of breast cancer progression. J Pathol. 2011 Jan;223(2):307–17. PMID:21125683

**193.** Bomeisl PE, Thompson CL, Harris LN, et al. Comparison of Oncotype DX recurrence score by histologic types of breast carcinoma. Arch Pathol Lab Med. 2015 Dec;139(12):1546–9. PMID:26619027

**194.** Bonadonna G, Valagussa P, Brambilla C, et al. Primary chemotherapy in operable breast cancer: eight-year experience at the Milan Cancer Institute. J Clin Oncol. 1998 Jan;16(1):93–100. PMID:9440728

**195.** Bondeson L, Lindholm K. Aspiration cytology of tubular breast carcinoma. Acta Cytol. 1990 Jan-Feb;34(1):15–20. PMID:2296836

**196.** Bongiorno MR, Doukaki S, Aricò M. Neurofibromatosis of the nipple-areolar area: a case series. J Med Case Rep. 2010 Jan 25;4:22. PMID:20205809

**197.** Bonnier P, Romain S, Giacalone PL, et al. Clinical and biologic prognostic factors in breast cancer diagnosed during postmenopausal hormone replacement therapy. Obstet Gynecol. 1995 Jan;85(1):11–7. PMID:7800305

**198.** Bonvalot S, Eldweny H, Haddad V, et al. Extra-abdominal primary fibromatosis: aggressive management could be avoided in a subgroup of patients. Eur J Surg Oncol. 2008 Apr;34(4):462–8. PMID:17709227

**199.** Borda LJ, Mervis JS, Romanelli P, et al. Clear cell acanthoma on the areola. Dermatol Online J. 2018 Jul 15;24(7):13030/qt9q47d056. PMID:30261576

**200.** Borden EC, Baker LH, Bell RS, et al. Soft tissue sarcomas of adults: state of the translational science. Clin Cancer Res. 2003 Jun;9(6):1941–56. PMID:12796356

**201.** Borst MJ, Ingold JA. Metastatic patterns of invasive lobular versus invasive ductal carcinoma of the breast. Surgery. 1993 Oct;114(4):637–41, discussion 641–2. PMID:8211676

**202.** Bosse K, Ott C, Biegner T, et al. 23-year-old female with an inflammatory myofibroblastic tumour of the breast: a case report and a review of the literature. Geburtshilfe Frauenheilkd. 2014 Feb;74(2):167–70. PMID:24741129

**203.** Bossuyt V. Processing and reporting of breast specimens in the neoadjuvant setting. Surg Pathol Clin. 2018 Mar;11(1):213–30. PMID:29413658

**204.** Bossuyt V, Provenzano E, Symmans WF, et al. Recommendations for standardized pathological characterization of residual disease for neoadjuvant clinical trials of breast cancer by the BIG-NABCG collaboration. Ann Oncol. 2015 Jul;26(7):1280–91. PMID:26019189

**205.** Boto A, Harigopal M. Strong androgen receptor expression can aid in distinguishing GATA3+ metastases. Hum Pathol. 2018 May;75:63–70. PMID:29408697

**206.** Botta G, Fessia L, Ghiringhello B. Juvenile milk protein secreting carcinoma. Virchows Arch A Pathol Anat Histol. 1982;395(2):145–52. PMID:7101723

**207.** Bottles K, Chan JS, Holly EA, et al. Cytologic criteria for fibroadenoma. A step-wise logistic regression analysis. Am J Clin Pathol. 1988 Jun;89(6):707–13. PMID:2835896

**208.** Bouaoun L, Sonkin D, Ardin M, et al. TP53 variations in human cancers: new lessons from the IARC TP53 Database and genomics data. Hum Mutat. 2016 Sep;37(9):865–76. PMID:27328919

**209.** Boudova L, Kazakov DV, Sima R, et al. Cutaneous lymphoid hyperplasia and other lymphoid infiltrates of the breast nipple: a retrospective clinicopathologic study of fifty-six patients. Am J Dermatopathol. 2005 Oct;27(5):375–86. PMID:16148405

**210.** Bougeard G, Renaux-Petel M, Flaman JM, et al. Revisiting Li-Fraumeni syndrome from TP53 mutation carriers. J Clin Oncol. 2015 Jul 20;33(21):2345–52. PMID:26014290

**211.** Boujelbene N, Khabir A, Boujelbene N, et al. Clinical review–breast adenoid cystic carcinoma. Breast. 2012 Apr;21(2):124–7. PMID:22154460

**212.** Boukhechba M, Kadiri H, El Khannoussi B. Invasive lobular carcinoma of the breast with extracellular mucin: case report of a new variant of lobular carcinoma of the breast. Case Rep Pathol. 2018 Apr 5;2018:5362951. PMID:29850340

**213.** Boulos FI, Dupont WD, Simpson JF, et al. Histologic associations and long-term cancer risk in columnar cell lesions of the breast: a retrospective cohort and a nested case-control study. Cancer. 2008 Nov 1;113(9):2415–21. PMID:18816618

**214.** Boulos FI, Granja NM, Simpson JF, et al. Intranodal papillary epithelial proliferations: a local process with a spectrum of morphologies and frequent association with papillomas in the breast. Am J Surg Pathol. 2014 Mar;38(3):383–8. PMID:24525508

**215.** Bourgeois JM, Knezevich SR, Mathers JA, et al. Molecular detection of the ETV6-NTRK3 gene fusion differentiates congenital fibrosarcoma from other childhood spindle cell tumors. Am J Surg Pathol. 2000 Jul;24(7):937–46. PMID:10895816

**216.** Bowman E, Oprea G, Okoli J, et al. Pseudoangiomatous stromal hyperplasia (PASH) of the breast: a series of 24 patients. Breast J. 2012 May-Jun;18(3):242–7. PMID:22583194

**217.** Bozovic-Spasojevic I, Zardavas D, Brohée S, et al. The prognostic role of androgen receptor in patients with early-stage breast cancer: a meta-analysis of clinical and gene expression data. Clin Cancer Res. 2017 Jun 1;23(11):2702–12. PMID:28151718

**218.** Brain E, Garrino C, Misset JL, et al. Long-term prognostic and predictive factors in 107 stage II/III breast cancer patients treated with anthracycline-based neoadjuvant chemotherapy. Br J Cancer. 1997;75(9):1360–7. PMID:9155059

**219.** Brankov N, Nino T, Hsiang D, et al. Utilizing Mohs surgery for tissue preservation in erosive adenomatosis of the nipple. Dermatol Surg. 2016 May;42(5):684–6. PMID:27045746

**220.** Bratthauer GL, Tavassoli FA. Lobular intraepithelial neoplasia: previously unexplored aspects assessed in 775 cases and their clinical implications. Virchows Arch. 2002 Feb;440(2):134–8. PMID:11964042

**221.** Bray F, Ferlay J, Soerjomataram I, et al. Global cancer statistics 2018: GLOBOCAN estimates of incidence and mortality worldwide for 36 cancers in 185 countries. CA Cancer J Clin. 2018 Nov;68(6):394–424. PMID:30207593

**222.** Bray F, McCarron P, Parkin DM. The changing global patterns of female breast cancer incidence and mortality. Breast Cancer Res. 2004;6(6):229–39. PMID:15535852

**223.** Breast Cancer Linkage Consortium. Cancer risks in BRCA2 mutation carriers. J Natl Cancer Inst. 1999 Aug 4;91(15):1310–6. PMID:10433620

**224.** Brenn T, Fletcher CD. Radiation-associated cutaneous atypical vascular lesions and angiosarcoma: clinicopathologic analysis of 42 cases. Am J Surg Pathol. 2005 Aug;29(8):983–96. PMID:16006792

**225.** Brennan MF, Antonescu CR, Moraco N, et al. Lessons learned from the study of 10,000 patients with soft tissue sarcoma. Ann Surg. 2014 Sep;260(3):416–21, discussion 421–2. PMID:25115417

**226.** Brents M, Hancock J. Ductal carcinoma in situ of the male breast. Breast Care (Basel). 2016 Aug;11(4):288–90. PMID:27721718

**227.** Breuer A, Kandel M, Fisseler-Eckhoff A, et al. BRCA1 germline mutation in a woman with metaplastic squamous cell breast cancer. Onkologie. 2007 Jun;30(6):316–8. PMID:17551255

**228.** Brieher WM, Yap AS. Cadherin junctions and their cytoskeleton(s). Curr Opin Cell Biol. 2013 Feb;25(1):39–46. PMID:23127608

**229.** Brierly JD, Gospodarowicz MK, Wittekind C, editors. TNM classification of malignant tumours. 8th ed. Oxford (UK): Wiley Blackwell; 2017.

**230.** Bright CJ, Rea DW, Francis A, et al. Comparison of quadrant-specific breast cancer incidence trends in the United States and England between 1975 and 2013. Cancer Epidemiol. 2016 Oct;44:186–94. PMID:27632243

**231.** Brinton LA, Cook MB, McCormack V, et al. Anthropometric and hormonal risk factors for male breast cancer: male breast cancer pooling project results. J Natl Cancer Inst. 2014 Mar;106(3):djt465. PMID:24552677

**232.** Briski LM, Jorns JM. Primary breast atypical lipomatous tumor/well-differentiated liposarcoma and dedifferentiated liposarcoma. Arch Pathol Lab Med. 2018 Feb;142(2):268–74. PMID:29372852

**233.** Britton P, Duffy SW, Sinnatamby R, et al. One-stop diagnostic breast clinics: How often are breast cancers missed? Br J Cancer. 2009 Jun 16;100(12):1873–8. PMID:19455145

**234.** Broeks A, Urbanus JH, Floore AN, et al. ATM-heterozygous germline mutations contribute to breast cancer-susceptibility. Am J Hum Genet. 2000 Feb;66(2):494–500. PMID:10677309

**235.** Broët P, de la Rochefordière A, Scholl SM, et al. Contralateral breast cancer: annual incidence and risk parameters. J Clin Oncol. 1995 Jul;13(7):1578–83. PMID:7602346

**236.** Brogi E, Oyama T, Koerner FC. Atypical cystic lobules in patients with lobular neoplasia. Int J Surg Pathol. 2001 Jul;9(3):201–6. PMID:11584316

**237.** Brookes MJ, Bourke AG. Radiological appearances of papillary breast lesions. Clin Radiol. 2008 Nov;63(11):1265–73. PMID:18929044

**237A.** Brooks MD, Burness ML, Wicha MS. Therapeutic implications of cellular heterogeneity and plasticity in breast cancer. Cell Stem Cell. 2015 Sep 3;17(3):260–71. PMID:26340526

**238.** Brosens LA, van Hattem WA, Jansen M, et al. Gastrointestinal polyposis syndromes. Curr Mol Med. 2007 Feb;7(1):29–46. PMID:17311531

**239.** Brosens LA, Wood LD, Offerhaus GJ, et al. Pathology and genetics of syndromic gastric polyps. Int J Surg Pathol. 2016 May;24(3):185–99. PMID:26721304

**240.** Brown AC, Audisio RA, Regitnig P. Granular cell tumour of the breast. Surg Oncol. 2011 Jun;20(2):97–105. PMID:20074934

**241.** Brown DC, Theaker JM, Banks PM, et al. Cytokeratin expression in smooth muscle and smooth muscle tumours. Histopathology. 1987 May;11(5):477–86. PMID:2440790

**242.** Brustein S, Filippa DA, Kimmel M, et al. Malignant lymphoma of the breast. A study of 53 patients. Ann Surg. 1987 Feb;205(2):144–50. PMID:3545107

**243.** Bubien V, Bonnet F, Brouste V, et al. High cumulative risks of cancer in patients with PTEN hamartoma tumour syndrome. J Med Genet. 2013 Apr;50(4):255–63. PMID:23335809

**244.** Buchanan CL, Flynn LW, Murray MP, et al. Is pleomorphic lobular carcinoma really a distinct clinical entity? J Surg Oncol. 2008 Oct 1;98(5):314–7. PMID:18668643

**245.** Buckle G, Maranda L, Skiles J, et al. Factors influencing survival among Kenyan children diagnosed with endemic Burkitt lymphoma between 2003 and 2011: a historical cohort study. Int J Cancer. 2016 Sep 15;139(6):1231–40. PMID:27136063

**246.** Budczies J, Bockmayr M, Denkert C, et al. Classical pathology and mutational load of breast cancer - integration of two worlds. J Pathol Clin Res. 2015 Jul 20;1(4):225–38. PMID:27499907

**247.** Buerger H, Otterbach F, Simon R, et al. Comparative genomic hybridization of ductal carcinoma in situ of the breast-evidence of multiple genetic pathways. J Pathol. 1999 Mar;187(4):396–402. PMID:10398097

**248.** Buerger H, Otterbach F, Simon R, et al. Different genetic pathways in the evolution of invasive breast cancer are associated with distinct morphological subtypes. J Pathol. 1999 Dec;189(4):521–6. PMID:10629552

**249.** Buisman FE, van Gelder L, Menke-Pluijmers MB, et al. Non-primary breast malignancies: a single institution's experience of a diagnostic challenge with important therapeutic consequences-a retrospective study. World J Surg Oncol. 2016 Jun 23;14(1):166. PMID:27337944

**250.** Buley ID, Gatter KC, Kelly PM, et al. Granular cell tumours revisited. An immunohistological and ultrastructural study. Histopathology. 1988 Mar;12(3):263–74. PMID:2452781

**251.** Bur ME, Zimarowski MJ, Schnitt SJ, et al. Estrogen receptor immunohistochemistry in carcinoma in situ of the breast. Cancer. 1992 Mar 1;69(5):1174–81. PMID:1739917

**252.** Burdick C, Rinehart RM, Matsumoto T, et al. Nipple adenoma and Paget's disease

in a man. Arch Surg. 1965 Nov;91(5):835–9. PMID:4284848
**253.** Burga AM, Tavassoli FA. Periductal stromal tumor: a rare lesion with low-grade sarcomatous behavior. Am J Surg Pathol. 2003 Mar;27(3):343–8. PMID:12604890
**254.** Bürger H, de Boer M, van Diest PJ, et al. Chromosome 16q loss–a genetic key to the understanding of breast carcinogenesis. Histol Histopathol. 2013 Mar;28(3):311–20. PMID:23348384
**255.** Burkitt D. A sarcoma involving the jaws in African children. Br J Surg. 1958 Nov;46(197):218–23. PMID:13628987
**256.** Burstein MD, Tsimelzon A, Poage GM, et al. Comprehensive genomic analysis identifies novel subtypes and targets of triple-negative breast cancer. Clin Cancer Res. 2015 Apr 1;21(7):1688–98. PMID:25208879
**257.** Bussolati G, Gugliotta P, Sapino A, et al. Chromogranin-reactive endocrine cells in argyrophilic carcinomas ("carcinoids") and normal tissue of the breast. Am J Pathol. 1985 Aug;120(2):186–92. PMID:4025508
**258.** Butler RS, Venta LA, Wiley EL, et al. Sonographic evaluation of infiltrating lobular carcinoma. AJR Am J Roentgenol. 1999 Feb;172(2):325–30. PMID:9930776
**259.** Buttitta F, Felicioni L, Barassi F, et al. PIK3CA mutation and histological type in breast carcinoma: high frequency of mutations in lobular carcinoma. J Pathol. 2006 Feb;208(3):350–5. PMID:16353168
**260.** Cabibi D, Cipolla C, Maria Florena A, et al. Solid variant of mammary "adenoid cystic carcinoma with basaloid features" merging with "small cell carcinoma". Pathol Res Pract. 2005;201(10):705–11. PMID:16325513
**261.** Cabras MG, Amichetti M, Nagliati M, et al. Primary non-Hodgkin's lymphoma of the breast: a report of 11 cases. Haematologica. 2004 Dec;89(12):1527–8. PMID:15590406
**262.** Cai Q, Long J, Lu W, et al. Genome-wide association study identifies breast cancer risk variant at 10q21.2: results from the Asia Breast Cancer Consortium. Hum Mol Genet. 2011 Dec 15;20(24):4991–9. PMID:21908515
**263.** Cai Q, Zhang B, Sung H, et al. Genome-wide association analysis in East Asians identifies breast cancer susceptibility loci at 1q32.1, 5q14.3 and 15q26.1. Nat Genet. 2014 Aug;46(8):886–90. PMID:25038754
**264.** Cai RZ, Tan PH. Adenomyoepithelioma of the breast with squamous and sebaceous metaplasia. Pathology. 2005 Dec;37(6):557–9. PMID:16373236
**265.** Cai Z, Chehab NH, Pavletich NP. Structure and activation mechanism of the CHK2 DNA damage checkpoint kinase. Mol Cell. 2009 Sep 24;35(6):818–29. PMID:19782031
**266.** Cakir A, Gonul II, Uluoglu O. A comprehensive morphological study for basal-like breast carcinomas with comparison to nonbasal-like carcinomas. Diagn Pathol. 2012 Oct 20;7:145. PMID:23082819
**267.** Calhoun BC. Core needle biopsy of the breast: an evaluation of contemporary data. Surg Pathol Clin. 2018 Mar;11(1):1–16. PMID:29413652
**268.** Calhoun BC, Booth CN. Atypical apocrine adenosis diagnosed on breast core biopsy: implications for management. Hum Pathol. 2014 Oct;45(10):2130–5. PMID:25106711
**269.** Calhoun BC, Collie AM, Lott-Limbach AA, et al. Lobular neoplasia diagnosed on breast core biopsy: frequency of carcinoma on excision and implications for management. Ann Diagn Pathol. 2016 Dec;25:20–5. PMID:27806840
**270.** Calhoun BC, Collins LC. Recommendations for excision following core needle biopsy of the breast: a contemporary evaluation of the literature. Histopathology. 2016 Jan;68(1):138–51. PMID:26768035
**271.** Caliskan M, Gatti G, Sosnovskikh I, et al. Paget's disease of the breast: the experience of the European Institute of Oncology and review of the literature. Breast Cancer Res Treat. 2008 Dec;112(3):513–21. PMID:18240020
**272.** Callari M, Cappelletti V, De Cecco L, et al. Gene expression analysis reveals a different transcriptomic landscape in female and male breast cancer. Breast Cancer Res Treat. 2011 Jun;127(3):601–10. PMID:20625818
**273.** Camelo-Piragua SI, Habib C, Kanumuri P, et al. Mucoepidermoid carcinoma of the breast shares cytogenetic abnormality with mucoepidermoid carcinoma of the salivary gland: a case report with molecular analysis and review of the literature. Hum Pathol. 2009 Jun;40(6):887–92. PMID:19200580
**274.** Cameselle-Teijeiro J, Abdulkader I, Barreiro-Morandeira F, et al. Breast tumor resembling the tall cell variant of papillary thyroid carcinoma: a case report. Int J Surg Pathol. 2006 Jan;14(1):79–84. PMID:16501842
**275.** Canas-Marques R, Schnitt SJ. E-cadherin immunohistochemistry in breast pathology: uses and pitfalls. Histopathology. 2016 Jan;68(1):57–69. PMID:26768029
**276.** Cancello G, Maisonneuve P, Rotmensz N, et al. Prognosis in women with small (T1mic,T1a,T1b) node-negative operable breast cancer by immunohistochemically selected subtypes. Breast Cancer Res Treat. 2011 Jun;127(3):713–20. PMID:21452022
**277.** Cancer Genome Atlas Network. Comprehensive molecular portraits of human breast tumours. Nature. 2012 Oct 4;490(7418):61–70. PMID:23000897
**278.** Cangiarella J, Guth A, Axelrod D, et al. Is surgical excision necessary for the management of atypical lobular hyperplasia and lobular carcinoma in situ diagnosed on core needle biopsy? A report of 38 cases and review of the literature. Arch Pathol Lab Med. 2008 Jun;132(6):979–83. PMID:18517282
**279.** Cantile M, Di Bonito M, Cerrone M, et al. Primary breast angiosarcoma in young women from the same geographic region in a short period of time: only a coincidence or an increased risk? Breast J. 2018 Jan;24(1):91–3. PMID:28597488
**280.** Capella C, Eusebi V, Mann B, et al. Endocrine differentiation in mucoid carcinoma of the breast. Histopathology. 1980 Nov;4(6):613–30. PMID:6254868
**281.** Capella C, Usellini L, Papotti M, et al. Ultrastructural features of neuroendocrine differentiated carcinomas of the breast. Ultrastruct Pathol. 1990 Jul-Aug;14(4):321–34. PMID:2200185
**282.** Caplain A, Drouet Y, Peyron M, et al. Management of patients diagnosed with atypical ductal hyperplasia by vacuum-assisted core biopsy: a prospective assessment of the guidelines used at our institution. Am J Surg. 2014 Aug;208(2):260–7. PMID:24680949
**283.** Carbognin L, Sperduti I, Fabi A, et al. Prognostic impact of proliferation for resected early stage 'pure' invasive lobular breast cancer: cut-off analysis of Ki67 according to histology and clinical validation. Breast. 2017 Oct;35:21–6. PMID:28628772
**284.** Cardoso F, Bartlett JMS, Slaets L, et al. Characterization of male breast cancer: results of the EORTC 10085/TBCRC/BIG/NABCG International Male Breast Cancer Program. Ann Oncol. 2018 Feb 1;29(2):405–17. PMID:29092024
**285.** Cardoso F, van't Veer LJ, Bogaerts J, et al. 70-gene signature as an aid to treatment decisions in early-stage breast cancer. N Engl J Med. 2016 Aug 25;375(8):717–29. PMID:27557300
**286.** Carey LA, Metzger R, Dees EC, et al. American Joint Committee on Cancer tumor-node-metastasis stage after neoadjuvant chemotherapy and breast cancer outcome. J Natl Cancer Inst. 2005 Aug 3;97(15):1137–42. PMID:16077072
**287.** Carey LA, Perou CM, Livasy CA, et al. Race, breast cancer subtypes, and survival in the Carolina Breast Cancer Study. JAMA. 2006 Jun 7;295(21):2492–502. PMID:16757721
**288.** Carley AM, Chivukula M, Carter GJ, et al. Frequency and clinical significance of simultaneous association of lobular neoplasia and columnar cell alterations in breast tissue specimens. Am J Clin Pathol. 2008 Aug;130(2):254–8. PMID:18628095
**289.** Carlson JW, Fletcher CD. Immunohistochemistry for beta-catenin in the differential diagnosis of spindle cell lesions: analysis of a series and review of the literature. Histopathology. 2007 Oct;51(4):509–14. PMID:17711447
**290.** Carney JA. The Carney complex (myxomas, spotty pigmentation, endocrine overactivity, and schwannomas). Dermatol Clin. 1995 Jan;13(1):19–26. PMID:7712644
**291.** Carney JA, Stratakis CA. Ductal adenoma of the breast and the Carney complex. Am J Surg Pathol. 1996 Sep;20(9):1154–5. PMID:8764753
**292.** Carney JA, Toorkey BC. Myxoid fibroadenoma and allied conditions (myxomatosis) of the breast. A heritable disorder with special associations including cardiac and cutaneous myxomas. Am J Surg Pathol. 1991 Aug;15(8):713–21. PMID:2069209
**293.** Carreira C, Romero C, Rodriguez R, et al. A cavernous haemangioma of breast in male: radiological-pathological correlation. Eur Radiol. 2001;11(2):292–4. PMID:11218030
**294.** Carter BA, Jensen RA, Simpson JF, et al. Benign transport of breast epithelium into axillary lymph nodes after biopsy. Am J Clin Pathol. 2000 Feb;113(2):259–65. PMID:10664628
**295.** Carter BA, Page DL, Schuyler P, et al. No elevation in long-term breast carcinoma risk for women with fibroadenomas that contain atypical hyperplasia. Cancer. 2001 Jul 1;92(1):30–6. PMID:11443606
**296.** Carter CS, Skala SL, Chinnaiyan AM, et al. Immunohistochemical characterization of fumarate hydratase (FH) and succinate dehydrogenase (SDH) in cutaneous leiomyomas for detection of familial cancer syndromes. Am J Surg Pathol. 2017 Jun;41(6):801–9. PMID:28288038
**297.** Carter D. Intraductal papillary tumors of the breast: a study of 78 cases. Cancer. 1977 Apr;39(4):1689–92. PMID:851947
**298.** Carter MR, Hornick JL, Lester S, et al. Spindle cell (sarcomatoid) carcinoma of the breast: a clinicopathologic and immunohistochemical analysis of 29 cases. Am J Surg Pathol. 2006 Mar;30(3):300–9. PMID:16538049
**299.** Casadei S, Norquist BM, Walsh T, et al. Contribution of inherited mutations in the BRCA2-interacting protein PALB2 to familial breast cancer. Cancer Res. 2011 Mar 15;71(6):2222–9. PMID:21285249
**300.** Castillo JJ, Winer ES, Olszewski AJ. Population-based prognostic factors for survival in patients with Burkitt lymphoma: an analysis from the Surveillance, Epidemiology, and End Results database. Cancer. 2013 Oct 15;119(20):3672–9. PMID:23913575
**301.** Castroviejo-Bermejo M, Cruz C, Llop-Guevara A, et al. A RAD51 assay feasible in routine tumor samples calls PARP inhibitor response beyond BRCA mutation. EMBO Mol Med. 2018 Dec;10(12):e9172. PMID:30377213
**302.** Catalina-Fernández I, Sáenz-Santamaria J. Lipid-rich carcinoma of breast: a case report with fine needle aspiration cytology. Diagn Cytopathol. 2009 Dec;37(12):935–6. PMID:19795489
**303.** Catena F, Santini D, Di Saverio S, et al. Adenomyoepithelioma of the breast: an intricate diagnostic problem. Breast Care (Basel). 2008;3(2):125–7. PMID:21373216
**304.** Catucci I, Milgrom R, Kushnir A, et al. Germline mutations in BRIP1 and PALB2 in Jewish high cancer risk families. Fam Cancer. 2012 Sep;11(3):483–91. PMID:22692731
**305.** Cavallaro U, Dejana E. Adhesion molecule signalling: not always a sticky business. Nat Rev Mol Cell Biol. 2011 Mar;12(3):189–97. PMID:21346732
**306.** Cawson JN, Law EM, Kavanagh AM. Invasive lobular carcinoma: sonographic features of cancers detected in a BreastScreen program. Australas Radiol. 2001 Feb;45(1):25–30. PMID:11259968
**307.** Cesarman E, Knowles DM. Kaposi's sarcoma-associated herpesvirus: a lymphotropic human herpesvirus associated with Kaposi's sarcoma, primary effusion lymphoma, and multicentric Castleman's disease. Semin Diagn Pathol. 1997 Feb;14(1):54–66. PMID:9044510
**308.** Chang CK, Jacobs IA, Calilao G, et al. Metastatic infiltrating syringomatous adenoma of the breast. Arch Pathol Lab Med. 2003 Mar;127(3):e155–6. PMID:12653606
**309.** Chang HL, Lerwill MF, Goldstein AM. Breast hamartomas in adolescent females. Breast J. 2009 Sep-Oct;15(5):515–20. PMID:19624414
**310.** Chang SY, Fleiszer DM, Mesurolle B, et al. Breast tumor resembling the tall cell variant of papillary thyroid carcinoma. Breast J. 2009 Sep-Oct;15(5):531–5. PMID:19594763
**311.** Charfi L, Driss M, Mrad K, et al. Primary well differentiated liposarcoma: an unusual tumor in the breast. Breast J. 2009 Mar-Apr;15(2):206–7. PMID:19292812
**312.** Charpin C, Mathoulin MP, Andrac L, et al. Reappraisal of breast hamartomas. A morphological study of 41 cases. Pathol Res Pract. 1994 Apr;190(4):362–71. PMID:8078805
**313.** Charu V, Cimino-Mathews A. Peripheral nerve sheath tumors of the breast. Semin Diagn Pathol. 2017 Sep;34(5):420–6. PMID:28647116
**314.** Chaudary MA, Millis RR, Lane EB, et al. Paget's disease of the nipple: a ten year review including clinical, pathological, and immunohistochemical findings. Breast Cancer Res Treat. 1986;8(2):139–46. PMID:2434164
**315.** Chaudhry A, Williams S, Cook J, et al. The real-time intra-operative evaluation of sentinel lymph nodes in breast cancer patients using One Step Nucleic Acid Amplification (OSNA) and implications for clinical decision-making. Eur J Surg Oncol. 2014 Feb;40(2):150–7. PMID:24378008
**316.** Chavez-Macgregor M, Clarke CA, Lichtensztajn D, et al. Male breast cancer according to tumor subtype and race: a population-based study. Cancer. 2013 May 1;119(9):1611–7. PMID:23341341
**316A.** Cheang MC, Chia SK, Voduc D, et al. Ki67 index, HER2 status, and prognosis of patients with luminal B breast cancer. J Natl Cancer Inst. 2009 May 20;101(10):736–50. PMID:19436038
**317.** Chehab NH, Malikzay A, Appel M, et al. Chk2/hCds1 functions as a DNA damage checkpoint in G(1) by stabilizing p53. Genes Dev. 2000 Feb 1;14(3):278–88. PMID:10673500
**318.** CHEK2 Breast Cancer Case-Control Consortium. CHEK2*1100delC and susceptibility to breast cancer: a collaborative

analysis involving 10,860 breast cancer cases and 9,065 controls from 10 studies. Am J Hum Genet. 2004 Jun;74(6):1175–82. PMID:15122511
**319.** Chen AC, Paulino AC, Schwartz MR, et al. Population-based comparison of prognostic factors in invasive micropapillary and invasive ductal carcinoma of the breast. Br J Cancer. 2014 Jul 29;111(3):619–22. PMID:24921921
**320.** Chen AM, Meric-Bernstam F, Hunt KK, et al. Breast conservation after neoadjuvant chemotherapy: the MD Anderson Cancer Center experience. J Clin Oncol. 2004 Jun 15;22(12):2303–12. PMID:15197191
**321.** Chen BJ, Mariño-Enríquez A, Fletcher CD, et al. Loss of retinoblastoma protein expression in spindle cell/pleomorphic lipomas and cytogenetically related tumors: an immunohistochemical study with diagnostic implications. Am J Surg Pathol. 2012 Aug;36(8):1119–28. PMID:22790852
**322.** Chen CY, Sun LM, Anderson BO. Paget disease of the breast: changing patterns of incidence, clinical presentation, and treatment in the U.S. Cancer. 2006 Oct 1;107(7):1448–58. PMID:16933329
**323.** Chen H, Wu J, Zhang Z, et al. Association between BRCA status and triple-negative breast cancer: a meta-analysis. Front Pharmacol. 2018 Aug 21;9:909. PMID:30186165
**324.** Chen H, Wu K, Wang M, et al. Invasive micropapillary carcinoma of the breast has a better long-term survival than invasive ductal carcinoma of the breast in spite of its aggressive clinical presentations: a comparison based on large population database and case-control analysis. Cancer Med. 2017 Dec;6(12):2775–86. PMID:29072365
**324A.** Chen HL, Zhou MQ, Tian W, et al. Effect of age on breast cancer patient prognoses: a population-based study using the SEER 18 database. PLoS One. 2016 Oct 31;11(10):e0165409. PMID:27798652
**325.** Chen L, Li CI, Tang MT, et al. Reproductive factors and risk of luminal, HER2-overexpressing, and triple-negative breast cancer among multiethnic women. Cancer Epidemiol Biomarkers Prev. 2016 Sep;25(9):1297–304. PMID:27307466
**326.** Chen QX, Li JJ, Wang XX, et al. Similar outcomes between adenoid cystic carcinoma of the breast and invasive ductal carcinoma: a population-based study from the SEER 18 database. Oncotarget. 2017 Jan 24;8(4):6206–15. PMID:28008158
**327.** Chen S, Parmigiani G. Meta-analysis of BRCA1 and BRCA2 penetrance. J Clin Oncol. 2007 Apr 10;25(11):1329–33. PMID:17416853
**328.** Chen Y, Thompson W, Semenciw R, et al. Epidemiology of contralateral breast cancer. Cancer Epidemiol Biomarkers Prev. 1999 Oct;8(10):855–61. PMID:10548312
**329.** Chen YL, Chen JJ, Chang C, et al. Sclerosing adenosis: ultrasonographic and mammographic findings and correlation with histopathology. Mol Clin Oncol. 2017 Feb;6(2):157–62. PMID:28357084
**330.** Chen YY, Hwang ES, Roy R, et al. Genetic and phenotypic characteristics of pleomorphic lobular carcinoma in situ of the breast. Am J Surg Pathol. 2009 Nov;33(11):1683–94. PMID:19701073
**331.** Chen Z, Yang J, Li S, et al. Invasive lobular carcinoma of the breast: a special histological type compared with invasive ductal carcinoma. PLoS One. 2017 Sep 1;12(9):e0182397. PMID:28863134
**332.** Chene A, Donati D, Orem J, et al. Endemic Burkitt's lymphoma as a polymicrobial disease: new insights on the interaction between Plasmodium falciparum and Epstein-Barr virus. Semin Cancer Biol. 2009 Dec;19(6):411–20. PMID:19897039
**333.** Chenevix-Trench G, Spurdle AB, Gatei M, et al. Dominant negative ATM mutations in breast cancer families. J Natl Cancer Inst. 2002 Feb 6;94(3):205–15. PMID:11830610
**334.** Cheng CW, Wu PE, Yu JC, et al. Mechanisms of inactivation of E-cadherin in breast carcinoma: modification of the two-hit hypothesis of tumor suppressor gene. Oncogene. 2001 Jun 28;20(29):3814–23. PMID:11439345
**335.** Cheng DT, Mitchell TN, Zehir A, et al. Memorial Sloan Kettering-Integrated Mutation Profiling of Actionable Cancer Targets (MSK-IMPACT): a hybridization capture-based next-generation sequencing clinical assay for solid tumor molecular oncology. J Mol Diagn. 2015 May;17(3):251–64. PMID:25801821
**336.** Cheng M, Geng C, Tang T, et al. Mucoepidermoid carcinoma of the breast: four case reports and review of the literature. Medicine (Baltimore). 2017 Dec;96(51):e9385. PMID:29390541
**337.** Chesebro AL, Rives AF, Shaffer K. Male breast disease: what the radiologist needs to know. Curr Probl Diagn Radiol. 2018 Jul 29;S0363-0188(18)30061-6. PMID:30122313
**338.** Cheson BD, Fisher RI, Barrington SF, et al. Recommendations for initial evaluation, staging, and response assessment of Hodgkin and non-Hodgkin lymphoma: the Lugano classification. J Clin Oncol. 2014 Sep 20;32(27):3059–68. PMID:25113753
**339.** Cheung KL, Wong AW, Parker H, et al. Pathological features of primary breast cancer in the elderly based on needle core biopsies–a large series from a single centre. Crit Rev Oncol Hematol. 2008 Sep;67(3):263–7. PMID:18524618
**340.** Chia Y, Thike AA, Cheok PY, et al. Stromal keratin expression in phyllodes tumours of the breast: a comparison with other spindle cell breast lesions. J Clin Pathol. 2012 Apr;65(4):339–47. PMID:22259180
**341.** Chiacchio R, Panico L, D'Antonio A, et al. Mammary hamartomas: an immunohistochemical study of ten cases. Pathol Res Pract. 1999;195(4):231–6. PMID:10337660
**342.** Chiang S, Weigelt B, Wen HC, et al. IDH2 mutations define a unique subtype of breast cancer with altered nuclear polarity. Cancer Res. 2016 Dec 15;76(24):7118–29. PMID:27913435
**343.** Chibon F, Lagarde P, Salas S, et al. Validated prediction of clinical outcome in sarcomas and multiple types of cancer on the basis of a gene expression signature related to genome complexity. Nat Med. 2010 Jul;16(7):781–7. PMID:20581836
**344.** Chng TW, Gudi M, Lim SH, et al. Validation of the Singapore nomogram for outcome prediction in breast phyllodes tumours in a large patient cohort. J Clin Pathol. 2018 Feb;71(2):125–8. PMID:28751520
**345.** Chng TW, Lee JY, Lee CS, et al. Validation of the Singapore nomogram for outcome prediction in breast phyllodes tumours: an Australian cohort. J Clin Pathol. 2016 Dec;69(12):1124–6. PMID:27466383
**346.** Cho KS, Choi HY, Lee SW, et al. Sonographic findings in solitary schwannoma of the breast. J Clin Ultrasound. 2001 Feb;29(2):99–101. PMID:11425095
**347.** Cho WK, Choi DH, Lee J, et al. Comparison of failure patterns between tubular breast carcinoma and invasive ductal carcinoma (KROG 14-25). Breast. 2018 Apr;38:165–70. PMID:29413404
**348.** Choi M, Kipps T, Kurzrock R. ATM mutations in cancer: therapeutic implications. Mol Cancer Ther. 2016 Aug;15(8):1781–91. PMID:27413114
**349.** Choi N, Kim K, Shin KH, et al. Malignant and borderline phyllodes tumors of the breast: a multicenter study of 362 patients (KROG 16-08). Breast Cancer Res Treat. 2018 Sep;171(2):335–44. PMID:29808288
**350.** Chou WYY, Veis DJ, Aft R. Radial scar on image-guided breast biopsy: Is surgical excision necessary? Breast Cancer Res Treat. 2018 Jul;170(2):313–20. PMID:29532340
**351.** Christgen M, Steinemann D, Kühnle E, et al. Lobular breast cancer: clinical, molecular and morphological characteristics. Pathol Res Pract. 2016 Jul;212(7):583–97. PMID:27233940
**352.** Christie M, Chin-Lenn L, Watts MM, et al. Primary small cell carcinoma of the breast with TTF-1 and neuroendocrine marker expressing carcinoma in situ. Int J Clin Exp Pathol. 2010 Jun 30;3(6):629–33. PMID:20661411
**353.** Christou CM, Kyriacou K. BRCA1 and its network of interacting partners. Biology (Basel). 2013 Jan 2;2(1):40–63. PMID:24832651
**354.** Chu KC, Anderson WF. Rates for breast cancer characteristics by estrogen and progesterone receptor status in the major racial/ethnic groups. Breast Cancer Res Treat. 2002 Jun;74(3):199–211. PMID:12206512
**355.** Chua CL, Thomas A, Ng BK. Cystosarcoma phyllodes–Asian variations. Aust N Z J Surg. 1988 Apr;58(4):301–5. PMID:2855393
**356.** Chuba PJ, Hamre MR, Yap J, et al. Bilateral risk for subsequent breast cancer after lobular carcinoma-in-situ: analysis of Surveillance, Epidemiology, and End Results data. J Clin Oncol. 2005 Aug 20;23(24):5534–41. PMID:16110014
**357.** Chulakadabba A, Denariyakoon S, Chakkabat P, et al. Preoperative radiation in large angiomatosis of the breast, attempting breast conserving surgery: multidisciplinary approach. J Surg Case Rep. 2018 Feb 14;2018(2):rjy024. PMID:29479420
**358.** Chun KA, Cohen PR. Basal cell carcinoma of the nipple-areola complex: a comprehensive review of the world literature. Dermatol Ther (Heidelb). 2016 Sep;6(3):379–95. PMID:27363851
**359.** Ciatto S, Bonardi R, Cataliotti L, et al. Sarcomas of the breast: a multicenter series of 70 cases. Neoplasma. 1992;39(6):375–9. PMID:1491728
**360.** Cimino-Mathews A, Hicks JL, Sharma R, et al. A subset of malignant phyllodes tumors harbors alterations in the Rb/p16 pathway. Hum Pathol. 2013 Nov;44(11):2494–500. PMID:23916291
**361.** Cimino-Mathews A, Sharma R, Illei PB, et al. A subset of malignant phyllodes tumors express p63 and p40: a diagnostic pitfall in breast core needle biopsies. Am J Surg Pathol. 2014 Dec;38(12):1689–96. PMID:25046342
**362.** Cimino-Mathews AM. Peripheral nerve sheath tumors. Surg Pathol Clin. 2011 Sep;4(3):761–82. PMID:26837647
**363.** Ciriello G, Gatza ML, Beck AH, et al. Comprehensive molecular portraits of invasive lobular breast cancer. Cell. 2015 Oct 8;163(2):506–19. PMID:26451490
**364.** Ciurea A, Dudea SM, Lebovici A, et al. Diffuse angiomatosis of the breast–sonographic appearance. J Clin Ultrasound. 2014 Oct;42(8):498–501. PMID:24965677
**365.** Clark SL, Rodriguez AM, Snyder RR, et al. Structure-function of the tumor suppressor BRCA1. Comput Struct Biotechnol J. 2012 Apr 1;1(1):e201204005. PMID:22737296
**366.** Claus EB, Petruzella S, Matloff E, et al. Prevalence of BRCA1 and BRCA2 mutations in women diagnosed with ductal carcinoma in situ. JAMA. 2005 Feb 23;293(8):964–9. PMID:15728167
**367.** Claus EB, Stowe M, Carter D. Breast carcinoma in situ: risk factors and screening patterns. J Natl Cancer Inst. 2001 Dec 5;93(23):1811–7. PMID:11734598
**368.** Claus EB, Stowe M, Carter D. Family history of breast and ovarian cancer and the risk of breast carcinoma in situ. Breast Cancer Res Treat. 2003 Mar;78(1):7–15. PMID:12611452
**369.** Clemens MW, Horwitz SM. NCCN consensus guidelines for the diagnosis and management of breast implant-associated anaplastic large cell lymphoma. Aesthet Surg J. 2017 Mar 1;37(3):285–9. PMID:28184418
**370.** Clemens MW, Medeiros LJ, Butler CE, et al. Complete surgical excision is essential for the management of patients with breast implant-associated anaplastic large-cell lymphoma. J Clin Oncol. 2016 Jan 10;34(2):160–8. PMID:26628470
**371.** Cloyd JM, Yang RL, Allison KH, et al. Impact of histological subtype on long-term outcomes of neuroendocrine carcinoma of the breast. Breast Cancer Res Treat. 2014 Dec;148(3):637–44. PMID:25399232
**372.** Co M, Chen C, Tsang JY, et al. Mammary phyllodes tumour: a 15-year multicentre clinical review. J Clin Pathol. 2018 Jun;71(6):493–7. PMID:29146885
**373.** Co M, Tse GM, Chen C, et al. Coexistence of ductal carcinoma within mammary phyllodes tumor: a review of 557 cases from a 20-year region-wide database in Hong Kong and southern China. Clin Breast Cancer. 2018 Jun;18(3):e421–5. PMID:28689011
**374.** Cocco E, Scaltriti M, Drilon A. NTRK fusion-positive cancers and TRK inhibitor therapy. Nat Rev Clin Oncol. 2018 Dec;15(12):731–47. PMID:30333516
**375.** Coffin CM, Hornick JL, Fletcher CD. Inflammatory myofibroblastic tumor: comparison of clinicopathologic, histologic, and immunohistochemical features including ALK expression in atypical and aggressive cases. Am J Surg Pathol. 2007 Apr;31(4):509–20. PMID:17414097
**376.** Coffin CM, Watterson J, Priest JR, et al. Extrapulmonary inflammatory myofibroblastic tumor (inflammatory pseudotumor). A clinicopathologic and immunohistochemical study of 84 cases. Am J Surg Pathol. 1995 Aug;19(8):859–72. PMID:7611533
**377.** Cohen JM, Nazarian RM, Ferry JA, et al. Rare presentation of secondary cutaneous involvement by splenic marginal zone lymphoma: report of a case and review of the literature. Am J Dermatopathol. 2015 Jan;37(1):e1–4. PMID:25238446
**378.** Cohen MA, Newell MS. Radial scars of the breast encountered at core biopsy: review of histologic, imaging, and management considerations. AJR Am J Roentgenol. 2017 Nov;209(5):1168–77. PMID:28813198
**379.** Coindre JM. Grading of soft tissue sarcomas: review and update. Arch Pathol Lab Med. 2006 Oct;130(10):1448–53. PMID:17090186
**380.** Colditz GA, Rosner B. Cumulative risk of breast cancer to age 70 years according to risk factor status: data from the Nurses' Health Study. Am J Epidemiol. 2000 Nov 15;152(10):950–64. PMID:11092437
**381.** Colella R, Guerriero A, Giansanti M, et al. An additional case of breast tumor resembling the tall cell variant of papillary thyroid carcinoma. Int J Surg Pathol. 2015 May;23(3):217–20. PMID:24868004
**382.** Collins LC. Precursor lesions of the low-grade breast neoplasia pathway. Surg Pathol Clin. 2018 Mar;11(1):177–97. PMID:29413656
**383.** Collins LC, Achacoso N, Haque R, et al. Risk prediction for local breast cancer recurrence among women with DCIS treated

in a community practice: a nested, case-control study. Ann Surg Oncol. 2015 Dec;22 Suppl 3:S502–8. PMID:26059650
384. Collins LC, Aroner SA, Connolly JL, et al. Breast cancer risk by extent and type of atypical hyperplasia: an update from the Nurses' Health Studies. Cancer. 2016 Feb 15;122(4):515–20. PMID:26565738
385. Collins LC, Baer HJ, Tamimi RM, et al. Magnitude and laterality of breast cancer risk according to histologic type of atypical hyperplasia: results from the Nurses' Health Study. Cancer. 2007 Jan 15;109(2):180–7. PMID:17154175
386. Collins LC, Baer HJ, Tamimi RM, et al. The influence of family history on breast cancer risk in women with biopsy-confirmed benign breast disease: results from the Nurses' Health Study. Cancer. 2006 Sep 15;107(6):1240–7. PMID:16902983
387. Collins LC, Carlo VP, Hwang H, et al. Intracystic papillary carcinomas of the breast: a reevaluation using a panel of myoepithelial cell markers. Am J Surg Pathol. 2006 Aug;30(8):1002–7. PMID:16861972
388. Collins LC, Cole KS, Marotti JD, et al. Androgen receptor expression in breast cancer in relation to molecular phenotype: results from the Nurses' Health Study. Mod Pathol. 2011 Jul;24(7):924–31. PMID:21552212
389. Collins LC, Connolly JL, Page DL, et al. Diagnostic agreement in the evaluation of image-guided breast core needle biopsies: results from a randomized clinical trial. Am J Surg Pathol. 2004 Jan;28(1):126–31. PMID:14707874
390. Collins LC, Martyniak A, Kandel MJ, et al. Basal cytokeratin and epidermal growth factor receptor expression are not predictive of BRCA1 mutation status in women with triple-negative breast cancers. Am J Surg Pathol. 2009 Jul;33(7):1093–7. PMID:19390427
391. Collins LC, Tamimi RM, Baer HJ, et al. Outcome of patients with ductal carcinoma in situ untreated after diagnostic biopsy: results from the Nurses' Health Study. Cancer. 2005 May 1;103(9):1778–84. PMID:15770688
392. Colombo C, Miceli R, Lazar AJ, et al. CTNNB1 45F mutation is a molecular prognosticator of increased postoperative primary desmoid tumor recurrence: an independent, multicenter validation study. Cancer. 2013 Oct 15;119(20):3696–702. PMID:23913621
393. Comer JD, Cui X, Eisen CS, et al. Myofibroblastoma of the male breast: a rare entity with radiologic-pathologic correlation. Clin Imaging. 2017 Mar-Apr;42:109–12. PMID:27936420
394. Concannon P, Gatti RA. Diversity of ATM gene mutations detected in patients with ataxia-telangiectasia. Hum Mutat. 1997;10(2):100–7. PMID:9259193
395. Conlon N, Ross DS, Howard J, et al. Is there a role for Oncotype DX testing in invasive lobular carcinoma? Breast J. 2015 Sep-Oct;21(5):514–9. PMID:26271749
396. Conlon N, Sadri N, Corben AD, et al. Acinic cell carcinoma of breast: morphologic and immunohistochemical review of a rare breast cancer subtype. Hum Pathol. 2016 May;51:16–24. PMID:27067778
397. Cook JR, Dehner LP, Collins MH, et al. Anaplastic lymphoma kinase (ALK) expression in the inflammatory myofibroblastic tumor: a comparative immunohistochemical study. Am J Surg Pathol. 2001 Nov;25(11):1364–71. PMID:11684952
398. Coopey SB, Mazzola E, Buckley JM, et al. The role of chemoprevention in modifying the risk of breast cancer in women with atypical breast lesions. Breast Cancer Res Treat. 2012 Dec;136(3):627–33. PMID:23117858
399. Copson ER, Maishman TC, Tapper WJ, et al. Germline BRCA mutation and outcome in young-onset breast cancer (POSH): a prospective cohort study. Lancet Oncol. 2018 Feb;19(2):169–80. PMID:29337092
400. Coriat R, Mozer M, Caux F, et al. Endoscopic findings in Cowden syndrome. Endoscopy. 2011 Aug;43(8):723–6. PMID:21437855
401. Corso G, Figueiredo J, La Vecchia C, et al. Hereditary lobular breast cancer with an emphasis on E-cadherin genetic defect. J Med Genet. 2018 Jul;55(7):431–41. PMID:29929997
402. Costanzo PR, Pacenza NA, Aszpis SM, et al. Clinical and etiological aspects of gynecomastia in adult males: a multicenter study. Biomed Res Int. 2018 May 29;2018:8364824. PMID:30003107
403. Couch FJ, Hart SN, Sharma P, et al. Inherited mutations in 17 breast cancer susceptibility genes among a large triple-negative breast cancer cohort unselected for family history of breast cancer. J Clin Oncol. 2015 Feb 1;33(4):304–11. PMID:25452441
404. Couch FJ, Kuchenbaecker KB, Michailidou K, et al. Identification of four novel susceptibility loci for oestrogen receptor negative breast cancer. Nat Commun. 2016 Apr 27;7:11375. PMID:27117709
405. Couch FJ, Shimelis H, Hu C, et al. Associations between cancer predisposition testing panel genes and breast cancer. JAMA Oncol. 2017 Sep 1;3(9):1190–6. PMID:28418444
406. Couch FJ, Wang X, McGuffog L, et al. Genome-wide association study in BRCA1 mutation carriers identifies novel loci associated with breast and ovarian cancer risk. PLoS Genet. 2013;9(3):e1003212. PMID:23544013
407. Couch FJ, Weber BL. Mutations and polymorphisms in the familial early-onset breast cancer (BRCA1) gene. Breast Cancer Information Core. Hum Mutat. 1996;8(1):8–18. PMID:8807330
408. Cowan ML, Argani P, Cimino-Mathews A. Benign and low-grade fibroepithelial neoplasms of the breast have low recurrence rate after positive surgical margins. Mod Pathol. 2016 Mar;29(3):259–65. PMID:26743469
409. Cowell CF, Weigelt B, Sakr RA, et al. Progression from ductal carcinoma in situ to invasive breast cancer: revisited. Mol Oncol. 2013 Oct;7(5):859–69. PMID:23890733
410. Crago AM, Chmielecki J, Rosenberg M, et al. Near universal detection of alterations in CTNNB1 and Wnt pathway regulators in desmoid-type fibromatosis by whole-exome sequencing and genomic analysis. Genes Chromosomes Cancer. 2015 Oct;54(10):606–15. PMID:26171757
411. Crisi GM, Mandavilli S, Cronin E, et al. Invasive mammary carcinoma after immediate and short-term follow-up for lobular neoplasia on core biopsy. Am J Surg Pathol. 2003 Mar;27(3):325–33. PMID:12604888
412. Cross AS, Azzopardi JG, Krausz T, et al. A morphological and immunocytochemical study of a distinctive variant of ductal carcinoma in-situ of the breast. Histopathology. 1985 Jan;9(1):21–37. PMID:2579885
413. Crozat A, Aman P, Mandahl N, et al. Fusion of CHOP to a novel RNA-binding protein in human myxoid liposarcoma. Nature. 1993 Jun 17;363(6430):640–4. PMID:8510758
414. Cserni G. Benign apocrine papillary lesions of the breast lacking or virtually lacking myoepithelial cells-potential pitfalls in diagnosing malignancy. APMIS. 2012 Mar;120(3):249–52. PMID:22339683
415. Cserni G. Lack of myoepithelium in apocrine glands of the breast does not necessarily imply malignancy. Histopathology. 2008 Jan;52(2):253–5. PMID:18184276
416. Cserni G. Presence of basement membrane material around the tubules of tubulolobular carcinoma. Breast Care (Basel). 2008;3(6):423–5. PMID:21048914
417. Cserni G. What is a positive sentinel lymph node in a breast cancer patient? A practical approach. Breast. 2007 Apr;16(2):152–60. PMID:17081752
418. Cserni G, Chmielik E, Cserni B, et al. The new TNM-based staging of breast cancer. Virchows Arch. 2018 May;472(5):697–703. PMID:29380126
419. Cserni G, Floris G, Koufopoulos N, et al. Invasive lobular carcinoma with extracellular mucin production-a novel pattern of lobular carcinomas of the breast. Clinico-pathological description of eight cases. Virchows Arch. 2017 Jul;471(1):3–12. PMID:28528509
420. Cserni G, Wells CA, Kaya H, et al. Consistency in recognizing microinvasion in breast carcinomas is improved by immunohistochemistry for myoepithelial markers. Virchows Arch. 2016 Apr;468(4):473–81. PMID:26818833
421. Curigliano G, Burstein HJP, P Winer E, et al. De-escalating and escalating treatments for early-stage breast cancer: the St. Gallen International Expert Consensus Conference on the Primary Therapy of Early Breast Cancer 2017. Ann Oncol. 2017 Aug 1;28(8):1700–12. PMID:28838210
422. Curigliano G, Burstein HJ, Winer EP, et al. De-escalating and escalating treatments for early-stage breast cancer: the St. Gallen International Expert Consensus Conference on the Primary Therapy of Early Breast Cancer 2017. Ann Oncol. 2018 Oct 1;29(10):2153. PMID:29733336
423. Curtis C, Shah SP, Chin SF, et al. The genomic and transcriptomic architecture of 2,000 breast tumours reveals novel subgroups. Nature. 2012 Apr 18;486(7403):346–52. PMID:22522925
424. Cutress RI, McDowell A, Gabriel FG, et al. Observational and cost analysis of the implementation of breast cancer sentinel node intraoperative molecular diagnosis. J Clin Pathol. 2010 Jun;63(6):522–9. PMID:20439323
425. Cutuli B, Dilhuydy JM, De Lafontan B, et al. Ductal carcinoma in situ of the male breast. Analysis of 31 cases. Eur J Cancer. 1997 Jan;33(1):35–8. PMID:9071896
426. Cuzick J, Dowsett M, Pineda S, et al. Prognostic value of a combined estrogen receptor, progesterone receptor, Ki-67, and human epidermal growth factor receptor 2 immunohistochemical score and comparison with the Genomic Health recurrence score in early breast cancer. J Clin Oncol. 2011 Nov 10;29(32):4273–8. PMID:21990413
427. Cuzick J, Sestak I, Pinder SE, et al. Effect of tamoxifen and radiotherapy in women with locally excised ductal carcinoma in situ: long-term results from the UK/ANZ DCIS trial. Lancet Oncol. 2011 Jan;12(1):21–9. PMID:21145284
428. Cybulski C, Huzarski T, Byrski T, et al. Estrogen receptor status in CHEK2-positive breast cancers: implications for chemoprevention. Clin Genet. 2009 Jan;75(1):72–8. PMID:19021634
429. Da Silva L, Parry S, Reid L, et al. Aberrant expression of E-cadherin in lobular carcinomas of the breast. Am J Surg Pathol. 2008 May;32(5):773–83. PMID:18379416
430. Dabbs DJ, Bhargava R, Chivukula M. Lobular versus ductal breast neoplasms: the diagnostic utility of p120 catenin. Am J Surg Pathol. 2007 Mar;31(3):427–37. PMID:17325485
431. Dabbs DJ, Carter G, Fudge M, et al. Molecular alterations in columnar cell lesions of the breast. Mod Pathol. 2006 Mar;19(3):344–9. PMID:16400324
432. Dabbs DJ, Grenko RT, Silverman JF. Fine needle aspiration cytology of pleomorphic lobular carcinoma of the breast. Duct carcinoma as a diagnostic pitfall. Acta Cytol. 1994 Nov-Dec;38(6):923–6. PMID:7992580
433. Dabbs DJ, Schnitt SJ, Geyer FC, et al. Lobular neoplasia of the breast revisited with emphasis on the role of E-cadherin immunohistochemistry. Am J Surg Pathol. 2013 Jul;37(7):e1–11. PMID:23759937
434. Dadmanesh F, Fan X, Dastane A, et al. Comparative analysis of size estimation by mapping and counting number of blocks with ductal carcinoma in situ in breast excision specimens. Arch Pathol Lab Med. 2009 Jan;133(1):26–30. PMID:19123732
435. Daemen A, Manning G. HER2 is not a cancer subtype but rather a pan-cancer event and is highly enriched in AR-driven breast tumors. Breast Cancer Res. 2018 Jan 30;20(1):8. PMID:29382369
436. Dahlin AM, Wibom C, Ghasimi S, et al. Relation between established glioma risk variants and DNA methylation in the tumor. PLoS One. 2016 Oct 25;11(10):e0163067. PMID:27780202
437. Dahlstrom JE, Tait N, Cranney BG, et al. Fine needle aspiration cytology and core biopsy histology in infiltrating syringomatous adenoma of the breast. A case report. Acta Cytol. 1999 Mar-Apr;43(2):303–7. PMID:10097731
438. Dal Cin P, Wanschura S, Christiaens MR, et al. Hamartoma of the breast with involvement of 6p21 and rearrangement of HMGIY. Genes Chromosomes Cancer. 1997 Sep;20(1):90–2. PMID:9290959
439. Dalal KM, Kattan MW, Antonescu CR, et al. Subtype specific prognostic nomogram for patients with primary liposarcoma of the retroperitoneum, extremity, or trunk. Ann Surg. 2006 Sep;244(3):381–91. PMID:16926564
440. Dalberg K, Hellborg H, Wärnberg F. Paget's disease of the nipple in a population based cohort. Breast Cancer Res Treat. 2008 Sep;111(2):313–9. PMID:17952590
441. D'Alfonso TM, Ginter PS, Liu YF, et al. Cystic hypersecretory (in situ) carcinoma of the breast: a clinicopathologic and immunohistochemical characterization of 10 cases with clinical follow-up. Am J Surg Pathol. 2014 Jan;38(1):45–53. PMID:24121179
442. D'Alfonso TM, Mosquera JM, MacDonald TY, et al. MYB-NFIB gene fusion in adenoid cystic carcinoma of the breast with special focus paid to the solid variant with basaloid features. Hum Pathol. 2014 Nov;45(11):2270–80. PMID:25217885
443. D'Alfonso TM, Shin SJ. Small glandular proliferations of the breast. Surg Pathol Clin. 2012 Sep;5(3):591–643. PMID:26838282
444. D'Alfonso TM, Wang K, Chiu YL, et al. Pathologic upgrade rates on subsequent excision when lobular carcinoma in situ is the primary diagnosis in the needle core biopsy with special attention to the radiographic target. Arch Pathol Lab Med. 2013 Jul;137(7):927–35. PMID:23808465
445. Daling JR, Malone KE, Doody DR, et al. Relation of regimens of combined hormone replacement therapy to lobular, ductal, and other histologic types of breast carcinoma. Cancer. 2002 Dec 15;95(12):2455–64. PMID:12467057
446. Damiani S, Eusebi V. Gynecomastia in type-1 neurofibromatosis with features of pseudoangiomatous stromal hyperplasia with giant cells. Report of two cases. Virchows Arch. 2001 May;438(5):513–6. PMID:11407482
447. Damiani S, Pasquinelli G, Lamovec J,

et al. Acinic cell carcinoma of the breast: an immunohistochemical and ultrastructural study. Virchows Arch. 2000 Jul;437(1):74–81. PMID:10963383
**448.** D'Angelo P, Carli M, Ferrari A, et al. Breast metastases in children and adolescents with rhabdomyosarcoma: experience of the Italian Soft Tissue Sarcoma Committee. Pediatr Blood Cancer. 2010 Dec 15;55(7):1306–9. PMID:20730885
**449.** Dangoor A, Seddon B, Gerrand C, et al. UK guidelines for the management of soft tissue sarcomas. Clin Sarcoma Res. 2016 Nov 15;6:20. PMID:27891213
**450.** Daniel BL, Gardner RW, Birdwell RL, et al. Magnetic resonance imaging of intraductal papilloma of the breast. Magn Reson Imaging. 2003 Oct;21(8):887–92. PMID:14599539
**451.** Daniels BH, Ko JS, Rowe JJ, et al. Radiation-associated angiosarcoma in the setting of breast cancer mimicking radiation dermatitis: a diagnostic pitfall. J Cutan Pathol. 2017 May;44(5):456–61. PMID:28169467
**452.** Darabi H, Beesley J, Droit A, et al. Fine scale mapping of the 17q22 breast cancer locus using dense SNPs, genotyped within the Collaborative Oncological Gene-Environment Study (COGS). Sci Rep. 2016 Sep 7;6:32512. PMID:27600471
**453.** Darabi H, McCue K, Beesley J, et al. Polymorphisms in a putative enhancer at the 10q21.2 breast cancer risk locus regulate NRBF2 expression. Am J Hum Genet. 2015 Jul 2;97(1):22–34. PMID:26073781
**454.** Daroca PJ Jr, Reed RJ, Love GL, et al. Myoid hamartomas of the breast. Hum Pathol. 1985 Mar;16(3):212–9. PMID:3972402
**455.** Das Gupta TK, Brasfield RD, Strong EW, et al. Benign solitary schwannomas (neurilemomas). Cancer. 1969 Aug;24(2):355–66. PMID:5796779
**456.** Da Silva L, Lakhani SR. Pathology of hereditary breast cancer. Mod Pathol. 2010 May;23 Suppl 2:S46–51. PMID:20436502
**457.** Dave SS, Fu K, Wright GW, et al. Molecular diagnosis of Burkitt's lymphoma. N Engl J Med. 2006 Jun 8;354(23):2431–42. PMID:16760443
**458.** Davies H, Glodzik D, Morganella S, et al. HRDetect is a predictor of BRCA1 and BRCA2 deficiency based on mutational signatures. Nat Med. 2017 Apr;23(4):517–25. PMID:28288110
**459.** Davis WG, Hennessy B, Babiera G, et al. Metaplastic sarcomatoid carcinoma of the breast with absent or minimal overt invasive carcinomatous component: a misnomer. Am J Surg Pathol. 2005 Nov;29(11):1456–63. PMID:16224212
**460.** Daya D, Trus T, D'Souza TJ, et al. Hamartoma of the breast, an underrecognized breast lesion. A clinicopathologic and radiographic study of 25 cases. Am J Clin Pathol. 1995 Jun;103(6):685–9. PMID:7785651
**461.** de Bock GH, Schutte M, Krol-Warmerdam EM, et al. Tumour characteristics and prognosis of breast cancer patients carrying the germline CHEK2*1100delC variant. J Med Genet. 2004 Oct;41(10):731–5. PMID:15466005
**462.** de Boer M, van Leeuwen FE, Hauptmann M, et al. Breast implants and the risk of anaplastic large-cell lymphoma in the breast. JAMA Oncol. 2018 Mar 1;4(3):335–41. PMID:29302687
**463.** De Brot M, Koslow Mautner S, Muhsen S, et al. Pleomorphic lobular carcinoma in situ of the breast: a single institution experience with clinical follow-up and centralized pathology review. Breast Cancer Res Treat. 2017 Sep;165(2):411–20. PMID:28612228
**464.** De Chiara A, Losito S, Terracciano L, et al. Primary plasmacytoma of the breast. Arch Pathol Lab Med. 2001 Aug;125(8):1078–80. PMID:11473462
**465.** de Groot JS, Ratze MA, van Amersfoort M, et al. αE-catenin is a candidate tumor suppressor for the development of E-cadherin-expressing lobular-type breast cancer. J Pathol. 2018 Aug;245(4):456–67. PMID:29774524
**466.** De Leeuw WJ, Berx G, Vos CB, et al. Simultaneous loss of E-cadherin and catenins in invasive lobular breast cancer and lobular carcinoma in situ. J Pathol. 1997 Dec;183(4):404–11. PMID:9496256
**467.** de Leng WW, Jansen M, Carvalho R, et al. Genetic defects underlying Peutz-Jeghers syndrome (PJS) and exclusion of the polarity-associated MARK/Par1 gene family as potential PJS candidates. Clin Genet. 2007 Dec;72(6):568–73. PMID:17924967
**468.** de Moraes Schenka NG, Schenka AA, de Souza Queiroz L, et al. p63 and CD10: reliable markers in discriminating benign sclerosing lesions from tubular carcinoma of the breast? Appl Immunohistochem Mol Morphol. 2006 Mar;14(1):71–7. PMID:16540734
**469.** Deb S, Do H, Byrne D, et al. PIK3CA mutations are frequently observed in BRCAX but not BRCA2-associated male breast cancer. Breast Cancer Res. 2013;15(4):R69. PMID:23971979
**470.** Deb S, Jene N, Fox SB, et al. Genotypic and phenotypic analysis of familial male breast cancer shows under representation of the HER2 and basal subtypes in BRCA-associated carcinomas. BMC Cancer. 2012 Nov 9;12:510. PMID:23146383
**471.** Deb S, Johansson I, Byrne D, et al. Nuclear HIF1A expression is strongly prognostic in sporadic but not familial male breast cancer. Mod Pathol. 2014 Sep;27(9):1223–30. PMID:24457463
**472.** Deen SA, McKee GT, Kissin MW. Differential cytologic features of fibroepithelial lesions of the breast. Diagn Cytopathol. 1999 Feb;20(2):53–6. PMID:9951596
**473.** Degnim AC, Dupont WD, Radisky DC, et al. Extent of atypical hyperplasia stratifies breast cancer risk in 2 independent cohorts of women. Cancer. 2016 Oct;122(19):2971–8. PMID:27352219
**474.** Degnim AC, Visscher DW, Berman HK, et al. Stratification of breast cancer risk in women with atypia: a Mayo cohort study. J Clin Oncol. 2007 Jul 1;25(19):2671–7. PMID:17563394
**475.** Del Castillo M, Chibon F, Arnould L, et al. Secretory breast carcinoma: a histopathologic and genomic spectrum characterized by a joint specific ETV6-NTRK3 gene fusion. Am J Surg Pathol. 2015 Nov;39(11):1458–67. PMID:26291510
**476.** DeLair DF, Corben AD, Catalano JP, et al. Non-mammary metastases to the breast and axilla: a study of 85 cases. Mod Pathol. 2013 Mar;26(3):343–9. PMID:23174933
**477.** de la Torre M, Lindholm K, Lindgren A. Fine needle aspiration cytology of tubular breast carcinoma and radial scar. Acta Cytol. 1994 Nov-Dec;38(6):884–90. PMID:7992574
**478.** Dellapasqua S, Maisonneuve P, Viale G, et al. Immunohistochemically defined subtypes and outcome of apocrine breast cancer. Clin Breast Cancer. 2013 Apr;13(2):95–102. PMID:23245877
**479.** Demicco EG, Torres KE, Ghadimi MP, et al. Involvement of the PI3K/Akt pathway in myxoid/round cell liposarcoma. Mod Pathol. 2012 Feb;25(2):212–21. PMID:22020193
**480.** Deng G, Lu Y, Zlotnikov G, et al. Loss of heterozygosity in normal tissue adjacent to breast carcinomas. Science. 1996 Dec 20;274(5295):2057–9. PMID:8953032
**481.** Deng Y, Xue D, Wang X, et al. Mucinous cystadenocarcinoma of the breast with a basal-like immunophenotype. Pathol Int. 2012 Jun;62(6):429–32. PMID:22612513
**482.** Denkert C, von Minckwitz G, Darb-Esfahani S, et al. Tumour-infiltrating lymphocytes and prognosis in different subtypes of breast cancer: a pooled analysis of 3771 patients treated with neoadjuvant therapy. Lancet Oncol. 2018 Jan;19(1):40–50. PMID:29233559
**483.** Derksen PW, Braumuller TM, van der Burg E, et al. Mammary-specific inactivation of E-cadherin and p53 impairs functional gland development and leads to pleomorphic invasive lobular carcinoma in mice. Dis Model Mech. 2011 May;4(3):347–58. PMID:21282721
**484.** Derksen PW, Liu X, Saridin F, et al. Somatic inactivation of E-cadherin and p53 in mice leads to metastatic lobular mammary carcinoma through induction of anoikis resistance and angiogenesis. Cancer Cell. 2006 Nov;10(5):437–49. PMID:17097565
**485.** DeSantis CE, Bray F, Ferlay J, et al. International variation in female breast cancer incidence and mortality rates. Cancer Epidemiol Biomarkers Prev. 2015 Oct;24(10):1495–506. PMID:26359465
**486.** Desmedt C, Haibe-Kains B, Wirapati P, et al. Biological processes associated with breast cancer clinical outcome depend on the molecular subtypes. Clin Cancer Res. 2008 Aug 15;14(16):5158–65. PMID:18698033
**487.** Desmedt C, Salgado R, Fornili M, et al. Immune infiltration in invasive lobular breast cancer. J Natl Cancer Inst. 2018 Jul 1;110(7):768–76. PMID:29471435
**488.** Desmedt C, Zoppoli G, Gundem G, et al. Genomic characterization of primary invasive lobular breast cancer. J Clin Oncol. 2016 Jun 1;34(16):1872–81. PMID:26926684
**489.** Desouki MM, Li Z, Hameed O, et al. Incidental atypical proliferative lesions in reduction mammoplasty specimens: analysis of 2498 cases from 2 tertiary women's health centers. Hum Pathol. 2013 Sep;44(9):1877–81. PMID:23656973
**490.** Destounis SV, Murphy PF, Seifert PJ, et al. Management of patients diagnosed with lobular carcinoma in situ at needle core biopsy at a community-based outpatient facility. AJR Am J Roentgenol. 2012 Feb;198(2):281–7. PMID:22268169
**491.** de-Thé G, Geser A, Day NE, et al. Epidemiological evidence for causal relationship between Epstein-Barr virus and Burkitt's lymphoma from Ugandan prospective study. Nature. 1978 Aug 24;274(5673):756–61. PMID:210392
**492.** Devouassoux-Shisheboran M, Schammel MD, Man YG, et al. Fibromatosis of the breast: age-correlated morphofunctional features of 33 cases. Arch Pathol Lab Med. 2000 Feb;124(2):276–80. PMID:10656738
**493.** Deyrup AT, Lee VK, Hill CE, et al. Epstein-Barr virus-associated smooth muscle tumors are distinctive mesenchymal tumors reflecting multiple infection events: a clinicopathologic and molecular analysis of 29 tumors from 19 patients. Am J Surg Pathol. 2006 Jan;30(1):75–82. PMID:16330945
**494.** Di Cristofano C, Mrad K, Zavaglia K, et al. Papillary lesions of the breast: a molecular progression? Breast Cancer Res Treat. 2005 Mar;90(1):71–6. PMID:15770529
**495.** Di Filippo F, Di Filippo S, Ferrari AM, et al. Elaboration of a nomogram to predict nonsentinel node status in breast cancer patients with positive sentinel node, intraoperatively assessed with one step nucleic amplification: retrospective and validation phase. J Exp Clin Cancer Res. 2016 Dec 8;35(1):193. PMID:27931238
**496.** Di Napoli A, De Cecco L, Piccaluga PP, et al. Transcriptional analysis distinguishes breast implant-associated anaplastic large cell lymphoma from other peripheral T-cell lymphomas. Mod Pathol. 2019 Feb;32(2):216–30. PMID:30206415
**497.** Di Oto E, Biserni GB, Varga Z, et al. X chromosome gain is related to increased androgen receptor expression in male breast cancer. Virchows Arch. 2018 Aug;473(2):155–63. PMID:29802469
**498.** Di Oto E, Monti V, Cucchi MC, et al. X chromosome gain in male breast cancer. Hum Pathol. 2015 Dec;46(12):1908–12. PMID:26475094
**499.** Di Tommaso L, Foschini MP, Ragazzini T, et al. Mucoepidermoid carcinoma of the breast. Virchows Arch. 2004 Jan;444(1):13–9. PMID:14634807
**500.** Di Tommaso L, Franchi G, Destro A, et al. Toker cells of the breast. Morphological and immunohistochemical characterization of 40 cases. Hum Pathol. 2008 Sep;39(9):1295–300. PMID:18614197
**501.** Diab SG, Clark GM, Osborne CK, et al. Tumor characteristics and clinical outcome of tubular and mucinous breast carcinomas. J Clin Oncol. 1999 May;17(5):1442–8. PMID:10334529
**502.** Dialani V, Venkataraman S, Frieling G, et al. Does isolated flat epithelial atypia on vacuum-assisted breast core biopsy require surgical excision? Breast J. 2014 Nov-Dec;20(6):606–14. PMID:25264188
**503.** Diallo R, Schaefer KL, Bankfalvi A, et al. Secretory carcinoma of the breast: a distinct variant of invasive ductal carcinoma assessed by comparative genomic hybridization and immunohistochemistry. Hum Pathol. 2003 Dec;34(12):1299–305. PMID:14691916
**504.** Diaz LK, Wiley EL, Venta LA. Are malignant cells displaced by large-gauge needle core biopsy of the breast? AJR Am J Roentgenol. 1999 Nov;173(5):1303–13. PMID:10541110
**505.** Diaz NM, McDivitt RW, Wick MR. Pleomorphic adenoma of the breast: a clinicopathologic and immunohistochemical study of 10 cases. Hum Pathol. 1991 Dec;22(12):1206–14. PMID:1660850
**506.** Diaz-Arias AA, Hurt MA, Loy TS, et al. Leiomyoma of the breast. Hum Pathol. 1989 Apr;20(4):396–9. PMID:2467872
**507.** Diaz-Cascajo C, Borghi S, Weyers W, et al. Benign lymphangiomatous papules of the skin following radiotherapy: a report of five new cases and review of the literature. Histopathology. 1999 Oct;35(4):319–27. PMID:10564386
**508.** DiCostanzo D, Rosen PP, Gareen I, et al. Prognosis in infiltrating lobular carcinoma. An analysis of "classical" and variant tumors. Am J Surg Pathol. 1990 Jan;14(1):12–23. PMID:2153007
**509.** Dieci MV, Smutná V, Scott V, et al. Whole exome sequencing of rare aggressive breast cancer histologies. Breast Cancer Res Treat. 2016 Feb;156(1):21–32. PMID:26907767
**510.** Dietrich CU, Pandis N, Andersen JA, et al. Chromosome abnormalities in adenolipomas of the breast: karyotypic evidence that the mesenchymal component constitutes the neoplastic parenchyma. Cancer Genet Cytogenet. 1994 Feb;72(2):146–50. PMID:8143274
**511.** Dietzel M, Baltzer PA, Vag T, et al. Magnetic resonance mammography of invasive lobular versus ductal carcinoma: systematic comparison of 811 patients reveals high diagnostic accuracy irrespective of typing. J Comput Assist Tomogr. 2010 Jul;34(4):587–95. PMID:20657229
**512.** Dillon DA, Lester SC. Lesions of the nipple. Surg Pathol Clin. 2009 Jun;2(2):391–412. PMID:26838328
**513.** Dillon MF, McDermott EW, Hill AD, et al.

Predictive value of breast lesions of "uncertain malignant potential" and "suspicious for malignancy" determined by needle core biopsy. Ann Surg Oncol. 2007 Feb;14(2):704–11. PMID:17151788

514. Dimitriadis G, Papadopoulos V, Mimidis K. Eplerenone reverses spironolactone-induced painful gynaecomastia in cirrhotics. Hepatol Int. 2011 Jun;5(2):738–9. PMID:21484105

515. Din NU, Idrees R, Fatima S, et al. Secretory carcinoma of breast: clinicopathologic study of 8 cases. Ann Diagn Pathol. 2013 Feb;17(1):54–7. PMID:22832018

516. Disanto MG, Ambrosio MR, Rocca BJ, et al. Optimal minimal panels of immunohistochemistry for diagnosis of B-cell lymphoma for application in countries with limited resources and for triaging cases before referral to specialist centers. Am J Clin Pathol. 2016 May;145(5):687–95. PMID:27247372

517. Di Saverio S, Gutierrez J, Avisar E. A retrospective review with long term follow-up of 11,400 cases of pure mucinous breast carcinoma. Breast Cancer Res Treat. 2008 Oct;111(3):541–7. PMID:18026874

518. Dischinger PS, Tovar EA, Essenburg CJ, et al. NF1 deficiency correlates with estrogen receptor signaling and diminished survival in breast cancer. NPJ Breast Cancer. 2018 Aug 30;4:29. PMID:30182054

519. Dite GS, MacInnis RJ, Bickerstaffe A, et al. Breast cancer risk prediction using clinical models and 77 independent risk-associated SNPs for women aged under 50 years: Australian Breast Cancer Family Registry. Cancer Epidemiol Biomarkers Prev. 2016 Feb;25(2):359–65. PMID:26677205

520. Di Tommaso L, Rosai J. The capillary lobule: a deceptively benign feature of post-radiation angiosarcoma of the skin: report of three cases. Am J Dermatopathol. 2005 Aug;27(4):301–5. PMID:16121049

521. Dixon JM, Anderson TJ, Page DL, et al. Infiltrating lobular carcinoma of the breast. Histopathology. 1982 Mar;6(2):149–61. PMID:7076138

522. Doane AS, Danso M, Lal P, et al. An estrogen receptor-negative breast cancer subset characterized by a hormonally regulated transcriptional program and response to androgen. Oncogene. 2006 Jun 29;25(28):3994–4008. PMID:16491124

523. Doctor VM, Sirsat MV. Florid papillomatosis (adenoma) and other benign tumours of the nipple and areola. Br J Cancer. 1971 Mar;25(1):1–9. PMID:5581295

524. Doebar SC, Krol NM, van Marion R, et al. Progression of ductal carcinoma in situ to invasive breast cancer: comparative genomic sequencing. Virchows Arch. 2019 Feb;474(2):247–51. PMID:30284611

525. Doebar SC, Slaets L, Cardoso F, et al. Male breast cancer precursor lesions: analysis of the EORTC 10085/TBCRC/BIG/NABCG International Male Breast Cancer Program. Mod Pathol. 2017 Apr;30(4):509–18. PMID:28084333

526. Dogan S, Wang L, Ptashkin RN, et al. Mammary analog secretory carcinoma of the thyroid gland: a primary thyroid adenocarcinoma harboring ETV6-NTRK3 fusion. Mod Pathol. 2016 Sep;29(9):985–95. PMID:27282352

527. Dolgin E. Olaparib keeps hereditary breast tumors in check. Cancer Discov. 2017 Aug;7(8):OF10. PMID:28583909

528. Domagala P, Wokolorczyk D, Cybulski C, et al. Different CHEK2 germline mutations are associated with distinct immunophenotypic molecular subtypes of breast cancer. Breast Cancer Res Treat. 2012 Apr;132(3):937–45. PMID:21701879

529. Domagala W, Harezga B, Szadowska A, et al. Nuclear p53 protein accumulates preferentially in medullary and high-grade ductal but rarely in lobular breast carcinomas. Am J Pathol. 1993 Mar;142(3):669–74. PMID:8384406

530. Domchek SM, Friebel TM, Singer CF, et al. Association of risk-reducing surgery in BRCA1 or BRCA2 mutation carriers with cancer risk and mortality. JAMA. 2010 Sep 1;304(9):967–75. PMID:20810374

531. Domchek SM, Hecht JL, Fleming MD, et al. Lymphomas of the breast: primary and secondary involvement. Cancer. 2002 Jan 1;94(1):6–13. PMID:11815954

532. Domfeh AB, Carley AL, Striebel JM, et al. WT1 immunoreactivity in breast carcinoma: selective expression in pure and mixed mucinous subtypes. Mod Pathol. 2008 Oct;21(10):1217–23. PMID:18469795

533. Dômont J, Salas S, Lacroix L, et al. High frequency of beta-catenin heterozygous mutations in extra-abdominal fibromatosis: a potential molecular tool for disease management. Br J Cancer. 2010 Mar 16;102(6):1032–6. PMID:20197769

534. Domoto H, Tsuda H, Miyakawa K, et al. Invasive ductal carcinoma associated with tubular adenoma of the breast. Pathol Int. 2002 Mar;52(3):244–8. PMID:11972869

535. Donaldson AR, Sieck L, Booth CN, et al. Radial scars diagnosed on breast core biopsy: frequency of atypia and carcinoma on excision and implications for management. Breast. 2016 Dec;30:201–7. PMID:27371970

536. Donnell RM, Rosen PP, Lieberman PH, et al. Angiosarcoma and other vascular tumors of the breast. Am J Surg Pathol. 1981 Oct;5(7):629–42. PMID:7199829

537. Doren EL, Miranda RN, Selber JC, et al. U.S. epidemiology of breast implant-associated anaplastic large cell lymphoma. Plast Reconstr Surg. 2017 May;139(5):1042–50. PMID:28157769

538. Dores GM, Qubaiah O, Mody A, et al. A population-based study of incidence and patient survival of small cell carcinoma in the United States, 1992-2010. BMC Cancer. 2015 Mar 27;15:185. PMID:25885914

539. Downs-Kelly E, Bell D, Perkins GH, et al. Clinical implications of margin involvement by pleomorphic lobular carcinoma in situ. Arch Pathol Lab Med. 2011 Jun;135(6):737–43. PMID:21631266

540. Downs-Kelly E, Nayeemuddin KM, Albarracin C, et al. Matrix-producing carcinoma of the breast: an aggressive subtype of metaplastic carcinoma. Am J Surg Pathol. 2009 Apr;33(4):534–41. PMID:19047898

541. Dowsett M, Cuzick J, Wale C, et al. Prediction of risk of distant recurrence using the 21-gene recurrence score in node-negative and node-positive postmenopausal patients with breast cancer treated with anastrozole or tamoxifen: a TransATAC study. J Clin Oncol. 2010 Apr 10;28(11):1829–34. PMID:20212256

542. Dowsett M, Nielsen TO, A'Hern R, et al. Assessment of Ki67 in breast cancer: recommendations from the International Ki67 in Breast Cancer working group. J Natl Cancer Inst. 2011 Nov 16;103(22):1656–64. PMID:21960707

543. Doyle LA, Hornick JL. Mesenchymal tumors of the gastrointestinal tract other than GIST. Surg Pathol Clin. 2013 Sep;6(3):425–73. PMID:26839096

545. Dreyer G, Vandorpe T, Smeets A, et al. Triple negative breast cancer: clinical characteristics in the different histological subtypes. Breast. 2013 Oct;22(5):761–6. PMID:23416046

546. Drilon A, Laetsch TW, Kummar S, et al. Efficacy of larotrectinib in TRK fusion-positive cancers in adults and children. N Engl J Med. 2018 Feb 22;378(8):731–9. PMID:29466156

547. Droufakou S, Deshmane V, Roylance R, et al. Multiple ways of silencing E-cadherin gene expression in lobular carcinoma of the breast. Int J Cancer. 2001 May 1;92(3):404–8. PMID:11291078

548. du Toit RS, Locker AP, Ellis IO, et al. Invasive lobular carcinomas of the breast–the prognosis of histopathological subtypes. Br J Cancer. 1989 Oct;60(4):605–9. PMID:2803932

549. Duan X, Sneige N, Gullett AE, et al. Invasive Paget disease of the breast: clinicopathologic study of an underrecognized entity in the breast. Am J Surg Pathol. 2012 Sep;36(9):1353–8. PMID:22895267

550. Duffy MJ, Harbeck N, Nap M, et al. Clinical use of biomarkers in breast cancer: updated guidelines from the European Group on Tumor Markers (EGTM). Eur J Cancer. 2017 Apr;75:284–98. PMID:28259011

551. Duman BB, Sahin B, Güvenç B, et al. Lymphoma of the breast in a male patient. Med Oncol. 2011 Dec;28 Suppl 1:S490–3. PMID:20830532

552. Dunning AM, Michailidou K, Kuchenbaecker KB, et al. Breast cancer risk variants at 6q25 display different phenotype associations and regulate ESR1, RMND1 and CCDC170. Nat Genet. 2016 Apr;48(4):374–86. PMID:26928228

553. Dupont WD, Page DL. Risk factors for breast cancer in women with proliferative breast disease. N Engl J Med. 1985 Jan 17;312(3):146–51. PMID:3965932

554. Dupont WD, Page DL, Parl FF, et al. Long-term risk of breast cancer in women with fibroadenoma. N Engl J Med. 1994 Jul 7;331(1):10–5. PMID:8202095

555. Duprez R, Wilkerson PM, Lacroix-Triki M, et al. Immunophenotypic and genomic characterization of papillary carcinomas of the breast. J Pathol. 2012 Feb;226(3):427–41. PMID:22025283

556. Dursun F, Su Dur ŞM, Şahin C, et al. A rare cause of prepubertal gynecomastia: Sertoli cell tumor. Case Rep Pediatr. 2015;2015:439239. PMID:26366315

557. Dye K, Saucedo M, Raju D, et al. A common cancer in an uncommon location: a case report of squamous cell carcinoma of the nipple. Int J Surg Case Rep. 2017;36:94–7. PMID:28551484

558. Dyrstad SW, Yan Y, Fowler AM, et al. Breast cancer risk associated with benign breast disease: systematic review and meta-analysis. Breast Cancer Res Treat. 2015 Feb;149(3):569–75. PMID:25636589

559. Correa C, McGale P, Taylor C, et al. Overview of the randomized trials of radiotherapy in ductal carcinoma in situ of the breast. J Natl Cancer Inst Monogr. 2010;2010(41):162–77. PMID:20956824

560. Easton DF, Pharoah PD, Antoniou AC, et al. Gene-panel sequencing and the prediction of breast-cancer risk. N Engl J Med. 2015 Jun 4;372(23):2243–57. PMID:26014596

561. Easton DF, Pooley KA, Dunning AM, et al. Genome-wide association study identifies novel breast cancer susceptibility loci. Nature. 2007 Jun 28;447(7148):1087–93. PMID:17529967

562. Ebrahim L, Parry J, Taylor DB. Fibromatosis of the breast: a pictorial review of the imaging and histopathology findings. Clin Radiol. 2014 Oct;69(10):1077–83. PMID:24990452

563. Eby PR, Ochsner JE, DeMartini WB, et al. Frequency and upgrade rates of atypical ductal hyperplasia diagnosed at stereotactic vacuum-assisted breast biopsy: 9- versus 11-gauge. AJR Am J Roentgenol. 2009 Jan;192(1):229–34. PMID:19098204

564. Edelweiss M, Corben AD, Liberman L, et al. Focal extravasated mucin in breast core needle biopsies: Is surgical excision always necessary? Breast J. 2013 May-Jun;19(3):302–9. PMID:23534893

565. Efared B, Sidibé IS, Abdoulaziz S, et al. Tubular adenoma of the breast: a clinicopathologic study of a series of 9 cases. Clin Med Insights Pathol. 2018 Feb 5;11:1179555718757499. PMID:29449780

566. El Aouni N, Laurent I, Terrier P, et al. Granular cell tumor of the breast. Diagn Cytopathol. 2007 Nov;35(11):725–7. PMID:17924412

567. El Hag IA, Aodah A, Kollur SM, et al. Cytological clues in the distinction between phyllodes tumor and fibroadenoma. Cancer Cytopathol. 2010 Feb 25;118(1):33–40. PMID:20094997

568. Elayat G, Selim AG, Wells CA. Cell turnover in apocrine metaplasia and apocrine adenosis of the breast. Ann Diagn Pathol. 2010 Feb;14(1):1–7. PMID:20123450

569. Elbendary A, Xue R, Valdebran M, et al. Diagnostic criteria in intraepithelial pagetoid neoplasms: a histopathologic study and evaluation of select features in Paget disease, Bowen disease, and melanoma in situ. Am J Dermatopathol. 2017 Jun;39(6):419–27. PMID:28525420

570. Elghobashy M, Basu N, Warner R, et al. Metaplastic breast cancer masquerading as liposarcoma of the breast: a case report following oncoplastic treatment. Pathobiology. 2018;85(4):261–5. PMID:29788010

571. Ellingjord-Dale M, Vos L, Hjerkind KV, et al. Alcohol, physical activity, smoking, and breast cancer subtypes in a large, nested case-control study from the Norwegian Breast Cancer Screening Program. Cancer Epidemiol Biomarkers Prev. 2017 Dec;26(12):1736–44. PMID:28877889

572. Ellingjord-Dale M, Vos L, Tretli S, et al. Parity, hormones and breast cancer subtypes - results from a large nested case-control study in a national screening program. Breast Cancer Res. 2017 Jan 23;19(1):10. PMID:28114999

573. Ellis IO, Al-Sam S, Anderson N, et al. Pathology reporting of breast disease in surgical excision specimens incorporating the dataset for histological reporting of breast cancer. London (UK): The Royal College of Pathologists; June 2016.

574. Ellis IO, Galea M, Broughton N, et al. Pathological prognostic factors in breast cancer. II. Histological type. Relationship with survival in a large study with long-term follow-up. Histopathology. 1992 Jun;20(6):479–89. PMID:1607149

574A. Ellis MJ, Perou CM. The genomic landscape of breast cancer as a therapeutic roadmap. Cancer Discov. 2013 Jan;3(1):27–34. PMID:23319768

575. Ellsworth RE, Ellsworth DL, Love B, et al. Correlation of levels and patterns of genomic instability with histological grading of DCIS. Ann Surg Oncol. 2007 Nov;14(11):3070–7. PMID:17549568

576. Elmi M, Sequeira S, Azin A, et al. Evolving surgical treatment decisions for male breast cancer: an analysis of the National Surgical Quality Improvement Program (NSQIP) database. Breast Cancer Res Treat. 2018 Sep;171(2):427–34. PMID:29808286

577. Elmore JG, Longton GM, Carney PA, et al. Diagnostic concordance among pathologists interpreting breast biopsy specimens. JAMA. 2015 Mar 17;313(11):1122–32. PMID:25781441

578. Elmore JG, Nelson HD, Pepe MS, et al. Variability in pathologists' interpretations of individual breast biopsy slides: a population perspective. Ann Intern Med. 2016 May

17;164(10):649–55. PMID:26999810
**579.** Elmore JG, Tosteson AN, Pepe MS, et al. Evaluation of 12 strategies for obtaining second opinions to improve interpretation of breast histopathology: simulation study. BMJ. 2016 Jun 22;353:i3069. PMID:27334105
**580.** El-Naggar AK, Chan JKC, Grandis JR, et al., editors. WHO classification of head and neck tumours. Lyon (France): International Agency for Research on Cancer; 2017. (WHO classification of tumours series, 4th ed.; vol. 9). http://publications.iarc.fr/548.
**581.** El Sharouni MA, Postma EL, van Diest PJ. Correlation between E-cadherin and p120 expression in invasive ductal breast cancer with a lobular component and MRI findings. Virchows Arch. 2017 Dec;471(6):707–12. PMID:28779344
**582.** Elsheikh TM, Silverman JF. Follow-up surgical excision is indicated when breast core needle biopsies show atypical lobular hyperplasia or lobular carcinoma in situ: a correlative study of 33 patients with review of the literature. Am J Surg Pathol. 2005 Apr;29(4):534–43. PMID:15767810
**583.** Elshof LE, Schmidt MK, Rutgers EJT, et al. Cause-specific mortality in a population-based cohort of 9799 women treated for ductal carcinoma in situ. Ann Surg. 2018 May;267(5):952–8. PMID:28375855
**584.** Elshof LE, Tryfonidis K, Slaets L, et al. Feasibility of a prospective, randomised, open-label, international multicentre, phase III, non-inferiority trial to assess the safety of active surveillance for low risk ductal carcinoma in situ - the LORD study. Eur J Cancer. 2015 Aug;51(12):1497–510. PMID:26025767
**585.** Elston CW, Ellis IO. Pathological prognostic factors in breast cancer. I. The value of histological grade in breast cancer: experience from a large study with long-term follow-up. Histopathology. 1991 Nov;19(5):403–10. PMID:1757079
**586.** Elston CW, Sloane JP, Amendoeira I, et al. Causes of inconsistency in diagnosing and classifying intraductal proliferations of the breast. Eur J Cancer. 2000 Sep;36(14):1769–72. PMID:10974624
**587.** Elzahaby IA, Saleh S, Metwally IH, et al. Huge lactating adenoma of the breast: case report. Breast Dis. 2017;37(1):37–42. PMID:28269736
**588.** Ende L, Mercado C, Axelrod D, et al. Intraparenchymal leiomyoma of the breast: a case report and review of the literature. Ann Clin Lab Sci. 2007 Summer;37(3):268–73. PMID:17709693
**589.** Eng C. PTEN hamartoma tumor syndrome. In: Adam MP, Ardinger HH, Pagon RA, et al., editors. GeneReviews. Seattle (WA): University of Washington, Seattle; 2001 Nov 29 [updated 2016 Jun 2]. PMID:20301661
**590.** Engstrøm MJ, Opdahl S, Vatten LJ, et al. Invasive lobular breast cancer: the prognostic impact of histopathological grade, E-cadherin and molecular subtypes. Histopathology. 2015 Feb;66(3):409–19. PMID:25283075
**591.** Eren E, Edgunlu T, Korkmaz HA, et al. Genetic variants of estrogen beta and leptin receptors may cause gynecomastia in adolescent. Gene. 2014 May 15;541(2):101–6. PMID:24625355
**592.** Erhan Y, Erhan Y, Zekioğlu O. Pure invasive micropapillary carcinoma of the male breast: report of a rare case. Can J Surg. 2005 Apr;48(2):156–7. PMID:15887800
**593.** Erickson-Johnson MR, Chou MM, Evers BR, et al. Nodular fasciitis: a novel model of transient neoplasia induced by MYH9-USP6 gene fusion. Lab Invest. 2011 Oct;91(10):1427–33. PMID:21826056
**594.** Erinanc H, Türk E. The rare benign lesion that mimics a malignant tumor in breast parenchyma: nodular fasciitis of the breast. Case Rep Pathol. 2018 Apr 30;2018:1612587. PMID:29854526
**595.** Ersahin C, Bandyopadhyay S, Bhargava R. Thyroid transcription factor-1 and "basal marker"–expressing small cell carcinoma of the breast. Int J Surg Pathol. 2009 Oct;17(5):368–72. PMID:19578049
**596.** Espinosa I, Gallardo A, D'Angelo E, et al. Simultaneous carcinomas of the breast and ovary: utility of Pax-8, WT-1, and GATA3 for distinguishing independent primary tumors from metastases. Int J Gynecol Pathol. 2015 May;34(3):257–65. PMID:25844549
**597.** Esposito NN, Dabbs DJ, Bhargava R. Are encapsulated papillary carcinomas of the breast in situ or invasive? A basement membrane study of 27 cases. Am J Clin Pathol. 2009 Feb;131(2):228–42. PMID:19141383
**598.** Etzell JE, Devries S, Chew K, et al. Loss of chromosome 16q in lobular carcinoma in situ. Hum Pathol. 2001 Mar;32(3):292–6. PMID:11274638
**599.** Eusebi V, Casadei GP, Bussolati G, et al. Adenomyoepithelioma of the breast with a distinctive type of apocrine adenosis. Histopathology. 1987 Mar;11(3):305–15. PMID:2828217
**599A.** Eusebi V, Damiani S, Ellis IO, et al. Breast tumor resembling the tall cell variant of papillary thyroid carcinoma: report of 5 cases. Am J Surg Pathol. 2003 Aug;27(8):1114–8. PMID:12883243
**600.** Eusebi V, Feudale E, Foschini MP, et al. Long-term follow-up of in situ carcinoma of the breast. Semin Diagn Pathol. 1994 Aug;11(3):223–35. PMID:7831534
**601.** Eusebi V, Foschini MP, Bussolati G, et al. Myoblastomatoid (histiocytoid) carcinoma of the breast. A type of apocrine carcinoma. Am J Surg Pathol. 1995 May;19(5):553–62. PMID:7726365
**602.** Eusebi V, Lamovec J, Cattani MG, et al. Acantholytic variant of squamous-cell carcinoma of the breast. Am J Surg Pathol. 1986 Dec;10(12):855–61. PMID:2431630
**603.** Eusebi V, Magalhaes F, Azzopardi JG. Pleomorphic lobular carcinoma of the breast: an aggressive tumor showing apocrine differentiation. Hum Pathol. 1992 Jun;23(6):655–62. PMID:1592388
**604.** Eusebi V, Millis RR. Epitheliosis, infiltrating epitheliosis, and radial scar. Semin Diagn Pathol. 2010 Feb;27(1):5–12. PMID:20306826
**605.** Eusebi V, Millis RR, Cattani MG, et al. Apocrine carcinoma of the breast. A morphologic and immunocytochemical study. Am J Pathol. 1986 Jun;123(3):532–41. PMID:3717305
**606.** Evans DG, O'Hara C, Wilding A, et al. Mortality in neurofibromatosis 1: in North West England: an assessment of actuarial survival in a region of the UK since 1989. Eur J Hum Genet. 2011 Nov;19(11):1187–91. PMID:21694737
**607.** Evans N, Lyons K. The use of ultrasound in the diagnosis of invasive lobular carcinoma of the breast less than 10 mm in size. Clin Radiol. 2000 Apr;55(4):261–3. PMID:10767184
**608.** Evers B, Speksnijder EN, Schut E, et al. A tissue reconstitution model to study cancer cell-intrinsic and -extrinsic factors in mammary tumourigenesis. J Pathol. 2010 Jan;220(1):34–44. PMID:19927317
**609.** Fackenthal JD, Marsh DJ, Richardson AL, et al. Male breast cancer in Cowden syndrome patients with germline PTEN mutations. J Med Genet. 2001 Mar;38(3):159–64. PMID:11238682
**610.** Fadare O, Dadmanesh F, Alvarado-Cabrero I, et al. Lobular intraepithelial neoplasia (lobular carcinoma in situ) with comedo-type necrosis: a clinicopathologic study of 18 cases. Am J Surg Pathol. 2006 Nov;30(11):1445–53. PMID:17063087
**611.** Fadare O, Wang SA, Hileeto D. The expression of cytokeratin 5/6 in invasive lobular carcinoma of the breast: evidence of a basal-like subset? Hum Pathol. 2008 Mar;39(3):331–6. PMID:18261623
**612.** Falconieri G, Della Libera D, Zanconati F, et al. Leiomyosarcoma of the female breast: report of two new cases and a review of the literature. Am J Clin Pathol. 1997 Jul;108(1):19–25. PMID:9208974
**613.** Falomo E, Adejumo C, Carson KA, et al. Variability in the management recommendations given for high-risk breast lesions detected on image-guided core needle biopsy at U.S. academic institutions. Curr Probl Diagn Radiol. 2018 Jun 27;S0363-0188(18)30067-7. PMID:30075881
**614.** Fanburg-Smith JC, Majidi M, Miettinen M. Keratin expression in schwannoma; a study of 115 retroperitoneal and 22 peripheral schwannomas. Mod Pathol. 2006 Jan;19(1):115–21. PMID:16357842
**615.** Fanburg-Smith JC, Meis-Kindblom JM, Fante R, et al. Malignant granular cell tumor of soft tissue: diagnostic criteria and clinicopathologic correlation. Am J Surg Pathol. 1998 Jul;22(7):779–94. PMID:9669341
**616.** Fang Y, Wu J, Wang W, et al. Biologic behavior and long-term outcomes of breast ductal carcinoma in situ with microinvasion. Oncotarget. 2016 Sep 27;7(39):64182–90. PMID:27577080
**617.** Farinha P, André S, Cabeçadas J, et al. High frequency of MALT lymphoma in a series of 14 cases of primary breast lymphoma. Appl Immunohistochem Mol Morphol. 2002 Jun;10(2):115–20. PMID:12051628
**618.** Farinha P, Gascoyne RD. Molecular pathogenesis of mucosa-associated lymphoid tissue lymphoma. J Clin Oncol. 2005 Sep 10;23(26):6370–8. PMID:16155022
**619.** Farkash EA, Ferry JA, Harris NL, et al. Rare lymphoid malignancies of the breast: a report of two cases illustrating potential diagnostic pitfalls. J Hematop. 2009 Aug 20;2(4):237–44. PMID:20309431
**620.** Farmer P, Bonnefoi H, Becette V, et al. Identification of molecular apocrine breast tumours by microarray analysis. Oncogene. 2005 Jul 7;24(29):4660–71. PMID:15897907
**621.** Farrow JH, Ashikari H. Breast lesions in young girls. Surg Clin North Am. 1969 Apr;49(2):261–9. PMID:5813207
**622.** Farshid G, Edwards S, Kollias J, et al. Active surveillance of women diagnosed with atypical ductal hyperplasia on core needle biopsy may spare many women potentially unnecessary surgery, but at the risk of undertreatment for a minority: 10-year surgical outcomes of 114 consecutive cases from a single center. Mod Pathol. 2018 Mar;31(3):395–405. PMID:29099502
**623.** Fasola CE, Chen JJ, Jensen KC, et al. Characteristics and clinical outcomes of pleomorphic lobular carcinoma in situ of the breast. Breast J. 2018 Jan;24(1):66–9. PMID:28929550
**624.** Fassan M, Baffa R, Palazzo JP, et al. MicroRNA expression profiling of male breast cancer. Breast Cancer Res. 2009;11(4):R58. PMID:19664288
**625.** Faverly DR, Burgers L, Bult P, et al. Three dimensional imaging of mammary ductal carcinoma in situ: clinical implications. Semin Diagn Pathol. 1994 Aug;11(3):193–8. PMID:7831530
**626.** Fechner RE. Histologic variants of infiltrating lobular carcinoma of the breast. Hum Pathol. 1975 May;6(3):373–8. PMID:166034
**627.** Fechner RE. Infiltrating lobular carcinoma without lobular carcinoma in situ. Cancer. 1972 Jun;29(6):1539–45. PMID:4337952
**628.** Fedko MG, Scow JS, Shah SS, et al. Pure tubular carcinoma and axillary nodal metastases. Ann Surg Oncol. 2010 Oct;17 Suppl 3:338–42. PMID:20853056
**629.** Felts JL, Zhu J, Han B, et al. An analysis of Oncotype DX recurrence scores and clinicopathologic characteristics in invasive lobular breast cancer. Breast J. 2017 Nov;23(6):677–86. PMID:28097781
**630.** Ferlay J, Colombet M, Bray F. Cancer Incidence in Five Continents, CI5plus: IARC CancerBase No. 9 [Internet]. Lyon (France): International Agency for Research on Cancer; 2018. Available from: http://ci5.iarc.fr.
**631.** Ferlay J, Ervik M, Lam F, et al. Global Cancer Observatory: Cancer Today [Internet]. Lyon (France): International Agency for Research on Cancer; 2018. Available from: https://gco.iarc.fr/today.
**632.** Ferlicot S, Vincent-Salomon A, Médioni J, et al. Wide metastatic spreading in infiltrating lobular carcinoma of the breast. Eur J Cancer. 2004 Feb;40(3):336–41. PMID:14746850
**633.** Fernandez AP, Sun Y, Tubbs RR, et al. FISH for MYC amplification and anti-MYC immunohistochemistry: useful diagnostic tools in the assessment of secondary angiosarcoma and atypical vascular proliferations. J Cutan Pathol. 2012 Feb;39(2):234–42. PMID:22121953
**634.** Ferner RE. Neurofibromatosis 1 and neurofibromatosis 2: a twenty first century perspective. Lancet Neurol. 2007 Apr;6(4):340–51. PMID:17362838
**635.** Ferreira AI, Borges S, Sousa A, et al. Radial scar of the breast: Is it possible to avoid surgery? Eur J Surg Oncol. 2017 Jul;43(7):1265–72. PMID:28215506
**636.** Ferrufino-Schmidt MC, Medeiros LJ, Liu H, et al. Clinicopathologic features and prognostic impact of lymph node involvement in patients with breast implant-associated anaplastic large cell lymphoma. Am J Surg Pathol. 2018 Mar;42(3):293–305. PMID:29194092
**637.** Ferzoco RM, Ruddy KJ. The epidemiology of male breast cancer. Curr Oncol Rep. 2016 Jan;18(1):1. PMID:26694922
**638.** Fillion MM, Glass KE, Hayek J, et al. Healthcare costs reduced after incorporating the results of the American College of Surgeons Oncology Group Z0011 trial into clinical practice. Breast J. 2017 May;23(3):275–81. PMID:27900818
**639.** Fineberg S, Rosen PP. Cutaneous angiosarcoma and atypical vascular lesions of the skin and breast after radiation therapy for breast carcinoma. Am J Clin Pathol. 1994 Dec;102(6):757–63. PMID:7801888
**640.** Fiore M, Rimareix F, Mariani L, et al. Desmoid-type fibromatosis: a front-line conservative approach to select patients for surgical treatment. Ann Surg Oncol. 2009 Sep;16(9):2587–93. PMID:19568815
**641.** Fisher B, Costantino JP. Response: Re: Tamoxifen for prevention of breast cancer: report of the National Surgical Adjuvant Breast and Bowel Project P-1 Study. J Natl Cancer Inst. 1999 Nov 3;91(21):1891A–1892. PMID:10547399
**642.** Fisher B, Land S, Mamounas E, et al. Prevention of invasive breast cancer in women with ductal carcinoma in situ: an update of the National Surgical Adjuvant Breast and Bowel Project experience. Semin Oncol. 2001 Aug;28(4):400–18. PMID:11498833
**643.** Fisher C. Unusual myoid, perivascular, and postradiation lesions, with emphasis on atypical vascular lesion, postradiation

cutaneous angiosarcoma, myoepithelial tumors, myopericytoma, and perivascular epithelioid cell tumor. Semin Diagn Pathol. 2013 Feb;30(1):73–84. PMID:23327731
644. Fisher C, Magnusson B, Hardarson S, et al. Myxoid variant of follicular dendritic cell sarcoma arising in the breast. Ann Diagn Pathol. 1999 Apr;3(2):92–8. PMID:10196389
645. Fisher CJ, Hanby AM, Robinson L, et al. Mammary hamartoma–a review of 35 cases. Histopathology. 1992 Feb;20(2):99–106. PMID:1559675
646. Fisher ER, Costantino J, Fisher B, et al. Pathologic findings from the National Surgical Adjuvant Breast Project (NSABP) Protocol B-17. Five-year observations concerning lobular carcinoma in situ. Cancer. 1996 Oct 1;78(7):1403–16. PMID:8839545
647. Fisher ER, Gregorio RM, Redmond C, et al. Tubulolobular invasive breast cancer: a variant of lobular invasive cancer. Hum Pathol. 1977 Nov;8(6):679–83. PMID:924431
648. Fisher ER, Land SR, Fisher B, et al. Pathologic findings from the National Surgical Adjuvant Breast and Bowel Project: twelve-year observations concerning lobular carcinoma in situ. Cancer. 2004 Jan 15;100(2):238–44. PMID:14716756
649. Fisher ER, Wang J, Bryant J, et al. Pathobiology of preoperative chemotherapy: findings from the National Surgical Adjuvant Breast and Bowel (NSABP) protocol B-18. Cancer. 2002 Aug 15;95(4):681–95. PMID:12209710
650. Fitzgibbons PL, Henson DE, Hutter RV. Benign breast changes and the risk for subsequent breast cancer: an update of the 1985 consensus statement. Arch Pathol Lab Med. 1998 Dec;122(12):1053–5. PMID:9870852
651. Flaherty DC, Bawa R, Burton C, et al. Breast cancer in male adolescents and young adults. Ann Surg Oncol. 2017 Jan;24(1):84–90. PMID:27650826
652. Flanagan MR, Rendi MH, Calhoun KE, et al. Pleomorphic lobular carcinoma in situ: radiologic-pathologic features and clinical management. Ann Surg Oncol. 2015 Dec;22(13):4263–9. PMID:25893410
653. Fletcher CD, Beham A, Bekir S, et al. Epithelioid angiosarcoma of deep soft tissue: a distinctive tumor readily mistaken for an epithelial neoplasm. Am J Surg Pathol. 1991 Oct;15(10):915–24. PMID:1718176
654. Fletcher CDM, Bridge JA, Hogendoorn PCW, et al., editors. WHO classification of tumours of soft tissue and bone. Lyon (France): International Agency for Research on Cancer; 2013. (WHO classification of tumours series, 4th ed.; vol. 5). http://publications.iarc.fr/15.
655. Fletcher O, Johnson N, Dos Santos Silva I, et al. Family history, genetic testing, and clinical risk prediction: pooled analysis of CHEK2 1100delC in 1,828 bilateral breast cancers and 7,030 controls. Cancer Epidemiol Biomarkers Prev. 2009 Jan;18(1):230–4. PMID:19124502
656. Fletcher O, Johnson N, Orr N, et al. Novel breast cancer susceptibility locus at 9q31.2: results of a genome-wide association study. J Natl Cancer Inst. 2011 Mar 2;103(5):425–35. PMID:21263130
657. Flint A, Oberman HA. Infarction and squamous metaplasia of intraductal papilloma: a benign breast lesion that may simulate carcinoma. Hum Pathol. 1984 Aug;15(8):764–7. PMID:6745916
658. Flucke U, Requena L, Mentzel T. Radiation-induced vascular lesions of the skin: an overview. Adv Anat Pathol. 2013 Nov;20(6):407–15. PMID:24113311
659. Folpe AL, Chand EM, Goldblum JR, et al. Expression of Fli-1, a nuclear transcription factor, distinguishes vascular neoplasms from potential mimics. Am J Surg Pathol. 2001 Aug;25(8):1061–6. PMID:11474291
660. Fong PC, Yap TA, Boss DS, et al. Poly(ADP)-ribose polymerase inhibition: frequent durable responses in BRCA carrier ovarian cancer correlating with platinum-free interval. J Clin Oncol. 2010 May 20;28(15):2512–9. PMID:20406929
661. Foote FW Jr, Stewart FW. A histologic classification of carcinoma of the breast. Surgery. 1946 Jan;19:74–99. PMID:21022022
662. Foote FW, Stewart FW. Lobular carcinoma in situ: a rare form of mammary cancer. Am J Pathol. 1941 Jul;17(4):491–6.3. PMID:19970575
663. Fortuno C, James PA, Spurdle AB. Current review of TP53 pathogenic germline variants in breast cancer patients outside Li-Fraumeni syndrome. Hum Mutat. 2018 Dec;39(12):1764–73. PMID:30240537
664. Foschini MP, Asioli S, Foreid S, et al. Solid papillary breast carcinomas resembling the tall cell variant of papillary thyroid neoplasms: a unique invasive tumor with indolent behavior. Am J Surg Pathol. 2017 Jul;41(7):887–95. PMID:28418993
665. Foschini MP, Eusebi V. Microglandular adenosis of the breast: a deceptive and still mysterious benign lesion. Hum Pathol. 2018 Dec;82:1–9. PMID:29949742
666. Foschini MP, Krausz T. Salivary gland-type tumors of the breast: a spectrum of benign and malignant tumors including "triple negative carcinomas" of low malignant potential. Semin Diagn Pathol. 2010 Feb;27(1):77–90. PMID:20306833
667. Foschini MP, Marucci G, Eusebi V. Low-grade mucoepidermoid carcinoma of salivary glands: characteristic immunohistochemical profile and evidence of striated duct differentiation. Virchows Arch. 2002 May;440(5):536–42. PMID:12021929
668. Foschini MP, Morandi L, Asioli S, et al. The morphological spectrum of salivary gland type tumours of the breast. Pathology. 2017 Feb;49(2):215–27. PMID:28043647
669. Foschini MP, Pizzicannella G, Peterse JL, et al. Adenomyoepithelioma of the breast associated with low-grade adenosquamous and sarcomatoid carcinomas. Virchows Arch. 1995;427(3):243–50. PMID:7496592
670. Foschini MP, Rizzo A, De Leo A, et al. Solid variant of adenoid cystic carcinoma of the breast: a case series with proposal of a new grading system. Int J Surg Pathol. 2016 Apr;24(2):97–102. PMID:26378056
671. Foster MC, Helvie MA, Gregory NE, et al. Lobular carcinoma in situ or atypical lobular hyperplasia at core-needle biopsy: Is excisional biopsy necessary? Radiology. 2004 Jun;231(3):813–9. PMID:15105449
672. Foulkes WD, Knoppers BM, Turnbull C. Population genetic testing for cancer susceptibility: founder mutations to genomes. Nat Rev Clin Oncol. 2016 Jan;13(1):41–54. PMID:26483301
673. Foulkes WD, Stefansson IM, Chappuis PO, et al. Germline BRCA1 mutations and a basal epithelial phenotype in breast cancer. J Natl Cancer Inst. 2003 Oct 1;95(19):1482–5. PMID:14519755
674. Fraga-Guedes C, Gobbi H, Mastropasqua MG, et al. Clinicopathological and immunohistochemical study of 30 cases of post-radiation atypical vascular lesion of the breast. Breast Cancer Res Treat. 2014 Jul;146(2):347–54. PMID:24943869
675. Franceschini G, Terribile D, Scafetta I, et al. Conservative treatment of a rare case of multifocal adenoid cystic carcinoma of the breast: case report and literature review. Med Sci Monit. 2010 Mar;16(3):CS33–9. PMID:20190690
676. Francis A, Thomas J, Fallowfield L, et al. Addressing overtreatment of screen detected DCIS; the LORIS trial. Eur J Cancer. 2015 Nov;51(16):2296–303. PMID:26296293
677. Franco F, González-Rincón J, Lavernia J, et al. Mutational profile of primary breast diffuse large B-cell lymphoma. Oncotarget. 2017 Oct 24;8(61):102888–97. PMID:29262531
678. Franco Pérez F, Lavernia J, Aguiar-Bujanda D, et al. Primary breast lymphoma: analysis of 55 cases of the Spanish Lymphoma Oncology Group. Clin Lymphoma Myeloma Leuk. 2017 Mar;17(3):186–91. PMID:27847267
679. Frayling IM, Mautner VF, van Minkelen R, et al. Breast cancer risk in neurofibromatosis type 1 is a function of the type of NF1 gene mutation: a new genotype-phenotype correlation. J Med Genet. 2019 Apr;56(4):209–19. PMID:30530636
680. Freeman C, Berg JW, Cutler SJ. Occurrence and prognosis of extranodal lymphomas. Cancer. 1972 Jan;29(1):252–60. PMID:5007387
681. French JD, Ghoussaini M, Edwards SL, et al. Functional variants at the 11q13 risk locus for breast cancer regulate cyclin D1 expression through long-range enhancers. Am J Hum Genet. 2013 Apr 4;92(4):489–503. PMID:23540573
682. Friebel TM, Domchek SM, Rebbeck TR. Modifiers of cancer risk in BRCA1 and BRCA2 mutation carriers: systematic review and meta-analysis. J Natl Cancer Inst. 2014 Jun;106(6):dju091. PMID:24824314
683. Frykberg ER. Lobular carcinoma in situ of the breast. Breast J. 1999 Sep;5(5):296–303. PMID:11348305
684. Fu W, Lobocki CA, Silberberg BK, et al. Molecular markers in Paget disease of the breast. J Surg Oncol. 2001 Jul;77(3):171–8. PMID:11455553
685. Fuehrer N, Hartmann L, Degnim A, et al. Atypical apocrine adenosis of the breast: long-term follow-up in 37 patients. Arch Pathol Lab Med. 2012 Feb;136(2):179–82. PMID:22288965
686. Fujii T, Yajima R, Morita H, et al. Adenoma of the nipple projecting out of the nipple: curative resection without excision of the nipple. World J Surg Oncol. 2014 Apr 10;12:91. PMID:24716784
687. Fukami M, Miyado M, Nagasaki K, et al. Aromatase excess syndrome: a rare autosomal dominant disorder leading to pre- or peri-pubertal onset gynecomastia. Pediatr Endocrinol Rev. 2014 Mar;11(3):298–305. PMID:24716396
688. Fukamizu H, Yamanaka K, Takemoto S, et al. An acquired giant vascular tumour of the breast. Scand J Plast Reconstr Surg Hand Surg. 2002;36(1):53–5. PMID:11925831
689. Fukunaga M, Ushigome S. Myofibroblastoma of the breast with diverse differentiations. Arch Pathol Lab Med. 1997 Jun;121(6):599–603. PMID:9199625
690. Fukuoka K, Hirokawa M, Shimizu M, et al. Basaloid type adenoid cystic carcinoma of the breast. APMIS. 1999 Aug;107(8):762–6. PMID:10515126
691. Fukuoka K, Kanahara T, Tamura M, et al. Basement membrane substance in adenomyoepithelioma of the breast. Acta Cytol. 2001 Mar-Apr;45(2):282–3. PMID:11284321
692. Fusco N, Geyer FC, De Filippo MR, et al. Genetic events in the progression of adenoid cystic carcinoma of the breast to high-grade triple-negative breast cancer. Mod Pathol. 2016 Nov;29(11):1292–305. PMID:27491809
693. Gall TM, Frampton AE. Gene of the month: E-cadherin (CDH1). J Clin Pathol. 2013 Nov;66(11):928–32. PMID:23940132
694. Gamallo C, Palacios J, Suarez A, et al. Correlation of E-cadherin expression with differentiation grade and histological type in breast carcinoma. Am J Pathol. 1993 Apr;142(4):987–93. PMID:7682767
695. Ganjoo K, Advani R, Mariappan MR, et al. Non-Hodgkin lymphoma of the breast. Cancer. 2007 Jul 1;110(1):25–30. PMID:17541937
696. Gao F, Carter G, Tseng G, et al. Clinical importance of histologic grading of lobular carcinoma in situ in breast core needle biopsy specimens: current issues and controversies. Am J Clin Pathol. 2010 May;133(5):767–71. PMID:20395524
697. Gao FF, Khalbuss WE, Austin RM, et al. Cytomorphology of crystal storing histiocytosis in the breast associated with lymphoma: a case report. Acta Cytol. 2011;55(3):302–6. PMID:21525745
698. Gao Y, Niu Y, Wang X, et al. Genetic changes at specific stages of breast cancer progression detected by comparative genomic hybridization. J Mol Med (Berl). 2009 Feb;87(2):145–52. PMID:18936904
699. Garcia-Closas M, Couch FJ, Lindstrom S, et al. Genome-wide association studies identify four ER negative-specific breast cancer risk loci. Nat Genet. 2013 Apr;45(4):392–8, e1–2. PMID:23535733
700. Gatalica Z. Immunohistochemical analysis of apocrine breast lesions. Consistent over-expression of androgen receptor accompanied by the loss of estrogen and progesterone receptors in apocrine metaplasia and apocrine carcinoma in situ. Pathol Res Pract. 1997;193(11-12):753–8. PMID:9521507
701. Gatalica Z, Xiu J, Swensen J, et al. Molecular characterization of cancers with NTRK gene fusions. Mod Pathol. 2019 Jan;32(1):147–53. PMID:30171197
702. Gatta G, van der Zwan JM, Casali PG, et al. Rare cancers are not so rare: the rare cancer burden in Europe. Eur J Cancer. 2011 Nov;47(17):2493–511. PMID:22033323
703. Gatti RA, Tward A, Concannon P. Cancer risk in ATM heterozygotes: a model of phenotypic and mechanistic differences between missense and truncating mutations. Mol Genet Metab. 1999 Dec;68(4):419–23. PMID:10607471
704. Gaudet MM, Gapstur SM, Sun J, et al. Active smoking and breast cancer risk: original cohort data and meta-analysis. J Natl Cancer Inst. 2013 Apr 17;105(8):515–25. PMID:23449445
705. Gaudet MM, Kuchenbaecker KB, Vijai J, et al. Identification of a BRCA2-specific modifier locus at 6p24 related to breast cancer risk. PLoS Genet. 2013;9(3):e1003173. PMID:23544012
706. Gengler C, Coindre JM, Leroux A, et al. Vascular proliferations of the skin after radiation therapy for breast cancer: clinicopathologic analysis of a series in favor of a benign process: a study from the French Sarcoma Group. Cancer. 2007 Apr 15;109(8):1584–98. PMID:17357996
707. Georgiannos SN, Chin J, Goode AW, et al. Secondary neoplasms of the breast: a survey of the 20th century. Cancer. 2001 Nov 1;92(9):2259–66. PMID:11745279
708. Gersell DJ, Katzenstein AL. Spindle cell carcinoma of the breast. A clinocopathologic and ultrastructural study. Hum Pathol. 1981 Jun;12(6):550–61. PMID:7275095
709. Gervais MK, Burtenshaw SM, Maxwell J, et al. Clinical outcomes in breast angiosarcoma patients: a rare tumor with unique challenges. J Surg Oncol. 2017 Dec;116(8):1056–61. PMID:29205355
710. Geyer FC, Berman SH, Marchiò C,

et al. Genetic analysis of microglandular adenosis and acinic cell carcinomas of the breast provides evidence for the existence of a low-grade triple-negative breast neoplasia family. Mod Pathol. 2017 Jan;30(1):69–84. PMID:27713419

**711.** Geyer FC, de Biase D, Lambros MB, et al. Genomic profiling of mitochondrion-rich breast carcinoma: chromosomal changes may be relevant for mitochondria accumulation and tumour biology. Breast Cancer Res Treat. 2012 Feb;132(1):15–28. PMID:21509527

**712.** Geyer FC, Lacroix-Triki M, Colombo PE, et al. Molecular evidence in support of the neoplastic and precursor nature of microglandular adenosis. Histopathology. 2012 May;60 6B:E115–30. PMID:22486256

**713.** Geyer FC, Lacroix-Triki M, Savage K, et al. β-Catenin pathway activation in breast cancer is associated with triple-negative phenotype but not with CTNNB1 mutation. Mod Pathol. 2011 Feb;24(2):209–31. PMID:21076461

**714.** Geyer FC, Lambros MB, Natrajan R, et al. Genomic and immunohistochemical analysis of adenosquamous carcinoma of the breast. Mod Pathol. 2010 Jul;23(7):951–60. PMID:20453835

**715.** Geyer FC, Li A, Papanastasiou AD, et al. Recurrent hotspot mutations in HRAS Q61 and PI3K-AKT pathway genes as drivers of breast adenomyoepitheliomas. Nat Commun. 2018 May 8;9(1):1816. PMID:29739933

**716.** Geyer FC, Pareja F, Weigelt B, et al. The spectrum of triple-negative breast disease: high- and low-grade lesions. Am J Pathol. 2017 Oct;187(10):2139–51. PMID:28736315

**717.** Geyer FC, Weigelt B, Natrajan R, et al. Molecular analysis reveals a genetic basis for the phenotypic diversity of metaplastic breast carcinomas. J Pathol. 2010 Apr;220(5):562–73. PMID:20099298

**718.** Ghabach B, Anderson WF, Curtis RE, et al. Adenoid cystic carcinoma of the breast in the United States (1977 to 2006): a population-based cohort study. Breast Cancer Res. 2010;12(4):R54. PMID:20653964

**719.** Ghadimi MP, Liu P, Peng T, et al. Pleomorphic liposarcoma: clinical observations and molecular variables. Cancer. 2011 Dec 1;117(23):5359–69. PMID:21598240

**720.** Gharehdaghi M, Hassani M, Khooei AR, et al. Multicentric myxoid liposarcoma; a case report and literature review. Arch Bone Jt Surg. 2014 Mar;2(1):79–81. PMID:25207321

**721.** Gherardi G, Bernardi C, Marveggio C. Microglandular adenosis of the breast: fine-needle aspiration biopsy of two cases. Diagn Cytopathol. 1993;9(1):72–6. PMID:8458288

**722.** Ghosh K, Vierkant RA, Frank RD, et al. Association between mammographic breast density and histologic features of benign breast disease. Breast Cancer Res. 2017 Dec 19;19(1):134. PMID:29258587

**723.** Ghoussaini M, Edwards SL, Michailidou K, et al. Evidence that breast cancer risk at the 2q35 locus is mediated through IGFBP5 regulation. Nat Commun. 2014 Sep 23;4:4999. PMID:25248036

**724.** Ghoussaini M, Fletcher O, Michailidou K, et al. Genome-wide association analysis identifies three new breast cancer susceptibility loci. Nat Genet. 2012 Jan 22;44(3):312–8. PMID:22267197

**725.** Giacinti L, Claudio PP, Lopez M, et al. Epigenetic information and estrogen receptor alpha expression in breast cancer. Oncologist. 2006 Jan;11(1):1–8. PMID:16401708

**726.** Giacomazzi J, Graudenz MS, Osorio CA, et al. Prevalence of the TP53 p.R337H mutation in breast cancer patients in Brazil. PLoS One. 2014 Jun 17;9(6):e99893. PMID:24936644

**727.** Giardiello FM, Brensinger JD, Tersmette AC, et al. Very high risk of cancer in familial Peutz-Jeghers syndrome. Gastroenterology. 2000 Dec;119(6):1447–53. PMID:11113065

**728.** Giardiello FM, Welsh SB, Hamilton SR, et al. Increased risk of cancer in the Peutz-Jeghers syndrome. N Engl J Med. 1987 Jun 11;316(24):1511–4. PMID:3587280

**729.** Gibbons D, Leitch M, Coscia J, et al. Fine needle aspiration cytology and histologic findings of granular cell tumor of the breast: review of 19 cases with clinical/radiologic correlation. Breast J. 2000 Jan;6(1):27–30. PMID:11348331

**730.** Ginter PS, McIntire PJ, Shin SJ. Vascular tumours of the breast: a comprehensive review with focus on diagnostic challenges encountered in the core biopsy setting. Pathology. 2017 Feb;49(2):197–214. PMID:28049578

**731.** Ginter PS, Mosquera JM, MacDonald TY, et al. Diagnostic utility of MYC amplification and anti-MYC immunohistochemistry in atypical vascular lesions, primary or radiation-induced mammary angiosarcomas, and primary angiosarcomas of other sites. Hum Pathol. 2014 Apr;45(4):709–16. PMID:24457083

**732.** Ginter PS, Scognamiglio T, Tauchi-Nishi P, et al. Pleomorphic adenoma of breast: a radiological and pathological study of a common tumor in an uncommon location. Case Rep Pathol. 2015;2015:172750. PMID:25830053

**733.** Giovanella L, Marelli M, Ceriani L, et al. Evaluation of chromogranin A expression in serum and tissues of breast cancer patients. Int J Biol Markers. 2001 Oct-Dec;16(4):268–72. PMID:11820723

**734.** Giovannelli P, Di Donato M, Galasso G, et al. The androgen receptor in breast cancer. Front Endocrinol (Lausanne). 2018 Aug 28;9:492. PMID:30210453

**735.** Giuliano AE, Connolly JL, Edge SB, et al. Breast cancer-major changes in the American Joint Committee on Cancer eighth edition cancer staging manual. CA Cancer J Clin. 2017 Jul 8;67(4):290–303. PMID:28294295

**736.** Giulino-Roth L, Wang K, MacDonald TY, et al. Targeted genomic sequencing of pediatric Burkitt lymphoma identifies recurrent alterations in antiapoptotic and chromatin-remodeling genes. Blood. 2012 Dec 20;120(26):5181–4. PMID:23091298

**737.** Gleason BC, Hornick JL. Inflammatory myofibroblastic tumours: Where are we now? J Clin Pathol. 2008 Apr;61(4):428–37. PMID:17938159

**738.** Gleason BC, Nascimento AF. HMB-45 and Melan-A are useful in the differential diagnosis between granular cell tumor and malignant melanoma. Am J Dermatopathol. 2007 Feb;29(1):22–7. PMID:17284958

**739.** Glubb DM, Maranian MJ, Michailidou K, et al. Fine-scale mapping of the 5q11.2 breast cancer locus reveals at least three independent risk variants regulating MAP3K1. Am J Hum Genet. 2015 Jan 8;96(1):5–20. PMID:25529635

**740.** Gnant M, Harbeck N, Thomssen C. St. Gallen/Vienna 2017: a brief summary of the consensus discussion about escalation and de-escalation of primary breast cancer treatment. Breast Care (Basel). 2017 May;12(2):102–7. PMID:28559767

**741.** Gobbi H, Jensen RA, Simpson JF, et al. Atypical ductal hyperplasia and ductal carcinoma in situ of the breast associated with perineural invasion. Hum Pathol. 2001 Aug;32(8):785–90. PMID:11521220

**741A.** Gobbi H, Simpson JF, Borowsky A, et al. Metaplastic breast tumors with a dominant fibromatosis-like phenotype have a high risk of local recurrence. Cancer. 1999 May 15;85(10):2170–82. PMID:10326695

**742.** Gobbi H, Simpson JF, Jensen RA, et al. Metaplastic spindle cell breast tumors arising within papillomas, complex sclerosing lesions, and nipple adenomas. Mod Pathol. 2003 Sep;16(9):893–901. PMID:13679453

**743.** Gojon H, Fawunmi D, Valachis A. Sentinel lymph node biopsy in patients with microinvasive breast cancer: a systematic review and meta-analysis. Eur J Surg Oncol. 2014 Jan;40(1):5–11. PMID:24238761

**744.** Goldgar DE, Healey S, Dowty JG, et al. Rare variants in the ATM gene and risk of breast cancer. Breast Cancer Res. 2011 Jul 25;13(4):R73. PMID:21787400

**745.** Goldhirsch A, Winer EP, Coates AS, et al. Personalizing the treatment of women with early breast cancer: highlights of the St Gallen International Expert Consensus on the Primary Therapy of Early Breast Cancer 2013. Ann Oncol. 2013 Sep;24(9):2206–23. PMID:23917950

**746.** Goldhirsch A, Wood WC, Coates AS, et al. Strategies for subtypes–dealing with the diversity of breast cancer: highlights of the St. Gallen International Expert Consensus on the Primary Therapy of Early Breast Cancer 2011. Ann Oncol. 2011 Aug;22(8):1736–47. PMID:21709140

**747.** Gomes DS, Balabram D, Porto SS, et al. Lobular neoplasia: frequency and association with other breast lesions. Diagn Pathol. 2011 Aug 9;6:74. PMID:21827679

**748.** Gomes DS, Porto SS, Balabram D, et al. Inter-observer variability between general pathologists and a specialist in breast pathology in the diagnosis of lobular neoplasia, columnar cell lesions, atypical ductal hyperplasia and ductal carcinoma in situ of the breast. Diagn Pathol. 2014 Jun 19;9:121. PMID:24948027

**749.** Gómez Macías GS, Pérez Saucedo JE, Cardona Huerta S, et al. Invasive lobular carcinoma of the breast with extracellular mucin: a case report. Int J Surg Case Rep. 2016;25:33–6. PMID:27315432

**750.** Gong G, DeVries S, Chew KL, et al. Genetic changes in paired atypical and usual ductal hyperplasia of the breast by comparative genomic hybridization. Clin Cancer Res. 2001 Aug;7(8):2410–4. PMID:11489820

**751.** Gong S, Crane GM, McCall CM, et al. Expanding the spectrum of EBV-positive marginal zone lymphomas: a lesion associated with diverse immunodeficiency settings. Am J Surg Pathol. 2018 Oct;42(10):1306–16. PMID:29957733

**752.** Gonzalez KD, Noltner KA, Buzin CH, et al. Beyond Li Fraumeni syndrome: clinical characteristics of families with p53 germline mutations. J Clin Oncol. 2009 Mar 10;27(8):1250–6. PMID:19204208

**753.** Gonzalez-Angulo AM, Barlow WE, Gralow J, et al. SWOG S1007: a phase III, randomized clinical trial of standard adjuvant endocrine therapy with or without chemotherapy in patients with one to three positive nodes, hormone receptor (HR)-positive, and HER2-negative breast cancer with recurrence score (RS) of 25 or less [abstract]. J Clin Oncol. 2016 Sep 22;29(15 suppl):TPS104. Abstract no. TPS104. doi:10.1200/jco.2011.29.15_suppl.tps104.

**754.** González-Rivera M, Lobo M, López-Tarruella S, et al. Erratum to: Frequency of germline DNA genetic findings in an unselected prospective cohort of triple-negative breast cancer patients participating in a platinum-based neoadjuvant chemotherapy trial. Breast Cancer Res Treat. 2017 Sep;165(2):471. PMID:28721639

**755.** Goodman ZD, Taxy JB. Fibroadenomas of the breast with prominent smooth muscle. Am J Surg Pathol. 1981 Jan;5(1):99–101. PMID:7246853

**756.** Gooren LJ, van Trotsenburg MA, Giltay EJ, et al. Breast cancer development in transsexual subjects receiving cross-sex hormone treatment. J Sex Med. 2013 Dec;10(12):3129–34. PMID:24010586

**757.** Gospodarowicz MK, Sutcliffe SB. The extranodal lymphomas. Semin Radiat Oncol. 1995 Oct;5(4):281–300. PMID:10717152

**758.** Gown AM, Fulton RS, Kandalaft PL. Markers of metastatic carcinoma of breast origin. Histopathology. 2016 Jan;68(1):86–95. PMID:26768031

**759.** Gradishar WJ, Anderson BO, Balassanian R, et al. NCCN Guidelines Insights: Breast Cancer, Version 1.2017. J Natl Compr Canc Netw. 2017 Apr;15(4):433–51. PMID:28404755

**760.** Grady I, Gorsuch H, Wilburn-Bailey S. Long-term outcome of benign fibroadenomas treated by ultrasound-guided percutaneous excision. Breast J. 2008 May-Jun;14(3):275–8. PMID:18397185

**761.** Grady WM, Willis J, Guilford PJ, et al. Methylation of the CDH1 promoter as the second genetic hit in hereditary diffuse gastric cancer. Nat Genet. 2000 Sep;26(1):16–7. PMID:10973239

**762.** Grant RC, Al-Sukhni W, Borgida AE, et al. Exome sequencing identifies nonsegregating nonsense ATM and PALB2 variants in familial pancreatic cancer. Hum Genomics. 2013 Apr 5;7:11. PMID:23561644

**763.** Green I, McCormick B, Cranor M, et al. A comparative study of pure tubular and tubulolobular carcinoma of the breast. Am J Surg Pathol. 1997 Jun;21(6):653–7. PMID:9199642

**764.** Greenberg ML, Camaris C, Psarianos T, et al. Is there a role for fine-needle aspiration in radial scar/complex sclerosing lesions of the breast? Diagn Cytopathol. 1997 Jun;16(6):537–42. PMID:9181322

**765.** Gresik CM, Godellas C, Aranha GV, et al. Pseudoangiomatous stromal hyperplasia of the breast: a contemporary approach to its clinical and radiologic features and ideal management. Surgery. 2010 Oct;148(4):752–7, discussion 757–8. PMID:20708765

**766.** Grimm EE, Schmidt RA, Swanson PE, et al. Achieving 95% cross-methodological concordance in HER2 testing: causes and implications of discordant cases. Am J Clin Pathol. 2010 Aug;134(2):284–92. PMID:20660333

**767.** Grimm LJ, Bookhout CE, Bentley RC, et al. Concordant, non-atypical breast papillomas do not require surgical excision: a 10-year multi-institution study and review of the literature. Clin Imaging. 2018 Sep-Oct;51:180–5. PMID:29859481

**768.** Grin A, Horne G, Ennis M, et al. Measuring extent of ductal carcinoma in situ in breast excision specimens: a comparison of 4 methods. Arch Pathol Lab Med. 2009 Jan;133(1):31–7. PMID:19123733

**769.** Grin A, O'Malley FP, Mulligan AM. Cytokeratin 5 and estrogen receptor immunohistochemistry as a useful adjunct in identifying atypical papillary lesions on breast needle core biopsy. Am J Surg Pathol. 2009 Nov;33(11):1615–23. PMID:19675450

**770.** Gronchi A, Casali PG, Mariani L, et al. Quality of surgery and outcome in extra-abdominal aggressive fibromatosis: a series of patients surgically treated at a single institution. J Clin Oncol. 2003 Apr 1;21(7):1390–7. PMID:12663732

**771.** Gronchi A, Miceli R, Shurell E, et al. Outcome prediction in primary resected retroperitoneal soft tissue sarcoma: histology-specific overall survival and disease-free survival nomograms built on major sarcoma center data sets. J Clin Oncol. 2013 May

1;31(13):1649–55. PMID:23530096
772. Gronwald J, Byrski T, Huzarski T, et al. Influence of selected lifestyle factors on breast and ovarian cancer risk in BRCA1 mutation carriers from Poland. Breast Cancer Res Treat. 2006 Jan;95(2):105–9. PMID:16261399
773. Grossman RA, Pedroso FE, Byrne MM, et al. Does surgery or radiation therapy impact survival for patients with extrapulmonary small cell cancers? J Surg Oncol. 2011 Nov 1;104(6):604–12. PMID:21618245
774. Gruel N, Benhamo V, Bhalshankar J, et al. Polarity gene alterations in pure invasive micropapillary carcinomas of the breast. Breast Cancer Res. 2014 May 8;16(3):R46. PMID:24887297
775. Gruel N, Fuhrmann L, Lodillinsky C, et al. LIN7A is a major determinant of cell-polarity defects in breast carcinomas. Breast Cancer Res. 2016 Feb 17;18(1):23. PMID:26887652
776. Gruel N, Lucchesi C, Raynal V, et al. Lobular invasive carcinoma of the breast is a molecular entity distinct from luminal invasive ductal carcinoma. Eur J Cancer. 2010 Sep;46(13):2399–407. PMID:20570624
778. Gualco G, Bacchi CE. B-cell and T-cell lymphomas of the breast: clinical–pathological features of 53 cases. Int J Surg Pathol. 2008 Oct;16(4):407–13. PMID:18480397
779. Gualco G, Weiss LM, Harrington WJ Jr, et al. BCL6, MUM1, and CD10 expression in mantle cell lymphoma. Appl Immunohistochem Mol Morphol. 2010 Mar;18(2):103–8. PMID:19826251
780. Guan B, Wang H, Cao S, et al. Lipid-rich carcinoma of the breast clinicopathologic analysis of 17 cases. Ann Diagn Pathol. 2011 Aug;15(4):225–32. PMID:21396871
781. Gudjónsdóttir A, Hägerstrand I, Ostberg G. Adenoma of the nipple with carcinomatous development. Acta Pathol Microbiol Scand A. 1971;79(6):676–80. PMID:5123518
782. Guerini-Rocco E, Hodi Z, Piscuoglio S, et al. The repertoire of somatic genetic alterations of acinic cell carcinomas of the breast: an exploratory, hypothesis-generating study. J Pathol. 2015 Oct;237(2):166–78. PMID:26011570
783. Guerini-Rocco E, Piscuoglio S, Ng CK, et al. Microglandular adenosis associated with triple-negative breast cancer is a neoplastic lesion of triple-negative phenotype harbouring TP53 somatic mutations. J Pathol. 2016 Apr;238(5):677–88. PMID:26806567
783A. Guidi AJ, Tworek JA, Mais DD, et al. Breast specimen processing and reporting with an emphasis on margin evaluation: a College of American Pathologists survey of 866 laboratories. Arch Pathol Lab Med. 2018 Apr;142(4):496–506. PMID:29328775
784. Gullett NP, Rizzo M, Johnstone PA. National surgical patterns of care for primary surgery and axillary staging of phyllodes tumors. Breast J. 2009 Jan-Feb;15(1):41–4. PMID:19141133
785. Gumy-Pause F, Wacker P, Sappino AP. ATM gene and lymphoid malignancies. Leukemia. 2004 Feb;18(2):238–42. PMID:14628072
786. Günhan-Bilgen I, Oktay A. Tubular carcinoma of the breast: mammographic, sonographic, clinical and pathologic findings. Eur J Radiol. 2007 Jan;61(1):158–62. PMID:16987629
787. Guo Q, Schmidt MK, Kraft P, et al. Identification of novel genetic markers of breast cancer survival. J Natl Cancer Inst. 2015 Apr 18;107(5):djv081. PMID:25890600
788. Guo S, Wang Y, Rohr J, et al. Solid papillary carcinoma of the breast: a special entity needs to be distinguished from conventional invasive carcinoma avoiding over-treatment. Breast. 2016 Apr;26:67–72. PMID:27017244
789. Guo T, Wang Y, Shapiro N, et al. Pleomorphic lobular carcinoma in situ diagnosed by breast core biopsy: clinicopathologic features and correlation with subsequent excision. Clin Breast Cancer. 2018 Aug;18(4):e449–54. PMID:29102711
790. Guo T, Zhang L, Chang NE, et al. Consistent MYC and FLT4 gene amplification in radiation-induced angiosarcoma but not in other radiation-associated atypical vascular lesions. Genes Chromosomes Cancer. 2011 Jan;50(1):25–33. PMID:20949568
791. Guo X, Chen L, Lang R, et al. Invasive micropapillary carcinoma of the breast: association of pathologic features with lymph node metastasis. Am J Clin Pathol. 2006 Nov;126(5):740–6. PMID:17050071
792. Gupta D, Croitoru CM, Ayala AG, et al. E-cadherin immunohistochemical analysis of histiocytoid carcinoma of the breast. Ann Diagn Pathol. 2002 Jun;6(3):141–7. PMID:12089723
793. Guss CE, Divasta AD. Adolescent gynecomastia. Pediatr Endocrinol Rev. 2017 Jun;14(4):371–7. PMID:28613047
794. Gustafson P. Soft tissue sarcoma. Epidemiology and prognosis in 508 patients. Acta Orthop Scand Suppl. 1994 Jun;259:1–31. PMID:8042499
795. Gutierrez Barrera AM, Fouad TM, Song J, et al. BRCA mutations in women with inflammatory breast cancer. Cancer. 2018 Feb 1;124(3):466–74. PMID:29044548
796. Gutmann DH, Ferner RE, Listernick RH, et al. Neurofibromatosis type 1. Nat Rev Dis Primers. 2017 Feb 23;3:17004. PMID:28230061
797. Ha D, Dialani V, Mehta TS, et al. Mucocele-like lesions in the breast diagnosed with percutaneous biopsy: Is surgical excision necessary? AJR Am J Roentgenol. 2015 Jan;204(1):204–10. PMID:25539258
798. Ha SM, Cha JH, Shin HJ, et al. Radial scars/complex sclerosing lesions of the breast: radiologic and clinicopathologic correlation. BMC Med Imaging. 2018 Nov 3;18(1):39. PMID:30390667
799. Ha SM, Chae EY, Cha JH, et al. Association of BRCA mutation types, imaging features, and pathologic findings in patients with breast cancer with BRCA1 and BRCA2 mutations. AJR Am J Roentgenol. 2017 Oct;209(4):920–8. PMID:28796549
800. Haagensen CD, editor. Diseases of the breast. 3rd ed. Philadelphia (PA): Saunders; 1986.
801. Haagensen CD, Lane N, Lattes R, et al. Lobular neoplasia (so-called lobular carcinoma in situ) of the breast. Cancer. 1978 Aug;42(2):737–69. PMID:209887
802. HaDuong JH, Martin AA, Skapek SX, et al. Sarcomas. Pediatr Clin North Am. 2015 Feb;62(1):179–200. PMID:25435119
803. Haiman CA, Chen GK, Vachon CM, et al. A common variant at the TERT-CLPTM1L locus is associated with estrogen receptor-negative breast cancer. Nat Genet. 2011 Oct 30;43(12):1210–4. PMID:22037553
804. Haj M, Weiss M, Loberant N, et al. Inflammatory pseudotumor of the breast: case report and literature review. Breast J. 2003 Sep-Oct;9(5):423–5. PMID:12968967
805. Hajdu SI, Urban JA. Cancers metastatic to the breast. Cancer. 1972 Jun;29(6):1691–6. PMID:4337956
806. Hall J, Marcel V, Bolin C, et al. The associations of sequence variants in DNA-repair and cell-cycle genes with cancer risk: genotype-phenotype correlations. Biochem Soc Trans. 2009 Jun;37(Pt 3):527–33. PMID:19442246
807. Haltas H, Bayrak R, Yenidunya S, et al. Invasive lobular carcinoma with extracellular mucin as a distinct variant of lobular carcinoma: a case report. Diagn Pathol. 2012 Aug 6;7:91. PMID:22867429
808. Halteh P, Patel A, Eskreis-Winkler S, et al. Schwannoma of the breast: a common tumor in an uncommon location. Breast J. 2018 Mar;24(2):206–7. PMID:28707768
809. Hamdi Y, Soucy P, Kuchenbaeker KB, et al. Association of breast cancer risk in BRCA1 and BRCA2 mutation carriers with genetic variants showing differential allelic expression: identification of a modifier of breast cancer risk at locus 11q22.3. Breast Cancer Res Treat. 2017 Jan;161(1):117–34. PMID:27796716
810. Hameed O, Perry A, Banerjee R, et al. Papillary carcinoma of the breast lacks evidence of RET rearrangements despite morphological similarities to papillary thyroid carcinoma. Mod Pathol. 2009 Sep;22(9):1236–42. PMID:19543246
811. Hamele-Bena D, Cranor ML, Rosen PP. Mammary mucocele-like lesions. Benign and malignant. Am J Surg Pathol. 1996 Sep;20(9):1081–5. PMID:8764744
812. Hamele-Bena D, Cranor ML, Sciotto C, et al. Uncommon presentation of mammary myofibroblastoma. Mod Pathol. 1996 Jul;9(7):786–90. PMID:8832563
813. Hamilton-Dutoit SJ, Raphael M, Audouin J, et al. In situ demonstration of Epstein-Barr virus small RNAs (EBER 1) in acquired immunodeficiency syndrome-related lymphomas: correlation with tumor morphology and primary site. Blood. 1993 Jul 15;82(2):619–24. PMID:8392401
814. Hammer P, White K, Mengden S, et al. Nipple leiomyoma: a rare neoplasm with a broad spectrum of histologic appearances. J Cutan Pathol. 2019 May;46(5):343–6. PMID:30663114
815. Hammond ME, Hayes DF, Dowsett M, et al. American Society of Clinical Oncology/College of American Pathologists guideline recommendations for immunohistochemical testing of estrogen and progesterone receptors in breast cancer (unabridged version). Arch Pathol Lab Med. 2010 Jul;134(7):e48–72. PMID:20586616
816. Hammond ME, Hayes DF, Dowsett M, et al. American Society of Clinical Oncology/College of American Pathologists guideline recommendations for immunohistochemical testing of estrogen and progesterone receptors in breast cancer. Arch Pathol Lab Med. 2010 Jun;134(6):907–22. PMID:20524868
817. Hamperl H. The myothelia (myoepithelial cells). Normal state; regressive changes; hyperplasia; tumors. Curr Top Pathol. 1970;53:161–220. PMID:4323195
818. Han B, Mori I, Nakamura M, et al. Myoepithelial carcinoma arising in an adenomyoepithelioma of the breast: case report with immunohistochemical and mutational analysis. Pathol Int. 2006 Apr;56(4):211–6. PMID:16634967
819. Hanrahan EO, Gonzalez-Angulo AM, Giordano SH, et al. Overall survival and cause-specific mortality of patients with stage T1a,bN0M0 breast carcinoma. J Clin Oncol. 2007 Nov 1;25(31):4952–60. PMID:17971593
820. Hansford S, Kaurah P, Li-Chang H, et al. Hereditary diffuse gastric cancer syndrome: CDH1 mutations and beyond. JAMA Oncol. 2015 Apr;1(1):23–32. PMID:26182300
821. Haralambieva E, Schuuring E, Rosati S, et al. Interphase fluorescence in situ hybridization for detection of 8q24/MYC breakpoints on routine histologic sections: validation in Burkitt lymphomas from three geographic regions. Genes Chromosomes Cancer. 2004 May;40(1):10–8. PMID:15034863
822. Hare F, Giri S, Patel JK, et al. A population-based analysis of outcomes for small cell carcinoma of the breast by tumor stage and the use of radiation therapy. Springerplus. 2015 Mar 21;4:138. PMID:25853028
823. Harigopal M, Park K, Chen X, et al. Pathologic quiz case: a rapidly increasing breast mass in a postmenopausal woman. Malignant adenomyoepithelioma. Arch Pathol Lab Med. 2004 Feb;128(2):235–6. PMID:14736274
824. Harris LN, Ismaila N, McShane LM, et al. Use of biomarkers to guide decisions on adjuvant systemic therapy for women with early-stage invasive breast cancer: American Society of Clinical Oncology Clinical Practice Guideline Summary. J Oncol Pract. 2016 Apr;12(4):384–9. PMID:26957642
825. Harris M, Howell A, Chrissohou M, et al. A comparison of the metastatic pattern of infiltrating lobular carcinoma and infiltrating duct carcinoma of the breast. Br J Cancer. 1984 Jul;50(1):23–30. PMID:6331484
826. Hart J, Gardner JM, Edgar M, et al. Epithelioid schwannomas: an analysis of 58 cases including atypical variants. Am J Surg Pathol. 2016 May;40(5):704–13. PMID:26752543
827. Hartley RL, Stone JP, Temple-Oberle C. Breast cancer in transgender patients: a systematic review. Part 1: Male to female. Eur J Surg Oncol. 2018 Oct;44(10):1455–62. PMID:30087072
828. Hartmann LC, Degnim AC, Santen RJ, et al. Atypical hyperplasia of the breast–risk assessment and management options. N Engl J Med. 2015 Jan 1;372(1):78–89. PMID:25551530
829. Hartmann LC, Radisky DC, Frost MH, et al. Understanding the premalignant potential of atypical hyperplasia through its natural history: a longitudinal cohort study. Cancer Prev Res (Phila). 2014 Feb;7(2):211–7. PMID:24480577
830. Hartmann LC, Sellers TA, Frost MH, et al. Benign breast disease and the risk of breast cancer. N Engl J Med. 2005 Jul 21;353(3):229–37. PMID:16034008
831. Harvey JM, Clark GM, Osborne CK, et al. Estrogen receptor status by immunohistochemistry is superior to the ligand-binding assay for predicting response to adjuvant endocrine therapy in breast cancer. J Clin Oncol. 1999 May;17(5):1474–81. PMID:10334533
832. Hasebe T, Tsuda H, Hirohashi S, et al. Fibrotic focus in invasive ductal carcinoma: an indicator of high tumor aggressiveness. Jpn J Cancer Res. 1996 Apr;87(4):385–94. PMID:8641970
833. Hasebe T, Tsuda H, Tsubono Y, et al. Fibrotic focus in invasive ductal carcinoma of the breast: a histopathological prognostic parameter for tumor recurrence and tumor death within three years after the initial operation. Jpn J Cancer Res. 1997 Jun;88(6):590–9. PMID:9263537
834. Hashmi AA, Aijaz S, Mahboob R, et al. Clinicopathologic features of invasive metaplastic and micropapillary breast carcinoma: comparison with invasive ductal carcinoma of breast. BMC Res Notes. 2018 Jul 31;11(1):531. PMID:30064485
835. Hauke J, Horvath J, Groß E, et al. Gene panel testing of 5589 BRCA1/2-negative index patients with breast cancer in a routine diagnostic setting: results of the German Consortium for Hereditary Breast and Ovarian Cancer. Cancer Med. 2018 Apr;7(4):1349–58. PMID:29522266
836. Hayes MM. Adenomyoepithelioma of the breast: a review stressing its propensity for malignant transformation. J Clin Pathol. 2011 Jun;64(6):477–84. PMID:21307156

**837.** Hayes MM, Lesack D, Girardet C, et al. Carcinoma ex-pleomorphic adenoma of the breast. Report of three cases suggesting a relationship to metaplastic carcinoma of matrix-producing type. Virchows Arch. 2005 Feb;446(2):142–9. PMID:15583933
**838.** Hearle N, Schumacher V, Menko FH, et al. Frequency and spectrum of cancers in the Peutz-Jeghers syndrome. Clin Cancer Res. 2006 May 15;12(10):3209–15. PMID:16707622
**839.** Hechtman JF, Benayed R, Hyman DM, et al. Pan-Trk immunohistochemistry is an efficient and reliable screen for the detection of NTRK fusions. Am J Surg Pathol. 2017 Nov;41(11):1547–51. PMID:28719467
**840.** Hegyi L, Thway K, Newton R, et al. Malignant myoepithelioma arising in adenomyoepithelioma of the breast and coincident multiple gastrointestinal stromal tumours in a patient with neurofibromatosis type 1. J Clin Pathol. 2009 Jul;62(7):653–5. PMID:19561236
**841.** Heller SL, Elias K, Gupta A, et al. Outcome of high-risk lesions at MRI-guided 9-gauge vacuum-assisted breast biopsy. AJR Am J Roentgenol. 2014 Jan;202(1):237–45. PMID:24370150
**842.** Hendry S, Pang JB, Byrne DJ, et al. Relationship of the breast ductal carcinoma in situ immune microenvironment with clinicopathological and genetic features. Clin Cancer Res. 2017 Sep 1;23(17):5210–7. PMID:28611201
**843.** Hennessy BT, Giordano S, Broglio K, et al. Biphasic metaplastic sarcomatoid carcinoma of the breast. Ann Oncol. 2006 Apr;17(4):605–13. PMID:16469754
**844.** Hennessy BT, Gonzalez-Angulo AM, Stemke-Hale K, et al. Characterization of a naturally occurring breast cancer subset enriched in epithelial-to-mesenchymal transition and stem cell characteristics. Cancer Res. 2009 May 15;69(10):4116–24. PMID:19435916
**845.** Hennessy BT, Krishnamurthy S, Giordano S, et al. Squamous cell carcinoma of the breast. J Clin Oncol. 2005 Nov 1;23(31):7827–35. PMID:16258085
**846.** Henry NL, Braun TM, Breslin TM, et al. Variation in the use of advanced imaging at the time of breast cancer diagnosis in a statewide registry. Cancer. 2017 Aug 1;123(15):2975–83. PMID:28301680
**847.** Herbert M, Sandbank J, Liokumovich P, et al. Breast hamartomas: clinicopathological and immunohistochemical studies of 24 cases. Histopathology. 2002 Jul;41(1):30–4. PMID:12121234
**848.** Herbert M, Schvimer M, Zehavi S, et al. Breast hamartoma: fine-needle aspiration cytologic finding. Cancer. 2003 Aug 25;99(4):255–8. PMID:12925988
**849.** Herrington CS, Tarin D, Buley I, et al. Osteosarcomatous differentiation in carcinoma of the breast: a case of 'metaplastic' carcinoma with osteoclasts and osteoclast-like giant cells. Histopathology. 1994 Mar;24(3):282–5. PMID:8200630
**850.** Herz H, Cooke B, Goldstein D. Metastatic secretory breast cancer. Non-responsiveness to chemotherapy: case report and review of the literature. Ann Oncol. 2000 Oct;11(10):1343–7. PMID:11106125
**851.** Heslin MJ, Lewis JJ, Woodruff JM, et al. Core needle biopsy for diagnosis of extremity soft tissue sarcoma. Ann Surg Oncol. 1997 Jul-Aug;4(5):425–31. PMID:9259971
**852.** Heymann JJ, Halligan AM, Hoda SA, et al. Fine needle aspiration of breast masses in pregnant and lactating women: experience with 28 cases emphasizing Thinprep findings. Diagn Cytopathol. 2015 Mar;43(3):188–94. PMID:24976078
**853.** Hill CB, Yeh IT. Myoepithelial cell staining patterns of papillary breast lesions: from intraductal papillomas to invasive papillary carcinomas. Am J Clin Pathol. 2005 Jan;123(1):36–44. PMID:15762278
**854.** Hilleren DJ, Andersson IT, Lindholm K, et al. Invasive lobular carcinoma: mammographic findings in a 10-year experience. Radiology. 1991 Jan;178(1):149–54. PMID:1984294
**855.** Hilson JB, Schnitt SJ, Collins LC. Phenotypic alterations in ductal carcinoma in situ-associated myoepithelial cells: biologic and diagnostic implications. Am J Surg Pathol. 2009 Feb;33(2):227–32. PMID:18936688
**856.** Hilson JB, Schnitt SJ, Collins LC. Phenotypic alterations in myoepithelial cells associated with benign sclerosing lesions of the breast. Am J Surg Pathol. 2010 Jun;34(6):896–900. PMID:20463570
**857.** Hirose T, Scheithauer BW, Sano T. Giant plexiform schwannoma: a report of two cases with soft tissue and visceral involvement. Mod Pathol. 1997 Nov;10(11):1075–81. PMID:9388056
**858.** Hisaoka M, Takamatsu Y, Hirano Y, et al. Sebaceous carcinoma of the breast: case report and review of the literature. Virchows Arch. 2006 Oct;449(4):484–8. PMID:16944238
**859.** Hittmair AP, Lininger RA, Tavassoli FA. Ductal carcinoma in situ (DCIS) in the male breast: a morphologic study of 84 cases of pure DCIS and 30 cases of DCIS associated with invasive carcinoma–a preliminary report. Cancer. 1998 Nov 15;83(10):2139–49. PMID:9827718
**860.** Ho SK, Thike AA, Cheok PY, et al. Phyllodes tumours of the breast: the role of CD34, vascular endothelial growth factor and β-catenin in histological grading and clinical outcome. Histopathology. 2013 Sep;63(3):393–406. PMID:23772632
**861.** Hobert JA, Eng C. PTEN hamartoma tumor syndrome: an overview. Genet Med. 2009 Oct;11(10):687–94. PMID:19668082
**862.** Hock AK, Vousden KH. Tumor suppression by p53: fall of the triumvirate? Cell. 2012 Jun 8;149(6):1183–5. PMID:22682240
**863.** Hock YL, Mohamid W. Myxoid neurofibroma of the male breast: fine needle aspiration cytodiagnosis. Cytopathology. 1995 Feb;6(1):44–7. PMID:7734701
**864.** Hoda SA, Brogi E, Koerner FC, et al., editors. Rosen's breast pathology. 4th ed. Philadelphia (PA): Lippincott Williams & Wilkins; 2014.
**865.** Hodges KB, Abdul-Karim FW, Wang M, et al. Evidence for transformation of fibroadenoma of the breast to malignant phyllodes tumor. Appl Immunohistochem Mol Morphol. 2009 Jul;17(4):345–50. PMID:19276971
**866.** Hofvander J, Arbajian E, Stenkula KG, et al. Frequent low-level mutations of protein kinase D2 in angiolipoma. J Pathol. 2017 Apr;241(5):578–82. PMID:28139834
**867.** Holm-Rasmussen EV, Jensen MB, Balslev E, et al. The use of sentinel lymph node biopsy in the treatment of breast ductal carcinoma in situ: a Danish population-based study. Eur J Cancer. 2017 Dec;87:1–9. PMID:29096155
**868.** Hoogerbrugge N, Jongmans MC. Finding all BRCA pathogenic mutation carriers: best practice models. Eur J Hum Genet. 2016 Sep;24 Suppl 1:S19–26. PMID:27514840
**869.** Hopper JL, Dite GS, MacInnis RJ, et al. Age-specific breast cancer risk by body mass index and familial risk: prospective family study cohort (ProF-SC). Breast Cancer Res. 2018 Nov 3;20(1):132. PMID:30390716
**870.** Horii R, Akiyama F, Ikenaga M, et al. Muco-epidermoid carcinoma of the breast. Pathol Int. 2006 Sep;56(9):549–53. PMID:16930336
**871.** Horlings HM, Weigelt B, Anderson EM, et al. Genomic profiling of histological special types of breast cancer. Breast Cancer Res Treat. 2013 Nov;142(2):257–69. PMID:24162157
**872.** Horne CH, Reid IN, Milne GD. Prognostic significance of inappropriate production of pregnancy proteins by breast cancers. Lancet. 1976 Aug 7;2(7980):279–82. PMID:59853
**873.** Hornick JL, Bosenberg MW, Mentzel T, et al. Pleomorphic liposarcoma: clinicopathologic analysis of 57 cases. Am J Surg Pathol. 2004 Oct;28(10):1257–67. PMID:15371941
**874.** Hornick JL, Fletcher CD. Immunohistochemical staining for KIT (CD117) in soft tissue sarcomas is very limited in distribution. Am J Clin Pathol. 2002 Feb;117(2):188–93. PMID:11865845
**875.** Hornick JL, Sholl LM, Dal Cin P, et al. Expression of ROS1 predicts ROS1 gene rearrangement in inflammatory myofibroblastic tumors. Mod Pathol. 2015 May;28(5):732–9. PMID:25612511
**876.** Horowitz DP, Sharma CS, Connolly E, et al. Secretory carcinoma of the breast: results from the Survival, Epidemiology and End Results database. Breast. 2012 Jun;21(3):350–3. PMID:22494666
**877.** Hosein PJ, Maragulia JC, Salzberg MP, et al. A multicentre study of primary breast diffuse large B-cell lymphoma in the rituximab era. Br J Haematol. 2014 May;165(3):358–63. PMID:24467658
**878.** Hou Y, Chaudhary S, Gao FF, et al. Surgical follow-up results for apocrine adenosis and atypical apocrine adenosis diagnosed on breast core biopsy. Ann Diagn Pathol. 2016 Oct;24:4–6. PMID:27649945
**879.** Hou Y, Shen R, Chaudhary S, et al. Utility of different immunostains for diagnosis of metastatic breast carcinomas in both surgical and cytological specimens. Ann Diagn Pathol. 2017 Oct;30:21–7. PMID:28965624
**880.** Hou Y, Zynger DL, Li X, et al. Comparison of Oncotype DX with modified Magee equation recurrence scores in low-grade invasive carcinoma of breast. Am J Clin Pathol. 2017 Aug 1;148(2):167–72. PMID:28898988
**881.** Houssami N, Macaskill P, Marinovich ML, et al. The association of surgical margins and local recurrence in women with early-stage invasive breast cancer treated with breast-conserving therapy: a meta-analysis. Ann Surg Oncol. 2014 Mar;21(3):717–30. PMID:24473640
**882.** Howat AJ, Campbell PE. Angiomatosis: a vascular malformation of infancy and childhood. Report of 17 cases. Pathology. 1987 Oct;19(4):377–82. PMID:3444663
**883.** Hoyer J, Vasileiou G, Uebe S, et al. Addition of triple negativity of breast cancer as an indicator for germline mutations in predisposing genes increases sensitivity of clinical selection criteria. BMC Cancer. 2018 Sep 26;18(1):926. PMID:30257646
**884.** Hu H, Johani K, Almatroudi A, et al. Bacterial biofilm infection detected in breast implant-associated anaplastic large-cell lymphoma. Plast Reconstr Surg. 2016 Jun;137(6):1659–69. PMID:26890506
**885.** Hu S, Song Y, Sun X, et al. Primary breast diffuse large B-cell lymphoma in the rituximab era: therapeutic strategies and patterns of failure. Cancer Sci. 2018 Dec;109(12):3943–52. PMID:30302857
**886.** Huang HC, Hang JF, Wu MH, et al. Lung adenocarcinoma with ipsilateral breast metastasis: a simple coincidence? J Thorac Oncol. 2013 Jul;8(7):974–9. PMID:23774384
**887.** Huang K, Fu H, Shi YQ, et al. Prognostic factors for extra-abdominal and abdominal wall desmoids: a 20-year experience at a single institution. J Surg Oncol. 2009 Dec 1;100(7):563–9. PMID:19722232
**888.** Huang SC, Zhang L, Sung YS, et al. Recurrent CIC gene abnormalities in angiosarcomas: a molecular study of 120 cases with concurrent investigation of PLCG1, KDR, MYC, and FLT4 gene alterations. Am J Surg Pathol. 2016 May;40(5):645–55. PMID:26735859
**889.** Huang Y, Zhang H, Zhou Q, et al. Giant tubular adenoma of the accessory breast in the anterior chest wall occurred in a pregnant woman. Diagn Pathol. 2015 Jun 4;10:60. PMID:26040320
**890.** Hugh J, Hanson J, Cheang MC, et al. Breast cancer subtypes and response to docetaxel in node-positive breast cancer: use of an immunohistochemical definition in the BCIRG 001 trial. J Clin Oncol. 2009 Mar 10;27(8):1168–76. PMID:19204205
**891.** Hugh JC, Jackson FI, Hanson J, et al. Primary breast lymphoma. An immunohistologic study of 20 new cases. Cancer. 1990 Dec 15;66(12):2602–11. PMID:2249200
**891A.** Hui Y, Wang Y, Nam G, et al. Differentiating breast carcinoma with signet ring features from gastrointestinal signet ring carcinoma: assessment of immunohistochemical markers. Hum Pathol. 2018 Jul;77:11–9. PMID:29317235
**892.** Huijts PE, Hollestelle A, Balliu B, et al. CHEK2*1100delC homozygosity in the Netherlands–prevalence and risk of breast and lung cancer. Eur J Hum Genet. 2014 Jan;22(1):46–51. PMID:23652375
**893.** Hulsebos TJ, Plomp AS, Wolterman RA, et al. Germline mutation of INI1/SMARCB1 in familial schwannomatosis. Am J Hum Genet. 2007 Apr;80(4):805–10. PMID:17357086
**894.** Hultborn R, Hanson C, Köpf I, et al. Prevalence of Klinefelter's syndrome in male breast cancer patients. Anticancer Res. 1997 Nov-Dec;17(6D):4293–7. PMID:9494523
**895.** Hummel M, Bentink S, Berger H, et al. A biologic definition of Burkitt's lymphoma from transcriptional and genomic profiling. N Engl J Med. 2006 Jun 8;354(23):2419–30. PMID:16760442
**896.** Humphries MP, Jordan VC, Speirs V. Obesity and male breast cancer: provocative parallels? BMC Med. 2015 Jun 4;13:134. PMID:26044503
**897.** Humphries MP, Sundara Rajan S, Honarpisheh H, et al. Characterisation of male breast cancer: a descriptive biomarker study from a large patient series. Sci Rep. 2017 Mar 28;7:45293. PMID:28350011
**898.** Hungermann D, Buerger H, Oehlschlegel C, et al. Adenomyoepithelial tumours and myoepithelial carcinomas of the breast–a spectrum of monophasic and biphasic tumours dominated by immature myoepithelial cells. BMC Cancer. 2005 Jul 28;5:92. PMID:16050957
**899.** Hussien M, Sivananthan S, Anderson N, et al. Primary leiomyosarcoma of the breast: diagnosis, management and outcome. A report of a new case and review of literature. Breast. 2001 Dec;10(6):530–4. PMID:14965634
**900.** Hutter S, Piro RM, Reuss DE, et al. Whole exome sequencing reveals that the majority of schwannomatosis cases remain unexplained after excluding SMARCB1 and LZTR1 germline variants. Acta Neuropathol. 2014 Sep;128(3):449–52. PMID:25008767
**901.** Huynh DP, Mautner V, Baser ME, et al. Immunohistochemical detection of schwannomin and neurofibromin in vestibular schwannomas, ependymomas and meningiomas. J Neuropathol Exp Neurol. 1997 Apr;56(4):382–90. PMID:9100669
**902.** Huzarski T, Cybulski C, Domagała W, et al. Pathology of breast cancer in women

with constitutional CHEK2 mutations. Breast Cancer Res Treat. 2005 Mar;90(2):187–9. PMID:15803365
**903.** Huzarski T, Cybulski C, Wokolorczyk D, et al. Survival from breast cancer in patients with CHEK2 mutations. Breast Cancer Res Treat. 2014 Apr;144(2):397–403. PMID:24557336
**904.** Hwang ES, DeVries S, Chew KL, et al. Patterns of chromosomal alterations in breast ductal carcinoma in situ. Clin Cancer Res. 2004 Aug 1;10(15):5160–7. PMID:15297420
**905.** Hwang ES, Nyante SJ, Yi Chen Y, et al. Clonality of lobular carcinoma in situ and synchronous invasive lobular carcinoma. Cancer. 2004 Jun 15;100(12):2562–72. PMID:15197797
**906.** Hwang H, Barke LD, Mendelson EB, et al. Atypical lobular hyperplasia and classic lobular carcinoma in situ in core biopsy specimens: routine excision is not necessary. Mod Pathol. 2008 Oct;21(10):1208–16. PMID:18660792
**907.** IARC TP53 Database [Internet]. Lyon (France): International Agency for Research on Cancer; 2018. Version R19, August 2018. Available from: http://p53.iarc.fr/.
**908.** IARC Working Group on the Evaluation of Carcinogenic Risks to Humans. Pharmaceuticals. Volume 100 A. A review of human carcinogens. IARC Monogr Eval Carcinog Risks Hum. 2012;100(Pt A):1–401. PMID:23189749
**909.** Iaria G, Pisani F, De Luca L, et al. Prospective study of switch from cyclosporine to tacrolimus for fibroadenomas of the breast in kidney transplantation. Transplant Proc. 2010 May;42(4):1169–70. PMID:20534252
**910.** Ibrahim AE, Bateman AC, Theaker JM, et al. The role and histological classification of needle core biopsy in comparison with fine needle aspiration cytology in the preoperative assessment of impalpable breast lesions. J Clin Pathol. 2001 Feb;54(2):121–5. PMID:11215280
**911.** Ibrahim N, Bessissow A, Lalonde L, et al. Surgical outcome of biopsy-proven lobular neoplasia: Is there any difference between lobular carcinoma in situ and atypical lobular hyperplasia? AJR Am J Roentgenol. 2012 Feb;198(2):288–91. PMID:22268170
**912.** Ichihara S, Fujimoto T, Hashimoto K, et al. Double immunostaining with p63 and high-molecular-weight cytokeratins distinguishes borderline papillary lesions of the breast. Pathol Int. 2007 Mar;57(3):126–32. PMID:17295644
**913.** Ichinokawa Y, Ohtuki A, Hattori M, et al. A case of syringomatous adenoma of the nipple. Case Rep Dermatol. 2012 Jan;4(1):98–103. PMID:22649338
**914.** Ihrler S, Guntinas-Lichius O, Agaimy A, et al. Histological, immunohistological and molecular characteristics of intraductal precursor of carcinoma ex pleomorphic adenoma support a multistep carcinogenic process. Virchows Arch. 2017 Jun;470(6):601–9. PMID:28353089
**916.** Ilkay TM, Gozde K, Ozgur S, et al. Diagnosis of adenoid cystic carcinoma of the breast using fine-needle aspiration cytology: a case report and review of the literature. Diagn Cytopathol. 2015 Sep;43(9):722–6. PMID:26183224
**917.** Imamovic D, Bilalovic N, Skenderi F, et al. A clinicopathologic study of invasive apocrine carcinoma of the breast: a single-center experience. Breast J. 2018 Nov;24(6):1105–8. PMID:30240079
**918.** Inno A, Bogina G, Turazza M, et al. Neuroendocrine carcinoma of the breast: current evidence and future perspectives. Oncologist. 2016 Jan;21(1):28–32. PMID:26659223
**919.** Inoue M, Nakagomi H, Nakada H, et al. Specific sites of metastases in invasive lobular carcinoma: a retrospective cohort study of metastatic breast cancer. Breast Cancer. 2017 Sep;24(5):667–72. PMID:28108967
**920.** Institute of Medicine (US) Committee on the Safety of Silicone Breast Implants; Bondurant S, Ernster V, Herdman R, editors. Safety of silicone breast implants. Washington, DC: National Academies Press (US); 1999. PMID:20669503
**921.** International Association of Cancer Registries (IACR) [Internet]. Lyon (France): International Agency for Research on Cancer; 2019. ICD-O-3.2; updated 2019 Apr 23. Available from: http://www.iacr.com.fr/index.php?option=com_content&view=article&id=149:icd-o-3-2&catid=80&Itemid=545
**922.** International Immuno-Oncology Biomarker Working Group on Breast Cancer [Internet]. 2018. Available from: https://www.tilsinbreastcancer.org/.
**923.** Inyang A, Thomas DG, Jorns J. Heterologous liposarcomatous differentiation in malignant phyllodes tumor is histologically similar but immunohistochemically and molecularly distinct from well-differentiated liposarcoma of soft tissue. Breast J. 2016 May;22(3):282–6. PMID:26843318
**924.** Iorfida M, Maiorano E, Orvieto E, et al. Invasive lobular breast cancer: subtypes and outcome. Breast Cancer Res Treat. 2012 Jun;133(2):713–23. PMID:22399188
**925.** Iqbal J, Ginsburg O, Rochon PA, et al. Differences in breast cancer stage at diagnosis and cancer-specific survival by race and ethnicity in the United States. JAMA. 2015 Jan 13;313(2):165–73. PMID:25585328
**926.** Itagaki H, Yamamoto T, Hiroi A, et al. Synchronous and bilateral oncocytic carcinoma of the breast: a case report and review of the literature. Oncol Lett. 2017 Mar;13(3):1714–8. PMID:28454314
**927.** Jabi M, Dardick I, Cardigos N. Adenomyoepithelioma of the breast. Arch Pathol Lab Med. 1988 Jan;112(1):73–6. PMID:2447854
**928.** Jacobs PA, Maloney V, Cooke R, et al. Male breast cancer, age and sex chromosome aneuploidy. Br J Cancer. 2013 Mar 5;108(4):959–63. PMID:23299533
**929.** Jacoby LB, MacCollin M, Barone R, et al. Frequency and distribution of NF2 mutations in schwannomas. Genes Chromosomes Cancer. 1996 Sep;17(1):45–55. PMID:8889506
**930.** Jahn SW, Kashofer K, Thüringer A, et al. Mutation profiling of usual ductal hyperplasia of the breast reveals activating mutations predominantly at different levels of the PI3K/AKT/mTOR pathway. Am J Pathol. 2016 Jan;186(1):15–23. PMID:26718977
**931.** Jain RK, Mehta R, Dimitrov R, et al. Atypical ductal hyperplasia: interobserver and intraobserver variability. Mod Pathol. 2011 Jul;24(7):917–23. PMID:21532546
**932.** Jain S, Fisher C, Smith P, et al. Patterns of metastatic breast cancer in relation to histological type. Eur J Cancer. 1993;29A(15):2155–7. PMID:8297656
**933.** Janatova M, Kleibl Z, Stribrna J, et al. The PALB2 gene is a strong candidate for clinical testing in BRCA1- and BRCA2-negative hereditary breast cancer. Cancer Epidemiol Biomarkers Prev. 2013 Dec;22(12):2323–32. PMID:24136930
**934.** Jansen M, de Leng WW, Baas AF, et al. Mucosal prolapse in the pathogenesis of Peutz-Jeghers polyposis. Gut. 2006 Jan;55(1):1–5. PMID:16344569
**935.** Jassar A, Pathania K. Tubular variant of mammary adenomyoepithelioma: diagnostic challenges and cytomorphological correlation in two cases. Cytojournal. 2017 Dec 27;14:29. PMID:29333189
**936.** Javed A, Jenkins SM, Labow B, et al. Intermediate and long-term outcomes of fibroadenoma excision in adolescent and young adult patients. Breast J. 2019 Jan;25(1):91–5. PMID:30444280
**937.** Javid SH, Smith BL, Mayer E, et al. Tubular carcinoma of the breast: results of a large contemporary series. Am J Surg. 2009 May;197(5):674–7. PMID:18789411
**938.** Jayaram G, Jayalakshmi P, Yip CH. Leiomyosarcoma of the breast: report of a case with fine needle aspiration cytologic, histologic and immunohistochemical features. Acta Cytol. 2005 Nov-Dec;49(6):656–60. PMID:16450908
**939.** Jayaram G, Swain M, Chew MT, et al. Cytology of mucinous carcinoma of breast: a report of 28 cases with histological correlation. Malays J Pathol. 2000 Dec;22(2):65–71. PMID:16329537
**940.** Jensen KC, Kong CS. Cytologic diagnosis of columnar-cell lesions of the breast. Diagn Cytopathol. 2007 Feb;35(2):73–9. PMID:17230565
**941.** Jensen ML, Johansen P, Noer H, et al. Ductal adenoma of the breast: the cytological features of six cases. Diagn Cytopathol. 1994;10(2):143–5. PMID:8187593
**942.** Jernström H, Lubinski J, Lynch HT, et al. Breast-feeding and the risk of breast cancer in BRCA1 and BRCA2 mutation carriers. J Natl Cancer Inst. 2004 Jul 21;96(14):1094–8. PMID:15265971
**943.** Jeruss JS, Mittendorf EA, Tucker SL, et al. Staging of breast cancer in the neoadjuvant setting. Cancer Res. 2008 Aug 15;68(16):6477–81. PMID:18701468
**944.** Jesinger RA, Lattin GE Jr, Ballard EA, et al. Vascular abnormalities of the breast: arterial and venous disorders, vascular masses, and mimic lesions with radiologic-pathologic correlation. Radiographics. 2011 Nov-Dec;31(7):E117–36. PMID:22084191
**945.** Jeyaretna DS, Oriolowo A, Smith ME, et al. Solitary neurofibroma in the male breast. World J Surg Oncol. 2007 Feb 27;5:23. PMID:17324294
**946.** Jia Y, Sun C, Liu Z, et al. Primary breast diffuse large B-cell lymphoma: a population-based study from 1975 to 2014. Oncotarget. 2017 Dec 8;9(3):3956–67. PMID:29423097
**947.** Jiao YF, Nakamura S, Oikawa T, et al. Sebaceous gland metaplasia in intraductal papilloma of the breast. Virchows Arch. 2001 May;438(5):505–8. PMID:11407480
**948.** Jo VY, Fletcher CDM. SMARCB1/INI1 loss in epithelioid schwannoma: a clinicopathologic and immunohistochemical study of 65 cases. Am J Surg Pathol. 2017 Aug;41(8):1013–22. PMID:28368924
**949.** João C, Farinha P, da Silva MG, et al. Cytogenetic abnormalities in MALT lymphomas and their precursor lesions from different organs. A fluorescence in situ hybridization (FISH) study. Histopathology. 2007 Jan;50(2):217–24. PMID:17222250
**950.** Johansson I, Nilsson C, Berglund P, et al. Gene expression profiling of primary male breast cancers reveals two unique subgroups and identifies N-acetyltransferase-1 (NAT1) as a novel prognostic biomarker. Breast Cancer Res. 2012 Feb 14;14(1):R31. PMID:22333393
**951.** Johansson I, Ringnér M, Hedenfalk I. The landscape of candidate driver genes differs between male and female breast cancer. PLoS One. 2013 Oct 23;8(10):e78299. PMID:24194916
**952.** John BJ, Griffiths C, Ebbs SR. Pleomorphic adenoma of the breast should be excised with a cuff of normal tissue. Breast J. 2007 Jul-Aug;13(4):418–20. PMID:17593049
**953.** Johnson JB, Emory TH. Intracystic papillary carcinoma in a man with gynecomastia. Radiol Case Rep. 2015 Dec 7;3(4):214. PMID:27303554
**954.** Johnston WT, Mutalima N, Sun D, et al. Relationship between Plasmodium falciparum malaria prevalence, genetic diversity and endemic Burkitt lymphoma in Malawi. Sci Rep. 2014 Jan 17;4:3741. PMID:24434689
**955.** Jones AM, Mitter R, Springall R, et al. A comprehensive genetic profile of phyllodes tumours of the breast detects important mutations, intra-tumoral genetic heterogeneity and new genetic changes on recurrence. J Pathol. 2008 Apr;214(5):533–44. PMID:18288784
**956.** Jones C, Damiani S, Wells D, et al. Molecular cytogenetic comparison of apocrine hyperplasia and apocrine carcinoma of the breast. Am J Pathol. 2001 Jan;158(1):207–14. PMID:11141494
**957.** Jones C, Merrett S, Thomas VA, et al. Comparative genomic hybridization analysis of bilateral hyperplasia of usual type of the breast. J Pathol. 2003 Feb;199(2):152–6. PMID:12533827
**958.** Jones EL. Primary squamous-cell carcinoma of breast with pseudosarcomatous stroma. J Pathol. 1969 Feb;97(2):383–5. PMID:5352811
**959.** Jones MW, Norris HJ, Snyder RC. Infiltrating syringomatous adenoma of the nipple. A clinical and pathological study of 11 cases. Am J Surg Pathol. 1989 Mar;13(3):197–201. PMID:2919717
**960.** Jones MW, Norris HJ, Wargotz ES. Hamartomas of the breast. Surg Gynecol Obstet. 1991 Jul;173(1):54–6. PMID:1866672
**961.** Jones MW, Tavassoli FA. Coexistence of nipple duct adenoma and breast carcinoma: a clinicopathologic study of five cases and review of the literature. Mod Pathol. 1995 Aug;8(6):633–6. PMID:8532696
**962.** Jones S, Hruban RH, Kamiyama M, et al. Exomic sequencing identifies PALB2 as a pancreatic cancer susceptibility gene. Science. 2009 Apr 10;324(5924):217. PMID:19264984
**963.** Joshi D, Singh P, Zonunfawni Y, et al. Metaplastic carcinoma of the breast: cytological diagnosis and diagnostic pitfalls. Acta Cytol. 2011;55(4):313–8. PMID:21791899
**964.** Jozefczyk MA, Rosen PP. Vascular tumors of the breast. II. Perilobular hemangiomas and hemangiomas. Am J Surg Pathol. 1985 Jul;9(7):491–503. PMID:4091183
**965.** Jung SY, Kim HY, Nam BH, et al. Worse prognosis of metaplastic breast cancer patients than other patients with triple-negative breast cancer. Breast Cancer Res Treat. 2010 Apr;120(3):627–37. PMID:20143153
**966.** Kabat GC, Jones JG, Olson N, et al. A multi-center prospective cohort study of benign breast disease and risk of subsequent breast cancer. Cancer Causes Control. 2010 Jun;21(6):821–8. PMID:20084540
**967.** Kader HA, Jackson J, Mates D, et al. Tubular carcinoma of the breast: a population-based study of nodal metastases at presentation and of patterns of relapse. Breast J. 2001 Jan-Feb;7(1):8–13. PMID:11348409
**968.** Kadin ME, Deva A, Xu H, et al. Biomarkers provide clues to early events in the pathogenesis of breast implant-associated anaplastic large cell lymphoma. Aesthet Surg J. 2016 Jul;36(7):773–81. PMID:26979456
**969.** Kadin ME, Morgan J, Xu H, et al. IL-13 is produced by tumor cells in breast implant-associated anaplastic large cell lymphoma: implications for pathogenesis. Hum Pathol. 2018 Aug;78:54–62. PMID:29689246
**970.** Kalambo M, Adrada BE, Adeyefa MM, et al. Phyllodes tumor of the breast: ultrasound-pathology correlation. AJR Am J Roentgenol.

2018 Apr;210(4):W173–9. PMID:29412020
**971.** Kambouchner M, Godmer P, Guillevin L, et al. Low grade marginal zone B cell lymphoma of the breast associated with localised amyloidosis and corpora amylacea in a woman with long standing primary Sjögren's syndrome. J Clin Pathol. 2003 Jan;56(1):74–7. PMID:12499440
**972.** Kamihara J, Rana HQ, Garber JE. Germline TP53 mutations and the changing landscape of Li-Fraumeni syndrome. Hum Mutat. 2014 Jun;35(6):654–62. PMID:24706533
**973.** Kamitani T, Matsuo Y, Yabuuchi H, et al. Differentiation between benign phyllodes tumors and fibroadenomas of the breast on MR imaging. Eur J Radiol. 2014 Aug;83(8):1344–9. PMID:24856515
**974.** Kang A, Kumar JB, Thomas A, et al. A spontaneously resolving breast lesion: imaging and cytological findings of nodular fasciitis of the breast with FISH showing USP6 gene rearrangement. BMJ Case Rep. 2015 Dec 23;2015. PMID:26698206
**975.** Kang H, Tan M, Bishop JA, et al. Whole-exome sequencing of salivary gland mucoepidermoid carcinoma. Clin Cancer Res. 2017 Jan 1;23(1):283–8. PMID:27340278
**976.** Kanhai RC, Hage JJ, van Diest PJ, et al. Short-term and long-term histologic effects of castration and estrogen treatment on breast tissue of 14 male-to-female transsexuals in comparison with two chemically castrated men. Am J Surg Pathol. 2000 Jan;24(1):74–80. PMID:10632490
**977.** Kanojia D, Nagata Y, Garg M, et al. Genomic landscape of liposarcoma. Oncotarget. 2015 Dec 15;6(40):42429–44. PMID:26643872
**978.** Karabakhtsian RG, Johnson R, Sumkin J, et al. The clinical significance of lobular neoplasia on breast core biopsy. Am J Surg Pathol. 2007 May;31(5):717–23. PMID:17460455
**979.** Karamchandani JR, Nielsen TO, van de Rijn M, et al. Sox10 and S100 in the diagnosis of soft-tissue neoplasms. Appl Immunohistochem Mol Morphol. 2012 Oct;20(5):445–50. PMID:22495377
**980.** Karim RZ, O'Toole SA, Scolyer RA, et al. Recent insights into the molecular pathogenesis of mammary phyllodes tumours. J Clin Pathol. 2013 Jun;66(6):496–505. PMID:23404800
**981.** Kas K, Voz ML, Röijer E, et al. Promoter swapping between the genes for a novel zinc finger protein and beta-catenin in pleiomorphic adenomas with t(3;8)(p21;q12) translocations. Nat Genet. 1997 Feb;15(2):170–4. PMID:9020842
**982.** Kasper B, Baumgarten C, Garcia J, et al. An update on the management of sporadic desmoid-type fibromatosis: a European Consensus Initiative between Sarcoma PAtients EuroNet (SPAEN) and European Organization for Research and Treatment of Cancer (EORTC)/Soft Tissue and Bone Sarcoma Group (STBSG). Ann Oncol. 2017 Oct 1;28(10):2399–408. PMID:28961825
**983.** Kast K, Krause M, Schuler M, et al. Late onset Li-Fraumeni syndrome with bilateral breast cancer and other malignancies: case report and review of the literature. BMC Cancer. 2012 Jun 6;12:217. PMID:22672556
**984.** Kawaguchi K, Shin SJ. Immunohistochemical staining characteristics of low-grade adenosquamous carcinoma of the breast. Am J Surg Pathol. 2012 Jul;36(7):1009–20. PMID:22446941
**985.** Kawase K, Dimaio DJ, Tucker SL, et al. Paget's disease of the breast: there is a role for breast-conserving therapy. Ann Surg Oncol. 2005 May;12(5):391–7. PMID:15915373
**986.** Kazakov DV, Bisceglia M, Mukensnabl P, et al. Pseudoangiomatous stromal hyperplasia in lesions involving anogenital mammary-like glands. Am J Surg Pathol. 2005 Sep;29(9):1243–6. PMID:16096415
**987.** Kebudi R, Koc DC, Gorgun O, et al. Breast metastases in children and adolescents with rhabdomyosarcoma: a large single-institution experience and literature review. J Pediatr Hematol Oncol. 2017 Jan;39(1):67–71. PMID:27820124
**988.** Kehr EL, Jorns JM, Ang D, et al. Mucinous breast carcinomas lack PIK3CA and AKT1 mutations. Hum Pathol. 2012 Dec;43(12):2207–12. PMID:22705004
**989.** Kelly GL, Stylianou J, Rasaiyaah J, et al. Different patterns of Epstein-Barr virus latency in endemic Burkitt lymphoma (BL) lead to distinct variants within the BL-associated gene expression signature. J Virol. 2013 Mar;87(5):2882–94. PMID:23269792
**990.** Kelten Talu C, Leblebici C, Kilicaslan Ozturk T, et al. Primary breast carcinomas with neuroendocrine features: clinicopathological features and analysis of tumor growth patterns in 36 cases. Ann Diagn Pathol. 2018 Jun;34:122–30. PMID:29661717
**991.** Kensler KH, Regan MM, Heng YJ, et al. Prognostic and predictive value of androgen receptor expression in postmenopausal women with estrogen receptor-positive breast cancer: results from the Breast International Group Trial 1-98. Breast Cancer Res. 2019 Feb 22;21(1):30. PMID:30795773
**992.** Kerlikowske K. Epidemiology of ductal carcinoma in situ. J Natl Cancer Inst Monogr. 2010;2010(41):139–41. PMID:20956818
**993.** Kerlikowske K, Barclay J, Grady D, et al. Comparison of risk factors for ductal carcinoma in situ and invasive breast cancer. J Natl Cancer Inst. 1997 Jan 1;89(1):76–82. PMID:8978410
**994.** Keung EZ, Chiang YJ, Voss RK, et al. Defining the incidence and clinical significance of lymph node metastasis in soft tissue sarcoma. Eur J Surg Oncol. 2018 Jan;44(1):170–7. PMID:29208319
**995.** Khalifeh IM, Albarracin C, Diaz LK, et al. Clinical, histopathologic, and immunohistochemical features of microglandular adenosis and transition into in situ and invasive carcinoma. Am J Surg Pathol. 2008 Apr;32(4):544–52. PMID:18300793
**996.** Khan HN, Rampaul R, Blamey RW. Management of physiological gynaecomastia with tamoxifen. Breast. 2004 Feb;13(1):61–5. PMID:14759718
**997.** Khanafshar E, Phillipson J, Schammel DP, et al. Inflammatory myofibroblastic tumor of the breast. Ann Diagn Pathol. 2005 Jun;9(3):123–9. PMID:15944952
**998.** Khanna KK, Chenevix-Trench G. ATM and genome maintenance: defining its role in breast cancer susceptibility. J Mammary Gland Biol Neoplasia. 2004 Jul;9(3):247–62. PMID:15557798
**999.** Kheder ES, Hong DS. Emerging targeted therapy for tumors with NTRK fusion proteins. Clin Cancer Res. 2018 Dec 1;24(23):5807–14. PMID:29986850
**1000.** Khoury T, Chen X, Wang D, et al. Nomogram to predict the likelihood of upgrade of atypical ductal hyperplasia diagnosed on a core needle biopsy in mammographically detected lesions. Histopathology. 2015 Jul;67(1):106–20. PMID:25529860
**1001.** Khoury T, Karabakhtsian RG, Mattson D, et al. Pleomorphic lobular carcinoma in situ of the breast: clinicopathological review of 47 cases. Histopathology. 2014 Jun;64(7):981–93. PMID:24372322
**1002.** Khoury T, Kumar PR, Li Z, et al. Lobular neoplasia detected in MRI-guided core biopsy carries a high risk for upgrade: a study of 63 cases from four different institutions. Mod Pathol. 2016 Jan;29(1):25–33. PMID:26564004
**1003.** Khoury T, Li Z, Sanati S, et al. The risk of upgrade for atypical ductal hyperplasia detected on magnetic resonance imaging-guided biopsy: a study of 100 cases from four academic institutions. Histopathology. 2016 Apr;68(5):713–21. PMID:26291517
**1004.** Khurana KK, Wilbur D, Dawson AE. Fine needle aspiration cytology of invasive micropapillary carcinoma of the breast. A report of two cases. Acta Cytol. 1997 Jul-Aug;41(4) Suppl:1394–8. PMID:9990283
**1005.** Kiaer H, Nielsen B, Paulsen S, et al. Adenomyoepithelial adenosis and low-grade malignant adenomyoepithelioma of the breast. Virchows Arch A Pathol Anat Histopathol. 1984;405(1):55–67. PMID:6438900
**1006.** Kiesewetter B, Lukas J, Dolak W, et al. Gender aspects in extranodal marginal zone B-cell lymphoma of the mucosa-associated lymphoid tissue: Does sex matter? Oncology. 2016;91(5):243–50. PMID:27548082
**1007.** Kilpivaara O, Vahteristo P, Falck J, et al. CHEK2 variant I157T may be associated with increased breast cancer risk. Int J Cancer. 2004 Sep 10;111(4):543–7. PMID:15239132
**1007A.** Kim A, Heo SH, Kim YA, et al. An examination of the local cellular immune response to examples of both ductal carcinoma in situ (DCIS) of the breast and DCIS with microinvasion, with emphasis on tertiary lymphoid structures and tumor infiltrating lymphoctytes. Am J Clin Pathol. 2016 Jul;146(1):137–44. PMID:27402610
**1008.** Kim DJ, Sun WY, Ryu DH, et al. Microglandular adenosis. J Breast Cancer. 2011 Mar;14(1):72–5. PMID:21847399
**1009.** Kim HM, Park BW, Han SH, et al. Infiltrating syringomatous adenoma presenting as microcalcification in the nipple on screening mammogram: case report and review of the literature of radiologic features. Clin Imaging. 2010 Nov-Dec;34(6):462–5. PMID:21092877
**1010.** Kim J, Geyer FC, Martelotto LG, et al. MYBL1 rearrangements and MYB amplification in breast adenoid cystic carcinomas lacking the MYB-NFIB fusion gene. J Pathol. 2018 Feb;244(2):143–50. PMID:29149504
**1011.** Kim JY, Moon HG, Kang YJ, et al. The effect of reproductive factors on breast cancer presentation in women who are BRCA mutation carrier. J Breast Cancer. 2017 Sep;20(3):279–85. PMID:28970854
**1012.** Kim M, Kim HJ, Chung YR, et al. Microinvasive carcinoma versus ductal carcinoma in situ: a comparison of clinicopathological features and clinical outcomes. J Breast Cancer. 2018 Jun;21(2):197–205. PMID:29963116
**1013.** Kim MJ, Gong G, Joo HJ, et al. Immunohistochemical and clinicopathologic characteristics of invasive ductal carcinoma of breast with micropapillary carcinoma component. Arch Pathol Lab Med. 2005 Oct;129(10):1277–82. PMID:16196516
**1014.** Kim S, Kim JY, Kim DH, et al. Analysis of phyllodes tumor recurrence according to the histologic grade. Breast Cancer Res Treat. 2013 Oct;141(3):353–63. PMID:24062207
**1015.** Kim S, Moon BI, Lim W, et al. Expression patterns of GATA3 and the androgen receptor are strongly correlated in patients with triple-negative breast cancer. Hum Pathol. 2016 Sep;55:190–5. PMID:27184484
**1016.** Kim SE, Koo JS, Jung WH. Immunophenotypes of glycogen rich clear cell carcinoma. Yonsei Med J. 2012 Nov 1;53(6):1142–6. PMID:23074114
**1017.** Kim SE, Park JH, Hong S, et al. Primary mucinous cystadenocarcinoma of the breast: cytologic finding and expression of MUC5 are different from mucinous carcinoma. Korean J Pathol. 2012 Dec;46(6):611–6. PMID:23323116
**1018.** Kim SM, Kim HH, Shin HJ, et al. Cavernous haemangioma of the breast. Br J Radiol. 2006 Nov;79(947):e177–80. PMID:17065282
**1019.** Kindblom LG, Meis-Kindblom JM, Havel G, et al. Benign epithelioid schwannoma. Am J Surg Pathol. 1998 Jun;22(6):762–70. PMID:9630185
**1020.** King MC, Levy-Lahad E, Lahad A. Population-based screening for BRCA1 and BRCA2: 2014 Lasker Award. JAMA. 2014 Sep 17;312(11):1091–2. PMID:25198398
**1021.** King TA, Pilewskie M, Muhsen S, et al. Lobular carcinoma in situ: a 29-year longitudinal experience evaluating clinicopathologic features and breast cancer risk. J Clin Oncol. 2015 Nov 20;33(33):3945–52. PMID:26371145
**1022.** Kirova YM, Vilcoq JR, Asselain B, et al. Radiation-induced sarcomas after radiotherapy for breast carcinoma: a large-scale single-institution review. Cancer. 2005 Aug 15;104(4):856–63. PMID:15981282
**1023.** Kirschner LS, Carney JA, Pack SD, et al. Mutations of the gene encoding the protein kinase A type I-alpha regulatory subunit in patients with the Carney complex. Nat Genet. 2000 Sep;26(1):89–92. PMID:10973256
**1024.** Kirshenbaum G, Rhone DP. Solitary extramedullary plasmacytoma of the breast with serum monoclonal protein: a case report and review of the literature. Am J Clin Pathol. 1985 Feb;83(2):230–2. PMID:3918437
**1025.** Kizy S, Huang JL, Marmor S, et al. Impact of the 21-gene recurrence score on outcome in patients with invasive lobular carcinoma of the breast. Breast Cancer Res Treat. 2017 Oct;165(3):757–63. PMID:28647915
**1026.** Klein ME, Dabbs DJ, Shuai Y, et al. Prediction of the Oncotype DX recurrence score: use of pathology-generated equations derived by linear regression analysis. Mod Pathol. 2013 May;26(5):658–64. PMID:23503643
**1027.** Knezevich SR, Garnett MJ, Pysher TJ, et al. ETV6-NTRK3 gene fusions and trisomy 11 establish a histogenetic link between mesoblastic nephroma and congenital fibrosarcoma. Cancer Res. 1998 Nov 15;58(22):5046–8. PMID:9823307
**1028.** Knezevich SR, McFadden DE, Tao W, et al. A novel ETV6-NTRK3 gene fusion in congenital fibrosarcoma. Nat Genet. 1998 Feb;18(2):184–7. PMID:9462753
**1029.** Knijnenburg TA, Wang L, Zimmermann MT, et al. Genomic and molecular landscape of DNA damage repair deficiency across The Cancer Genome Atlas. Cell Rep. 2018 Apr 3;23(1):239–254.e6. PMID:29617664
**1030.** Knoop AS, Lænkholm AV, Jensen MB, et al. Estrogen receptor, progesterone receptor, HER2 status and Ki67 index and responsiveness to adjuvant tamoxifen in postmenopausal high-risk breast cancer patients enrolled in the DBCG 77C trial. Eur J Cancer. 2014 May;50(8):1412–21. PMID:24675287
**1031.** Kocjan G, Bourgain C, Fassina A, et al. The role of breast FNAC in diagnosis and clinical management: a survey of current practice. Cytopathology. 2008 Oct;19(5):271–8. PMID:18821945
**1032.** Koçyiğit C, Sarıtaş S, Çatlı G, et al. A novel mutation in human androgen receptor gene causing partial androgen insensitivity syndrome in a patient presenting with gynecomastia at puberty. J Clin Res Pediatr Endocrinol. 2016 Jun 5;8(2):232–5. PMID:27087292
**1033.** Koehl RH, Snyder RE, Hutter RV. The use of specimen roentgenography to detect small carcinomas not found by routine pathologic examination. CA Cancer J Clin. 1971 Jan-Feb;21(1):2–10. PMID:4993751

1034. Koenig C, Tavassoli FA. Mucinous cystadenocarcinoma of the breast. Am J Surg Pathol. 1998 Jun;22(6):698–703. PMID:9630176
1034A. Koh VCY, Ng CCY, Bay BH, et al. The utility of a targeted gene mutation panel in refining the diagnosis of breast phyllodes tumours. Pathology. 2019 Aug;51(5):531–4. PMID:31272781
1035. Koh VCY, Thike AA, Nasir NDM, et al. Size and heterologous elements predict metastases in malignant phyllodes tumours of the breast. Virchows Arch. 2018 Apr;472(4):615–21. PMID:29127495
1036. Kollmorgen DR, Varanasi JS, Edge SB, et al. Paget's disease of the breast: a 33-year experience. J Am Coll Surg. 1998 Aug;187(2):171–7. PMID:9704964
1037. Komaki K, Sakamoto G, Sugano H, et al. Mucinous carcinoma of the breast in Japan. A prognostic analysis based on morphologic features. Cancer. 1988 Mar 1;61(5):989–96. PMID:2827884
1038. Kondi-Pafitis A, Kairi-Vassilatou E, Grapsa D, et al. A large benign vascular neoplasm of the male breast. A case report and review of the literature. Eur J Gynaecol Oncol. 2005;26(4):454–6. PMID:16122203
1039. Kondis-Pafitis A, Psyhogios J, Spanidou-Carvouni H, et al. Clinicopathological study of vascular tumors of the breast: a series of ten patients with a long follow-up. Eur J Gynaecol Oncol. 2004;25(3):324–6. PMID:15171310
1040. Korhonen T, Huhtala H, Holli K. A comparison of the biological and clinical features of invasive lobular and ductal carcinomas of the breast. Breast Cancer Res Treat. 2004 May;85(1):23–9. PMID:15039595
1041. Korhonen T, Kuukasjärvi T, Huhtala H, et al. The impact of lobular and ductal breast cancer histology on the metastatic behavior and long term survival of breast cancer patients. Breast. 2013 Dec;22(6):1119–24. PMID:23863867
1042. Kornegoor R, Moelans CB, Verschuur-Maes AH, et al. Oncogene amplification in male breast cancer: analysis by multiplex ligation-dependent probe amplification. Breast Cancer Res Treat. 2012 Aug;135(1):49–58. PMID:22527098
1043. Kornegoor R, Moelans CB, Verschuur-Maes AH, et al. Promoter hypermethylation in male breast cancer: analysis by multiplex ligation-dependent probe amplification. Breast Cancer Res. 2012 Jul 5;14(4):R101. PMID:22765268
1044. Kornegoor R, van Diest PJ, Buerger H, et al. Tracing differences between male and female breast cancer: both diseases own a different biology. Histopathology. 2015 Dec;67(6):888–97. PMID:25941088
1045. Kornegoor R, Verschuur-Maes AH, Buerger H, et al. Fibrotic focus and hypoxia in male breast cancer. Mod Pathol. 2012 Oct;25(10):1397–404. PMID:22684218
1046. Kornegoor R, Verschuur-Maes AH, Buerger H, et al. Immunophenotyping of male breast cancer. Histopathology. 2012 Dec;61(6):1145–55. PMID:22958056
1047. Kornegoor R, Verschuur-Maes AH, Buerger H, et al. Molecular subtyping of male breast cancer by immunohistochemistry. Mod Pathol. 2012 Mar;25(3):398–404. PMID:22056953
1048. Kornegoor R, Verschuur-Maes AH, Buerger H, et al. The 3-layered ductal epithelium in gynecomastia. Am J Surg Pathol. 2012 May;36(5):762–8. PMID:22314184
1049. Korolczuk A, Amarowicz M, Bąk K, et al. Adenomyoepithelioma of the breast with late pulmonary metastases - case report and review of the literature. J Cardiothorac Surg. 2016 Aug 4;11(1):121. PMID:27487934
1050. Kothari AS, Beechey-Newman N, Hamed H, et al. Paget disease of the nipple: a multifocal manifestation of higher-risk disease. Cancer. 2002 Jul 1;95(1):1–7. PMID:12115309
1051. Kotsopoulos J, Lubinski J, Lynch HT, et al. Oophorectomy after menopause and the risk of breast cancer in BRCA1 and BRCA2 mutation carriers. Cancer Epidemiol Biomarkers Prev. 2012 Jul;21(7):1089–96. PMID:22564871
1052. Koufopoulos N, Goudeli C, Syrios J, et al. Mucinous cystadenocarcinoma of the breast: the challenge of diagnosing a rare entity. Rare Tumors. 2017 Oct 3;9(3):7016. PMID:29081926
1053. Kovács A, Máthé G, Mattsson J, et al. ALK-positive inflammatory myofibroblastic tumor of the nipple during pregnancy-an unusual presentation of a rare disease. Breast J. 2015 May-Jun;21(3):297–302. PMID:25772857
1054. Kővári B, Báthori Á, Cserni G. CD10 immunohistochemical expression in apocrine lesions of the breast. Pathobiology. 2015;82(6):259–63. PMID:26562027
1055. Kovárová M, Kubis M. Primary tumours of the heart. Acta Univ Palacki Olomuc Fac Med. 1987;117:409–12. PMID:2977705
1056. Kraft S, Fletcher CD. Atypical intradermal smooth muscle neoplasms: clinicopathologic analysis of 84 cases and a reappraisal of cutaneous "leiomyosarcoma". Am J Surg Pathol. 2011 Apr;35(4):599–607. PMID:21358302
1057. Krammer J, Pinker-Domenig K, Robson ME, et al. Breast cancer detection and tumor characteristics in BRCA1 and BRCA2 mutation carriers. Breast Cancer Res Treat. 2017 Jun;163(3):565–71. PMID:28343309
1058. Krausz T, Jenkins D, Grontoft O, et al. Secretory carcinoma of the breast in adults: emphasis on late recurrence and metastasis. Histopathology. 1989 Jan;14(1):25–36. PMID:2925177
1059. Krecke KN, Gisvold JJ. Invasive lobular carcinoma of the breast: mammographic findings and extent of disease at diagnosis in 184 patients. AJR Am J Roentgenol. 1993 Nov;161(5):957–60. PMID:8273634
1060. Kriege M, Hollestelle A, Jager A, et al. Survival and contralateral breast cancer in CHEK2 1100delC breast cancer patients: impact of adjuvant chemotherapy. Br J Cancer. 2014 Aug 26;111(5):1004–13. PMID:24918820
1061. Krings G, Bean GR, Chen YY. Fibroepithelial lesions; the WHO spectrum. Semin Diagn Pathol. 2017 Sep;34(5):438–52. PMID:28688536
1062. Krings G, Chen YY. Genomic profiling of metaplastic breast carcinomas reveals genetic heterogeneity and relationship to ductal carcinoma. Mod Pathol. 2018 Nov;31(11):1661–74. PMID:29946183
1063. Krings G, Joseph NM, Bean GR, et al. Genomic profiling of breast secretory carcinomas reveals distinct genetics from other breast cancers and similarity to mammary analog secretory carcinomas. Mod Pathol. 2017 Aug;30(8):1086–99. PMID:28548128
1064. Krings G, McIntire P, Shin SJ. Myofibroblastic, fibroblastic and myoid lesions of the breast. Semin Diagn Pathol. 2017 Sep;34(5):427–37. PMID:28751104
1065. Krop I, Ismaila N, Stearns V. Use of biomarkers to guide decisions on adjuvant systemic therapy for women with early-stage invasive breast cancer: American Society of Clinical Oncology clinical practice focused update guideline summary. J Oncol Pract. 2017 Nov;13(11):763–6. PMID:28696818
1066. Kryvenko ON, Chitale DA, VanEgmond EM, et al. Angiolipoma of the female breast: clinicomorphological correlation of 52 cases. Int J Surg Pathol. 2011 Feb;19(1):35–43. PMID:21087987
1067. Ku J, Campbell C, Bennett I. Leiomyoma of the nipple. Breast J. 2006 Jul-Aug;12(4):377–80. PMID:16848853
1068. Kuba MG, Lester SC, Giess CS, et al. Fibromatosis of the breast: diagnostic accuracy of core needle biopsy. Am J Clin Pathol. 2017 Sep 1;148(3):243–50. PMID:28821190
1069. Kuchenbaecker KB, McGuffog L, Barrowdale D, et al. Evaluation of polygenic risk scores for breast and ovarian cancer risk prediction in BRCA1 and BRCA2 mutation carriers. J Natl Cancer Inst. 2017 Jul 1;109(7):djw302. PMID:28376175
1070. Kuchenbaecker KB, Neuhausen SL, Robson M, et al. Associations of common breast cancer susceptibility alleles with risk of breast cancer subtypes in BRCA1 and BRCA2 mutation carriers. Breast Cancer Res. 2014 Dec 31;16(6):3416. PMID:25919761
1071. Kucukzeybek BB, Yigit S, Sari AA, et al. Primary mucinous cystadenocarcinoma of the breast with amplification of the HER2 gene confirmed by FISH - case report and review of the literature. Pol J Pathol. 2014 Mar;65(1):70–3. PMID:25119013
1072. Kuijper A, Buerger H, Simon R, et al. Analysis of the progression of fibroepithelial tumours of the breast by PCR-based clonality assay. J Pathol. 2002 Aug;197(5):575–81. PMID:12210075
1073. Kuijper A, Mommers EC, van der Wall E, et al. Histopathology of fibroadenoma of the breast. Am J Clin Pathol. 2001 May;115(5):736–42. PMID:11345838
1074. Kulkarni N, Pezzi CM, Greif JM, et al. Rare breast cancer: 933 adenoid cystic carcinomas from the National Cancer Data Base. Ann Surg Oncol. 2013 Jul;20(7):2236–41. PMID:23456318
1075. Kulshreshtha B, Arpita A, Rajesh PT, et al. Adolescent gynecomastia is associated with a high incidence of obesity, dysglycemia, and family background of diabetes mellitus. Indian J Endocrinol Metab. 2017 Jan-Feb;21(1):160–4. PMID:28217517
1076. Kumar E, Patel NR, Demicco EG, et al. Cutaneous nodular fasciitis with genetic analysis: a case series. J Cutan Pathol. 2016 Dec;43(12):1143–9. PMID:27686647
1077. Kumar H, Narasimha A, Bhaskaran, et al. Concurrent lactating adenoma and infiltrating ductal carcinoma: a case report. J Clin Diagn Res. 2015 Aug;9(8):ED14–5. PMID:26435957
1078. Kundu UR, Guo M, Landon G, et al. Fine-needle aspiration cytology of sclerosing adenosis of the breast: a retrospective review of cytologic features in conjunction with corresponding histologic features and radiologic findings. Am J Clin Pathol. 2012 Jul;138(1):96–102. PMID:22706864
1079. Kuo F, Lally K, Lewis M, et al. Granular cell tumour in male breast mimicking breast carcinoma. BMJ Case Rep. 2019 Mar 5;12(3):e227805. PMID:30842135
1080. Kurebayashi J, Izuo M, Ishida T, et al. Two cases of lipid-secreting carcinoma of the breast: case reports with an electron microscopic study. Jpn J Clin Oncol. 1988 Sep;18(3):249–54. PMID:3045374
1081. Kurozumi S, Matsumoto H, Hayashi Y, et al. Power of PgR expression as a prognostic factor for ER-positive/HER2-negative breast cancer patients at intermediate risk classified by the Ki67 labeling index. BMC Cancer. 2017 May 22;17(1):354. PMID:28532429
1082. Kwast AB, Groothuis-Oudshoorn KC, Grandjean I, et al. Histological type is not an independent prognostic factor for the risk pattern of breast cancer recurrences. Breast Cancer Res Treat. 2012 Aug;135(1):271–80. PMID:22810087
1083. La Vecchia C, Parazzini F, Franceschi S, et al. Risk factors for benign breast disease and their relation with breast cancer risk. Pooled information from epidemiologic studies. Tumori. 1985 Apr 30;71(2):167–78. PMID:4002347
1084. Lack EE, Worsham GF, Callihan MD, et al. Granular cell tumor: a clinicopathologic study of 110 patients. J Surg Oncol. 1980;13(4):301–16. PMID:6246310
1085. Lacle MM, Kornegoor R, Moelans CB, et al. Analysis of copy number changes on chromosome 16q in male breast cancer by multiplex ligation-dependent probe amplification. Mod Pathol. 2013 Nov;26(11):1461–7. PMID:23743929
1086. Lacle MM, Moelans CB, Kornegoor R, et al. Chromosome 17 copy number changes in male breast cancer. Cell Oncol (Dordr). 2015 Jun;38(3):237–45. PMID:25906114
1087. Lacle MM, van der Pol C, Witkamp A, et al. Prognostic value of mitotic index and Bcl2 expression in male breast cancer. PLoS One. 2013;8(4):e60138. PMID:23573235
1088. Lacle MM, van Diest PJ, Goldschmeding R, et al. Expression of connective tissue growth factor in male breast cancer: clinicopathologic correlations and prognostic value. PLoS One. 2015 Mar 4;10(3):e0118957. PMID:25738829
1089. Lacroix-Triki M, Geyer FC, Lambros MB, et al. β-catenin/Wnt signalling pathway in fibromatosis, metaplastic carcinomas and phyllodes tumours of the breast. Mod Pathol. 2010 Nov;23(11):1438–48. PMID:20693983
1090. Lacroix-Triki M, Lambros MB, Geyer FC, et al. Absence of microsatellite instability in mucinous carcinomas of the breast. Int J Clin Exp Pathol. 2010 Nov 27;4(1):22–31. PMID:21228925
1091. Lacroix-Triki M, Suarez PH, MacKay A, et al. Mucinous carcinoma of the breast is genomically distinct from invasive ductal carcinomas of no special type. J Pathol. 2010 Nov;222(3):282–98. PMID:20815046
1092. Laé M, Fréneaux P, Sastre-Garau X, et al. Secretory breast carcinomas with ETV6-NTRK3 fusion gene belong to the basal-like carcinoma spectrum. Mod Pathol. 2009 Feb;22(2):291–8. PMID:19011601
1093. Laé M, La Rosa P, Mandel J, et al. Whole-genome profiling helps to classify phyllodes tumours of the breast. J Clin Pathol. 2016 Dec;69(12):1081–7. PMID:27207013
1094. Lahat G, Lazar A, Lev D. Sarcoma epidemiology and etiology: potential environmental and genetic factors. Surg Clin North Am. 2008 Jun;88(3):451–81, v. PMID:18514694
1095. Lai R, Weiss LM, Chang KL, et al. Frequency of CD43 expression in non-Hodgkin lymphoma. A survey of 742 cases and further characterization of rare CD43+ follicular lymphomas. Am J Clin Pathol. 1999 Apr;111(4):488–94. PMID:10191768
1096. Lakhani SR, Chaggar R, Davies S, et al. Genetic alterations in 'normal' luminal and myoepithelial cells of the breast. J Pathol. 1999 Dec;189(4):496–503. PMID:10629549
1097. Lakhani SR, Collins N, Stratton MR, et al. Atypical ductal hyperplasia of the breast: clonal proliferation with loss of heterozygosity on chromosomes 16q and 17p. J Clin Pathol. 1995 Jul;48(7):611–5. PMID:7560165
1098. Lakhani SR, Ellis IO, Schnitt SJ, et al., editors. WHO classification of tumours of the breast. Lyon (France): International Agency for Research on Cancer; 2012. (WHO classification of tumours series, 4th ed.; vol. 4). http://publications.iarc.fr/14.
1099. Lakhani SR, Jacquemier J, Sloane JP, et al. Multifactorial analysis of differences between sporadic breast cancers and cancers

involving BRCA1 and BRCA2 mutations. J Natl Cancer Inst. 1998 Aug 5;90(15):1138–45. PMID:9701363
1100. Lakhani SR, O'Hare MJ. The mammary myoepithelial cell–Cinderella or ugly sister? Breast Cancer Res. 2001;3(1):1–4. PMID:11250738
1101. Lakhani SR, Slack DN, Hamoudi RA, et al. Detection of allelic imbalance indicates that a proportion of mammary hyperplasia of usual type are clonal, neoplastic proliferations. Lab Invest. 1996 Jan;74(1):129–35. PMID:8569175
1102. Lale S, Kure K, Lingamfelter D. Challenges to diagnose metaplastic carcinoma of the breast through cytologic methods: an eight-case series. Diagn Pathol. 2011 Jan 18;6:7. PMID:21244696
1102A. Lalloo F, Varley J, Ellis D, et al. Prediction of pathogenic mutations in patients with early-onset breast cancer by family history. Lancet. 2003 Mar 29;361(9363):1101–2. PMID:12672316
1103. Lamb J, McGoogan E. Fine needle aspiration cytology of breast in invasive carcinoma of tubular type and in radial scar/complex sclerosing lesions. Cytopathology. 1994 Feb;5(1):17–26. PMID:8173027
1104. Lamb LR, Bahl M, Hughes KS, et al. Pathologic upgrade rates of high-risk breast lesions on digital two-dimensional vs tomosynthesis mammography. J Am Coll Surg. 2018 May;226(5):858–67. PMID:29410346
1105. Lambertini M, Santoro L, Del Mastro L, et al. Reproductive behaviors and risk of developing breast cancer according to tumor subtype: a systematic review and meta-analysis of epidemiological studies. Cancer Treat Rev. 2016 Sep;49:65–76. PMID:27529149
1106. Lambird PA, Shelley WM. The spatial distribution of lobular in situ mammary carcinoma. Implications for size and site of breast biopsy. JAMA. 1969 Oct 27;210(4):689–93. PMID:5394401
1107. Lammie GA, Millis RR. Ductal adenoma of the breast–a review of fifteen cases. Hum Pathol. 1989 Sep;20(9):903–8. PMID:2550351
1108. Lamovec J, Bracko M. Metastatic pattern of infiltrating lobular carcinoma of the breast: an autopsy study. J Surg Oncol. 1991 Sep;48(1):28–33. PMID:1653879
1109. Lamovec J, Jancar J. Primary malignant lymphoma of the breast. Lymphoma of the mucosa-associated lymphoid tissue. Cancer. 1987 Dec 15;60(12):3033–41. PMID:3315180
1110. Lamovec J, Us-Krasovec M, Zidar A, et al. Adenoid cystic carcinoma of the breast: a histologic, cytologic, and immunohistochemical study. Semin Diagn Pathol. 1989 May;6(2):153–64. PMID:2474845
1111. Landrum ML, Ornstein DL. Hypertrophic osteoarthropathy associated with metastatic phyllodes tumor. Am J Clin Oncol. 2003 Apr;26(2):146–50. PMID:12714885
1112. Langeveld D, Jansen M, de Boer DV, et al. Aberrant intestinal stem cell lineage dynamics in Peutz-Jeghers syndrome and familial adenomatous polyposis consistent with protracted clonal evolution in the crypt. Gut. 2012 Jun;61(6):839–46. PMID:21940722
1113. Langlands F, Cornford E, Rakha E, et al. Imaging overview of metaplastic carcinomas of the breast: a large study of 71 cases. Br J Radiol. 2016 Aug;89(1064):20140644. PMID:27245135
1114. Lanng C, Eriksen BØ, Hoffmann J. Lipoma of the breast: a diagnostic dilemma. Breast. 2004 Oct;13(5):408–11. PMID:15454196
1115. Lapid O, van Wingerden JJ, Perlemuter L. Tamoxifen therapy for the management of pubertal gynecomastia: a systematic review. J Pediatr Endocrinol Metab. 2013;26(9-10):803–7. PMID:23729603
1116. Larson PS, de las Morenas A, Cerda SR, et al. Quantitative analysis of allele imbalance supports atypical ductal hyperplasia lesions as direct breast cancer precursors. J Pathol. 2006 Jul;209(3):307–16. PMID:16604511
1117. Laskin WB, Fetsch JF, Lasota J, et al. Benign epithelioid peripheral nerve sheath tumors of the soft tissues: clinicopathologic spectrum of 33 cases. Am J Surg Pathol. 2005 Jan;29(1):39–51. PMID:15613855
1118. Laucirica R, Bentz JS, Khalbuss WE, et al. Performance characteristics of mucinous (colloid) carcinoma of the breast in fine-needle aspirates: observations from the College of American Pathologists Interlaboratory Comparison Program in Nongynecologic Cytopathology. Arch Pathol Lab Med. 2011 Dec;135(12):1533–8. PMID:22129179
1118A. Laurent E, Begueret H, Bonhomme B, et al. SOX10, GATA3, GCDFP15, androgen receptor, and mammaglobin for the differential diagnosis between triple-negative breast cancer and TTF1-negative lung adenocarcinoma. Am J Surg Pathol. 2019 Mar;43(3):293–302. PMID:30628926
1118B. Lavigne M, Menet E, Tille JC, et al. Comprehensive clinical and molecular analyses of neuroendocrine carcinomas of the breast. Mod Pathol. 2018 Jan;31(1):68–82. PMID:28884749
1119. Lavoué V, Fritel X, Antoine M, et al. Clinical practice guidelines from the French College of Gynecologists and Obstetricians (CNGOF): benign breast tumors - short text. Eur J Obstet Gynecol Reprod Biol. 2016 May;200:16–23. PMID:26967341
1120. Lawrenson K, Kar S, McCue K, et al. Functional mechanisms underlying pleiotropic risk alleles at the 19p13.1 breast-ovarian cancer susceptibility locus. Nat Commun. 2016 Sep 7;7:12675. PMID:27601076
1121. Lazar AJ, Tuvin D, Hajibashi S, et al. Specific mutations in the beta-catenin gene (CTNNB1) correlate with local recurrence in sporadic desmoid tumors. Am J Pathol. 2008 Nov;173(5):1518–27. PMID:18832571
1122. Le BH, Boyer PJ, Lewis JE, et al. Granular cell tumor: immunohistochemical assessment of inhibin-alpha, protein gene product 9.5, S100 protein, CD68, and Ki-67 proliferative index with clinical correlation. Arch Pathol Lab Med. 2004 Jul;128(7):771–5. PMID:15214825
1123. Le Gal M, Ollivier L, Asselain B, et al. Mammographic features of 455 invasive lobular carcinomas. Radiology. 1992 Dec;185(3):705–8. PMID:1438749
1124. Le Guellec S, Soubeyran I, Rochaix P, et al. CTNNB1 mutation analysis is a useful tool for the diagnosis of desmoid tumors: a study of 260 desmoid tumors and 191 potential morphologic mimics. Mod Pathol. 2012 Dec;25(12):1551–8. PMID:22766794
1125. Leal C, Costa I, Fonseca D, et al. Intracystic (encysted) papillary carcinoma of the breast: a clinical, pathological, and immunohistochemical study. Hum Pathol. 1998 Oct;29(10):1097–104. PMID:9781648
1126. Lechner MG, Megiel C, Church CH, et al. Survival signals and targets for therapy in breast implant-associated ALK–anaplastic large cell lymphoma. Clin Cancer Res. 2012 Sep 1;18(17):4549–59. PMID:22791880
1127. Lecuit T, Yap AS. E-cadherin junctions as active mechanical integrators in tissue dynamics. Nat Cell Biol. 2015 May;17(5):533–9. PMID:25925582
1128. Lee AH. The histological diagnosis of metastases to the breast from extramammary malignancies. J Clin Pathol. 2007 Dec;60(12):1333–41. PMID:18042689
1129. Lee AH. Use of immunohistochemistry in the diagnosis of problematic breast lesions. J Clin Pathol. 2013 Jun;66(6):471–7. PMID:23486609
1130. Lee C, Boughey J. Case report of a synchronous nipple adenoma and breast carcinoma with current multi-modality radiologic imaging. Breast J. 2016 Jan-Feb;22(1):105–10. PMID:26548327
1131. Lee EK, Kook SH, Kwag HJ, et al. Schwannoma of the breast showing massive exophytic growth: a case report. Breast. 2006 Aug;15(4):562–6. PMID:16844378
1132. Lee HW, Kim TE, Cho SY, et al. Invasive Paget disease of the breast: 20 years of experience at a single institution. Hum Pathol. 2014 Dec;45(12):2480–7. PMID:25288235
1133. Lee JEA, Li N, Rowley SM, et al. Molecular analysis of PALB2-associated breast cancers. J Pathol. 2018 May;245(1):53–60. PMID:29431189
1134. Lee JH, Kim SH, Kang BJ, et al. Ultrasonographic features of benign adenomyoepithelioma of the breast. Korean J Radiol. 2010 Sep-Oct;11(5):522–7. PMID:20808695
1135. Lee JY, Schizas M, Geyer FC, et al. Lobular carcinomas in situ display intralesion genetic heterogeneity and clonal evolution in the progression to invasive lobular carcinoma. Clin Cancer Res. 2019 Jan 15;25(2):674–86. PMID:30185420
1136. Lee SH, Park JM, Kook SH, et al. Metastatic tumors to the breast: mammographic and ultrasonographic findings. J Ultrasound Med. 2000 Apr;19(4):257–62. PMID:10759349
1137. Lee YS, Filie A, Arthur D, et al. Breast implant-associated anaplastic large cell lymphoma in a patient with Li-Fraumeni syndrome. Histopathology. 2015 Dec;67(6):925–7. PMID:25974645
1138. Leekha N, Muralee M, Mathews A, et al. Pleomorphic adenoma of breast-a case report and review of literature. Indian J Surg Oncol. 2014 Jun;5(2):152–4. PMID:25114471
1139. Lefkowitz M, Lefkowitz W, Wargotz ES. Intraductal (intracystic) papillary carcinoma of the breast and its variants: a clinicopathological study of 77 cases. Hum Pathol. 1994 Aug;25(8):802–9. PMID:8056421
1140. Lehmann BD, Bauer JA, Chen X, et al. Identification of human triple-negative breast cancer subtypes and preclinical models for selection of targeted therapies. J Clin Invest. 2011 Jul;121(7):2750–67. PMID:21633166
1140A. Lehmann BD, Jovanović B, Chen X, et al. Refinement of triple-negative breast cancer molecular subtypes: implications for neoadjuvant chemotherapy selection. PLoS One. 2016 Jun 16;11(6):e0157368. PMID:27310713
1141. Lehmann U, Streichert T, Otto B, et al. Identification of differentially expressed microRNAs in human male breast cancer. BMC Cancer. 2010 Mar 23;10:109. PMID:20331864
1142. Lehmann-Che J, Hamy AS, Porcher R, et al. Molecular apocrine breast cancers are aggressive estrogen receptor negative tumors overexpressing either HER2 or GCDFP15. Breast Cancer Res. 2013 May 11;15(3):R37. PMID:23663520
1143. Leibl S, Regitnig P, Moinfar F. Flat epithelial atypia (DIN 1a, atypical columnar change): an underdiagnosed entity very frequently coexisting with lobular neoplasia. Histopathology. 2007 Jun;50(7):859–65. PMID:17543075
1144. Leithner A, Gapp M, Radl R, et al. Immunohistochemical analysis of desmoid tumours. J Clin Pathol. 2005 Nov;58(11):1152–6. PMID:16254103
1145. Lempiäinen H, Halazonetis TD. Emerging common themes in regulation of PIKKs and PI3Ks. EMBO J. 2009 Oct 21;28(20):3067–73. PMID:19779456
1146. Lenze D, Leoncini L, Hummel M, et al. The different epidemiologic subtypes of Burkitt lymphoma share a homogenous micro RNA profile distinct from diffuse large B-cell lymphoma. Leukemia. 2011 Dec;25(12):1869–76. PMID:21701491
1147. Lepe M, Kalife ET, Ou J, et al. 'Inside-out' p120 immunostaining pattern in invasive micropapillary carcinoma of the breast; additional unequivocal evidence of reversed polarity. Histopathology. 2017 Apr;70(5):832–4. PMID:27862202
1148. Leroy B, Ballinger ML, Baran-Marszak F, et al. Recommended guidelines for validation, quality control, and reporting of TP53 variants in clinical practice. Cancer Res. 2017 Mar 15;77(6):1250–60. PMID:28254861
1149. Leroy B, Fournier JL, Ishioka C, et al. The TP53 website: an integrative resource centre for the TP53 mutation database and TP53 mutant analysis. Nucleic Acids Res. 2013 Jan;41(Database issue):D962–9. PMID:23161690
1150. Lerwill MF. Current practical applications of diagnostic immunohistochemistry in breast pathology. Am J Surg Pathol. 2004 Aug;28(8):1076–91. PMID:15252316
1151. Lesluyes T, Pérot G, Largeau MR, et al. RNA sequencing validation of the Complexity INdex in SARComas prognostic signature. Eur J Cancer. 2016 Apr;57:104–11. PMID:26916546
1152. Lesser ML, Rosen PP, Kinne DW. Multicentricity and bilaterality in invasive breast carcinoma. Surgery. 1982 Feb;91(2):234–40. PMID:6277027
1153. Lesseur C, Diergaarde B, Olshan AF, et al. Genome-wide association analyses identify new susceptibility loci for oral cavity and pharyngeal cancer. Nat Genet. 2016 Dec;48(12):1544–50. PMID:27749845
1155. Lester SC, Bose S, Chen YY, et al. Protocol for the examination of specimens from patients with ductal carcinoma in situ of the breast. Arch Pathol Lab Med. 2009 Jan;133(1):15–25. PMID:19123730
1156. Lester SC, Bose S, Chen YY, et al. Protocol for the examination of specimens from patients with invasive carcinoma of the breast. Arch Pathol Lab Med. 2009 Oct;133(10):1515–38. PMID:19792042
1157. Lesueur GC, Brown RW, Bhathal PS. Incidence of perilobular hemangioma in the female breast. Arch Pathol Lab Med. 1983 Jun;107(6):308–10. PMID:6687795
1158. Leucci E, Cocco M, Onnis A, et al. MYC translocation-negative classical Burkitt lymphoma cases: an alternative pathogenetic mechanism involving miRNA deregulation. J Pathol. 2008 Dec;216(4):440–50. PMID:18802929
1159. Leung AKC, Leung AAC. Gynecomastia in infants, children, and adolescents. Recent Pat Endocr Metab Immune Drug Discov. 2017;10(2):127–37. PMID:28260521
1160. Levi Z, Baris HN, Kedar I, et al. Upper and lower gastrointestinal findings in PTEN mutation-positive Cowden syndrome patients participating in an active surveillance program. Clin Transl Gastroenterol. 2011 Nov 17;2:e5. PMID:23238744
1161. Levy A, Lang AE. Ataxia-telangiectasia: a review of movement disorders, clinical features, and genotype correlations. Mov Disord. 2018 Aug;33(8):1238–47. PMID:29436738
1162. Levy-Lahad E, Catane R, Eisenberg S, et al. Founder BRCA1 and BRCA2 mutations in Ashkenazi Jews in Israel: frequency and differential penetrance in ovarian cancer and in breast-ovarian cancer families. Am J Hum Genet. 1997 May;60(5):1059–67.

PMID:9150153

**1163.** Lew M, Pang JC, Jing X, et al. Young investigator challenge: the utility of GATA3 immunohistochemistry in the evaluation of metastatic breast carcinomas in malignant effusions. Cancer Cytopathol. 2015 Oct;123(10):576–81. PMID:26465236

**1164.** Lewis JT, Hartmann LC, Vierkant RA, et al. An analysis of breast cancer risk in women with single, multiple, and atypical papilloma. Am J Surg Pathol. 2006 Jun;30(6):665–72. PMID:16723843

**1165.** Li CI. Risk of mortality by histologic type of breast cancer in the United States. Horm Cancer. 2010 Jun;1(3):156–65. PMID:21761358

**1166.** Li CI, Anderson BO, Daling JR, et al. Changing incidence of lobular carcinoma in situ of the breast. Breast Cancer Res Treat. 2002 Oct;75(3):259–68. PMID:12353815

**1167.** Li CI, Anderson BO, Daling JR, et al. Trends in incidence rates of invasive lobular and ductal breast carcinoma. JAMA. 2003 Mar 19;289(11):1421–4. PMID:12636465

**1168.** Li CI, Anderson BO, Porter P, et al. Changing incidence rate of invasive lobular breast carcinoma among older women. Cancer. 2000 Jun 1;88(11):2561–9. PMID:10861434

**1169.** Li CI, Chlebowski RT, Freiberg M, et al. Alcohol consumption and risk of postmenopausal breast cancer by subtype: the Women's Health Initiative Observational Study. J Natl Cancer Inst. 2010 Sep 22;102(18):1422–31. PMID:20733117

**1170.** Li CI, Daling JR, Malone KE. Age-specific incidence rates of in situ breast carcinomas by histologic type, 1980 to 2001. Cancer Epidemiol Biomarkers Prev. 2005 Apr;14(4):1008–11. PMID:15824180

**1171.** Li CI, Daling JR, Malone KE, et al. Relationship between established breast cancer risk factors and risk of seven different histologic types of invasive breast cancer. Cancer Epidemiol Biomarkers Prev. 2006 May;15(5):946–54. PMID:16702375

**1172.** Li CI, Malone KE, Saltzman BS, et al. Risk of invasive breast carcinoma among women diagnosed with ductal carcinoma in situ and lobular carcinoma in situ, 1988-2001. Cancer. 2006 May 15;106(10):2104–12. PMID:16604564

**1173.** Li CI, Moe RE, Daling JR. Risk of mortality by histologic type of breast cancer among women aged 50 to 79 years. Arch Intern Med. 2003 Oct 13;163(18):2149–53. PMID:14557212

**1174.** Li CI, Uribe DJ, Daling JR. Clinical characteristics of different histologic types of breast cancer. Br J Cancer. 2005 Oct 31;93(9):1046–52. PMID:16175185

**1175.** Li CI, Weiss NS, Stanford JL, et al. Hormone replacement therapy in relation to risk of lobular and ductal breast carcinoma in middle-aged women. Cancer. 2000 Jun 1;88(11):2570–7. PMID:10861435

**1176.** Li D, Deng J, He H, et al. Primary breast diffuse large B-cell lymphoma shows an activated B-cell-like phenotype. Ann Diagn Pathol. 2012 Oct;16(5):335–43. PMID:22569408

**1177.** Li D, Xiao X, Yang W, et al. Secretory breast carcinoma: a clinicopathological and immunophenotypic study of 15 cases with a review of the literature. Mod Pathol. 2012 Apr;25(4):567–75. PMID:22157932

**1178.** Li H, Sun X, Miller E, et al. BMI, reproductive factors, and breast cancer molecular subtypes: a case-control study and meta-analysis. J Epidemiol. 2017 Apr;27(4):143–51. PMID:28142040

**1179.** Li J, Meeks H, Feng BJ, et al. Targeted massively parallel sequencing of a panel of putative breast cancer susceptibility genes in a large cohort of multiple-case breast and ovarian cancer families. J Med Genet. 2016 Jan;53(1):34–42. PMID:26534844

**1180.** Li M, Du J, Wang LJ, et al. A case of nipple adenoma detected by sonography. Chin Med J (Engl). 2016 Oct 5;129(19):2386–7. PMID:27647201

**1181.** Li N, Wang X, Zhang H, et al. Young male breast cancer, a small crowd, the survival, and prognosis? A population-based study. Medicine (Baltimore). 2018 Oct;97(40):e12686. PMID:30290658

**1182.** Li W, Han Y, Wang C, et al. Precise pathologic diagnosis and individualized treatment improve the outcomes of invasive micropapillary carcinoma of the breast: a 12-year prospective clinical study. Mod Pathol. 2018 Jun;31(6):956–64. PMID:29403084

**1183.** Li X, Peng J, Zhang Z, et al. Mammary mucinous cystadenocarcinoma. Breast J. 2012 May-Jun;18(3):282–3. PMID:22489551

**1184.** Li X, Xu Y, Ye H, et al. Encapsulated papillary carcinoma of the breast: a clinicopathological study of 49 cases. Curr Probl Cancer. 2018 May-Jun;42(3):291–301. PMID:29731165

**1185.** Li Y, Zhang S, Wei X, et al. The clinical features and management of women with ductal carcinoma in situ with microinvasion: a retrospective cohort study. Int J Surg. 2015 Jul;19:91–4. PMID:26013173

**1186.** Li YF, Lv MH, Chen LF, et al. Giant lipoma of the breast: a case report and review of the literature. Clin Breast Cancer. 2011 Dec;11(6):420–2. PMID:21729672

**1187.** Lian D, Cheah E, Tan PH, et al. Phyllodes tumour with intraductal growth: a rare cause of nipple discharge. Histopathology. 2007 Apr;50(5):666–9. PMID:17394506

**1188.** Liang M, Zhang Y, Sun C, et al. Association between CHEK2*1100delC and breast cancer: a systematic review and meta-analysis. Mol Diagn Ther. 2018 Aug;22(4):397–407. PMID:29909568

**1189.** Liao HY, Zhang WW, Sun JY, et al. The clinicopathological features and survival outcomes of different histological subtypes in triple-negative breast cancer. J Cancer. 2018 Jan 1;9(2):296–303. PMID:29344276

**1190.** Liau JY, Lee YH, Tsai JH, et al. Frequent PIK3CA activating mutations in nipple adenomas. Histopathology. 2017 Jan;70(2):195–202. PMID:27441415

**1191.** Liaw D, Marsh DJ, Li J, et al. Germline mutations of the PTEN gene in Cowden disease, an inherited breast and thyroid cancer syndrome. Nat Genet. 1997 May;16(1):64–7. PMID:9140396

**1192.** Liberman L, Sama M, Susnik B, et al. Lobular carcinoma in situ at percutaneous breast biopsy: surgical biopsy findings. AJR Am J Roentgenol. 1999 Aug;173(2):291–9. PMID:10430122

**1193.** Lien HC, Chen YL, Juang YL, et al. Frequent alterations of HER2 through mutation, amplification, or overexpression in pleomorphic lobular carcinoma of the breast. Breast Cancer Res Treat. 2015 Apr;150(2):447–55. PMID:25773929

**1194.** Lien HC, Huang CS, Yang YW, et al. Mutational analysis of MED12 exon 2 in a spectrum of fibroepithelial tumours of the breast: implications for pathogenesis and histogenesis. Histopathology. 2016 Feb;68(3):433–41. PMID:26109290

**1195.** Lien HC, Lin CW, Mao TL, et al. p53 overexpression and mutation in metaplastic carcinoma of the breast: genetic evidence for a monoclonal origin of both the carcinomatous and the heterogeneous sarcomatous components. J Pathol. 2004 Oct;204(2):131–9.

PMID:15376261

**1196.** Liguori G, Cantile M, Cerrone M, et al. Breast MALT lymphomas: a clinicopathological and cytogenetic study of 9 cases. Oncol Rep. 2012 Oct;28(4):1211–6. PMID:22842723

**1197.** Lim HS, Kuzmiak CM, Jeong SI, et al. Invasive micropapillary carcinoma of the breast: MR imaging findings. Korean J Radiol. 2013 Jul-Aug;14(4):551–8. PMID:23901311

**1198.** Lim J, Govindarajulu S, Sahu A, et al. Multiple Step-section Frozen Section sentinel lymph node biopsy–a review of 717 patients. Breast. 2013 Oct;22(5):639–42. PMID:23953247

**1199.** Lim SZ, Selvarajan S, Thike AA, et al. Breast sarcomas and malignant phyllodes tumours: comparison of clinicopathological features, treatment strategies, prognostic factors and outcomes. Breast Cancer Res Treat. 2016 Sep;159(2):229–44. PMID:27541020

**1200.** Lim WK, Ong CK, Tan J, et al. Exome sequencing identifies highly recurrent MED12 somatic mutations in breast fibroadenoma. Nat Genet. 2014 Aug;46(8):877–80. PMID:25038752

**1201.** Lim-Co RY, Gisser SD. Unusual variant of lipid-rich mammary carcinoma. Arch Pathol Lab Med. 1978 Apr;102(4):193–5. PMID:580713

**1202.** Limite G, Di Micco R, Esposito E, et al. Acinic cell carcinoma of the breast: review of the literature. Int J Surg. 2014;12 Suppl 1:S35–9. PMID:24859406

**1203.** Limite G, Di Micco R, Esposito E, et al. The first case of acinic cell carcinoma of the breast within a fibroadenoma: case report. Int J Surg. 2014;12 Suppl 1:S232–5. PMID:24859396

**1204.** Lin FdeM, Pincerato KM, Bacchi CE, et al. Coordinated expression of oestrogen and androgen receptors in HER2-positive breast carcinomas: impact on proliferative activity. J Clin Pathol. 2012 Jan;65(1):64–8. PMID:22039288

**1205.** Lin WY, Camp NJ, Ghoussaini M, et al. Identification and characterization of novel associations in the CASP8/ALS2CR12 region on chromosome 2 with breast cancer risk. Hum Mol Genet. 2015 Jan 1;24(1):285–98. PMID:25168388

**1206.** Lin X, Yan C, Gao Y, et al. Genetic variants at 9p21.3 are associated with risk of esophageal squamous cell carcinoma in a Chinese population. Cancer Sci. 2017 Feb;108(2):250–5. PMID:27960044

**1207.** Lindström S, Thompson DJ, Paterson AD, et al. Genome-wide association study identifies multiple loci associated with both mammographic density and breast cancer risk. Nat Commun. 2014 Oct 24;5:5303. PMID:25342443

**1208.** Lininger RA, Park WS, Man YG, et al. LOH at 16p13 is a novel chromosomal alteration detected in benign and malignant microdissected papillary neoplasms of the breast. Hum Pathol. 1998 Oct;29(10):1113–8. PMID:9781650

**1209.** Lips EH, Mukhtar RA, Yau C, et al. Lobular histology and response to neoadjuvant chemotherapy in invasive breast cancer. Breast Cancer Res Treat. 2012 Nov;136(1):35–43. PMID:22961065

**1210.** Lipsa A, Kowtal P, Sarin R. Novel germline STK11 variants and breast cancer phenotype identified in an Indian cohort of Peutz-Jeghers syndrome. Hum Mol Genet. 2019 Jun 1;28(11):1885–93. PMID:30689838

**1211.** Liu C, Chang H, Li XH, et al. Network meta-analysis on the effects of DNA damage response-related gene mutations on overall survival of breast cancer based on TCGA database. J Cell Biochem. 2017 Dec;118(12):4728–34. PMID:28513990

**1212.** Liu F, Yang M, Li Z, et al. Invasive micropapillary mucinous carcinoma of the breast is associated with poor prognosis. Breast Cancer Res Treat. 2015 Jun;151(2):443–51. PMID:25953688

**1213.** Liu GF, Yang Q, Haffty BG, et al. Clinical-pathologic features and long-term outcomes of tubular carcinoma of the breast compared with invasive ductal carcinoma treated with breast conservation therapy. Int J Radiat Oncol Biol Phys. 2009 Dec 1;75(5):1304–8. PMID:19386432

**1214.** Liu H, Tan H, Cheng Y, et al. Imaging findings in mucinous breast carcinoma and correlating factors. Eur J Radiol. 2011 Dec;80(3):706–12. PMID:20615642

**1215.** Liu J, Jia W, Zeng Y, et al. Adolescent male adenoid cystic breast carcinoma. Am Surg. 2012 May;78(5):E288–9. PMID:22691333

**1216.** Liu J, Liu X, Feng X, et al. C-kit overexpression correlates with KIT gene copy numbers increases in phyllodes tumors of the breast. Breast Cancer Res Treat. 2015 Jan;149(2):395–401. PMID:25534827

**1217.** Liu L, Chi YY, Wang AA, et al. Marital status and survival of patients with hormone receptor-positive male breast cancer: a Surveillance, Epidemiology, and End Results (SEER) population-based study. Med Sci Monit. 2018 May 24;24:3425–41. PMID:29795054

**1218.** Liu N, Johnson KJ, Ma CX. Male breast cancer: an updated Surveillance, Epidemiology, and End Results data analysis. Clin Breast Cancer. 2018 Oct;18(5):e997–1002. PMID:30007834

**1219.** Liu SY, Joseph NM, Ravindranathan A, et al. Genomic profiling of malignant phyllodes tumors reveals aberrations in FGFR1 and PI-3 kinase/RAS signaling pathways and provides insights into intratumoral heterogeneity. Mod Pathol. 2016 Sep;29(9):1012–27. PMID:27255162

**1220.** Liu X, Wu H, Teng L, et al. High-grade encapsulated papillary carcinoma of the breast is clinicopathologically distinct from low/intermediate-grade neoplasms in Chinese patients. Histol Histopathol. 2019 Feb;34(2):137–47. PMID:30004109

**1221.** Liu XY, Jiang YZ, Liu YR, et al. Clinicopathological characteristics and survival outcomes of invasive cribriform carcinoma of breast: a SEER population-based study. Medicine (Baltimore). 2015 Aug;94(31):e1309. PMID:26252312

**1222.** Livasy CA, Karaca G, Nanda R, et al. Phenotypic evaluation of the basal-like subtype of invasive breast carcinoma. Mod Pathol. 2006 Feb;19(2):264–71. PMID:16341146

**1223.** Lloyd J, Flanagan AM. Mammary and extramammary Paget's disease. J Clin Pathol. 2000 Oct;53(10):742–9. PMID:11064666

**1223A.** Lloyd-Lewis B, Harris OB, Watson CJ, et al. Mammary stem cells: premise, properties, and perspectives. Trends Cell Biol. 2017 Aug;27(8):556–67. PMID:28487183

**1224.** Lodding P, Kindblom LG, Angervall L, et al. Cellular schwannoma. A clinicopathologic study of 29 cases. Virchows Arch A Pathol Anat Histopathol. 1990;416(3):237–48. PMID:2105560

**1225.** Loghavi S, Khoury JD. Unusual breast mass: lymphoma with crystal-storing histiocytosis. Blood. 2015 Apr 9;125(15):2445. PMID:26038772

**1226.** Loghavi S, Medeiros LJ, Javadi S, et al. Breast implant-associated anaplastic large cell lymphoma with bone marrow involvement. Aesthet Surg J. 2018 Jun 13;38(7):NP 92–6. PMID:29635424

**1227.** Loi S, Michiels S, Salgado R, et al. Tumor infiltrating lymphocytes are prognostic in triple negative breast cancer and predictive

for trastuzumab benefit in early breast cancer: results from the FinHER trial. Ann Oncol. 2014 Aug;25(8):1544–50. PMID:24608200
1228. Loi S, Sirtaine N, Piette F, et al. Prognostic and predictive value of tumor-infiltrating lymphocytes in a phase III randomized adjuvant breast cancer trial in node-positive breast cancer comparing the addition of docetaxel to doxorubicin with doxorubicin-based chemotherapy: BIG 02-98. J Clin Oncol. 2013 Mar 1;31(7):860–7. PMID:23341518
1229. Loibl S, Volz C, Mau C, et al. Response and prognosis after neoadjuvant chemotherapy in 1,051 patients with infiltrating lobular breast carcinoma. Breast Cancer Res Treat. 2014 Feb;144(1):153–62. PMID:24504379
1230. Loke BN, Md Nasir ND, Thike AA, et al. Genetics and genomics of breast fibroadenomas. J Clin Pathol. 2018 May;71(5):381–7. PMID:29248888
1231. Londero V, Zuiani C, Linda A, et al. Lobular neoplasia: core needle breast biopsy underestimation of malignancy in relation to radiologic and pathologic features. Breast. 2008 Dec;17(6):623–30. PMID:18619840
1232. Long J, Cai Q, Sung H, et al. Genome-wide association study in east Asians identifies novel susceptibility loci for breast cancer. PLoS Genet. 2012;8(2):e1002532. PMID:22383897
1233. Long J, Zhang B, Signorello LB, et al. Evaluating genome-wide association study-identified breast cancer risk variants in African-American women. PLoS One. 2013 Apr 8;8(4):e58350. PMID:23593120
1234. Loose JH, Patchefsky AS, Hollander IJ, et al. Adenomyoepithelioma of the breast. A spectrum of biologic behavior. Am J Surg Pathol. 1992 Sep;16(9):868–76. PMID:1384377
1235. Lopes S, Vide J, Moreira E, et al. Paget disease of the male breast. Dermatol Online J. 2017 Apr 15;23(4):13030/qt0t89d5dg. PMID:28541881
1236. López-Bonet E, Alonso-Ruano M, Barraza G, et al. Solid neuroendocrine breast carcinomas: incidence, clinico-pathological features and immunohistochemical profiling. Oncol Rep. 2008 Dec;20(6):1369–74. PMID:19020716
1237. Lopez-Garcia MA, Geyer FC, Lacroix-Triki M, et al. Breast cancer precursors revisited: molecular features and progression pathways. Histopathology. 2010 Aug;57(2):171–92. PMID:20500230
1238. Lopez-Garcia MA, Geyer FC, Natrajan R, et al. Transcriptomic analysis of tubular carcinomas of the breast reveals similarities and differences with molecular subtype-matched ductal and lobular carcinomas. J Pathol. 2010 Sep;222(1):64–75. PMID:20593406
1239. López-Urrutia E, Salazar-Rojas V, Brito-Elías L, et al. BRCA mutations: Is everything said? Breast Cancer Res Treat. 2019 Jan;173(1):49–54. PMID:30293211
1240. Louwman MW, Vriezen M, van Beek MW, et al. Uncommon breast tumors in perspective: incidence, treatment and survival in the Netherlands. Int J Cancer. 2007 Jul 1;121(1):127–35. PMID:17330844
1241. Love C, Sun Z, Jima D, et al. The genetic landscape of mutations in Burkitt lymphoma. Nat Genet. 2012 Dec;44(12):1321–5. PMID:23143597
1242. Lovly CM, Gupta A, Lipson D, et al. Inflammatory myofibroblastic tumors harbor multiple potentially actionable kinase fusions. Cancer Discov. 2014 Aug;4(8):889–95. PMID:24875859
1243. Lozada JR, Basili T, Pareja F, et al. Solid papillary breast carcinomas resembling the tall cell variant of papillary thyroid neoplasms (solid papillary carcinomas with reverse polarity) harbour recurrent mutations affecting IDH2 and PIK3CA: a validation cohort. Histopathology. 2018 Aug;73(2):339–44. PMID:29603332
1244. Lozada JR, Burke KA, Maguire A, et al. Myxoid fibroadenomas differ from conventional fibroadenomas: a hypothesis-generating study. Histopathology. 2017 Oct;71(4):626–34. PMID:28513873
1245. Lu HM, Li S, Black MH, et al. Association of breast and ovarian cancers with predisposition genes identified by large-scale sequencing. JAMA Oncol. 2019 Jan 1;5(1):51–7. PMID:30128536
1246. Lu YJ, Osin P, Lakhani SR, et al. Comparative genomic hybridization analysis of lobular carcinoma in situ and atypical lobular hyperplasia and potential roles for gains and losses of genetic material in breast neoplasia. Cancer Res. 1998 Oct 15;58(20):4721–7. PMID:9788628
1247. Lüchtrath H, Moll R. Mucoepidermoid mammary carcinoma. Immunohistochemical and biochemical analyses of intermediate filaments. Virchows Arch A Pathol Anat Histopathol. 1989;416(2):105–13. PMID:2480681
1248. Ludmir EB, Milgrom SA, Pinnix CC, et al. Primary breast diffuse large B-cell lymphoma: treatment strategies and patterns of failure. Leuk Lymphoma. 2018 Dec;59(12):2896–903. PMID:29697005
1249. Lui PC, Lau PP, Tse GM, et al. Fine needle aspiration cytology of invasive micropapillary carcinoma of the breast. Pathology. 2007 Aug;39(4):401–5. PMID:17676481
1250. Luini A, Aguilar M, Gatti G, et al. Metaplastic carcinoma of the breast, an unusual disease with worse prognosis: the experience of the European Institute of Oncology and review of the literature. Breast Cancer Res Treat. 2007 Mar;101(3):349–53. PMID:17009109
1251. Luk PP, Wykes J, Selinger CI, et al. Diagnostic and prognostic utility of mastermind-like 2 (MAML2) gene rearrangement detection by fluorescent in situ hybridization (FISH) in mucoepidermoid carcinoma of the salivary glands. Oral Surg Oral Med Oral Pathol Oral Radiol. 2016 May;121(5):530–41. PMID:27068311
1252. Luna-Moré S, Casquero S, Pérez-Mellado A, et al. Importance of estrogen receptors for the behavior of invasive micropapillary carcinoma of the breast. Review of 68 cases with follow-up of 54. Pathol Res Pract. 2000;196(1):35–9. PMID:10674270
1253. Luna-Moré S, Gonzalez B, Acedo C, et al. Invasive micropapillary carcinoma of the breast. A new special type of invasive mammary carcinoma. Pathol Res Pract. 1994 Aug;190(7):668–74. PMID:7808965
1254. Luo J, Margolis KL, Wactawski-Wende J, et al. Association of active and passive smoking with risk of breast cancer among postmenopausal women: a prospective cohort study. BMJ. 2011 Mar 1;342:d1016. PMID:21363864
1255. Ly D, Forman D, Ferlay J, et al. An international comparison of male and female breast cancer incidence rates. Int J Cancer. 2013 Apr 15;132(8):1918–26. PMID:22987302
1256. Lyle PL, Bridge JA, Simpson JF, et al. Liposarcomatous differentiation in malignant phyllodes tumours is unassociated with MDM2 or CDK4 amplification. Histopathology. 2016 Jun;68(7):1040–5. PMID:26542423
1257. Lyons TG, Robson ME. Resurrection of PARP inhibitors in breast cancer. J Natl Compr Canc Netw. 2018 Sep;16(9):1150–6. PMID:30181424
1258. Ma CX, Bose R, Gao F, et al. Neratinib efficacy and circulating tumor DNA detection of HER2 mutations in HER2 nonamplified metastatic breast cancer. Clin Cancer Res. 2017 Oct 1;23(19):5687–95. PMID:28679771
1258A. Ma X, Han Y, Fan Y, et al. Clinicopathologic characteristics and prognosis of glycogen-rich clear cell carcinoma of the breast. Breast J. 2014 Mar-Apr;20(2):166–73. PMID:24400866
1259. Ma XJ, Dahiya S, Richardson E, et al. Gene expression profiling of the tumor microenvironment during breast cancer progression. Breast Cancer Res. 2009;11(1):R7. PMID:19187537
1260. Ma XJ, Salunga R, Tuggle JT, et al. Gene expression profiles of human breast cancer progression. Proc Natl Acad Sci U S A. 2003 May 13;100(10):5974–9. PMID:12714683
1261. MacGrogan G, Tavassoli FA. Central atypical papillomas of the breast: a clinicopathological study of 119 cases. Virchows Arch. 2003 Nov;443(5):609–17. PMID:13680220
1263. MacPherson G, Healey CS, Teare MD, et al. Association of a common variant of the CASP8 gene with reduced risk of breast cancer. J Natl Cancer Inst. 2004 Dec 15;96(24):1866–9. PMID:15601643
1264. Madanikia SA, Bergner A, Ye X, et al. Increased risk of breast cancer in women with NF1. Am J Med Genet A. 2012 Dec;158A(12):3056–60. PMID:23165953
1265. Magnusson M, Beath K, Cooter R, et al. The epidemiology of breast implant-associated anaplastic large cell lymphoma in Australia and New Zealand confirms the highest risk for grade 4 surface breast implants. Plast Reconstr Surg. 2019 May;143(5):1285–92. PMID:30789476
1266. Magrath I. Epidemiology: clues to the pathogenesis of Burkitt lymphoma. Br J Haematol. 2012 Mar;156(6):744–56. PMID:22260300
1267. Magro G. Differential diagnosis of benign spindle cell lesions. Surg Pathol Clin. 2018 Mar;11(1):91–121. PMID:29413661
1268. Magro G. Mammary myofibroblastoma: a tumor with a wide morphologic spectrum. Arch Pathol Lab Med. 2008 Nov;132(11):1813–20. PMID:18976021
1269. Magro G. Mammary myofibroblastoma: an update with emphasis on the most diagnostically challenging variants. Histol Histopathol. 2016 Jan;31(1):1–23. PMID:26328916
1270. Magro G, Angelico G, Righi A, et al. Utility of STAT6 and 13q14 deletion in the classification of the benign spindle cell stromal tumors of the breast. Hum Pathol. 2018 Nov;81:55–64. PMID:29940288
1271. Magro G, Bisceglia M, Michal M, et al. Spindle cell lipoma-like tumor, solitary fibrous tumor and myofibroblastoma of the breast: a clinico-pathological analysis of 13 cases in favor of a unifying histogenetic concept. Virchows Arch. 2002 Mar;440(3):249–60. PMID:11889594
1272. Magro G, Michal M, Bisceglia M. Benign spindle cell tumors of the mammary stroma: diagnostic criteria, classification, and histogenesis. Pathol Res Pract. 2001;197(7):453–66. PMID:11482575
1273. Magro G, Righi A, Casorzo L, et al. Mammary and vaginal myofibroblastomas are genetically related lesions: fluorescence in situ hybridization analysis shows deletion of 13q14 region. Hum Pathol. 2012 Nov;43(11):1887–93. PMID:22575260
1274. Mahoney MC, Robinson-Smith TM, Shaughnessy EA. Lobular neoplasia at 11-gauge vacuum-assisted stereotactic biopsy: correlation with surgical excisional biopsy and mammographic follow-up. AJR Am J Roentgenol. 2006 Oct;187(4):949–54. PMID:16985141
1275. Maia T, Amendoeira I. Breast sebaceous carcinoma-a rare entity. Clinico-pathological description of two cases and brief review. Virchows Arch. 2018 May;472(5):877–80. PMID:29556777
1276. Maiorano E, Regan MM, Viale G, et al. Prognostic and predictive impact of central necrosis and fibrosis in early breast cancer: results from two International Breast Cancer Study Group randomized trials of chemoendocrine adjuvant therapy. Breast Cancer Res Treat. 2010 May;121(1):211–8. PMID:19280340
1277. Makhlouf HR, Sobin LH. Inflammatory myofibroblastic tumors (inflammatory pseudotumors) of the gastrointestinal tract: How closely are they related to inflammatory fibroid polyps? Hum Pathol. 2002 Mar;33(3):307–15. PMID:11979371
1278. Makretsov N. Now, later of never: multicenter randomized controlled trial call–Is surgery necessary after atypical breast core biopsy results in mammographic screening settings? Int J Surg Oncol. 2015;2015:192579. PMID:25977821
1279. Makretsov N, He M, Hayes M, et al. A fluorescence in situ hybridization study of ETV6-NTRK3 fusion gene in secretory breast carcinoma. Genes Chromosomes Cancer. 2004 Jun;40(2):152–7. PMID:15101049
1280. Malberger E, Yerushalmi R, Tamir A, et al. Diagnosis of fibroadenoma in breast fine needle aspirates devoid of typical stroma. Acta Cytol. 1997 Sep-Oct;41(5):1483–8. PMID:9305388
1281. Malcolm TI, Hodson DJ, Macintyre EA, et al. Challenging perspectives on the cellular origins of lymphoma. Open Biol. 2016 Sep;6(9):160232. PMID:27683157
1282. Malkin D. Li-Fraumeni syndrome. Genes Cancer. 2011 Apr;2(4):475–84. PMID:21779515
1283. Malkin D, Li FP, Strong LC, et al. Germ line p53 mutations in a familial syndrome of breast cancer, sarcomas, and other neoplasms. Science. 1990 Nov 30;250(4985):1233–8. PMID:1978757
1284. Maluf HM, Koerner FC. Solid papillary carcinoma of the breast. A form of intraductal carcinoma with endocrine differentiation frequently associated with mucinous carcinoma. Am J Surg Pathol. 1995 Nov;19(11):1237–44. PMID:7573685
1285. Man S, Ellis IO, Sibbering M, et al. High levels of allele loss at the FHIT and ATM genes in non-comedo ductal carcinoma in situ and grade I tubular invasive breast cancers. Cancer Res. 1996 Dec 1;56(23):5484–9. PMID:8968105
1286. Mandelker D, Zhang L, Kemel Y, et al. Mutation detection in patients with advanced cancer by universal sequencing of cancer-related genes in tumor and normal DNA vs guideline-based germline testing. JAMA. 2017 Sep 5;318(9):825–35. PMID:28873162
1287. Manders JB, Kuerer HM, Smith BD, et al. Clinical utility of the 12-gene DCIS score assay: impact on radiotherapy recommendations for patients with ductal carcinoma in situ. Ann Surg Oncol. 2017 Mar;24(3):660–8. PMID:27704370
1288. Manipadam MT, Jacob A, Rajnikanth J. Giant lactating adenoma of the breast. J Surg Case Rep. 2010 Nov 1;2010(9):8. PMID:24946360
1289. Mann RM, Kuhl CK, Kinkel K, et al. Breast MRI: guidelines from the European Society of Breast Imaging. Eur Radiol. 2008 Jul;18(7):1307–18. PMID:18389253
1290. Manner J, Radlwimmer B, Hohenberger P, et al. MYC high level gene amplification is a distinctive feature of angiosarcomas after irradiation or chronic lymphedema. Am J Pathol. 2010 Jan;176(1):34–9. PMID:20008140
1291. Mantilla JG, Koenigsberg T, Reig B, et al. Core biopsy of vascular neoplasms

of the breast: pathologic features, imaging, and clinical findings. Am J Surg Pathol. 2016 Oct;40(10):1424–34. PMID:27340752
1292. Marchese C, Montera M, Torrini M, et al. Granular cell tumor in a PHTS patient with a novel germline PTEN mutation. Am J Med Genet A. 2003 Jul 15;120A(2):286–8. PMID:12833416
1293. Marchiò C, Geyer FC, Ng CK, et al. The genetic landscape of breast carcinomas with neuroendocrine differentiation. J Pathol. 2017 Feb;241(3):405–19. PMID:27925203
1294. Marchiò C, Iravani M, Natrajan R, et al. Genomic and immunophenotypical characterization of pure micropapillary carcinomas of the breast. J Pathol. 2008 Aug;215(4):398–410. PMID:18484683
1295. Marchiò C, Iravani M, Natrajan R, et al. Mixed micropapillary-ductal carcinomas of the breast: a genomic and immunohistochemical analysis of morphologically distinct components. J Pathol. 2009 Jul;218(3):301–15. PMID:19479727
1296. Marchiò C, Pietribiasi F, Castiglione R, et al. "Giants in a microcosm": multinucleated giant cells populating an invasive micropapillary carcinoma of the breast. Int J Surg Pathol. 2015 Dec;23(8):654–5. PMID:26370736
1297. Marian C, Boila A, Soanca D, et al. Malignant transformation of adenomyoepithelioma of the breast by a monophasic population: a report of two cases and review of literature. APMIS. 2013 Apr;121(4):272–9. PMID:23030630
1298. Mariño-Enríquez A, Dal Cin P. ALK as a paradigm of oncogenic promiscuity: different mechanisms of activation and different fusion partners drive tumors of different lineages. Cancer Genet. 2013 Nov;206(11):357–73. PMID:24091028
1299. Mariño-Enríquez A, Fletcher CD, Dal Cin P, et al. Dedifferentiated liposarcoma with "homologous" lipoblastic (pleomorphic liposarcoma-like) differentiation: clinicopathologic and molecular analysis of a series suggesting revised diagnostic criteria. Am J Surg Pathol. 2010 Aug;34(8):1122–31. PMID:20588177
1300. Maritz RM, Michelow PM. Cytological criteria to distinguish phyllodes tumour of the breast from fibroadenoma. Acta Cytol. 2017;61(6):418–24. PMID:28738381
1300A. Markopoulos C, Mantas D, Philipidis T, et al. Glycogen-rich clear cell carcinoma of the breast. World J Surg Oncol. 2008 Apr 29;6:44. PMID:18442419
1301. Marshall LM, Hunter DJ, Connolly JL, et al. Risk of breast cancer associated with atypical hyperplasia of lobular and ductal types. Cancer Epidemiol Biomarkers Prev. 1997 May;6(5):297–301. PMID:9149887
1302. Martin RW 3rd, Neldner KH, Boyd AS, et al. Multiple cutaneous granular cell tumors and neurofibromatosis in childhood. A case report and review of the literature. Arch Dermatol. 1990 Aug;126(8):1051–6. PMID:2166484
1303. Martinelli G, Ryan G, Seymour JF, et al. Primary follicular and marginal-zone lymphoma of the breast: clinical features, prognostic factors and outcome: a study by the International Extranodal Lymphoma Study Group. Ann Oncol. 2009 Dec;20(12):1993–9. PMID:19570964
1304. Martinelli G, Ryan G. Primary breast lymphoma. In: Cavalli F, Stein H, Zucca E, editors. Extranodal lymphomas: pathology and management. London (UK): Informa; 2008. pp. 168–73.
1305. Martinez V, Azzopardi JG. Invasive lobular carcinoma of the breast: incidence and variants. Histopathology. 1979 Nov;3(6):467–88. PMID:229072
1306. Marucci G, Betts CM, Golouh R, et al. Toker cells are probably precursors of Paget cell carcinoma: a morphological and ultrastructural description. Virchows Arch. 2002 Aug;441(2):117–23. PMID:12189500
1307. Marzullo F, Zito FA, Marzullo A, et al. Infiltrating cribriform carcinoma of the breast. A clinico-pathologic and immunohistochemical study of 5 cases. Eur J Gynaecol Oncol. 1996;17(3):228–31. PMID:8780923
1308. Masciari S, Dillon DA, Rath M, et al. Breast cancer phenotype in women with TP53 germline mutations: a Li-Fraumeni syndrome consortium effort. Breast Cancer Res Treat. 2012 Jun;133(3):1125–30. PMID:22392042
1309. Masood S, Davis C, Kubik MJ. Changing the term "breast tumor resembling the tall cell variant of papillary thyroid carcinoma" to "tall cell variant of papillary breast carcinoma". Adv Anat Pathol. 2012 Mar;19(2):108–10. PMID:22313838
1310. Mastracci TL, Shadeo A, Colby SM, et al. Genomic alterations in lobular neoplasia: a microarray comparative genomic hybridization signature for early neoplastic proliferationin the breast. Genes Chromosomes Cancer. 2006 Nov;45(11):1007–17. PMID:16897748
1311. Mastracci TL, Tjan S, Bane AL, et al. E-cadherin alterations in atypical lobular hyperplasia and lobular carcinoma in situ of the breast. Mod Pathol. 2005 Jun;18(6):741–51. PMID:15696125
1312. Mastrangelo G, Coindre JM, Ducimetière F, et al. Incidence of soft tissue sarcoma and beyond: a population-based prospective study in 3 European regions. Cancer. 2012 Nov 1;118(21):5339–48. PMID:22517534
1313. Mastropasqua MG, Maiorano E, Pruneri G, et al. Immunoreactivity for c-kit and p63 as an adjunct in the diagnosis of adenoid cystic carcinoma of the breast. Mod Pathol. 2005 Oct;18(10):1277–82. PMID:15846389
1314. Masuda H, Baggerly KA, Wang Y, et al. Differential response to neoadjuvant chemotherapy among 7 triple-negative breast cancer molecular subtypes. Clin Cancer Res. 2013 Oct 1;19(19):5533–40. PMID:23948975
1315. Matoso A, Easley SE, Gnepp DR, et al. Salivary gland acinar-like differentiation of the breast. Histopathology. 2009 Jan;54(2):262–3. PMID:19207954
1316. Matsubayashi RN, Adachi A, Yasumori K, et al. Adenoma of the nipple: correlation of magnetic resonance imaging findings with histologic features. J Comput Assist Tomogr. 2006 Jan-Feb;30(1):148–50. PMID:16365591
1317. Mattia AR, Ferry JA, Harris NL. Breast lymphoma. A B-cell spectrum including the low grade B-cell lymphoma of mucosa associated lymphoid tissue. Am J Surg Pathol. 1993 Jun;17(6):574–87. PMID:8333556
1318. Mattoch IW, Robbins JB, Kempson RL, et al. Post-radiotherapy vascular proliferations in mammary skin: a clinicopathologic study of 11 cases. J Am Acad Dermatol. 2007 Jul;57(1):126–33. PMID:17572278
1319. Mavaddat N, Barrowdale D, Andrulis IL, et al. Pathology of breast and ovarian cancers among BRCA1 and BRCA2 mutation carriers: results from the Consortium of Investigators of Modifiers of BRCA1/2 (CIMBA). Cancer Epidemiol Biomarkers Prev. 2012 Jan;21(1):134–47. PMID:22144499
1320. Mavaddat N, Peock S, Frost D, et al. Cancer risks for BRCA1 and BRCA2 mutation carriers: results from prospective analysis of EMBRACE. J Natl Cancer Inst. 2013 Jun 5;105(11):812–22. PMID:23628597
1321. Mavaddat N, Pharoah PD, Michailidou K, et al. Prediction of breast cancer risk based on profiling with common genetic variants. J Natl Cancer Inst. 2015 Apr 8;107(5):djv036. PMID:25855707
1322. Maxwell AJ, Clements K, Dodwell DJ, et al. The radiological features, diagnosis and management of screen-detected lobular neoplasia of the breast: findings from the Sloane Project. Breast. 2016 Jun;27:109–15. PMID:27060553
1323. Maxwell AJ, Clements K, Hilton B, et al. Risk factors for the development of invasive cancer in unresected ductal carcinoma in situ. Eur J Surg Oncol. 2018 Apr;44(4):429–35. PMID:29398324
1324. Mazzella FM, Sieber SC, Braza F. Ductal carcinoma of male breast with prominent lipid-rich component. Pathology. 1995 Jul;27(3):280–3. PMID:8532397
1325. Mazzola E, Cheng SC, Parmigiani G. The penetrance of ductal carcinoma in situ among BRCA1 and BRCA2 mutation carriers. Breast Cancer Res Treat. 2013 Jan;137(1):315–8. PMID:23184082
1326. Mbulaiteye SM, Anderson WF, Ferlay J, et al. Pediatric, elderly, and emerging adult-onset peaks in Burkitt's lymphoma incidence diagnosed in four continents, excluding Africa. Am J Hematol. 2012 Jun;87(6):573–8. PMID:22488262
1327. McBoyle MF, Razek HA, Carter JL, et al. Tubular carcinoma of the breast: an institutional review. Am Surg. 1997 Jul;63(7):639–44, discussion 644–5. PMID:9202540
1328. McCart Reed AE, Kalaw E, Nones K, et al. Phenotypic and molecular dissection of metaplastic breast cancer and the prognostic implications. J Pathol. 2019 Feb;247(2):214–27. PMID:30350370
1329. McCart Reed AE, Kutasovic JR, Nones K, et al. Mixed ductal-lobular carcinomas: evidence for progression from ductal to lobular morphology. J Pathol. 2018 Apr;244(4):460–8. PMID:29344954
1330. McClatchey AI. Neurofibromatosis. Annu Rev Pathol. 2007;2:191–216. PMID:18039098
1331. McCullar B, Pandey M, Yaghmour G, et al. Genomic landscape of small cell carcinoma of the breast contrasted to small cell carcinoma of the lung. Breast Cancer Res Treat. 2016 Jul;158(1):195–202. PMID:27329168
1332. McDermott KM, Crocker PR, Harris A, et al. Overexpression of MUC1 reconfigures the binding properties of tumor cells. Int J Cancer. 2001 Dec 15;94(6):783–91. PMID:11745478
1333. McDivitt RW, Boyce W, Gersell D. Tubular carcinoma of the breast. Clinical and pathological observations concerning 135 cases. Am J Surg Pathol. 1982 Jul;6(5):401–11. PMID:6289683
1334. McDivitt RW, Stewart FW. Breast carcinoma in children. JAMA. 1966 Jan 31;195(5):388–90. PMID:4285563
1335. McGowan TS, Cummings BJ, O'Sullivan B, et al. An analysis of 78 breast sarcoma patients without distant metastases at presentation. Int J Radiat Oncol Biol Phys. 2000 Jan 15;46(2):383–90. PMID:10661345
1336. McKeever K, Shepherd CW, Crawford H, et al. An epidemiological, clinical and genetic survey of neurofibromatosis type 1 in children under sixteen years of age. Ulster Med J. 2008 Sep;77(3):160–3. PMID:18956796
1337. McKinnon PJ. ATM and ataxia telangiectasia. EMBO Rep. 2004 Aug;5(8):772–6. PMID:15289825
1338. McLaren BK, Smith J, Schuyler PA, et al. Adenomyoepithelioma: clinical, histologic, and immunohistologic evaluation of a series of related lesions. Am J Surg Pathol. 2005 Oct;29(10):1294–9. PMID:16160470
1339. Meares AL, Frank RD, Degnim AC, et al. Mucocele-like lesions of the breast: a clinical outcome and histologic analysis of 102 cases. Hum Pathol. 2016 Mar;49:33–8. PMID:26826407
1340. Meattini I, Pezzulla D, Saieva C, et al. Triple negative apocrine carcinomas as a distinct subtype of triple negative breast cancer: a case-control study. Clin Breast Cancer. 2018 Oct;18(5):e773–80. PMID:29573977
1341. Meijers-Heijboer H, van den Ouweland A, Klijn J, et al. Low-penetrance susceptibility to breast cancer due to CHEK2(*)1100delC in noncarriers of BRCA1 or BRCA2 mutations. Nat Genet. 2002 May;31(1):55–9. PMID:11967536
1342. Meiss AE, Thomas M, Modesitt SC, et al. Clinicopathologic characterization of breast carcinomas in patients with non-BRCA germline mutations: results from a single institution's high-risk population. Hum Pathol. 2018 Dec;82:20–31. PMID:29958926
1343. Mekhail Y, Prather A, Hanna C, et al. Focal angiomatosis of the breast with MRI and histologic features. Radiol Case Rep. 2017 Mar 18;12(2):219–22. PMID:28491155
1344. Melchor L, Benítez J. The complex genetic landscape of familial breast cancer. Hum Genet. 2013 Aug;132(8):845–63. PMID:23552954
1345. Melhem-Bertrandt A, Bojadzieva J, Ready KJ, et al. Early onset HER2-positive breast cancer is associated with germline TP53 mutations. Cancer. 2012 Feb 15;118(4):908–13. PMID:21761402
1346. Menen RS, Ganesan N, Bevers T, et al. Long-term safety of observation in selected women following core biopsy diagnosis of atypical ductal hyperplasia. Ann Surg Oncol. 2017 Jan;24(1):70–6. PMID:27573525
1347. Menes TS, Rosenberg R, Balch S, et al. Upgrade of high-risk breast lesions detected on mammography in the Breast Cancer Surveillance Consortium. Am J Surg. 2014 Jan;207(1):24–31. PMID:24112677
1348. Menet E, Becette V, Briffod M. Cytologic diagnosis of lobular carcinoma of the breast: experience with 555 patients in the Rene Huguenin Cancer Center. Cancer. 2008 Apr 25;114(2):111–7. PMID:18300231
1349. Mentha G, Meyer P, Huber O, et al. [Liver transplantation. Preliminary results in the district University Hospital of Geneva]. Schweiz Med Wochenschr. 1990 Jul 21;120(29):1037–44. French. PMID:2374894
1350. Mentzel T, Kiss K. Reduced H3K27me3 expression in radiation-associated angiosarcoma of the breast. Virchows Arch. 2018 Mar;472(3):361–8. PMID:28983701
1351. Mentzel T, Schildhaus HU, Palmedo G, et al. Postradiation cutaneous angiosarcoma after treatment of breast carcinoma is characterized by MYC amplification in contrast to atypical vascular lesions after radiotherapy and control cases: clinicopathological, immunohistochemical and molecular analysis of 66 cases. Mod Pathol. 2012 Jan;25(1):75–85. PMID:21909081
1352. Mercado CL, Toth HK, Axelrod D, et al. Fine-needle aspiration biopsy of benign adenomyoepithelioma of the breast: radiologic and pathologic correlation in four cases. Diagn Cytopathol. 2007 Nov;35(11):690–4. PMID:17924402
1353. Merchant NB, Lewis JJ, Woodruff JM, et al. Extremity and trunk desmoid tumors: a multifactorial analysis of outcome. Cancer. 1999 Nov 15;86(10):2045–52. PMID:10570430
1354. Merino MJ. Plasmacytoma of the breast. Arch Pathol Lab Med. 1984 Aug;108(8):676–8. PMID:6378141
1355. Mersch J, Jackson MA, Park M, et al. Erratum to: Mersch J, Jackson MA, Park M, Nebgen D, Peterson SK, Singletary C, Arun BK and Litton JK. Cancers associated with BRCA1 and BRCA2 mutations other than breast and ovarian. Cancer. 2015;121:269-275. Cancer.

2015 Jul;121(14):2474–5. PMID:26132389
1356. Mester J, Eng C. When overgrowth bumps into cancer: the PTEN-opathies. Am J Med Genet C Semin Med Genet. 2013 May;163C(2):114–21. PMID:23613428
1357. Mesurolle B, Sygal V, Lalonde L, et al. Sonographic and mammographic appearances of breast hemangioma. AJR Am J Roentgenol 2008 Jul;191(1):W17-22. PMID:18562711
1358. Metovic J, Gallino C, Zanon E, et al. Eccrine spiradenoma of the nipple: case report, differential diagnosis and literature review. Histol Histopathol. 2019 Aug;34(8):909–15. PMID:30806477
1359. Metzger-Filho O, Michiels S, Bertucci F, et al. Genomic grade adds prognostic value in invasive lobular carcinoma. Ann Oncol. 2013 Feb;24(2):377–84. PMID:23028037
1360. Metzger-Filho O, Tutt A, de Azambuja E, et al. Dissecting the heterogeneity of triple-negative breast cancer. J Clin Oncol. 2012 May 20;30(15):1879–87. PMID:22454417
1361. Meyer A, Dörk T, Sohn C, et al. Breast cancer in patients carrying a germ-line CHEK2 mutation: outcome after breast conserving surgery and adjuvant radiotherapy. Radiother Oncol. 2007 Mar;82(3):349–53. PMID:17250914
1362. Meyer KB, O'Reilly M, Michailidou K, et al. Fine-scale mapping of the FGFR2 breast cancer risk locus: putative functional variants differentially bind FOXA1 and E2F1. Am J Hum Genet. 2013 Dec 5;93(6):1046–60. PMID:24290378
1363. Michailidou K, Beesley J, Lindstrom S, et al. Genome-wide association analysis of more than 120,000 individuals identifies 15 new susceptibility loci for breast cancer. Nat Genet. 2015 Apr;47(4):373–80. PMID:25751625
1364. Michailidou K, Hall P, Gonzalez-Neira A, et al. Large-scale genotyping identifies 41 new loci associated with breast cancer risk. Nat Genet. 2013 Apr;45(4):353–61, e1–2. PMID:23535729
1365. Michailidou K, Lindström S, Dennis J, et al. Association analysis identifies 65 new breast cancer risk loci. Nature. 2017 Nov 2;551(7678):92–4. PMID:29059683
1366. Michal M, Baumruk L, Burger J, et al. Adenomyoepithelioma of the breast with undifferentiated carcinoma component. Histopathology. 1994 Mar;24(3):274–6. PMID:7515373
1367. Michaut M, Chin SF, Majewski I, et al. Integration of genomic, transcriptomic and proteomic data identifies two biologically distinct subtypes of invasive lobular breast cancer. Sci Rep. 2016 Jan 5;6:18517. PMID:26729235
1368. Middleton LP, Grant S, Stephens T, et al. Lobular carcinoma in situ diagnosed by core needle biopsy: When should it be excised? Mod Pathol. 2003 Feb;16(2):120–9. PMID:12591964
1369. Middleton LP, Palacios DM, Bryant BR, et al. Pleomorphic lobular carcinoma: morphology, immunohistochemistry, and molecular analysis. Am J Surg Pathol. 2000 Dec;24(12):1650–6. PMID:11117786
1370. Miettinen M. Immunoreactivity for cytokeratin and epithelial membrane antigen in leiomyosarcoma. Arch Pathol Lab Med. 1988 Jun;112(6):637–40. PMID:2454091
1371. Miettinen M, McCue PA, Sarlomo-Rikala M, et al. Sox10–a marker for not only schwannian and melanocytic neoplasms but also myoepithelial cell tumors of soft tissue: a systematic analysis of 5134 tumors. Am J Surg Pathol. 2015 Jun;39(6):826–35. PMID:25724000
1372. Miettinen MM, Antonescu CR, Fletcher CDM, et al. Histopathologic evaluation of atypical neurofibromatous tumors and their transformation into malignant peripheral nerve sheath tumor in patients with neurofibromatosis 1-a consensus overview. Hum Pathol. 2017 Sep;67:1–10. PMID:28551330
1373. Milanezi MF, Saggioro FP, Zanati SG, et al. Pseudoangiomatous hyperplasia of mammary stroma associated with gynaecomastia. J Clin Pathol. 1998 Mar;51(3):204–6. PMID:9659260
1374. Miles RR, Arnold S, Cairo MS. Risk factors and treatment of childhood and adolescent Burkitt lymphoma/leukaemia. Br J Haematol. 2012 Mar;156(6):730–43. PMID:22260323
1375. Miller MC, Johnson P, Kim S, et al. Tubular adenomas of the breast: a rare diagnosis. BMJ Case Rep. 2018 Aug 27;2018. PMID:30150335
1376. Mills AME, E Gottlieb C, M Wendroth S, et al. Pure apocrine carcinomas represent a clinicopathologically distinct androgen receptor-positive subset of triple-negative breast cancers. Am J Surg Pathol. 2016 Aug;40(8):1109–16. PMID:27259012
1377. Mills MN, Yang GQ, Oliver DE, et al. Histologic heterogeneity of triple negative breast cancer: a National Cancer Centre Database analysis. Eur J Cancer. 2018 Jul;98:48–58. PMID:29870876
1378. Milne RL, Antoniou AC. Genetic modifiers of cancer risk for BRCA1 and BRCA2 mutation carriers. Ann Oncol. 2011 Jan;22 Suppl 1:i11–7. PMID:21285145
1379. Milne RL, Burwinkel B, Michailidou K, et al. Common non-synonymous SNPs associated with breast cancer susceptibility: findings from the Breast Cancer Association Consortium. Hum Mol Genet. 2014 Nov 15;23(22):6096–111. PMID:24943594
1380. Milne RL, Kuchenbaecker KB, Michailidou K, et al. Identification of ten variants associated with risk of estrogen-receptor-negative breast cancer. Nat Genet. 2017 Dec;49(12):1767–78. PMID:29058716
1381. Minami S, Matsuo S, Azuma T, et al. Parenchymal leiomyoma of the breast: a case report with special reference to magnetic resonance imaging findings and an update review of literature. Breast Cancer. 2011 Jul;18(3):231–6. PMID:21416339
1382. Miranda RN, Aladily TN, Prince HM, et al. Breast implant-associated anaplastic large-cell lymphoma: long-term follow-up of 60 patients. J Clin Oncol. 2014 Jan 10;32(2):114–20. PMID:24323027
1383. Miremadi A, Pinder SE, Lee AH, et al. Neuroendocrine differentiation and prognosis in breast adenocarcinoma. Histopathology. 2002 Mar;40(3):215–22. PMID:11895486
1384. Mirza IA, Shahab N. Small cell carcinoma of the breast. Semin Oncol. 2007 Feb;34(1):64–6. PMID:17270668
1385. Mishima C, Kagara N, Tanei T, et al. Mutational analysis of MED12 in fibroadenomas and phyllodes tumors of the breast by means of targeted next-generation sequencing. Breast Cancer Res Treat. 2015 Jul;152(2):305–12. PMID:26093648
1386. Mitchell JS, Li N, Weinhold N, et al. Genome-wide association study identifies multiple susceptibility loci for multiple myeloma. Nat Commun. 2016 Jul 1;7:12050. PMID:27363682
1387. Mitnick JS, Gianutsos R, Pollack AH, et al. Tubular carcinoma of the breast: sensitivity of diagnostic techniques and correlation with histopathology. AJR Am J Roentgenol. 1999 Feb;172(2):319–23. PMID:9930775
1388. Mito JK, Mitra D, Barysauskas CM, et al. A comparison of outcomes and prognostic features for radiation-associated angiosarcoma of the breast and other radiation-associated sarcomas. Int J Radiat Oncol Biol Phys. 2019 Jun 1;104(2):425–35. PMID:30703514
1389. Moelans CB, de Wegers RA, Monsuurs HN, et al. Molecular differences between ductal carcinoma in situ and adjacent invasive breast carcinoma: a multiplex ligation-dependent probe amplification study. Cell Oncol (Dordr). 2011 Oct;34(5):475–82. PMID:21547576
1390. Moelans CB, Verschuur-Maes AH, van Diest PJ. Frequent promoter hypermethylation of BRCA2, CDH13, MGMT, PAX5, PAX6 and WT1 in ductal carcinoma in situ and invasive breast cancer. J Pathol. 2011 Oct;225(2):222–31. PMID:21710692
1391. Mogal H, Brown DR, Isom S, et al. Intracystic papillary carcinoma of the breast: a SEER database analysis of implications for therapy. Breast. 2016 Jun;27:87–92. PMID:27054753
1392. Mohammadi A, Rosa M. Carcinoma of the breast with choriocarcinomatous features. Arch Pathol Lab Med. 2011 Sep;135(9):1097–100. PMID:21877993
1393. Mohanty SK, Kim SA, DeLair DF, et al. Comparison of metastatic neuroendocrine neoplasms to the breast and primary invasive mammary carcinomas with neuroendocrine differentiation. Mod Pathol. 2016 Aug;29(8):788–98. PMID:27125358
1394. Mohsin SK, Weiss H, Havighurst T, et al. Progesterone receptor by immunohistochemistry and clinical outcome in breast cancer: a validation study. Mod Pathol. 2004 Dec;17(12):1545–54. PMID:15272277
1395. Moinfar F. Flat ductal intraepithelial neoplasia of the breast: evolution of Azzopardi's "clinging" concept. Semin Diagn Pathol. 2010 Feb;27(1):37–48. PMID:20306829
1396. Moinfar F, Man YG, Arnould L, et al. Concurrent and independent genetic alterations in the stromal and epithelial cells of mammary carcinoma: implications for tumorigenesis. Cancer Res. 2000 May 1;60(9):2562–6. PMID:10811140
1397. Moinfar F, Man YG, Bratthauer GL, et al. Genetic abnormalities in mammary ductal intraepithelial neoplasia-flat type ("clinging ductal carcinoma in situ"): a simulator of normal mammary epithelium. Cancer. 2000 May 1;88(9):2072–81. PMID:10813719
1398. Mokbel K. Grading of infiltrating lobular carcinoma. Eur J Surg Oncol. 2001 Sep;27(6):609–10. PMID:11520101
1399. Moll R, Mitze M, Frixen UH, et al. Differential loss of E-cadherin expression in infiltrating ductal and lobular breast carcinomas. Am J Pathol. 1993 Dec;143(6):1731–42. PMID:8256859
1400. Moll UM, Chumas J. Morphologic effects of neoadjuvant chemotherapy in locally advanced breast cancer. Pathol Res Pract. 1997;193(3):187–96. PMID:9198104
1401. Molland JG, Donnellan M, Janu NC, et al. Infiltrating lobular carcinoma–a comparison of diagnosis, management and outcome with infiltrating duct carcinoma. Breast. 2004 Oct;13(5):389–96. PMID:15454194
1402. Møller P, Hagen AI, Apold J, et al. Genetic epidemiology of BRCA mutations–family history detects less than 50% of the mutation carriers. Eur J Cancer. 2007 Jul;43(11):1713–7. PMID:17574839
1403. Møller P, Seppälä T, Bernstein I, et al. Cancer incidence and survival in Lynch syndrome patients receiving colonoscopic and gynaecological surveillance: first report from the Prospective Lynch Syndrome Database. Gut. 2017 Mar;66(3):464–72. PMID:26657901
1404. Møller P, Seppälä T, Bernstein I, et al. Incidence of and survival after subsequent cancers in carriers of pathogenic MMR variants with previous cancer: a report from the Prospective Lynch Syndrome Database. Gut. 2017 Sep;66(9):1657–64. PMID:27261338
1405. Møller P, Seppälä TT, Bernstein I, et al. Cancer risk and survival in path_MMR carriers by gene and gender up to 75 years of age: a report from the Prospective Lynch Syndrome Database. Gut. 2018 Jul;67(7):1306–16. PMID:28754778
1406. Molyneux EM, Rochford R, Griffin B, et al. Burkitt's lymphoma. Lancet. 2012 Mar 31;379(9822):1234–44. PMID:22333947
1407. Montagna E, Maisonneuve P, Rotmensz N, et al. Heterogeneity of triple-negative breast cancer: histologic subtyping to inform the outcome. Clin Breast Cancer. 2013 Feb;13(1):31–9. PMID:23098574
1408. Monteiro JC, Ferguson KM, McKinna JA, et al. Ectopic production of human chorionic gonadotrophin-like material by breast cancer. Cancer. 1984 Feb 15;53(4):957–62. PMID:6692294
1409. Montgomery E, Torbenson MS, Kaushal M, et al. Beta-catenin immunohistochemistry separates mesenteric fibromatosis from gastrointestinal stromal tumor and sclerosing mesenteritis. Am J Surg Pathol. 2002 Oct;26(10):1296–301. PMID:12360044
1410. Montgomery ND, Bianchi GD, Klauber-Demore N, et al. Bilateral syringomatous adenomas of the nipple: case report with immunohistochemical characterization of a rare tumor mimicking malignancy. Am J Clin Pathol. 2014 May;141(5):727–31. PMID:24713747
1411. Moo TA, Alabdulkareem H, Tam A, et al. Association between recurrence and re-excision for close and positive margins versus observation in patients with benign phyllodes tumors. Ann Surg Oncol. 2017 Oct;24(10):3088–92. PMID:28766221
1412. Mooney KL, Bassett LW, Apple SK. Upgrade rates of high-risk breast lesions diagnosed on core needle biopsy: a single-institution experience and literature review. Mod Pathol. 2016 Dec;29(12):1471–84. PMID:27538687
1413. Moore KH, Thaler HT, Tan LK, et al. Immunohistochemically detected tumor cells in the sentinel lymph nodes of patients with breast carcinoma: biologic metastasis or procedural artifact? Cancer. 2004 Mar 1;100(5):929–34. PMID:14983487
1414. Moran MS, Schnitt SJ, Giuliano AE, et al. Society of Surgical Oncology-American Society for Radiation Oncology consensus guideline on margins for breast-conserving surgery with whole-breast irradiation in stages I and II invasive breast cancer. Int J Radiat Oncol Biol Phys. 2014 Mar 1;88(3):553–64. PMID:24521674
1415. Morandi L, Pession A, Marucci GL, et al. Intraepidermal cells of Paget's carcinoma of the breast can be genetically different from those of the underlying carcinoma. Hum Pathol. 2003 Dec;34(12):1321–30. PMID:14691919
1415A. Morita M, Yamaguchi R, Tanaka M, et al. Two progressive pathways of microinvasive carcinoma: low-grade luminal pathway and high-grade HER2 pathway based on high tumour-infiltrating lymphocytes. J Clin Pathol. 2016 Oct;69(10):890–8. PMID:27030304
1416. Moritani S, Ichihara S, Hasegawa M, et al. Uniqueness of ductal carcinoma in situ of the breast concurrent with papilloma: implications from a detailed topographical and histopathological study of 50 cases treated by mastectomy and wide local excision. Histopathology. 2013 Sep;63(3):407–17. PMID:23829486
1417. Moritani S, Ichihara S, Yatabe Y, et al. Immunohistochemical expression of myoepithelial markers in adenomyoepithelioma of the breast: a unique paradoxical staining pattern of high-molecular weight cytokeratins. Virchows Arch. 2015 Feb;466(2):191–8.

PMID:25479938

**1418.** Moritani S, Kushima R, Sugihara H, et al. Availability of CD10 immunohistochemistry as a marker of breast myoepithelial cells on paraffin sections. Mod Pathol. 2002 Apr;15(4):397–405. PMID:11950913

**1419.** Moritz AW, Wiedenhoefer JF, Profit AP, et al. Breast adenomyoepithelioma and adenomyoepithelioma with carcinoma (malignant adenomyoepithelioma) with associated breast malignancies: a case series emphasizing histologic, radiologic, and clinical correlation. Breast. 2016 Oct;29:132–9. PMID:27494340

**1420.** Moriya T, Sakamoto K, Sasano H, et al. Immunohistochemical analysis of Ki-67, p53, p21, and p27 in benign and malignant apocrine lesions of the breast: its correlation to histologic findings in 43 cases. Mod Pathol. 2000 Jan;13(1):13–8. PMID:10658905

**1421.** Morrogh M, Andrade VP, Giri D, et al. Cadherin-catenin complex dissociation in lobular neoplasia of the breast. Breast Cancer Res Treat. 2012 Apr;132(2):641–52. PMID:22080244

**1422.** Morrow M, Berger D, Thelmo W. Diffuse cystic angiomatosis of the breast. Cancer. 1988 Dec 1;62(11):2392–6. PMID:3179956

**1423.** Morrow M, Van Zee KJ, Solin LJ, et al. Society of Surgical Oncology-American Society for Radiation Oncology-American Society of Clinical Oncology consensus guideline on margins for breast-conserving surgery with whole-breast irradiation in ductal carcinoma in situ. J Clin Oncol. 2016 Nov 20;34(33):4040–6. PMID:27528719

**1424.** Moy L, Slanetz PJ, Moore R, et al. Specificity of mammography and US in the evaluation of a palpable abnormality: retrospective review. Radiology. 2002 Oct;225(1):176–81. PMID:12355002

**1425.** Mulligan AM, O'Malley FP. Metastatic potential of encapsulated (intracystic) papillary carcinoma of the breast: a report of 2 cases with axillary lymph node micrometastases. Int J Surg Pathol. 2007 Apr;15(2):143–7. PMID:17478767

**1426.** Mulligan S, Hu P, Murphy A, et al. Variations in MALT1 gene disruptions detected by FISH in 109 MALT lymphomas occurring in different primary sites. J Assoc Genet Technol. 2011;37(2):76–9. PMID:21654070

**1427.** Mullooly M, Khodr ZG, Dallal CM, et al. Epidemiologic risk factors for in situ and invasive breast cancers among postmenopausal women in the National Institutes of Health-AARP Diet and Health Study. Am J Epidemiol. 2017 Dec 15;186(12):1329–40. PMID:28637226

**1428.** Mun SH, Ko EY, Han BK, et al. Secretory carcinoma of the breast: sonographic features. J Ultrasound Med. 2008 Jun;27(6):947–54. PMID:18499854

**1429.** Mundo L, Ambrosio MR, Picciolini M, et al. Unveiling another missing piece in EBV-driven lymphomagenesis: EBV-encoded microRNAs expression in EBER-negative Burkitt lymphoma cases. Front Microbiol. 2017 Mar 1;8:229. PMID:28298901

**1430.** Murakami A, Kawachi K, Sasaki T, et al. Sebaceous carcinoma of the breast. Pathol Int. 2009 Mar;59(3):188–92. PMID:19261098

**1431.** Muranen TA, Blomqvist C, Dörk T, et al. Patient survival and tumor characteristics associated with CHEK2:p.I157T - findings from the Breast Cancer Association Consortium. Breast Cancer Res. 2016 Oct 3;18(1):98. PMID:27716369

**1432.** Muranen TA, Greco D, Blomqvist C, et al. Genetic modifiers of CHEK2*1100delC-associated breast cancer risk. Genet Med. 2017 May;19(5):599–603. PMID:27711073

**1433.** Muranen TA, Greco D, Fagerholm R, et al. Breast tumors from CHEK2 1100delC-mutation

carriers: genomic landscape and clinical implications. Breast Cancer Res. 2011 Sep 20;13(5):R90. PMID:21542898

**1434.** Murat A, Kansiz F, Kabakus N, et al. Neurofibroma of the breast in a boy with neurofibromatosis type 1. Clin Imaging. 2004 Nov-Dec;28(6):415–7. PMID:15531141

**1435.** Murphy SB, Hustu HO. A randomized trial of combined modality therapy of childhood non-Hodgkin's lymphoma. Cancer. 1980 Feb 15;45(4):630–7. PMID:6986967

**1436.** Murray MP, Luedtke C, Liberman L, et al. Classic lobular carcinoma in situ and atypical lobular hyperplasia at percutaneous breast core biopsy: outcomes of prospective excision. Cancer. 2013 Mar 1;119(5):1073–9. PMID:23132235

**1437.** Myhre-Jensen O. A consecutive 7-year series of 1331 benign soft tissue tumours. Clinicopathologic data. Comparison with sarcomas. Acta Orthop Scand. 1981 Jun;52(3):287–93. PMID:7282321

**1438.** Nadelman CM, Leslie KO, Fishbein MC. "Benign," metastasizing adenomyoepithelioma of the breast: a report of 2 cases. Arch Pathol Lab Med. 2006 Sep;130(9):1349–53. PMID:16948523

**1439.** Nagao T, Kinoshita T, Hojo T, et al. The differences in the histological types of breast cancer and the response to neoadjuvant chemotherapy: the relationship between the outcome and the clinicopathological characteristics. Breast. 2012 Jun;21(3):289–95. PMID:22277312

**1440.** Nagar H, Marmor S, Hammar B. Haemangiomas of the breast in children. Eur J Surg. 1992 Sep;158(9):503–5. PMID:1358220

**1441.** Nagata Y, Yoshioka M, Uramoto H, et al. Malignant melanoma of the nipple: a case report. J Breast Cancer. 2018 Mar;21(1):96–101. PMID:29628990

**1442.** Nagel JH, Peeters JK, Smid M, et al. Gene expression profiling assigns CHEK2 1100delC breast cancers to the luminal intrinsic subtypes. Breast Cancer Res Treat. 2012 Apr;132(2):439–48. PMID:21614566

**1443.** Nagi C, Bleiweiss I, Jaffer S. Epithelial displacement in breast lesions: a papillary phenomenon. Arch Pathol Lab Med. 2005 Nov;129(11):1465–9. PMID:16253028

**1444.** Nagi CS, O'Donnell JE, Tismenetsky M, et al. Lobular neoplasia on core needle biopsy does not require excision. Cancer. 2008 May 15;112(10):2152–8. PMID:18348299

**1445.** Nakagawa S, Miki Y, Miyashita M, et al. Tumor microenvironment in invasive lobular carcinoma: possible therapeutic targets. Breast Cancer Res Treat. 2016 Jan;155(1):65–75. PMID:26715212

**1446.** Nakai T, Ichihara S, Kada A, et al. The unique luminal staining pattern of cytokeratin 5/6 in adenoid cystic carcinoma of the breast may aid in differentiating it from its mimickers. Virchows Arch. 2016 Aug;469(2):213–22. PMID:27240462

**1447.** Nakhlis F, Gilmore L, Gelman R, et al. Incidence of adjacent synchronous invasive carcinoma and/or ductal carcinoma in-situ in patients with lobular neoplasia on core biopsy: results from a prospective multi-institutional registry (TBCRC 020). Ann Surg Oncol. 2016 Mar;23(3):722–8. PMID:26542585

**1448.** Nakhlis F, Harrison BT, Giess CS, et al. Evaluating the rate of upgrade to invasive breast cancer and/or ductal carcinoma in situ following a core biopsy diagnosis of non-classic lobular carcinoma in situ. Ann Surg Oncol. 2019 Jan;26(1):55–61. PMID:30362065

**1449.** Nakken S, Hovig E, Møller P, editors. Prospective Lynch Syndrome Database [Internet]. Edinburgh (UK): European Hereditary Tumour Group & Middlesex (UK):

International Society for Gastrointestinal Hereditary Tumours; 2019. Available from http://www.lscarisk.org.

**1450.** Nalwa A, Nath D, Suri V, et al. Myeloid sarcoma of the breast in an aleukemic patient: a rare entity in an uncommon location. Malays J Pathol. 2015 Apr;37(1):63–6. PMID:25890617

**1451.** Nangal JK, Kapoor A, Narayan S, et al. A case of CD68 negative histiocytic sarcoma of axilla masquerading as metastatic breast cancer. J Surg Case Rep. 2014 Jul 16;2014(7):rju071. PMID:25031040

**1452.** Naresh KN, Ibrahim HA, Lazzi S, et al. Diagnosis of Burkitt lymphoma using an algorithmic approach–applicable in both resource-poor and resource-rich countries. Br J Haematol. 2011 Sep;154(6):770–6. PMID:21718280

**1453.** Narod SA. Modifiers of risk of hereditary breast cancer. Oncogene. 2006 Sep 25;25(43):5832–6. PMID:16998497

**1454.** Narod SA, Huzarski T, Gronwald J, et al. Predictors of survival for breast cancer patients with a BRCA1 mutation. Breast Cancer Res Treat. 2018 Apr;168(2):513–21. PMID:29247441

**1455.** Narula HS, Carlson HE. Gynaecomastia–pathophysiology, diagnosis and treatment. Nat Rev Endocrinol. 2014 Nov;10(11):684–98. PMID:25112235

**1456.** Nascimento AF, Raut CP, Fletcher CD. Primary angiosarcoma of the breast: clinicopathologic analysis of 49 cases, suggesting that grade is not prognostic. Am J Surg Pathol. 2008 Dec;32(12):1896–904. PMID:18813119

**1457.** Nascimento AG, Karas M, Rosen PP, et al. Leiomyoma of the nipple. Am J Surg Pathol. 1979 Apr;3(2):151–4. PMID:532847

**1458.** Näslund-Koch C, Nordestgaard BG, Bojesen SE. Increased risk for other cancers in addition to breast cancer for CHEK2*1100delC heterozygotes estimated from the Copenhagen General Population Study. J Clin Oncol. 2016 Apr 10;34(11):1208–16. PMID:26884562

**1459.** Nasrallah MP, Nasrallah IM, Yu GH. Fine-needle aspiration of superficial myxoid neurofibroma in the region of the breast. Diagn Cytopathol. 2015 May;43(5):427–31. PMID:25722038

**1460.** Nassar A. Core needle biopsy versus fine needle aspiration biopsy in breast–a historical perspective and opportunities in the modern era. Diagn Cytopathol. 2011 May;39(5):380–8. PMID:20949457

**1461.** Nassar A, Conners AL, Celik B, et al. Radial scar/complex sclerosing lesions: a clinicopathologic correlation study from a single institution. Ann Diagn Pathol. 2015 Feb;19(1):24–8. PMID:25578683

**1462.** Nassar A, Visscher DW, Degnim AC, et al. Complex fibroadenoma and breast cancer risk: a Mayo Clinic Benign Breast Disease Cohort study. Breast Cancer Res Treat. 2015 Sep;153(2):397–405. PMID:26264469

**1463.** Nassar H. Carcinomas with micropapillary morphology: clinical significance and current concepts. Adv Anat Pathol. 2004 Nov;11(6):297–303. PMID:15505530

**1464.** Nassar H, Elieff MP, Kronz JD, et al. Pseudoangiomatous stromal hyperplasia (PASH) of the breast with foci of morphologic malignancy: a case of PASH with malignant transformation? Int J Surg Pathol. 2010 Dec;18(6):564–9. PMID:18611932

**1465.** Nassar H, Pansare V, Zhang H, et al. Pathogenesis of invasive micropapillary carcinoma: role of MUC1 glycoprotein. Mod Pathol. 2004 Sep;17(9):1045–50. PMID:15154007

**1466.** Nassar H, Qureshi H, Adsay NV, et al. Clinicopathologic analysis of solid papillary

carcinoma of the breast and associated invasive carcinomas. Am J Surg Pathol. 2006 Apr;30(4):501–7. PMID:16625097

**1467.** Nassif S, Ozdemirli M. EBV-positive low-grade marginal zone lymphoma in the breast with massive amyloid deposition arising in a heart transplant patient: a report of an unusual case. Pediatr Transplant. 2013 Sep;17(6):E141–5. PMID:23773403

**1468.** National Comprehensive Cancer Network (NCCN). Genetic/familial high-risk assessment: breast and ovarian. Plymouth Meeting (PA): NCCN; 2018 [accessed 2018 Nov 4]. Available from: https://www.nccn.org/professionals/physician_gls/default.aspx.

**1469.** National Comprehensive Cancer Network (NCCN). NCCN clinical practice guidelines in oncology (NCCN guidelines): breast cancer. Version 1.2018. Fort Washington (PA): NCCN; 2018 [accessed 2018 Nov 1]. Available from: https://www.nccn.org/professionals/physician_gls/default.aspx.

**1470.** Natrajan R, Lambros MB, Geyer FC, et al. Loss of 16q in high grade breast cancer is associated with estrogen receptor status: evidence for progression in tumors with a luminal phenotype? Genes Chromosomes Cancer. 2009 Apr;48(4):351–65. PMID:19156836

**1471.** Natrajan R, Wilkerson PM, Marchiò C, et al. Characterization of the genomic features and expressed fusion genes in micropapillary carcinomas of the breast. J Pathol. 2014 Apr;232(5):553–65. PMID:24395524

**1472.** Natsiopoulos I, Liappis T, Demiri E, et al. Diffuse breast angiomatosis with involvement of overlying skin: a case report. Clin Breast Cancer. 2016 Feb;16(1):e7–10. PMID:26456034

**1473.** Nayak A, Bleiweiss IJ, Dumoff K, et al. Mucinous cystadenocarcinoma of the breast: report of 2 cases including one with long-term local recurrence. Int J Surg Pathol. 2018 Dec;26(8):749–57. PMID:29745281

**1474.** Nayar R, Zhuang Z, Merino MJ, et al. Loss of heterozygosity on chromosome 11q13 in lobular lesions of the breast using tissue microdissection and polymerase chain reaction. Hum Pathol. 1997 Mar;28(3):277–82. PMID:9042790

**1475.** Neal L, Sandhu NP, Hieken TJ, et al. Diagnosis and management of benign, atypical, and indeterminate breast lesions detected on core needle biopsy. Mayo Clin Proc. 2014 Apr;89(4):536–47. PMID:24684875

**1476.** Negahban S, Ahmadi N, Oryan A, et al. Primary bilateral Burkitt lymphoma of the lactating breast: a case report and review of the literature. Mol Diagn Ther. 2010 Aug 1;14(4):243–50. PMID:20799767

**1477.** Nelen MR, Kremer H, Konings IB, et al. Novel PTEN mutations in patients with Cowden disease: absence of clear genotype-phenotype correlations. Eur J Hum Genet. 1999 Apr;7(3):267–73. PMID:10234502

**1478.** Nelen MR, Padberg GW, Peeters EA, et al. Localization of the gene for Cowden disease to chromosome 10q22-23. Nat Genet. 1996 May;13(1):114–6. PMID:8673088

**1479.** Nelson ER, Sharma R, Argani P, et al. Utility of Sox10 labeling in metastatic breast carcinomas. Hum Pathol. 2017 Sep;67:205–10. PMID:28843711

**1480.** Nelson RA, Guye ML, Luu T, et al. Survival outcomes of metaplastic breast cancer patients: results from a US population-based analysis. Ann Surg Oncol. 2015 Jan;22(1):24–31. PMID:25012264

**1481.** Neuhaus T, Hess T. Bilateral extramedullary plasmacytoma of the breast. Breast J. 2014 May-Jun;20(3):315–8. PMID:24673829

**1482.** Neuman HB, Brogi E, Ebrahim A, et al.

Desmoid tumors (fibromatoses) of the breast: a 25-year experience. Ann Surg Oncol. 2008 Jan;15(1):274–80. PMID:17896146
**1483.** Neuman JF. Evaluation and treatment of gynecomastia. Am Fam Physician. 1997 Apr;55(5):1835–44, 1849–50. PMID:9105209
**1484.** Neuville A, Chibon F, Coindre JM. Grading of soft tissue sarcomas: from histological to molecular assessment. Pathology. 2014 Feb;46(2):113–20. PMID:24378389
**1485.** Nevanlinna H, Bartek J. The CHEK2 gene and inherited breast cancer susceptibility. Oncogene. 2006 Sep 25;25(43):5912–9. PMID:16998506
**1486.** Newcomb PA, Trentham-Dietz A, Hampton JM, et al. Late age at first full term birth is strongly associated with lobular breast cancer. Cancer. 2011 May 1;117(9):1946–56. PMID:21509772
**1487.** Newman PL, Fletcher CD. Smooth muscle tumours of the external genitalia: clinicopathological analysis of a series. Histopathology. 1991 Jun;18(6):523–9. PMID:1879812
**1488.** Newman W. Lobular carcinoma of the female breast. Report of 73 cases. Ann Surg. 1966 Aug;164(2):305–14. PMID:5915941
**1489.** Ng CKY, Piscuoglio S, Geyer FC, et al. The landscape of somatic genetic alterations in metaplastic breast carcinomas. Clin Cancer Res. 2017 Jul 15;23(14):3859–70. PMID:28153863
**1490.** Ng WK. Fine needle aspiration cytology of invasive cribriform carcinoma of the breast with osteoclastlike giant cells: a case report. Acta Cytol. 2001 Jul-Aug;45(4):593–8. PMID:11480724
**1491.** Ng WK. Fine-needle aspiration cytology findings of an uncommon micropapillary variant of pure mucinous carcinoma of the breast: review of patients over an 8-year period. Cancer. 2002 Oct 25;96(5):280–8. PMID:12378595
**1492.** Ngeow J, Sesock K, Eng C. Clinical implications for germline PTEN spectrum disorders. Endocrinol Metab Clin North Am. 2017 Jun;46(2):503–17. PMID:28476234
**1493.** Ngoma T, Adde M, Durosinmi M, et al. Treatment of Burkitt lymphoma in equatorial Africa using a simple three-drug combination followed by a salvage regimen for patients with persistent or recurrent disease. Br J Haematol. 2012 Sep;158(6):749–62. PMID:22844968
**1494.** Nguyen B, Veys I, Leduc S, et al. Genomic, transcriptomic, epigenetic, and immune profiling of mucinous breast cancer. J Natl Cancer Inst. 2019 Feb 21;djz023. PMID:30789657
**1495.** Nguyen CV, Falcón-Escobedo R, Hunt KK, et al. Pleomorphic ductal carcinoma of the breast: predictors of decreased overall survival. Am J Surg Pathol. 2010 Apr;34(4):486–93. PMID:20154588
**1496.** Nguyen GK, Neifer R. Aspiration biopsy cytology of secretory carcinoma of the breast. Diagn Cytopathol. 1987 Sep;3(3):234–7. PMID:2822366
**1497.** Ni M, Chen Y, Lim E, et al. Targeting androgen receptor in estrogen receptor-negative breast cancer. Cancer Cell. 2011 Jul 12;20(1):119–31. PMID:21741601
**1498.** Ni Y, Zbuk KM, Sadler T, et al. Germline mutations and variants in the succinate dehydrogenase genes in Cowden and Cowden-like syndromes. Am J Hum Genet. 2008 Aug;83(2):261–8. PMID:18678321
**1499.** Ni YB, Tsang JYS, Shao MM, et al. GATA-3 is superior to GCDFP-15 and mammaglobin to identify primary and metastatic breast cancer. Breast Cancer Res Treat. 2018 May;169(1):25–32. PMID:29340880
**1500.** Nichols KE, Malkin D. Genotype versus phenotype: the yin and yang of germline TP53 mutations in Li-Fraumeni syndrome. J Clin Oncol. 2015 Jul 20;33(21):2331–3. PMID:26101242
**1501.** Nicholson S, Hanby A, Clements K, et al. Variations in the management of the axilla in screen-detected ductal carcinoma in situ: evidence from the UK NHS breast screening programme audit of screen detected DCIS. Eur J Surg Oncol. 2015 Jan;41(1):86–93. PMID:25441934
**1502.** Nicolas MM, Wu Y, Middleton LP, et al. Loss of myoepithelium is variable in solid papillary carcinoma of the breast. Histopathology. 2007 Nov;51(5):657–65. PMID:17927587
**1503.** Nicolis GL, Modlinger RS, Gabrilove JL. A study of the histopathology of human gynecomastia. J Clin Endocrinol Metab. 1971 Feb;32(2):173–8. PMID:5539033
**1504.** Niell B, Specht M, Gerade B, et al. Is excisional biopsy required after a breast core biopsy yields lobular neoplasia? AJR Am J Roentgenol. 2012 Oct;199(4):929–35. PMID:22997389
**1505.** Nielsen TO, Parker JS, Leung S, et al. A comparison of PAM50 intrinsic subtyping with immunohistochemistry and clinical prognostic factors in tamoxifen-treated estrogen receptor-positive breast cancer. Clin Cancer Res. 2010 Nov 1;16(21):5222–32. PMID:20837693
**1506.** Nigro DM, Organ CH Jr. Fibroadenoma of the female breast. Some epidemiologic surprises. Postgrad Med. 1976 May;59(5):113–7. PMID:177964
**1507.** Nik-Zainal S, Davies H, Staaf J, et al. Landscape of somatic mutations in 560 breast cancer whole-genome sequences. Nature. 2016 Jun 2;534(7605):47–54. PMID:27135926
**1508.** Nindrea RD, Harahap WA, Aryandono T, et al. Association of BRCA1 promoter methylation with breast cancer in Asia: a meta-analysis. Asian Pac J Cancer Prev. 2018 Apr 25;19(4):885–9. PMID:29693332
**1509.** Nishimura R, Tan PH, Thike AA, et al. Utility of the Singapore nomogram for predicting recurrence-free survival in Japanese women with breast phyllodes tumours. J Clin Pathol. 2014 Aug;67(8):748–50. PMID:24811489
**1510.** Nishizaki T, Chew K, Chu L, et al. Genetic alterations in lobular breast cancer by comparative genomic hybridization. Int J Cancer. 1997 Oct 21;74(5):513–7. PMID:9355973
**1511.** Nobukawa B, Fujii H, Hirai S, et al. Breast carcinoma diverging to aberrant melanocytic differentiation: a case report with histopathologic and loss of heterozygosity analyses. Am J Surg Pathol. 1999 Oct;23(10):1280–7. PMID:10524531
**1512.** Noel JC, Van Geertruyden J, Engohan-Aloghe C. Angiolipoma of the breast in a male: a case report and review of the literature. Int J Surg Pathol. 2011 Dec;19(6):813–6. PMID:20034977
**1513.** Noguchi S, Motomura K, Inaji H, et al. Clonal analysis of solitary intraductal papilloma of the breast by means of polymerase chain reaction. Am J Pathol. 1994 Jun;144(6):1320–5. PMID:7911274
**1514.** Noguchi S, Yokouchi H, Aihara T, et al. Progression of fibroadenoma to phyllodes tumor demonstrated by clonal analysis. Cancer. 1995 Nov 15;76(10):1779–85. PMID:8625047
**1515.** Nolan E, Savas P, Policheni AN, et al. Combined immune checkpoint blockade as a therapeutic strategy for BRCA1-mutated breast cancer. Sci Transl Med. 2017 Jun 7;9(393):eaal4922. PMID:28592566
**1516.** Nonaka D, Chiriboga L, Rubin BP. Sox10: a pan-schwannian and melanocytic marker. Am J Surg Pathol. 2008 Sep;32(9):1291–8. PMID:18636017
**1517.** Nonaka D, Chiriboga L, Soslow RA. Expression of Pax8 as a useful marker in distinguishing ovarian carcinomas from mammary carcinomas. Am J Surg Pathol. 2008 Oct;32(10):1566–71. PMID:18724243
**1518.** Nones K, Johnson J, Newell F, et al. Whole-genome sequencing reveals clinically relevant insights into the aetiology of familial breast cancers. Ann Oncol. 2019 May 15;mdz132. PMID:31090900
**1519.** Nordenskjöld A, Fohlin H, Fornander T, et al. Progesterone receptor positivity is a predictor of long-term benefit from adjuvant tamoxifen treatment of estrogen receptor positive breast cancer. Breast Cancer Res Treat. 2016 Nov;160(2):313–22. PMID:27722840
**1520.** Norris HJ, Taylor HB. Prognosis of mucinous (gelatinous) carcinoma of the breast. Cancer. 1965 Jul;18:879–85. PMID:14308235
**1521.** Northridge ME, Rhoads GG, Wartenberg D, et al. The importance of histologic type on breast cancer survival. J Clin Epidemiol. 1997 Mar;50(3):283–90. PMID:9120527
**1522.** Noske A, Schwabe M, Pahl S, et al. Report of a metaplastic carcinoma of the breast with multi-directional differentiation: an adenoid cystic carcinoma, a spindle cell carcinoma and melanoma. Virchows Arch. 2008 May;452(5):575–9. PMID:18283489
**1523.** Nuttall FQ, Warrier RS, Gannon MC. Gynecomastia and drugs: a critical evaluation of the literature. Eur J Clin Pharmacol. 2015 May;71(5):569–78. PMID:25827472
**1524.** Oakley GJ 3rd, Tubbs RR, Crowe J, et al. HER-2 amplification in tubular carcinoma of the breast. Am J Clin Pathol. 2006 Jul;126(1):55–8. PMID:16753605
**1525.** Oba T, Ono M, Iesato A, et al. Lipid-rich carcinoma of the breast that is strongly positive for estrogen receptor: a case report and literature review. Onco Targets Ther. 2016 Mar 18;9:1641–6. PMID:27051299
**1526.** Oberman HA. Hamartomas and hamartoma variants of the breast. Semin Diagn Pathol. 1989 May;6(2):135–45. PMID:2669070
**1527.** Oberman HA. Metaplastic carcinoma of the breast. A clinicopathologic study of 29 patients. Am J Surg Pathol. 1987 Dec;11(12):918–29. PMID:2825549
**1528.** Oberman HA. Secretory carcinoma of the breast in adults. Am J Surg Pathol. 1980 Oct;4(5):465–70. PMID:7435774
**1529.** Obiorah IE, Ozdemirli M. Myeloid sarcoma with megakaryoblastic differentiation presenting as a breast mass. Hematol Oncol Stem Cell Ther. 2018 Sep;11(3):178–82. PMID:29684340
**1530.** O'Connell P, Pekkel V, Fuqua SA, et al. Analysis of loss of heterozygosity in 399 premalignant breast lesions at 15 genetic loci. J Natl Cancer Inst. 1998 May 6;90(9):697–703. PMID:9586667
**1531.** O'Connor IF, Shembekar MV, Shousha S. Breast carcinoma developing in patients on hormone replacement therapy: a histological and immunohistological study. J Clin Pathol. 1998 Dec;51(12):935–8. PMID:10070338
**1532.** Odashiro AN, Odashiro Miiji LN, Odashiro DN, et al. Mammary myofibroblastoma: report of two cases with fine-needle aspiration cytology and review of the cytology literature. Diagn Cytopathol. 2004 Jun;30(6):406–10. PMID:15176028
**1534.** Ogwang MD, Bhatia K, Biggar RJ, et al. Incidence and geographic distribution of endemic Burkitt lymphoma in northern Uganda revisited. Int J Cancer. 2008 Dec 1;123(11):2658–63. PMID:18767045
**1535.** Oh M, McBride A, Yun S, et al. BRCA1 and BRCA2 gene mutations and colorectal cancer risk: systematic review and meta-analysis. J Natl Cancer Inst. 2018 Nov 1;110(11):1178–89. PMID:30380096
**1536.** Ohashi R, Matsubara M, Watarai Y, et al. Pleomorphic lobular carcinoma of the breast: a comparison of cytopathological features with other lobular carcinoma variants. Cytopathology. 2017 Apr;28(2):122–30. PMID:27489086
**1537.** Ohta M, Mori M, Kawada T, et al. Collagenous spherulosis associated with adenomyoepithelioma of the breast: a case report. Acta Cytol. 2010 May-Jun;54(3):314–8. PMID:20518417
**1538.** Ohtake T, Abe R, Kimijima I, et al. Intraductal extension of primary invasive breast carcinoma treated by breast-conservative surgery. Computer graphic three-dimensional reconstruction of the mammary duct-lobular systems. Cancer. 1995 Jul 1;76(1):32–45. PMID:8630874
**1539.** Ohuchi N. Breast-conserving surgery for invasive cancer: a principle based on segmental anatomy. Tohoku J Exp Med. 1999 Jun;188(2):103–18. PMID:10526872
**1540.** Ohuchi N, Abe R, Kasai M. Possible cancerous change of intraductal papillomas of the breast. A 3-D reconstruction study of 25 cases. Cancer. 1984 Aug 15;54(4):605–11. PMID:6331624
**1541.** Ohuchi N, Furuta A, Mori S. Management of ductal carcinoma in situ with nipple discharge. Intraductal spreading of carcinoma is an unfavorable pathologic factor for breast-conserving surgery. Cancer. 1994 Aug 15;74(4):1294–302. PMID:8055451
**1542.** Oishi N, Brody GS, Ketterling RP, et al. Genetic subtyping of breast implant-associated anaplastic large cell lymphoma. Blood. 2018 Aug 2;132(5):544–7. PMID:29921615
**1543.** Oiwa M, Endo T, Ichihara S, et al. Sclerosing adenosis as a predictor of breast cancer bilaterality and multicentricity. Virchows Arch. 2015 Jul;467(1):71–8. PMID:25838080
**1544.** Oka H, Shiozaki H, Kobayashi K, et al. Expression of E-cadherin cell adhesion molecules in human breast cancer tissues and its relationship to metastasis. Cancer Res. 1993 Apr 1;53(7):1696–701. PMID:8453644
**1545.** Okada K, Suzuki Y, Saito Y, et al. Two cases of ductal adenoma of the breast. Breast Cancer. 2006;13(4):354–9. PMID:17146162
**1546.** Oliveira C, Sousa S, Pinheiro H, et al. Quantification of epigenetic and genetic 2nd hits in CDH1 during hereditary diffuse gastric cancer syndrome progression. Gastroenterology. 2009 Jun;136(7):2137–48. PMID:19269290
**1547.** Olivier M, Goldgar DE, Sodha N, et al. Li-Fraumeni and related syndromes: correlation between tumor type, family structure, and TP53 genotype. Cancer Res. 2003 Oct 15;63(20):6643–50. PMID:14583457
**1548.** Olivier M, Hollstein M, Hainaut P. TP53 mutations in human cancers: origins, consequences, and clinical use. Cold Spring Harb Perspect Biol. 2010 Jan;2(1):a001008. PMID:20182602
**1549.** O'Malley FP, Bane A. An update on apocrine lesions of the breast. Histopathology. 2008 Jan;52(1):3–10. PMID:18171412
**1550.** O'Malley FP, Bane AL. The spectrum of apocrine lesions of the breast. Adv Anat Pathol. 2004 Jan;11(1):1–9. PMID:14676636
**1551.** O'Malley FP, Mohsin SK, Badve S, et al. Interobserver reproducibility in the diagnosis of flat epithelial atypia of the breast. Mod Pathol. 2006 Feb;19(2):172–9. PMID:16424892
**1552.** Omar L, Pfeifer CM, Kulkarni S, et al. Granular cell tumor in a premenstrual female breast. Clin Imaging. 2018 Nov-Dec;52:334–6. PMID:30241035
**1553.** O'Neil M, Madan R, Tawfik OW, et al. Lobular carcinoma in situ/atypical lobular

hyperplasia on breast needle biopsies: Does it warrant surgical excisional biopsy? A study of 27 cases. Ann Diagn Pathol. 2010 Aug;14(4):251–5. PMID:20637429
**1554.** Onnis A, De Falco G, Antonicelli G, et al. Alteration of microRNAs regulated by c-Myc in Burkitt lymphoma. PLoS One. 2010 Sep 24;5(9):e12960. PMID:20930934
**1555.** Ono M, Yoshikawa K, Yamaguchi T, et al. A case of breast cancer coexisting with florid papillomatosis of the nipple. Breast Cancer. 1998 Jun 30;5(1):87–91. PMID:11091632
**1556.** Organ CH Jr, Organ BC. Fibroadenoma of the female breast: a critical clinical assessment. J Natl Med Assoc. 1983 Jul;75(7):701–4. PMID:6887274
**1557.** Orguc S, Akin M, Aydogdu I, et al. Bilateral plasmacytoma of the breast. Breast J. 2018 Mar;24(2):210–1. PMID:28805290
**1558.** Orloff MS, Eng C. Genetic and phenotypic heterogeneity in the PTEN hamartoma tumour syndrome. Oncogene. 2008 Sep 18;27(41):5387–97. PMID:18794875
**1559.** Orr N, Dudbridge F, Dryden N, et al. Fine-mapping identifies two additional breast cancer susceptibility loci at 9q31.2. Hum Mol Genet. 2015 May 15;24(10):2966–84. PMID:25652398
**1560.** Orvieto E, Maiorano E, Bottiglieri L, et al. Clinicopathologic characteristics of invasive lobular carcinoma of the breast: results of an analysis of 530 cases from a single institution. Cancer. 2008 Oct 1;113(7):1511–20. PMID:18704988
**1561.** Orzalesi L, Casella D, Criscenti V, et al. Microinvasive breast cancer: pathological parameters, cancer subtypes distribution, and correlation with axillary lymph nodes invasion. Results of a large single-institution series. Breast Cancer. 2016 Jul;23(4):640–8. PMID:25981971
**1562.** Osborn G, Wilton F, Stevens G, et al. A review of needle core biopsy diagnosed radial scars in the Welsh Breast Screening Programme. Ann R Coll Surg Engl. 2011 Mar;93(2):123–6. PMID:21073820
**1563.** O'Shea R, Clarke R, Berkley E, et al. Next generation sequencing is informing phenotype: a TP53 example. Fam Cancer. 2018 Jan;17(1):123–8. PMID:28509937
**1564.** Oshida K, Miyauchi M, Yamamoto N, et al. Phyllodes tumor arising in ectopic breast tissue of the axilla. Breast Cancer. 2003;10(1):82–4. PMID:12525768
**1564A.** O'Sullivan CC, Swain SM. Pertuzumab: evolving therapeutic strategies in the management of HER2-overexpressing breast cancer. Expert Opin Biol Ther. 2013 May;13(5):779–90. PMID:23530718
**1565.** Otsuki Y, Yamada M, Shimizu S, et al. Solid-papillary carcinoma of the breast: clinicopathological study of 20 cases. Pathol Int. 2007 Jul;57(7):421–9. PMID:17587241
**1566.** Ozaki S, Mizukami Y, Kawahara E. Cytologic features of nipple adenoma: a report of four cases of adenoma of the nipple. Diagn Cytopathol. 2015 Aug;43(8):664–8. PMID:26011103
**1567.** Ozerdem U, McNiff JM, Tavassoli FA. Cytokeratin 7-negative mammary Paget's disease: a diagnostic pitfall. Pathol Res Pract. 2016 Apr;212(4):279–81. PMID:26944832
**1568.** Ozerdem U, Swistel A, Antonio LB, et al. Invasive Paget disease of the nipple: a brief review of the literature and report of the first case with axillary nodal metastases. Int J Surg Pathol. 2014 Sep;22(6):566–9. PMID:24583835
**1569.** Pacioles T, Seth R, Orellana C, et al. Malignant phyllodes tumor of the breast presenting with hypoglycemia: a case report and literature review. Cancer Manag Res. 2014 Dec 8;6:467–73. PMID:25525388
**1570.** Padmore RF, Lara JF, Ackerman DJ, et al. Primary combined malignant melanoma and ductal carcinoma of the breast. A report of two cases. Cancer. 1996 Dec 15;78(12):2515–25. PMID:8952560
**1571.** Pagani A, Sapino A, Eusebi V, et al. PIP/GCDFP-15 gene expression and apocrine differentiation in carcinomas of the breast. Virchows Arch. 1994;425(5):459–65. PMID:7850069
**1572.** Page DL. Apocrine carcinomas of the breast. Breast. 2005 Feb;14(1):1–2. PMID:15695073
**1573.** Page DL, Dixon JM, Anderson TJ, et al. Invasive cribriform carcinoma of the breast. Histopathology. 1983 Jul;7(4):525–36. PMID:6884999
**1574.** Page DL, Dupont WD, Rogers LW. Ductal involvement by cells of atypical lobular hyperplasia in the breast: a long-term follow-up study of cancer risk. Hum Pathol. 1988 Feb;19(2):201–7. PMID:3343034
**1575.** Page DL, Dupont WD, Rogers LW, et al. Atypical hyperplastic lesions of the female breast. A long-term follow-up study. Cancer. 1985 Jun 1;55(11):2698–708. PMID:2986821
**1576.** Page DL, Kidd TE Jr, Dupont WD, et al. Lobular neoplasia of the breast: higher risk for subsequent invasive cancer predicted by more extensive disease. Hum Pathol. 1991 Dec;22(12):1232–9. PMID:1748429
**1577.** Page DL, Salhany KE, Jensen RA, et al. Subsequent breast carcinoma risk after biopsy with atypia in a breast papilloma. Cancer. 1996 Jul 15;78(2):258–66. PMID:8674001
**1578.** Page DL, Schuyler PA, Dupont WD, et al. Atypical lobular hyperplasia as a unilateral predictor of breast cancer risk: a retrospective cohort study. Lancet. 2003 Jan 11;361(9352):125–9. PMID:12531579
**1579.** Paik S, Shak S, Tang G, et al. A multigene assay to predict recurrence of tamoxifen-treated, node-negative breast cancer. N Engl J Med. 2004 Dec 30;351(27):2817–26. PMID:15591335
**1580.** Paik S, Tang G, Shak S, et al. Gene expression and benefit of chemotherapy in women with node-negative, estrogen receptor-positive breast cancer. J Clin Oncol. 2006 Aug 10;24(23):3726–34. PMID:16720680
**1581.** Pailoor K, Fernandes H, Cs J, et al. Fine needle aspiration cytology of male breast lesions - a retrospective study over a six year period. J Clin Diagn Res. 2014 Oct;8(10):FC13–5. PMID:25478347
**1582.** Palacios J, Benito N, Pizarro A, et al. Anomalous expression of P-cadherin in breast carcinoma. Correlation with E-cadherin expression and pathological features. Am J Pathol. 1995 Mar;146(3):605–12. PMID:7534041
**1583.** Palacios J, Sarrió D, García-Macias MC, et al. Frequent E-cadherin gene inactivation by loss of heterozygosity in pleomorphic lobular carcinoma of the breast. Mod Pathol. 2003 Jul;16(7):674–8. PMID:12861063
**1584.** Palazzo JP, Hyslop T. Hyperplastic ductal and lobular lesions and carcinomas in situ of the breast: reproducibility of current diagnostic criteria among community- and academic-based pathologists. Breast J. 1998 Jul;4(4):230–7. PMID:21223441
**1585.** Palermo MH, Pinto MB, Zanetti JS, et al. Primary mucoepidermoid carcinoma of the breast: a case report with immunohistochemical analysis and comparison with salivary gland mucoepidermoid carcinomas. Pol J Pathol. 2013 Oct;64(3):210–5. PMID:24166608
**1586.** Paliogiannis P, Cossu A, Palmieri G, et al. Breast nodular fasciitis: a comprehensive review. Breast Care (Basel). 2016 Aug;11(4):270–4. PMID:27721715
**1587.** Palli D, Galli M, Bianchi S, et al. Reproducibility of histological diagnosis of breast lesions: results of a panel in Italy. Eur J Cancer. 1996 Apr;32A(4):603–7. PMID:8695260
**1588.** Pallis L, Wilking N, Cedermark B, et al. Receptors for estrogen and progesterone in breast carcinoma in situ. Anticancer Res. 1992 Nov-Dec;12 6B:2113–5. PMID:1295456
**1589.** Panagopoulos I, Gorunova L, Bjerkehagen B, et al. The recurrent chromosomal translocation t(12;18)(q14~15;q12~21) causes the fusion gene HMGA2-SETBP1 and HMGA2 expression in lipoma and osteochondrolipoma. Int J Oncol. 2015 Sep;47(3):884–90. PMID:26202160
**1590.** Panagopoulos I, Höglund M, Mertens F, et al. Fusion of the EWS and CHOP genes in myxoid liposarcoma. Oncogene. 1996 Feb 1;12(3):489–94. PMID:8637704
**1591.** Pang JM, Deb S, Takano EA, et al. Methylation profiling of ductal carcinoma in situ and its relationship to histopathological features. Breast Cancer Res. 2014 Oct 21;16(5):423. PMID:25331261
**1592.** Pang JM, Gorringe KL, Wong SQ, et al. Appraisal of the technologies and review of the genomic landscape of ductal carcinoma in situ of the breast. Breast Cancer Res. 2015 Jun 16;17:80. PMID:26078038
**1593.** Pant I, Kaur G, Joshi SC, et al. Myxoid liposarcoma of the breast in a 25-year-old female as a diagnostic pitfall in fine needle aspiration cytology: report of a rare case. Diagn Cytopathol. 2008 Sep;36(9):674–7. PMID:18677756
**1594.** Pantziarka P. Li Fraumeni syndrome, cancer and senescence: a new hypothesis. Cancer Cell Int. 2013 Apr 15;13(1):35. PMID:23587008
**1595.** Papachristou DN, Kinne D, Ashikari R, et al. Melanoma of the nipple and areola. Br J Surg. 1979 Apr;66(4):287–8. PMID:455001
**1596.** Papadatos G, Rangan AM, Psarianos T, et al. Probability of axillary node involvement in patients with tubular carcinoma of the breast. Br J Surg. 2001 Jun;88(6):860–4. PMID:11412259
**1597.** Papalas JA, Wylie JD, Dash RC. Recurrence risk and margin status in granular cell tumors of the breast: a clinicopathologic study of 13 patients. Arch Pathol Lab Med. 2011 Jul;135(7):890–5. PMID:21732779
**1598.** Pardoll DM. The blockade of immune checkpoints in cancer immunotherapy. Nat Rev Cancer. 2012 Mar 22;12(4):252–64. PMID:22437870
**1599.** Pareja F, Brandes AH, Basili T, et al. Loss-of-function mutations in ATP6AP1 and ATP6AP2 in granular cell tumors. Nat Commun. 2018 Aug 30;9(1):3533. PMID:30166553
**1600.** Pareja F, Corben AD, Brennan SB, et al. Breast intraductal papillomas without atypia in radiologic-pathologic concordant core-needle biopsies: rate of upgrade to carcinoma at excision. Cancer. 2016 Sep 15;122(18):2819–27. PMID:27315013
**1601.** Pareja F, Geyer FC, Kumar R, et al. Phyllodes tumors with and without fibroadenoma-like areas display distinct genomic features and may evolve through distinct pathways. NPJ Breast Cancer. 2017 Oct 12;3:40. PMID:29043292
**1602.** Pareja F, Lee JY, Brown DN, et al. The genomic landscape of mucinous breast cancer. J Natl Cancer Inst. 2019 Jul;111(7):737–41. PMID:30649385
**1603.** Parham DM, Fisher C. Angiosarcomas of the breast developing post radiotherapy. Histopathology. 1997 Aug;31(2):189–95. PMID:9279573
**1604.** Parise CA, Bauer KR, Caggiano V. Variation in breast cancer subtypes with age and race/ethnicity. Crit Rev Oncol Hematol. 2010 Oct;76(1):44–52. PMID:19800812
**1605.** Park B, Hopper JL, Win AK, et al. Reproductive factors as risk modifiers of breast cancer in BRCA mutation carriers and high-risk non-carriers. Oncotarget. 2017 Oct 31;8(60):102110–8. PMID:29254229
**1606.** Park JS, Lee ST, Han JW, et al. Difference in risk of breast and ovarian cancer according to putative functional domain regions in Korean BRCA1/2 mutation carriers. Clin Breast Cancer. 2018 Oct;18(5):362–373.e1. PMID:29673794
**1607.** Park S, Koo JS, Kim MS, et al. Characteristics and outcomes according to molecular subtypes of breast cancer as classified by a panel of four biomarkers using immunohistochemistry. Breast. 2012 Feb;21(1):50–7. PMID:21865043
**1608.** Parker JS, Mullins M, Cheang MC, et al. Supervised risk predictor of breast cancer based on intrinsic subtypes. J Clin Oncol. 2009 Mar 10;27(8):1160–7. PMID:19204204
**1609.** Pasquale-Styles MA, Milikowski C. Three-millimeter apocrine adenoma in a man: a case report and review of the literature. Arch Pathol Lab Med. 2003 Nov;127(11):1498–500. PMID:14567753
**1610.** Pasquali P, Freites-Martinez A, Fortuño A. Nipple adenoma: new images and cryosurgery treatment. Breast J. 2016 Sep;22(5):584–5. PMID:27345934
**1611.** Pastorello RG, D'Almeida Costa F, Osório CABT, et al. Breast implant-associated anaplastic large cell lymphoma in a Li-Fraumeni patient: a case report. Diagn Pathol. 2018 Jan 25;13(1):10. PMID:29370815
**1612.** Patel A, D'Alfonso T, Cheng E, et al. Sentinel lymph nodes in classic invasive lobular carcinoma of the breast: cytokeratin immunostain ensures detection, and precise determination of extent, of involvement. Am J Surg Pathol. 2017 Nov;41(11):1499–505. PMID:28877063
**1613.** Paterakos M, Watkin WG, Edgerton SM, et al. Invasive micropapillary carcinoma of the breast: a prognostic study. Hum Pathol. 1999 Dec;30(12):1459–63. PMID:10667424
**1614.** Pathmanathan N, Renthawa J, French JR, et al. Intraoperative sentinel lymph node assessment in breast cancer: a comparison of rapid diagnostic method based on CK19 mRNA expression and imprint cytology. ANZ J Surg. 2014 Oct;84(10):730–4. PMID:24899463
**1615.** Patil T, Bernard B. Complications of androgen deprivation therapy in men with prostate cancer. Oncology (Williston Park). 2018 Sep 15;32(9):470–4, CV3. PMID:30248169
**1616.** Patton KT, Deyrup AT, Weiss SW. Atypical vascular lesions after surgery and radiation of the breast: a clinicopathologic study of 32 cases analyzing histologic heterogeneity and association with angiosarcoma. Am J Surg Pathol. 2008 Jun;32(6):943–50. PMID:18551753
**1617.** Patwardhan UM, Vu MT, Soballe PW. Multiple schwannomas in a patient with gynecomastia. Breast J. 2017 May;23(3):360–2. PMID:27988983
**1618.** Patzelt M, Zarubova L, Klener P, et al. Anaplastic large-cell lymphoma associated with breast implants: a case report of a transgender female. Aesthetic Plast Surg. 2018 Apr;42(2):451–5. PMID:29101436
**1619.** Paul Wright G, Davis AT, Koehler TJ, et al. Hormone receptor status does not affect prognosis in metaplastic breast cancer: a population-based analysis with comparison to infiltrating ductal and lobular carcinomas. Ann Surg Oncol. 2014 Oct;21(11):3497–503. PMID:24838367
**1620.** Pauwels P, Sciot R, Croiset F, et al.

Myofibroblastoma of the breast: genetic link with spindle cell lipoma. J Pathol. 2000 Jul;191(3):282–5. PMID:10878550
**1621.** Peiro G, Bornstein BA, Connolly JL, et al. The influence of infiltrating lobular carcinoma on the outcome of patients treated with breast-conserving surgery and radiation therapy. Breast Cancer Res Treat. 2000 Jan;59(1):49–54. PMID:10752679
**1622.** Peña A, Shah SS, Fazzio RT, et al. Multivariate model to identify women at low risk of cancer upgrade after a core needle biopsy diagnosis of atypical ductal hyperplasia. Breast Cancer Res Treat. 2017 Jul;164(2):295–304. PMID:28474262
**1623.** Penault-Llorca F, Radosevic-Robin N. Biomarkers of residual disease after neoadjuvant therapy for breast cancer. Nat Rev Clin Oncol. 2016 Aug;13(8):487–503. PMID:26856744
**1624.** Penkert J, Schmidt G, Hofmann W, et al. Breast cancer patients suggestive of Li-Fraumeni syndrome: mutational spectrum, candidate genes, and unexplained heredity. Breast Cancer Res. 2018 Aug 7;20(1):87. PMID:30086788
**1625.** Pereira B, Chin SF, Rueda OM, et al. The somatic mutation profiles of 2,433 breast cancers refines their genomic and transcriptomic landscapes. Nat Commun. 2016 May 10;7:11479. PMID:27161491
**1626.** Pereira H, Pinder SE, Sibbering DM, et al. Pathological prognostic factors in breast cancer. IV: Should you be a typer or a grader? A comparative study of two histological prognostic features in operable breast carcinoma. Histopathology. 1995 Sep;27(3):219–26. PMID:8522285
**1626A.** Perez AA, Balabram D, Salles Mde A, et al. Ductal carcinoma in situ of the breast: correlation between histopathological features and age of patients. Diagn Pathol. 2014 Dec 3;9:227. PMID:25471940
**1627.** Perez EA, Romond EH, Suman VJ, et al. Trastuzumab plus adjuvant chemotherapy for human epidermal growth factor receptor 2-positive breast cancer: planned joint analysis of overall survival from NSABP B-31 and NCCTG N9831. J Clin Oncol. 2014 Nov 20;32(33):3744–52. PMID:25332249
**1628.** Perez-Montiel MD, Plaza JA, Dominguez-Malagon H, et al. Differential expression of smooth muscle myosin, smooth muscle actin, h-caldesmon, and calponin in the diagnosis of myofibroblastic and smooth muscle lesions of skin and soft tissue. Am J Dermatopathol. 2006 Apr;28(2):105–11. PMID:16625070
**1629.** Perlman S, Becker-Catania S, Gatti RA. Ataxia-telangiectasia: diagnosis and treatment. Semin Pediatr Neurol. 2003 Sep;10(3):173–82. PMID:14653405
**1630.** Perou CM, Sørlie T, Eisen MB, et al. Molecular portraits of human breast tumours. Nature. 2000 Aug 17;406(6797):747–52. PMID:10963602
**1631.** Perry A, Roth KA, Banerjee R, et al. NF1 deletions in S-100 protein-positive and negative cells of sporadic and neurofibromatosis 1 (NF1)-associated plexiform neurofibromas and malignant peripheral nerve sheath tumors. Am J Pathol. 2001 Jul;159(1):57–61. PMID:11438454
**1632.** Persson F, Andrén Y, Winnes M, et al. High-resolution genomic profiling of adenomas and carcinomas of the salivary glands reveals amplification, rearrangement, and fusion of HMGA2. Genes Chromosomes Cancer. 2009 Jan;48(1):69–82. PMID:18828159
**1633.** Pestalozzi BC, Zahrieh D, Mallon E, et al. Distinct clinical and prognostic features of infiltrating lobular carcinoma of the breast: combined results of 15 International Breast Cancer Study Group clinical trials. J Clin Oncol. 2008 Jun 20;26(18):3006–14. PMID:18458044
**1634.** Peters GN, Wolff M, Haagensen CD. Tubular carcinoma of the breast. Clinical pathologic correlations based on 100 cases. Ann Surg. 1981 Feb;193(2):138–49. PMID:7469549
**1635.** Petersson F, Ivan D, Kazakov DV, et al. Pigmented Paget disease–a diagnostic pitfall mimicking melanoma. Am J Dermatopathol. 2009 May;31(3):223–6. PMID:19384061
**1636.** Petersson F, Pang B, Thamboo TP, et al. Mucinous cystadenocarcinoma of the breast with amplification of the HER2-gene confirmed by FISH: the first case reported. Hum Pathol. 2010 Jun;41(6):910–3. PMID:20338619
**1637.** Petrelli F, Barni S. Response to neoadjuvant chemotherapy in ductal compared to lobular carcinoma of the breast: a meta-analysis of published trials including 1,764 lobular breast cancer. Breast Cancer Res Treat. 2013 Nov;142(2):227–35. PMID:24177758
**1638.** Petridis C, Brook MN, Shah V, et al. Genetic predisposition to ductal carcinoma in situ of the breast. Breast Cancer Res. 2016 Feb 17;18(1):22. PMID:26884359
**1639.** Petridis C, Shinomiya I, Kohut K, et al. Germline CDH1 mutations in bilateral lobular carcinoma in situ. Br J Cancer. 2014 Feb 18;110(4):1053–7. PMID:24366306
**1640.** Pettinato G, Manivel CJ, Panico L, et al. Invasive micropapillary carcinoma of the breast: clinicopathologic study of 62 cases of a poorly recognized variant with highly aggressive behavior. Am J Clin Pathol. 2004 Jun;121(6):857–66. PMID:15198358
**1641.** Pétursson HI, Kovács A, Mattsson J, et al. Evaluation of intraoperative touch imprint cytology on axillary sentinel lymph nodes in invasive breast carcinomas, a retrospective study of 1227 patients comparing sensitivity in the different tumor subtypes. PLoS One. 2018 Apr 12;13(4):e0195560. PMID:29649327
**1642.** Pfaff CL, Parra EJ, Bonilla C, et al. Population structure in admixed populations: effect of admixture dynamics on the pattern of linkage disequilibrium. Am J Hum Genet. 2001 Jan;68(1):198–207. PMID:11112661
**1643.** Philip J, Harris WG, Rustage JH. Radiography of breast biopsy specimens. Br J Surg. 1982 Mar;69(3):126–7. PMID:7066650
**1644.** Phillips SR, A'Hern R, Thomas JM. Aggressive fibromatosis of the abdominal wall, limbs and limb girdles. Br J Surg. 2004 Dec;91(12):1624–9. PMID:15505878
**1645.** Philpott C, Tovell H, Frayling IM, et al. The NF1 somatic mutational landscape in sporadic human cancers. Hum Genomics. 2017 Jun 21;11(1):13. PMID:28637487
**1646.** Piccaluga PP, De Falco G, Kustagi M, et al. Gene expression analysis uncovers similarity and differences among Burkitt lymphoma subtypes. Blood. 2011 Mar 31;117(13):3596–608. PMID:21245480
**1647.** Piccaluga PP, Navari M, De Falco G, et al. Virus-encoded microRNA contributes to the molecular profile of EBV-positive Burkitt lymphomas. Oncotarget. 2016 Jan 5;7(1):224–40. PMID:26325594
**1648.** Pickett JL, Chou A, Andrici JA, et al. Inflammatory myofibroblastic tumors of the female genital tract are under-recognized: a low threshold for ALK immunohistochemistry is required. Am J Surg Pathol. 2017 Oct;41(10):1433–42. PMID:28731868
**1649.** Picouleau E, Denis M, Lavoue V, et al. Atypical hyperplasia of the breast: the black hole of routine breast cancer screening. Anticancer Res. 2012 Dec;32(12):5441–6. PMID:23225449
**1650.** Pilarski R, Burt R, Kohlman W, et al. Cowden syndrome and the PTEN hamartoma tumor syndrome: systematic review and revised diagnostic criteria. J Natl Cancer Inst. 2013 Nov 6;105(21):1607–16. PMID:24136893
**1651.** Pimiento JM, Gadgil PV, Santillan AA, et al. Phyllodes tumors: race-related differences. J Am Coll Surg. 2011 Oct;213(4):537–42. PMID:21856184
**1652.** Pinder SE, Reis-Filho JS. Non-operative breast pathology: columnar cell lesions. J Clin Pathol. 2007 Dec;60(12):1307–12. PMID:17182657
**1653.** Pirie A, Guo Q, Kraft P, et al. Common germline polymorphisms associated with breast cancer-specific survival. Breast Cancer Res. 2015 Apr 22;17:58. PMID:25897948
**1654.** Pisano ED, Fajardo LL, Tsimikas J, et al. Rate of insufficient samples for fine-needle aspiration for nonpalpable breast lesions in a multicenter clinical trial: the Radiologic Diagnostic Oncology Group 5 Study. The RDOG5 investigators. Cancer. 1998 Feb 15;82(4):679–88. PMID:9477100
**1655.** Piscuoglio S, Geyer FC, Burke KA, et al. Massively parallel sequencing analysis of synchronous fibroepithelial lesions supports the concept of progression from fibroadenoma to phyllodes tumor. NPJ Breast Cancer. 2016 Nov 16;2:16035. PMID:28721388
**1656.** Piscuoglio S, Hodi Z, Katabi N, et al. Are acinic cell carcinomas of the breast and salivary glands distinct diseases? Histopathology. 2015 Oct;67(4):529–37. PMID:25688711
**1657.** Piscuoglio S, Murray M, Fusco N, et al. MED12 somatic mutations in fibroadenomas and phyllodes tumours of the breast. Histopathology. 2015 Nov;67(5):719–29. PMID:25855048
**1658.** Piscuoglio S, Ng CK, Martelotto LG, et al. Integrative genomic and transcriptomic characterization of papillary carcinomas of the breast. Mol Oncol. 2014 Dec;8(8):1588–602. PMID:25041824
**1659.** Piscuoglio S, Ng CK, Murray M, et al. Massively parallel sequencing of phyllodes tumours of the breast reveals actionable mutations, and TERT promoter hotspot mutations and TERT gene amplification as likely drivers of progression. J Pathol. 2016 Mar;238(4):508–18. PMID:26832993
**1660.** Piscuoglio S, Ng CK, Murray MP, et al. The genomic landscape of male breast cancers. Clin Cancer Res. 2016 Aug 15;22(16):4045–56. PMID:26960396
**1661.** Piscuoglio S, Ng CKY, Geyer FC, et al. Genomic and transcriptomic heterogeneity in metaplastic carcinomas of the breast. NPJ Breast Cancer. 2017 Dec 1;3:48. PMID:29214215
**1662.** Pitanguy I, Torres E, Salgado F, et al. Breast pathology and reduction mammaplasty. Plast Reconstr Surg. 2005 Mar;115(3):729–34, discussion 735. PMID:15731670
**1663.** Pitino A, Squillaci S, Spairani C, et al. Tall cell variant of papillary breast carcinoma: an additional case with review of the literature. Pathologica. 2017 Sep;109(3):162–7. PMID:29154377
**1664.** Podetta M, D'Ambrosio G, Ferrari A, et al. Low-grade fibromatosis-like spindle cell metaplastic carcinoma: a basal-like tumor with a favorable clinical outcome. Report of two cases. Tumori. 2009 Mar-Apr;95(2):264–7. PMID:19579879
**1665.** Poling JS, Yonescu R, Subhawong AP, et al. MYB labeling by immunohistochemistry is more sensitive and specific for breast adenoid cystic carcinoma than MYB labeling by FISH. Am J Surg Pathol. 2017 Jul;41(7):973–9. PMID:28498281
**1666.** Popnikolov NK, Cavone SM, Schultz PM, et al. Diagnostic utility of p75 neurotrophin receptor (p75NTR) as a marker of breast myoepithelial cells. Mod Pathol. 2005 Dec;18(12):1535–41. PMID:16258511
**1667.** Porter PL, Garcia R, Moe R, et al. C-erbB-2 oncogene protein in in situ and invasive lobular breast neoplasia. Cancer. 1991 Jul 15;68(2):331–4. PMID:1676930
**1668.** Posner MC, Shiu MH, Newsome JL, et al. The desmoid tumor. Not a benign disease. Arch Surg. 1989 Feb;124(2):191–6. PMID:2916941
**1669.** Pouysségur J, Pastan I. Mutants of mouse fibroblasts altered in the synthesis of cell surface glycoproteins. Preliminary evidence for a defect in the acetylation of glucosamine 6-phosphate. J Biol Chem. 1977 Mar 10;252(5):1639–46. PMID:838733
**1670.** Powell CM, Cranor ML, Rosen PP. Multinucleated stromal giant cells in mammary fibroepithelial neoplasms. A study of 11 patients. Arch Pathol Lab Med. 1994 Sep;118(9):912–6. PMID:8080361
**1671.** Powell CM, Cranor ML, Rosen PP. Pseudoangiomatous stromal hyperplasia (PASH). A mammary stromal tumor with myofibroblastic differentiation. Am J Surg Pathol. 1995 Mar;19(3):270–7. PMID:7872425
**1672.** Powell CM, Rosen PP. Adipose differentiation in cystosarcoma phyllodes. A study of 14 cases. Am J Surg Pathol. 1994 Jul;18(7):720–7. PMID:8017566
**1673.** Prasad ML, Osborne MP, Giri DD, et al. Microinvasive carcinoma (T1mic) of the breast: clinicopathologic profile of 21 cases. Am J Surg Pathol. 2000 Mar;24(3):422–8. PMID:10716157
**1674.** Prat A, Parker JS, Karginova O, et al. Phenotypic and molecular characterization of the claudin-low intrinsic subtype of breast cancer. Breast Cancer Res. 2010;12(5):R68. PMID:20813035
**1675.** Prescott RJ, Eyden BP, Reeve NL. Sebaceous differentiation in a breast carcinoma with ductal, myoepithelial and squamous elements. Histopathology. 1992 Aug;21(2):181–4. PMID:1324221
**1676.** Pritzlaff M, Summerour P, McFarland R, et al. Male breast cancer in a multi-gene panel testing cohort: insights and unexpected results. Breast Cancer Res Treat. 2017 Feb;161(3):575–86. PMID:28008555
**1677.** Provenzano E, Bossuyt V, Viale G, et al. Standardization of pathologic evaluation and reporting of postneoadjuvant specimens in clinical trials of breast cancer: recommendations from an international working group. Mod Pathol. 2015 Sep;28(9):1185–201. PMID:26205180
**1678.** Pruneri G, Masullo M, Renne G, et al. Follicular dendritic cell sarcoma of the breast. Virchows Arch. 2002 Aug;441(2):194–9. PMID:12189511
**1679.** Puri S, Mohindroo S, Gulati A. Collagenous spherulosis: an interesting cytological finding in breast lesion. Cytojournal. 2015 Nov 30;12:25. PMID:26681973
**1680.** Purrington KS, Visscher DW, Wang C, et al. Genes associated with histopathologic features of triple negative breast tumors predict molecular subtypes. Breast Cancer Res Treat. 2016 May;157(1):117–31. PMID:27083182
**1681.** Qian F, Wang S, Mitchell J, et al. Height and body mass index as modifiers of breast cancer risk in BRCA1/2 mutation carriers: a Mendelian randomization study. J Natl Cancer Inst. 2019 Apr 1;111(4):350–64. PMID:30312457
**1682.** Quesada AE, Medeiros LJ, Clemens MW, et al. Breast implant-associated anaplastic large cell lymphoma: a review. Mod Pathol. 2019 Feb;32(2):166–88. PMID:30206414
**1683.** Quincey C, Raitt N, Bell J, et al. Intracytoplasmic lumina–a useful diagnostic feature of adenocarcinomas. Histopathology. 1991 Jul;19(1):83–7. PMID:1916690

1684. Quinn CM, Ostrowski JL. Cytological and architectural heterogeneity in ductal carcinoma in situ of the breast. J Clin Pathol. 1997 Jul;50(7):596–9. PMID:9306942

1685. Rabban JT, Sgroi DC. Sclerosing lesions of the breast. Semin Diagn Pathol. 2004 Feb;21(1):42–7. PMID:15074558

1686. Rabban JT, Swain RS, Zaloudek CJ, et al. Immunophenotypic overlap between adenoid cystic carcinoma and collagenous spherulosis of the breast: potential diagnostic pitfalls using myoepithelial markers. Mod Pathol. 2006 Oct;19(10):1351–7. PMID:16810311

1687. Rabbitts TH, Forster A, Larson R, et al. Fusion of the dominant negative transcription regulator CHOP with a novel gene FUS by translocation t(12;16) in malignant liposarcoma. Nat Genet. 1993 Jun;4(2):175–80. PMID:7503811

1688. Racz JM, Degnim AC. When does atypical ductal hyperplasia require surgical excision? Surg Oncol Clin N Am. 2018 Jan;27(1):23–32. PMID:29132563

1689. Radhi JM. Immunohistochemical analysis of pleomorphic lobular carcinoma: higher expression of p53 and chromogranin and lower expression of ER and PgR. Histopathology. 2000 Feb;36(2):156–60. PMID:10672061

1690. Ragazzi M, de Biase D, Betts CM, et al. Oncocytic carcinoma of the breast: frequency, morphology and follow-up. Hum Pathol. 2011 Feb;42(2):166–75. PMID:21111455

1691. Rageth CJ, O'Flynn EA, Comstock C, et al. First International Consensus Conference on lesions of uncertain malignant potential in the breast (B3 lesions). Breast Cancer Res Treat. 2016 Sep;159(2):203–13. PMID:27522516

1692. Rageth CJ, Rubenov R, Bronz C, et al. Atypical ductal hyperplasia and the risk of underestimation: tissue sampling method, multifocality, and associated calcification significantly influence the diagnostic upgrade rate based on subsequent surgical specimens. Breast Cancer. 2019 Jul;26(4):452–8. PMID:30591993

1693. Rahman N, Seal S, Thompson D, et al. PALB2, which encodes a BRCA2-interacting protein, is a breast cancer susceptibility gene. Nat Genet. 2007 Feb;39(2):165–7. PMID:17200668

1694. Rahmani S, Turton P, Shaaban A, et al. Overview of gynecomastia in the modern era and the Leeds Gynaecomastia Investigation algorithm. Breast J. 2011 May-Jun;17(3):246–55. PMID:21477170

1695. Rainey JJ, Omenah D, Sumba PO, et al. Spatial clustering of endemic Burkitt's lymphoma in high-risk regions of Kenya. Int J Cancer. 2007 Jan 1;120(1):121–7. PMID:17019706

1696. Raj SD, Sahani VG, Adrada BE, et al. Pseudoangiomatous stromal hyperplasia of the breast: multimodality review with pathologic correlation. Curr Probl Diagn Radiol. 2017 Mar-Apr;46(2):130–5. PMID:26949063

1697. Rakha EA, Aleskandarany M, El-Sayed ME, et al. The prognostic significance of inflammation and medullary histological type in invasive carcinoma of the breast. Eur J Cancer. 2009 Jul;45(10):1780–7. PMID:19286369

1698. Rakha EA, Aleskandarany MA, Lee AH, et al. An approach to the diagnosis of spindle cell lesions of the breast. Histopathology. 2016 Jan;68(1):33–44. PMID:26768028

1699. Rakha EA, Aleskandarany MA, Samaka RM, et al. Pleomorphic adenoma-like tumour of the breast. Histopathology. 2016 Feb;68(3):405–10. PMID:26096183

1700. Rakha EA, Badve S, Eusebi V, et al. Breast lesions of uncertain malignant nature and limited metastatic potential: proposals to improve their recognition and clinical management. Histopathology. 2016 Jan;68(1):45–56. PMID:26348644

1701. Rakha EA, Coimbra ND, Hodi Z, et al. Immunoprofile of metaplastic carcinomas of the breast. Histopathology. 2017 May;70(6):975–85. PMID:28029685

1702. Rakha EA, El-Sayed ME, Green AR, et al. Prognostic markers in triple-negative breast cancer. Cancer. 2007 Jan 1;109(1):25–32. PMID:17146782

1703. Rakha EA, El-Sayed ME, Lee AH, et al. Prognostic significance of Nottingham histologic grade in invasive breast carcinoma. J Clin Oncol. 2008 Jul 1;26(19):3153–8. PMID:18490649

1704. Rakha EA, El-Sayed ME, Menon S, et al. Histologic grading is an independent prognostic factor in invasive lobular carcinoma of the breast. Breast Cancer Res Treat. 2008 Sep;111(1):121–7. PMID:17929165

1705. Rakha EA, El-Sayed ME, Powe DG, et al. Invasive lobular carcinoma of the breast: response to hormonal therapy and outcomes. Eur J Cancer. 2008 Jan;44(1):73–83. PMID:18035533

1706. Rakha EA, Gandhi N, Climent F, et al. Encapsulated papillary carcinoma of the breast: an invasive tumor with excellent prognosis. Am J Surg Pathol. 2011 Aug;35(8):1093–103. PMID:21753694

1707. Rakha EA, Ho BC, Naik V, et al. Outcome of breast lesions diagnosed as lesion of uncertain malignant potential (B3) or suspicious of malignancy (B4) on needle core biopsy, including detailed review of epithelial atypia. Histopathology. 2011 Mar;58(4):626–32. PMID:21371081

1708. Rakha EA, Lee AH, Evans AJ, et al. Tubular carcinoma of the breast: further evidence to support its excellent prognosis. J Clin Oncol. 2010 Jan 1;28(1):99–104. PMID:19917872

1709. Rakha EA, Lee AH, Jenkins JA, et al. Characterization and outcome of breast needle core biopsy diagnoses of lesions of uncertain malignant potential (B3) in abnormalities detected by mammographic screening. Int J Cancer. 2011 Sep 15;129(6):1417–24. PMID:21128240

1710. Rakha EA, Martin S, Lee AH, et al. The prognostic significance of lymphovascular invasion in invasive breast carcinoma. Cancer. 2012 Aug 1;118(15):3670–80. PMID:22180017

1711. Rakha EA, Miligy IM, Gorringe KL, et al. Invasion in breast lesions: the role of the epithelial-stroma barrier. Histopathology. 2018 Jun;72(7):1075–83. PMID:29197112

1712. Rakha EA, Patel A, Powe DG, et al. Clinical and biological significance of E-cadherin protein expression in invasive lobular carcinoma of the breast. Am J Surg Pathol. 2010 Oct;34(10):1472–9. PMID:20871222

1713. Rakha EA, Putti TC, Abd El-Rehim DM, et al. Morphological and immunophenotypic analysis of breast carcinomas with basal and myoepithelial differentiation. J Pathol. 2006 Mar;208(4):495–506. PMID:16429394

1714. Rakha EA, Reis-Filho JS, Baehner F, et al. Breast cancer prognostic classification in the molecular era: the role of histological grade. Breast Cancer Res. 2010;12(4):207. PMID:20804570

1715. Rakha EA, Shaaban AM, Haider SA, et al. Outcome of pure mucocele-like lesions diagnosed on breast core biopsy. Histopathology. 2013 May;62(6):894–8. PMID:23402386

1716. Rakha EA, Tan PH, Varga Z, et al. Prognostic factors in metaplastic carcinoma of the breast: a multi-institutional study. Br J Cancer. 2015 Jan 20;112(2):283–9. PMID:25422911

1717. Rakha EA, van Deurzen CH, Paish EC, et al. Pleomorphic lobular carcinoma of the breast: Is it a prognostically significant pathological subtype independent of histological grade? Mod Pathol. 2013 Apr;26(4):496–501. PMID:23238630

1718. Rakha EA, Varga Z, Elsheik S, et al. High-grade encapsulated papillary carcinoma of the breast: an under-recognized entity. Histopathology. 2015 Apr;66(5):740–6. PMID:25382726

1719. Ramachandra S, Machin L, Ashley S, et al. Immunohistochemical distribution of c-erbB-2 in in situ breast carcinoma–a detailed morphological analysis. J Pathol. 1990 May;161(1):7–14. PMID:1973459

1720. Ramljak V, Sarcević B, Vrdoljak DV, et al. Fine needle aspiration cytology in diagnosing rare breast carcinoma–two case reports. Coll Antropol. 2010 Mar;34(1):201–5. PMID:20432752

1721. Ranade A, Batra R, Sandhu G, et al. Clinicopathological evaluation of 100 cases of mucinous carcinoma of breast with emphasis on axillary staging and special reference to a micropapillary pattern. J Clin Pathol. 2010 Dec;63(12):1043–7. PMID:20962055

1722. Rao P, Lahat G, Arnold C, et al. Angiosarcoma: a tissue microarray study with diagnostic implications. Am J Dermatopathol. 2013 Jun;35(4):432–7. PMID:23689692

1723. Rao P, Shousha S. Male nipple adenoma with DCIS followed 9 years later by invasive carcinoma. Breast J. 2010 May-Jun;16(3):317–8. PMID:20408826

1724. Rao VK, Weiss SW. Angiomatosis of soft tissue. An analysis of the histologic features and clinical outcome in 51 cases. Am J Surg Pathol. 1992 Aug;16(8):764–71. PMID:1497117

1725. Raphael M, Gentilhomme O, Tulliez M, et al. Histopathologic features of high-grade non-Hodgkin's lymphomas in acquired immunodeficiency syndrome. Arch Pathol Lab Med. 1991 Jan;115(1):15–20. PMID:1987908

1726. Rasbridge SA, Gillett CE, Sampson SA, et al. Epithelial (E-) and placental (P-) cadherin cell adhesion molecule expression in breast carcinoma. J Pathol. 1993 Feb;169(2):245–50. PMID:8383197

1727. Rasbridge SA, Millis RR. Adenomyoepithelioma of the breast with malignant features. Virchows Arch. 1998 Feb;432(2):123–30. PMID:9504856

1728. Rasmussen BB, Rose C, Christensen IB. Prognostic factors in primary mucinous breast carcinoma. Am J Clin Pathol. 1987 Feb;87(2):155–60. PMID:3028120

1729. Rasmussen BB, Rose C, Thorpe SM, et al. Argyrophilic cells in 202 human mucinous breast carcinomas. Relation to histopathologic and clinical factors. Am J Clin Pathol. 1985 Dec;84(6):737–40. PMID:2416216

1730. Rathod J, Taori K, Disawal A, et al. A rare case of male primary breast lymphoma. J Breast Cancer. 2011 Dec;14(4):333–6. PMID:22323922

1731. Raut CP, Miceli R, Strauss DC, et al. External validation of a multi-institutional retroperitoneal sarcoma nomogram. Cancer. 2016 May 1;122(9):1417–24. PMID:26916507

1732. Rebbeck TR, Friebel TM, Friedman E, et al. Mutational spectrum in a worldwide study of 29,700 families with BRCA1 or BRCA2 mutations. Hum Mutat. 2018 May;39(5):593–620. PMID:29446198

1733. Rebbeck TR, Mitra N, Wan F, et al. Association of type and location of BRCA1 and BRCA2 mutations with risk of breast and ovarian cancer. JAMA. 2015 Apr 7;313(13):1347–61. PMID:25849179

1734. Recine MA, Deavers MT, Middleton LP, et al. Serous carcinoma of the ovary and peritoneum with metastases to the breast and axillary lymph nodes: a potential pitfall. Am J Surg Pathol. 2004 Dec;28(12):1646–51. PMID:15577686

1735. Reeves GK, Beral V, Green J, et al. Hormonal therapy for menopause and breast-cancer risk by histological type: a cohort study and meta-analysis. Lancet Oncol. 2006 Nov;7(11):910–8. PMID:17081916

1736. Reeves GK, Pirie K, Green J, et al. Reproductive factors and specific histological types of breast cancer: prospective study and meta-analysis. Br J Cancer. 2009 Feb 10;100(3):538–44. PMID:19190634

1737. Regan MM, Francis PA, Pagani O, et al. Absolute benefit of adjuvant endocrine therapies for premenopausal women with hormone receptor-positive, human epidermal growth factor receptor 2-negative early breast cancer: TEXT and SOFT trials. J Clin Oncol. 2016 Jul 1;34(19):2221–31. PMID:27044936

1738. Reid S, Schindler D, Hanenberg H, et al. Biallelic mutations in PALB2 cause Fanconi anemia subtype FA-N and predispose to childhood cancer. Nat Genet. 2007 Feb;39(2):162–4. PMID:17200671

1739. Reinhardt F, Mathys B, Reinecke P, et al. Magnetic resonance imaging findings of high-grade ductal carcinoma in situ of the male breast: a case report. SAGE Open Med Case Rep. 2018 Jun 12;6:X18781727. PMID:29977557

1740. Reis-Filho JS, Faoro LN, Gasparetto EL, et al. Mammary epithelioid myofibroblastoma arising in bilateral gynecomastia: case report with immunohistochemical profile. Int J Surg Pathol. 2001 Oct;9(4):331–4. PMID:12574852

1741. Reis-Filho JS, Fulford LG, Crebassa B, et al. Collagenous spherulosis in an adenomyoepithelioma of the breast. J Clin Pathol. 2004 Jan;57(1):83–6. PMID:14693844

1742. Reis-Filho JS, Fulford LG, Lakhani SR, et al. Pathologic quiz case: a 62-year-old woman with a 4.5-cm nodule in the right breast. Lipid-rich breast carcinoma. Arch Pathol Lab Med. 2003 Sep;127(9):e396–8. PMID:12951994

1743. Reis-Filho JS, Lakhani SR. The diagnosis and management of pre-invasive breast disease: genetic alterations in pre-invasive lesions. Breast Cancer Res. 2003;5(6):313–9. PMID:14580249

1744. Reis-Filho JS, Milanezi F, Carvalho S, et al. Metaplastic breast carcinomas exhibit EGFR, but not HER2, gene amplification and overexpression: immunohistochemical and chromogenic in situ hybridization analysis. Breast Cancer Res. 2005;7(6):R1028–35. PMID:16280056

1745. Reis-Filho JS, Milanezi F, Steele D, et al. Metaplastic breast carcinomas are basal-like tumours. Histopathology. 2006 Jul;49(1):10–21. PMID:16842242

1746. Reis-Filho JS, Natrajan R, Vatcheva R, et al. Is acinic cell carcinoma a variant of secretory carcinoma? A FISH study using ETV6 'split apart' probes. Histopathology. 2008 Jun;52(7):840–6. PMID:18462362

1747. Reis-Filho JS, Pinheiro C, Lambros MB, et al. EGFR amplification and lack of activating mutations in metaplastic breast carcinomas. J Pathol. 2006 Aug;209(4):445–53. PMID:16739104

1748. Reis-Filho JS, Simpson PT, Jones C, et al. Pleomorphic lobular carcinoma of the breast: role of comprehensive molecular pathology in characterization of an entity. J Pathol. 2005 Sep;207(1):1–13. PMID:15957152

1749. Rekhtman N, Pietanza MC, Hellmann MD, et al. Next-generation sequencing of pulmonary large cell neuroendocrine carcinoma reveals small cell carcinoma-like and non-small cell carcinoma-like subsets. Clin Cancer Res.

2016 Jul 15;22(14):3618–29. PMID:26960398
**1750.** Renault AL, Mebirouk N, Fuhrmann L, et al. Morphology and genomic hallmarks of breast tumours developed by ATM deleterious variant carriers. Breast Cancer Res. 2018 Apr 17;20(1):28. PMID:29665859
**1751.** Renaux-Petel M, Charbonnier F, Théry JC, et al. Contribution of de novo and mosaic TP53 mutations to Li-Fraumeni syndrome. J Med Genet. 2018 Mar;55(3):173–80. PMID:29070607
**1752.** Rendi MH, Dintzis SM, Lehman CD, et al. Lobular in-situ neoplasia on breast core needle biopsy: imaging indication and pathologic extent can identify which patients require excisional biopsy. Ann Surg Oncol. 2012 Mar;19(3):914–21. PMID:21861212
**1753.** Renshaw AA, Derhagopian RP, Martinez P, et al. Lobular neoplasia in breast core needle biopsy specimens is associated with a low risk of ductal carcinoma in situ or invasive carcinoma on subsequent excision. Am J Clin Pathol. 2006 Aug;126(2):310–3. PMID:16891208
**1754.** Requena L, Kutzner H, Mentzel T, et al. Benign vascular proliferations in irradiated skin. Am J Surg Pathol. 2002 Mar;26(3):328–37. PMID:11859204
**1755.** Resetkova E, Sahin A, Ayala AG, et al. Breast carcinoma with choriocarcinomatous features. Ann Diagn Pathol. 2004 Apr;8(2):74–9. PMID:15060884
**1756.** Reusche R, Winocour S, Degnim A, et al. Diffuse dermal angiomatosis of the breast: a series of 22 cases from a single institution. Gland Surg. 2015 Dec;4(6):554–60. PMID:26645009
**1757.** Reynolds RD, Pajak TF, Greenberg BR, et al. Lung cancer as a second primary. Cancer. 1978 Dec;42(6):2887–93. PMID:215300
**1758.** Ribelles N, Santonja A, Pajares B, et al. The seed and soil hypothesis revisited: current state of knowledge of inherited genes on prognosis in breast cancer. Cancer Treat Rev. 2014 Mar;40(2):293–9. PMID:24112814
**1759.** Ribrag V, Bibeau F, El Weshi A, et al. Primary breast lymphoma: a report of 20 cases. Br J Haematol. 2001 Nov;115(2):253–6. PMID:11703318
**1760.** Richter J, Schlesner M, Hoffmann S, et al. Recurrent mutation of the ID3 gene in Burkitt lymphoma identified by integrated genome, exome and transcriptome sequencing. Nat Genet. 2012 Dec;44(12):1316–20. PMID:23143595
**1761.** Riegert-Johnson DL, Gleeson FC, Roberts M, et al. Cancer and Lhermitte-Duclos disease are common in Cowden syndrome patients. Hered Cancer Clin Pract. 2010 Jun 17;8(1):6. PMID:20565722
**1762.** Riener MO, Nikolopoulos E, Herr A, et al. Microarray comparative genomic hybridization analysis of tubular breast carcinoma shows recurrent loss of the CDH13 locus on 16q. Hum Pathol. 2008 Nov;39(11):1621–9. PMID:18656243
**1763.** Righi A, Lenzi M, Morandi L, et al. Adenoid cystic carcinoma of the breast associated with invasive duct carcinoma: a case report. Int J Surg Pathol. 2011 Apr;19(2):230–4. PMID:19233861
**1764.** Rindi G, Klimstra DS, Abedi-Ardekani B, et al. A common classification framework for neuroendocrine neoplasms: an International Agency for Research on Cancer (IARC) and World Health Organization (WHO) expert consensus proposal. Mod Pathol. 2018 Dec;31(12):1770–86. PMID:30140036
**1765.** Ripamonti CB, Colombo M, Mondini P, et al. First description of an acinic cell carcinoma of the breast in a BRCA1 mutation carrier: a case report. BMC Cancer. 2013 Feb 1;13:46. PMID:23374397
**1766.** Rissanen T, Tikkakoski T, Autio AL, et al. Ultrasonography of invasive lobular breast carcinoma. Acta Radiol. 1998 May;39(3):285–91. PMID:9571945
**1767.** Rivandi M, Martens JWM, Hollestelle A. Elucidating the underlying functional mechanisms of breast cancer susceptibility through post-GWAS analyses. Front Genet. 2018 Aug 2;9:280. PMID:30116257
**1768.** Rizzolo P, Silvestri V, Tommasi S, et al. Male breast cancer: genetics, epigenetics, and ethical aspects. Ann Oncol. 2013 Nov;24 Suppl 8:viii75–82. PMID:24131976
**1769.** Ro JY, Silva EG, Gallager HS. Adenoid cystic carcinoma of the breast. Hum Pathol. 1987 Dec;18(12):1276–81. PMID:2824330
**1770.** Robbe P, Popitsch N, Knight SJL, et al. Clinical whole-genome sequencing from routine formalin-fixed, paraffin-embedded specimens: pilot study for the 100,000 Genomes Project. Genet Med. 2018 Oct;20(10):1196–205. PMID:29388947
**1771.** Robbiani DF, Deroubaix S, Feldhahn N, et al. Plasmodium infection promotes genomic instability and AID-dependent B cell lymphoma. Cell. 2015 Aug 13;162(4):727–37. PMID:26276629
**1772.** Robens J, Goldstein L, Gown AM, et al. Thyroid transcription factor-1 expression in breast carcinomas. Am J Surg Pathol. 2010 Dec;34(12):1881–5. PMID:21107096
**1773.** Roberts NJ, Jiao Y, Yu J, et al. ATM mutations in patients with hereditary pancreatic cancer. Cancer Discov. 2012 Jan;2(1):41–6. PMID:22585167
**1773A.** Robson M, Im SA, Senkus E, et al. Olaparib for metastatic breast cancer in patients with a germline BRCA mutation. N Engl J Med. 2017 Aug 10;377(6):523–33. PMID:28578601
**1773B.** Robson ME, Tung N, Conte P, et al. OlympiAD final overall survival and tolerability results: olaparib versus chemotherapy treatment of physician's choice in patients with a germline BRCA mutation and HER2-negative metastatic breast cancer. Ann Oncol. 2019 Apr 1;30(4):558–66. PMID:30689707
**1774.** Roden AC, Macon WR, Keeney GL, et al. Seroma-associated primary anaplastic large-cell lymphoma adjacent to breast implants: an indolent T-cell lymphoproliferative disorder. Mod Pathol. 2008 Apr;21(4):455–63. PMID:18223553
**1776.** Rogers D, Karki C, Bartlett C, et al. The motor disorders of mental handicap. An overlap with the motor disorders of severe psychiatric illness. Br J Psychiatry. 1991 Jan;158:97–102. PMID:2015458
**1777.** Rohayem J, Nieschlag E, Zitzmann M, et al. Testicular function during puberty and young adulthood in patients with Klinefelter's syndrome with and without spermatozoa in seminal fluid. Andrology. 2016 Nov;4(6):1178–86. PMID:27611179
**1778.** Rohen C, Caselitz J, Stern C, et al. A hamartoma of the breast with an aberration of 12q mapped to the MAR region by fluorescence in situ hybridization. Cancer Genet Cytogenet. 1995 Oct 1;84(1):82–4. PMID:7497449
**1779.** Roithmann S, Toledano M, Tourani JM, et al. HIV-associated non-Hodgkin's lymphomas: clinical characteristics and outcome. The experience of the French Registry of HIV-Associated Tumors. Ann Oncol. 1991 Apr;2(4):289–95. PMID:1868025
**1780.** Rombouts AJM, Huising J, Hugen N, et al. Assessment of radiotherapy-associated angiosarcoma after breast cancer treatment in a Dutch population-based study. JAMA Oncol. 2019 Feb 1;5(2):267–9. PMID:30676608
**1780A.** Romero P, Benhamo V, Deniziaut G, et al. Medullary breast carcinoma, a triple-negative breast cancer associated with BCLG overexpression. Am J Pathol. 2018 Oct;188(10):2378–91. PMID:30075151
**1781.** Roncaroli F, Lamovec J, Zidar A, et al. Acinic cell-like carcinoma of the breast. Virchows Arch. 1996 Sep;429(1):69–74. PMID:8865856
**1782.** Rosa M, Masood S. Cytomorphology of male breast lesions: diagnostic pitfalls and clinical implications. Diagn Cytopathol. 2012 Feb;40(2):179–84. PMID:22246937
**1783.** Rosa M, Mohammadi A, Masood S. Lobular carcinoma of the breast with extracellular mucin: new variant of mucin-producing carcinomas? Pathol Int. 2009 Jun;59(6):405–9. PMID:19490472
**1784.** Rosai J. Borderline epithelial lesions of the breast. Am J Surg Pathol. 1991 Mar;15(3):209–21. PMID:1847606
**1785.** Rosen PP. Adenomyoepithelioma of the breast. Hum Pathol. 1987 Dec;18(12):1232–7. PMID:2824328
**1786.** Rosen PP. Syringomatous adenoma of the nipple. Am J Surg Pathol. 1983 Dec;7(8):739–45. PMID:6660349
**1787.** Rosen PP. Vascular tumors of the breast. III. Angiomatosis. Am J Surg Pathol. 1985 Sep;9(9):652–8. PMID:4051097
**1788.** Rosen PP. Vascular tumors of the breast. V. Nonparenchymal hemangiomas of mammary subcutaneous tissues. Am J Surg Pathol. 1985 Oct;9(10):723–9. PMID:4061730
**1789.** Rosen PP, Caicco JA. Florid papillomatosis of the nipple. A study of 51 patients, including nine with mammary carcinoma. Am J Surg Pathol. 1986 Feb;10(2):87–101. PMID:3006526
**1790.** Rosen PP, Cranor ML. Secretory carcinoma of the breast. Arch Pathol Lab Med. 1991 Feb;115(2):141–4. PMID:1992979
**1791.** Rosen PP, editor. Rosen's breast pathology. 3rd ed. Philadelphia (PA): Lippincott Williams & Wilkins; 2008.
**1792.** Rosen PP, Ernsberger D. Mammary fibromatosis. A benign spindle-cell tumor with significant risk for local recurrence. Cancer. 1989 Apr 1;63(7):1363–9. PMID:2920364
**1793.** Rosen PP, Jozefczyk MA, Boram LH. Vascular tumors of the breast. IV. The venous hemangioma. Am J Surg Pathol. 1985 Sep;9(9):659–65. PMID:4051098
**1794.** Rosen PP, Kimmel M, Ernsberger D. Mammary angiosarcoma. The prognostic significance of tumor differentiation. Cancer. 1988 Nov 15;62(10):2145–51. PMID:3179927
**1795.** Rosen PP, Kosloff C, Lieberman PH, et al. Lobular carcinoma in situ of the breast. Detailed analysis of 99 patients with average follow-up of 24 years. Am J Surg Pathol. 1978 Sep;2(3):225–51. PMID:210682
**1796.** Rosen PP, Ridolfi RL. The perilobular hemangioma. A benign microscopic vascular lesion of the breast. Am J Clin Pathol. 1977 Jul;68(1):21–3. PMID:868802
**1797.** Rosen PP, Senie R, Schottenfeld D, et al. Noninvasive breast carcinoma: frequency of unsuspected invasion and implications for treatment. Ann Surg. 1979 Mar;189(3):377–82. PMID:218506
**1798.** Rosenbohm A, Hirsch S, Volk AE, et al. The metabolic and endocrine characteristics in spinal and bulbar muscular atrophy. J Neurol. 2018 May;265(5):1026–36. PMID:29464380
**1799.** Rosolen A, Perkins SL, Pinkerton CR, et al. Revised international pediatric non-Hodgkin lymphoma staging system. J Clin Oncol. 2015 Jun 20;33(18):2112–8. PMID:25940716
**1800.** Ross DS, Giri DD, Akram MM, et al. Fibroepithelial lesions in the breast of adolescent females: a clinicopathological study of 54 cases. Breast J. 2017 Mar;23(2):182–92. PMID:28299887
**1801.** Ross DS, Hoda SA. Microinvasive (T1mic) lobular carcinoma of the breast: clinicopathologic profile of 16 cases. Am J Surg Pathol. 2011 May;35(5):750–6. PMID:21415700
**1802.** Ross JS, Gay LM, Wang K, et al. Nonamplification ERBB2 genomic alterations in 5605 cases of recurrent and metastatic breast cancer: an emerging opportunity for anti-HER2 targeted therapies. Cancer. 2016 Sep 1;122(17):2654–62. PMID:27284958
**1803.** Rosso R, Scelsi M, Carnevali L. Granular cell traumatic neuroma: a lesion occurring in mastectomy scars. Arch Pathol Lab Med. 2000 May;124(5):709–11. PMID:10782152
**1804.** Rossouw JE, Anderson GL, Prentice RL, et al. Risks and benefits of estrogen plus progestin in healthy postmenopausal women: principal results from the Women's Health Initiative randomized controlled trial. JAMA. 2002 Jul 17;288(3):321–33. PMID:12117397
**1805.** Rothblum-Oviatt C, Wright J, Lefton-Greif MA, et al. Ataxia telangiectasia: a review. Orphanet J Rare Dis. 2016 Nov 25;11(1):159. PMID:27884168
**1806.** Rowe JJ, Cheah AL, Calhoun BC. Lipomatous tumors of the breast: a contemporary review. Semin Diagn Pathol. 2017 Sep;34(5):453–61. PMID:28662999
**1807.** Royal College of Pathologists [Internet]. London (UK): Royal College of Pathologists; 2019. Cancer datasets and tissue pathways. Available from: https://www.rcpath.org/profession/guidelines/cancer-datasets-and-tissue-pathways.html.
**1808.** Rozan S, Vincent-Salomon A, Zafrani B, et al. No significant predictive value of c-erbB-2 or p53 expression regarding sensitivity to primary chemotherapy or radiotherapy in breast cancer. Int J Cancer. 1998 Feb 20;79(1):27–33. PMID:9495354
**1809.** Rudas M, Neumayer R, Gnant MF, et al. p53 protein expression, cell proliferation and steroid hormone receptors in ductal and lobular in situ carcinomas of the breast. Eur J Cancer. 1997 Jan;33(1):39–44. PMID:9071897
**1810.** Ruddy KJ, Winer EP. Male breast cancer: risk factors, biology, diagnosis, treatment, and survivorship. Ann Oncol. 2013 Jun;24(6):1434–43. PMID:23425944
**1811.** Ruffolo EF, Koerner FC, Maluf HM. Metaplastic carcinoma of the breast with melanocytic differentiation. Mod Pathol. 1997 Jun;10(6):592–6. PMID:9195577
**1812.** Rugo HS, Olopade OI, DeMichele A, et al. Adaptive randomization of veliparib-carboplatin treatment in breast cancer. N Engl J Med. 2016 Jul 7;375(1):23–34. PMID:27406347
**1813.** Rungta S, Kleer CG. Metaplastic carcinomas of the breast: diagnostic challenges and new translational insights. Arch Pathol Lab Med. 2012 Aug;136(8):896–900. PMID:22849737
**1814.** Ryan G, Martinelli G, Kuper-Hommel M, et al. Primary diffuse large B-cell lymphoma of the breast: prognostic factors and outcomes of a study by the International Extranodal Lymphoma Study Group. Ann Oncol. 2008 Feb;19(2):233–41. PMID:17932394
**1815.** Saad RS, Richmond L, Nofech-Mozes S, et al. Fine-needle aspiration biopsy of breast adenomyoepithelioma: a potential false positive pitfall and presence of intranuclear cytoplasmic inclusions. Diagn Cytopathol. 2012 Nov;40(11):1005–9. PMID:21548117
**1816.** Sadanaga N, Okada S, Shiotani S, et al. Clinical characteristics of small cell carcinoma of the breast. Oncol Rep. 2008 Apr;19(4):981–5. PMID:18357385
**1817.** Saglam A, Can B. Coexistence of lactating adenoma and invasive ductal adenocarcinoma of the breast in a pregnant woman. J Clin Pathol. 2005 Jan;58(1):87–9.

PMID:15623491
1818. Sahin S, Karatas F, Erdem GU, et al. Invasive pleomorphic lobular histology is an adverse prognostic factor on survival in patients with breast cancer. Am Surg. 2017 Apr 1;83(4):359–64. PMID:28424130
1819. Sahoo S, Green I, Rosen PP. Bilateral Paget disease of the nipple associated with lobular carcinoma in situ. Arch Pathol Lab Med. 2002 Jan;126(1):90–2. PMID:11800657
1820. Said SM, Visscher DW, Nassar A, et al. Flat epithelial atypia and risk of breast cancer: a Mayo cohort study. Cancer. 2015 May 15;121(10):1548–55. PMID:25639678
1821. Sai-Giridhar P, Al-Ramadhani S, George D, et al. A multicentre validation of Metasin: a molecular assay for the intraoperative assessment of sentinel lymph nodes from breast cancer patients. Histopathology. 2016 May;68(6):875–87. PMID:26383172
1822. Saimura M, Anan K, Mitsuyama S, et al. Ductal carcinoma in situ arising in tubular adenoma of the breast. Breast Cancer. 2015 Jul;22(4):428–31. PMID:22700460
1823. Saito T, Ryu M, Fukumura Y, et al. A case of myxoid liposarcoma of the breast. Int J Clin Exp Pathol. 2013 Jun 15;6(7):1432–6. PMID:23826427
1824. Sakharpe A, Lahat G, Gulamhusein T, et al. Epithelioid sarcoma and unclassified sarcoma with epithelioid features: clinicopathological variables, molecular markers, and a new experimental model. Oncologist. 2011;16(4):512–22. PMID:21357725
1825. Sakr RA, Schizas M, Carniello JV, et al. Targeted capture massively parallel sequencing analysis of LCIS and invasive lobular cancer: repertoire of somatic genetic alterations and clonal relationships. Mol Oncol. 2016 Feb;10(2):360–70. PMID:26643573
1826. Sakuma T, Mimura A, Tanigawa N, et al. Fine needle aspiration cytology of acinic cell carcinoma of the breast. Cytopathology. 2013 Dec;24(6):403–5. PMID:22734799
1827. Sakuma T, Mori M, Kokubo C, et al. Cytology of breast pleomorphic adenoma associated with extensive apocrine metaplasia. Diagn Cytopathol. 2018 Jan;46(1):56–8. PMID:28994509
1828. Salemis NS. Florid papillomatosis of the nipple: a rare presentation and review of the literature. Breast Dis. 2015;35(2):153–6. PMID:25585841
1829. Salemis NS, Gemenetzis G, Karagkiouzis G, et al. Tubular adenoma of the breast: a rare presentation and review of the literature. J Clin Med Res. 2012 Feb;4(1):64–7. PMID:22383931
1830. Salgado R, Denkert C, Campbell C, et al. Tumor-infiltrating lymphocytes and associations with pathological complete response and event-free survival in HER2-positive early-stage breast cancer treated with lapatinib and trastuzumab: a secondary analysis of the NeoALTTO trial. JAMA Oncol. 2015 Jul;1(4):448–54. PMID:26181252
1831. Salgado R, Denkert C, Demaria S, et al. The evaluation of tumor-infiltrating lymphocytes (TILs) in breast cancer: recommendations by an International TILs Working Group 2014. Ann Oncol. 2015 Feb;26(2):259–71. PMID:25214542
1832. Salhany KE, Page DL. Fine-needle aspiration of mammary lobular carcinoma in situ and atypical lobular hyperplasia. Am J Clin Pathol. 1989 Jul;92(1):22–6. PMID:2750704
1834. Samani NJ, Erdmann J, Hall AS, et al. Genomewide association analysis of coronary artery disease. N Engl J Med. 2007 Aug 2;357(5):443–53. PMID:17634449
1835. Sander S, Calado DP, Srinivasan L, et al. Synergy between PI3K signaling and MYC in Burkitt lymphomagenesis. Cancer Cell. 2012 Aug 14;22(2):167–79. PMID:22897848
1836. Sanders MA, Brock JE, Harrison BT, et al. Nipple-invasive primary carcinomas: clinical, imaging, and pathologic features of breast carcinomas originating in the nipple. Arch Pathol Lab Med. 2018 May;142(5):598–605. PMID:29431468
1837. Sanders MA, Dominici L, Denison C, et al. Paget disease of the breast with invasion from nipple skin into the dermis: an unusual type of skin invasion not associated with an adverse outcome. Arch Pathol Lab Med. 2013 Jan;137(1):72–6. PMID:23276177
1838. Sanders ME, Schuyler PA, Simpson JF, et al. Continued observation of the natural history of low-grade ductal carcinoma in situ reaffirms proclivity for local recurrence even after more than 30 years of follow-up. Mod Pathol. 2015 May;28(5):662–9. PMID:25502729
1839. Sandison AT. Metastatic tumours in the breast. Br J Surg. 1959 Jul;47:54–8. PMID:14441414
1840. Sangoi AR, Shrestha B, Yang G, et al. The novel marker GATA3 is significantly more sensitive than traditional markers mammaglobin and GCDFP15 for identifying breast cancer in surgical and cytology specimens of metastatic and matched primary tumors. Appl Immunohistochem Mol Morphol. 2016 Apr;24(4):229–37. PMID:25906123
1841. Sapino A, Papotti M, Pietribiasi F, et al. Diagnostic cytological features of neuroendocrine differentiated carcinoma of the breast. Virchows Arch. 1998 Sep;433(3):217–22. PMID:9769124
1842. Sapino A, Papotti M, Righi L, et al. Clinical significance of neuroendocrine carcinoma of the breast. Ann Oncol. 2001;12 Suppl 2:S115–7. PMID:11762336
1843. Sapino A, Righi L, Cassoni P, et al. Expression of apocrine differentiation markers in neuroendocrine breast carcinomas of aged women. Mod Pathol. 2001 Aug;14(8):768–76. PMID:11504836
1844. Sapino A, Righi L, Cassoni P, et al. Expression of the neuroendocrine phenotype in carcinomas of the breast. Semin Diagn Pathol. 2000 May;17(2):127–37. PMID:10839613
1845. Sapino A, Roepman P, Linn SC, et al. MammaPrint molecular diagnostics on formalin-fixed, paraffin-embedded tissue. J Mol Diagn. 2014 Mar;16(2):190–7. PMID:24378251
1846. Sarrió D, Moreno-Bueno G, Hardisson D, et al. Epigenetic and genetic alterations of APC and CDH1 genes in lobular breast cancer: relationships with abnormal E-cadherin and catenin expression and microsatellite instability. Int J Cancer. 2003 Aug 20;106(2):208–15. PMID:12800196
1847. Sarrió D, Pérez-Mies B, Hardisson D, et al. Cytoplasmic localization of p120ctn and E-cadherin loss characterize lobular breast carcinoma from preinvasive to metastatic lesions. Oncogene. 2004 Apr 22;23(19):3272–83. PMID:15077190
1848. Sastre-Garau X, Jouve M, Asselain B, et al. Infiltrating lobular carcinoma of the breast. Clinicopathologic analysis of 975 cases with reference to data on conservative therapy and metastatic patterns. Cancer. 1996 Jan 1;77(1):113–20. PMID:8630916
1849. Satou A, Asano N, Nakazawa A, et al. Epstein-Barr virus (EBV)-positive sporadic Burkitt lymphoma: an age-related lymphoproliferative disorder? Am J Surg Pathol. 2015 Feb;39(2):227–35. PMID:25321330
1850. Sau P, Solis J, Lupton GP, et al. Pigmented breast carcinoma. A clinical and histopathologic simulator of malignant melanoma. Arch Dermatol. 1989 Apr;125(4):536–9. PMID:2930211
1851. Savitsky K, Bar-Shira A, Gilad S, et al. A single ataxia telangiectasia gene with a product similar to PI-3 kinase. Science. 1995 Jun 23;268(5218):1749–53. PMID:7792600
1852. Sawhney N, Garrahan N, Douglas-Jones AG, et al. Epithelial–stromal interactions in tumors. A morphologic study of fibroepithelial tumors of the breast. Cancer. 1992 Oct 15;70(8):2115–20. PMID:1327488
1853. Sawyer E, Roylance R, Petridis C, et al. Genetic predisposition to in situ and invasive lobular carcinoma of the breast. PLoS Genet. 2014 Apr 17;10(4):e1004285. PMID:24743323
1854. Sawyer EJ, Hanby AM, Poulsom R, et al. Beta-catenin abnormalities and associated insulin-like growth factor overexpression are important in phyllodes tumours and fibroadenomas of the breast. J Pathol. 2003 Aug;200(5):627–32. PMID:12898599
1855. Sawyer EJ, Hanby AM, Rowan AJ, et al. The Wnt pathway, epithelial-stromal interactions, and malignant progression in phyllodes tumours. J Pathol. 2002 Apr;196(4):437–44. PMID:11920740
1856. Sawyer S, Mitchell G, McKinley J, et al. A role for common genomic variants in the assessment of familial breast cancer. J Clin Oncol. 2012 Dec 10;30(35):4330–6. PMID:23109704
1857. Scheffzek K, Ahmadian MR, Wiesmüller L, et al. Structural analysis of the GAP-related domain from neurofibromin and its implications. EMBO J. 1998 Aug 3;17(15):4313–27. PMID:9687500
1858. Schelfout K, Van Goethem M, Kersschot E, et al. Preoperative breast MRI in patients with invasive lobular breast cancer. Eur Radiol. 2004 Jul;14(7):1209–16. PMID:15024602
1859. Schmid P, Adams S, Rugo HS, et al. Atezolizumab and nab-paclitaxel in advanced triple-negative breast cancer. N Engl J Med. 2018 Nov 29;379(22):2108–21. PMID:30345906
1860. Schmidt MK, Hogervorst F, van Hien R, et al. Age- and tumor subtype-specific breast cancer risk estimates for CHEK2*1100delC carriers. J Clin Oncol. 2016 Aug 10;34(23):2750–60. PMID:27269948
1861. Schmidt MK, Tollenaar RA, de Kemp SR, et al. Breast cancer survival and tumor characteristics in premenopausal women carrying the CHEK2*1100delC germline mutation. J Clin Oncol. 2007 Jan 1;25(1):64–9. PMID:17132695
1862. Schmitt FC, Reis-Filho JS. Oncogenes, granules and breast cancer: What has c-myc to do with apocrine changes? Breast. 2002 Dec;11(6):463–5. PMID:14965710
1863. Schmitz R, Young RM, Ceribelli M, et al. Burkitt lymphoma pathogenesis and therapeutic targets from structural and functional genomics. Nature. 2012 Oct 4;490(7418):116–20. PMID:22885699
1864. Schnitt SJ. Benign breast disease and breast cancer risk: morphology and beyond. Am J Surg Pathol. 2003 Jun;27(6):836–41. PMID:12766590
1865. Schnitt SJ. Clinging carcinoma: an American perspective. Semin Diagn Pathol. 2010 Feb;27(1):31–6. PMID:20306828
1866. Schnitt SJ. Spindle cell lesions of the breast. Surg Pathol Clin. 2009 Jun;2(2):375–90. PMID:26838327
1867. Schnitt SJ, Connolly JL. Processing and evaluation of breast excision specimens. A clinically oriented approach. Am J Clin Pathol. 1992 Jul;98(1):125–37. PMID:1615916
1868. Schnitt SJ, Connolly JL, Tavassoli FA, et al. Interobserver reproducibility in the diagnosis of ductal proliferative breast lesions using standardized criteria. Am J Surg Pathol. 1992 Dec;16(12):1133–43. PMID:1463092
1869. Schnitt SJ, Morrow M. Lobular carcinoma in situ: current concepts and controversies. Semin Diagn Pathol. 1999 Aug;16(3):209–23. PMID:10490198
1870. Schnitt SJ, Vincent-Salomon A. Columnar cell lesions of the breast. Adv Anat Pathol. 2003 May;10(3):113–24. PMID:12717115
1871. Schoenmakers EF, Wanschura S, Mols R, et al. Recurrent rearrangements in the high mobility group protein gene, HMGI-C, in benign mesenchymal tumours. Nat Genet. 1995 Aug;10(4):436–44. PMID:7670494
1872. Scholtysik R, Kreuz M, Klapper W, et al. Detection of genomic aberrations in molecularly defined Burkitt's lymphoma by array-based, high resolution, single nucleotide polymorphism analysis. Haematologica. 2010 Dec;95(12):2047–55. PMID:20823134
1873. Schon K, Tischkowitz M. Clinical implications of germline mutations in breast cancer: TP53. Breast Cancer Res Treat. 2018 Jan;167(2):417–23. PMID:29039119
1874. Schoolmeester JK, Lastra RR. Granular cell tumors overexpress TFE3 without corollary gene rearrangement. Hum Pathol. 2015 Aug;46(8):1242–3. PMID:26009539
1875. Schoolmeester JK, Moyer AM, Goodenberger ML, et al. Pathologic findings in breast, fallopian tube, and ovary specimens in non-BRCA hereditary breast and/or ovarian cancer syndromes: a study of 18 patients with deleterious germline mutations in RAD51C, BARD1, BRIP1, PALB2, MUTYH, or CHEK2. Hum Pathol. 2017 Dec;70:14–26. PMID:28709830
1876. Schrader KA, Masciari S, Boyd N, et al. Germline mutations in CDH1 are infrequent in women with early-onset or familial lobular breast cancers. J Med Genet. 2011 Jan;48(1):64–8. PMID:20921021
1877. Schrader KA, Nelson TN, De Luca A, et al. Multiple granular cell tumors are an associated feature of LEOPARD syndrome caused by mutation in PTPN11. Clin Genet. 2009 Feb;75(2):185–9. PMID:19054014
1878. Schrager CA, Schneider D, Gruener AC, et al. Clinical and pathological features of breast disease in Cowden's syndrome: an underrecognized syndrome with an increased risk of breast cancer. Hum Pathol. 1998 Jan;29(1):47–53. PMID:9445133
1879. Schroeder MC, Rastogi P, Geyer CE Jr, et al. Early and locally advanced metaplastic breast cancer: presentation and survival by receptor status in Surveillance, Epidemiology, and End Results (SEER) 2010-2014. Oncologist. 2018 Apr;23(4):481–8. PMID:29330212
1880. Schwartz GF, Patchefsky AS, Finklestein SD, et al. Nonpalpable in situ ductal carcinoma of the breast. Predictors of multicentricity and microinvasion and implications for treatment. Arch Surg. 1989 Jan;124(1):29–32. PMID:2535928
1881. Schwentner L, Kurzeder C, Kreienberg R, et al. Focus on haematogenous dissemination of the malignant cystosarcoma phylloides: institutional experience. Arch Gynecol Obstet. 2011 Mar;283(3):591–6. PMID:21069366
1882. Scoggins M, Krishnamurthy S, Santiago L, et al. Lobular carcinoma in situ of the breast: clinical, radiological, and pathological correlation. Acad Radiol. 2013 Apr;20(4):463–70. PMID:23498988
1883. Scolyer RA, McKenzie PR, Achmed D, et al. Can phyllodes tumours of the breast be distinguished from fibroadenomas using fine needle aspiration cytology? Pathology. 2001 Nov;33(4):437–43. PMID:11827409
1884. Scopsi L, Andreola S, Pilotti S, et al. Mucinous carcinoma of the breast. A clinicopathologic, histochemical, and

immunocytochemical study with special reference to neuroendocrine differentiation. Am J Surg Pathol. 1994 Jul;18(7):702–11. PMID:8017565

**1885.** Screening & Immunisations Team, NHS Digital. NHS Breast Screening Programme: England 2016-17. Leeds (UK): Health and Social Care Information Centre; 2018 Jan 31 [updated 2018 Apr 4, cited 2018 Oct 11]. Available from: https://files.digital.nhs.uk/pdf/m/f/breast_screening_programme__england__2016-17_-_report__v2.pdf.

**1886.** Sebastiano C, Gennaro L, Brogi E, et al. Benign vascular lesions of the breast diagnosed by core needle biopsy do not require excision. Histopathology. 2017 Nov;71(5):795–804. PMID:28644513

**1887.** Seethala RR, Hunt JL, Baloch ZW, et al. Adenoid cystic carcinoma with high-grade transformation: a report of 11 cases and a review of the literature. Am J Surg Pathol. 2007 Nov;31(11):1683–94. PMID:18059225

**1888.** Seifert G. Are adenomyoepithelioma of the breast and epithelial-myoepithelial carcinoma of the salivary glands identical tumours? Virchows Arch. 1998 Sep;433(3):285–8. PMID:9769134

**1889.** Sek P, Zawrocki A, Biernat W, et al. HER2 molecular subtype is a dominant subtype of mammary Paget's cells. An immunohistochemical study. Histopathology. 2010 Oct;57(4):564–71. PMID:20955381

**1890.** Sekimizu M, Yoshida A, Mitani S, et al. Frequent mutations of genes encoding vacuolar H+-ATPase components in granular cell tumors. Genes Chromosomes Cancer. 2019 Jun;58(6):373–80. PMID:30597645

**1891.** Selim AG, El-Ayat G, Naase M, et al. C-myc oncoprotein expression and gene amplification in apocrine metaplasia and apocrine change within sclerosing adenosis of the breast. Breast. 2002 Dec;11(6):466–72. PMID:14965711

**1892.** Selim AG, El-Ayat G, Wells CA. c-erbB2 oncoprotein expression, gene amplification, and chromosome 17 aneusomy in apocrine adenosis of the breast. J Pathol. 2000 Jun;191(2):138–42. PMID:10861572

**1893.** Selim AG, Ryan A, El-Ayat GA, et al. Loss of heterozygosity and allelic imbalance in apocrine adenosis of the breast. Cancer Detect Prev. 2001;25(3):262–7. PMID:11425268

**1894.** Selinko VL, Middleton LP, Dempsey PJ. Role of sonography in diagnosing and staging invasive lobular carcinoma. J Clin Ultrasound. 2004 Sep;32(7):323–32. PMID:15293298

**1895.** Seminog OO, Goldacre MJ. Risk of benign tumours of nervous system, and of malignant neoplasms, in people with neurofibromatosis: population-based record-linkage study. Br J Cancer. 2013 Jan 15;108(1):193–8. PMID:23257896

**1896.** Sengupta S, Pal S, Biswas BK, et al. Evaluation of clinico-radio-pathological features of tubular adenoma of breast: a study of ten cases with histopathological differential diagnosis. Iran J Pathol. 2015 Winter;10(1):17–22. PMID:26516321

**1897.** Sengupta S, Pal S, Biswas BK, et al. Preoperative diagnosis of tubular adenoma of breast - 10 years of experience. N Am J Med Sci. 2014 May;6(5):219–23. PMID:24926447

**1898.** Senkus E, Kyriakides S, Ohno S, et al. Primary breast cancer: ESMO Clinical Practice Guidelines for diagnosis, treatment and follow-up. Ann Oncol. 2015 Sep;26 Suppl 5:v8–30. PMID:26314782

**1899.** Senkus E, Kyriakides S, Penault-Llorca F, et al. Primary breast cancer: ESMO Clinical Practice Guidelines for diagnosis, treatment and follow-up. Ann Oncol. 2013 Oct;24 Suppl 6:vi7–23. PMID:23970019

**1900.** Sentani K, Tashiro T, Uraoka N, et al. Primary mammary mucinous cystadenocarcinoma: cytological and histological findings. Diagn Cytopathol. 2012 Jul;40(7):624–8. PMID:21472867

**1901.** Seo IS, Min KW. Postirradiation epithelioid angiosarcoma of the breast: a case report with immunohistochemical and electron microscopic study. Ultrastruct Pathol. 2003 May-Jun;27(3):197–203. PMID:12775509

**1902.** Seong M, Ko EY, Han BK, et al. Radiologic findings of primary mucinous cystadenocarcinoma of the breast: a report of two cases and a literature review. J Breast Cancer. 2016 Sep;19(3):330–3. PMID:27721884

**1903.** Severson TM, Zwart W. A review of estrogen receptor/androgen receptor genomics in male breast cancer. Endocr Relat Cancer. 2017 Mar;24(3):R27–34. PMID:28062545

**1904.** Sevim Y, Kocaay AF, Eker T, et al. Breast hamartoma: a clinicopathologic analysis of 27 cases and a literature review. Clinics (Sao Paulo). 2014 Aug;69(8):515–23. PMID:25141109

**1905.** Shaaban AM, Ball GR, Brannan RA, et al. A comparative biomarker study of 514 matched cases of male and female breast cancer reveals gender-specific biological differences. Breast Cancer Res Treat. 2012 Jun;133(3):949–58. PMID:22094935

**1906.** Shabaik A, Lin G, Peterson M, et al. Reliability of Her2/neu, estrogen receptor, and progesterone receptor testing by immunohistochemistry on cell block of FNA and serous effusions from patients with primary and metastatic breast carcinoma. Diagn Cytopathol. 2011 May;39(5):328–32. PMID:21488175

**1907.** Shah V, Nowinski S, Levi D, et al. PIK3CA mutations are common in lobular carcinoma in situ, but are not a biomarker of progression. Breast Cancer Res. 2017 Jan 17;19(1):7. PMID:28095868

**1908.** Shah-Khan MG, Geiger XJ, Reynolds C, et al. Long-term follow-up of lobular neoplasia (atypical lobular hyperplasia/lobular carcinoma in situ) diagnosed on core needle biopsy. Ann Surg Oncol. 2012 Oct;19(10):3131–8. PMID:22847124

**1909.** Shakya R, Reid LJ, Reczek CR, et al. BRCA1 tumor suppression depends on BRCT phosphoprotein binding, but not its E3 ligase activity. Science. 2011 Oct 28;334(6055):525–8. PMID:22034435

**1910.** Shamir ER, Chen YY, Chu T, et al. Pleomorphic and florid lobular carcinoma in situ variants of the breast: a clinicopathologic study of 85 cases with and without invasive carcinoma from a single academic center. Am J Surg Pathol. 2019 Mar;43(3):399–408. PMID:30489319

**1911.** Sharif S, Moran A, Huson SM, et al. Women with neurofibromatosis 1 are at a moderately increased risk of developing breast cancer and should be considered for early screening. J Med Genet. 2007 Aug;44(8):481–4. PMID:17369502

**1912.** Sharma-Oates A, Shaaban AM, Tomlinson I, et al. Heterogeneity of germline variants in high risk breast and ovarian cancer susceptibility genes in India. Precis Clin Med. 2018 Sep;1(2):75–87. doi:10.1093/pcmedi/pby010.

**1913.** Sheffield BS, Kos Z, Asleh-Aburaya K, et al. Molecular subtype profiling of invasive breast cancers weakly positive for estrogen receptor. Breast Cancer Res Treat. 2016 Feb;155(3):483–90. PMID:26846986

**1914.** Shehata BM, Fishman I, Collings MH, et al. Pseudoangiomatous stromal hyperplasia of the breast in pediatric patients: an underrecognized entity. Pediatr Dev Pathol. 2009 Nov-Dec;12(6):450–4. PMID:19606909

**1915.** Sher T, Hennessy BT, Valero V, et al. Primary angiosarcomas of the breast. Cancer. 2007 Jul 1;110(1):173–8. PMID:17541936

**1916.** Sheth NA, Saruiya JN, Ranadive KJ, et al. Ectopic production of human chorionic gonadotrophin by human breast tumours. Br J Cancer. 1974 Dec;30(6):566–70. PMID:4374964

**1917.** Shi P, Wang M, Zhang Q, et al. Lipid-rich carcinoma of the breast. A clinicopathological study of 49 cases. Tumori. 2008 May-Jun;94(3):342–6. PMID:18705401

**1918.** Shiloh Y. ATM and related protein kinases: safeguarding genome integrity. Nat Rev Cancer. 2003 Mar;3(3):155–68. PMID:12612651

**1919.** Shimao K, Haga S, Shimizu T, et al. Acinic cell adenocarcinoma arising in the breast of a young male: a clinicopathological, immunohistochemical and ultrastructural study. Breast Cancer. 1998 Jun 30;5(1):77–81. PMID:11091630

**1920.** Shin C, Low I, Ng D, et al. USP6 gene rearrangement in nodular fasciitis and histological mimics. Histopathology. 2016 Nov;69(5):784–91. PMID:27271298

**1921.** Shin HJ, Kim HH, Kim SM, et al. Pure and mixed tubular carcinoma of the breast: mammographic and sonographic differential features. Korean J Radiol. 2007 Mar-Apr;8(2):103–10. PMID:17420627

**1922.** Shin SJ, DeLellis RA, Ying L, et al. Small cell carcinoma of the breast: a clinicopathologic and immunohistochemical study of nine patients. Am J Surg Pathol. 2000 Sep;24(9):1231–8. PMID:10976697

**1923.** Shin SJ, Kanomata N, Rosen PP. Mammary carcinoma with prominent cytoplasmic lipofuscin granules mimicking melanocytic differentiation. Histopathology. 2000 Nov;37(5):456–9. PMID:11119128

**1924.** Shin SJ, Lal A, De Vries S, et al. Florid lobular carcinoma in situ: molecular profiling and comparison to classic lobular carcinoma in situ and pleomorphic lobular carcinoma in situ. Hum Pathol. 2013 Oct;44(10):1998–2009. PMID:23809857

**1925.** Shin SJ, Rosen PP. Excisional biopsy should be performed if lobular carcinoma in situ is seen on needle core biopsy. Arch Pathol Lab Med. 2002 Jun;126(6):697–701. PMID:12033958

**1926.** Shin SJ, Rosen PP. Solid variant of mammary adenoid cystic carcinoma with basaloid features: a study of nine cases. Am J Surg Pathol. 2002 Apr;26(4):413–20. PMID:11914618

**1927.** Shin SJ, Sheikh FS, Allenby PA, et al. Invasive secretory (juvenile) carcinoma arising in ectopic breast tissue of the axilla. Arch Pathol Lab Med. 2001 Oct;125(10):1372–4. PMID:11570920

**1928.** Shin SJ, Simpson PT, Da Silva L, et al. Molecular evidence for progression of microglandular adenosis (MGA) to invasive carcinoma. Am J Surg Pathol. 2009 Apr;33(4):496–504. PMID:19047897

**1929.** Shintaku M, Yamamoto Y, Kono F, et al. Chondrolipoma of the breast as a rare variant of myofibroblastoma: an immunohistochemical study of two cases. Virchows Arch. 2017 Oct;471(4):531–5. PMID:28653201

**1930.** Shirah BH, Shirah HA. Incidental unilateral and bilateral ductal carcinoma in situ encountered in the surgical management of young male gynecomastia. Breast Dis. 2016 Jul 28;36(2-3):103–10. PMID:27612041

**1931.** Shirley SE, Duncan ND, Escoffery CT, et al. Angiomatosis of the breast in a male child. A case report with immunohistochemical analysis. West Indian Med J. 2002 Dec;51(4):254–6.

PMID:12632645

**1932.** Shousha S. Glandular Paget's disease of the nipple. Histopathology. 2007 May;50(6):812–4. PMID:17376174

**1933.** Shousha S, Backhous CM, Alaghband-Zadeh J, et al. Alveolar variant of invasive lobular carcinoma of the breast. A tumor rich in estrogen receptors. Am J Clin Pathol. 1986 Jan;85(1):1–5. PMID:3940412

**1934.** Shousha S, Schoenfeld A, Moss J, et al. Light and electron microscopic study of an invasive cribriform carcinoma with extensive microcalcification developing in a breast with silicone augmentation. Ultrastruct Pathol. 1994 Sep-Oct;18(5):519–23. PMID:7810003

**1935.** Shousha S, Tisdall M, Sinnett HD. Paget's disease of the nipple occurring after conservative surgery for ductal carcinoma in situ of the breast. Histopathology. 2004 Oct;45(4):416–8. PMID:15469484

**1936.** Shukla N, Roberts SS, Baki MO, et al. Successful targeted therapy of refractory pediatric ETV6-NTRK3 fusion-positive secretory breast carcinoma. JCO Precis Oncol. 2017;2017. PMID:29623306

**1937.** Siddiq A, Couch FJ, Chen GK, et al. A meta-analysis of genome-wide association studies of breast cancer identifies two novel susceptibility loci at 6q14 and 20q11. Hum Mol Genet. 2012 Dec 15;21(24):5373–84. PMID:22976474

**1938.** Siddiqui NH, Cabay RJ, Salem F. Fine-needle aspiration biopsy of a case of breast carcinoma with choriocarcinomatous features. Diagn Cytopathol. 2006 Oct;34(10):694–7. PMID:16955470

**1939.** Siegel RL, Miller KD, Jemal A. Cancer statistics, 2016. CA Cancer J Clin. 2016 Jan-Feb;66(1):7–30. PMID:26742998

**1940.** Siegel RL, Miller KD, Jemal A. Cancer statistics, 2017. CA Cancer J Clin. 2017 Jan;67(1):7–30. PMID:28055103

**1941.** Silver SA, Tavassoli FA. Pleomorphic carcinoma of the breast: clinicopathological analysis of 26 cases of an unusual high-grade phenotype of ductal carcinoma. Histopathology. 2000 Jun;36(6):505–14. PMID:10849092

**1942.** Silverman EM, Oberman HA. Metastatic neoplasms in the breast. Surg Gynecol Obstet. 1974 Jan;138(1):26–8. PMID:4809000

**1943.** Silverman JF, Masood S, Ducatman BS, et al. Can FNA biopsy separate atypical hyperplasia, carcinoma in situ, and invasive carcinoma of the breast? Cytomorphologic criteria and limitations in diagnosis. Diagn Cytopathol. 1993 Dec;9(6):713–28. PMID:8143551

**1944.** Silverstein MJ, Lewinsky BS, Waisman JR, et al. Infiltrating lobular carcinoma. Is it different from infiltrating duct carcinoma? Cancer. 1994 Mar 15;73(6):1673–7. PMID:8156495

**1945.** Silverstein MJ, Waisman JR, Gamagami P, et al. Intraductal carcinoma of the breast (208 cases). Clinical factors influencing treatment choice. Cancer. 1990 Jul 1;66(1):102–8. PMID:2162238

**1946.** Silvestri V, Barrowdale D, Mulligan AM, et al. Male breast cancer in BRCA1 and BRCA2 mutation carriers: pathology data from the Consortium of Investigators of Modifiers of BRCA1/2. Breast Cancer Res. 2016 Feb 9;18(1):15. PMID:26857456

**1947.** Simha MR, Doctor VM, Udwadia TE. Mixed tumour of salivary gland type of the male breast. Indian J Cancer. 1992 Mar;29(1):14–7. PMID:1328037

**1948.** Simpson J, Page D. Lobular neoplasia. In: Elston CW, Ellis IO, editors. The breast. London (UK): Churchill Livingstone; 1998. (Systematic pathology series, 3rd ed.; vol. 13).

**1949.** Simpson PT, Gale T, Fulford LG, et

al. The diagnosis and management of pre-invasive breast disease: pathology of atypical lobular hyperplasia and lobular carcinoma in situ. Breast Cancer Res. 2003;5(5):258–62. PMID:12927036
**1950.** Simpson PT, Gale T, Reis-Filho JS, et al. Columnar cell lesions of the breast: the missing link in breast cancer progression? A morphological and molecular analysis. Am J Surg Pathol. 2005 Jun;29(6):734–46. PMID:15897740
**1951.** Simpson PT, Reis-Filho JS, Lambros MB, et al. Molecular profiling pleomorphic lobular carcinomas of the breast: evidence for a common molecular genetic pathway with classic lobular carcinomas. J Pathol. 2008 Jul;215(3):231–44. PMID:18473330
**1952.** Simpson RH, Cope N, Skálová A, et al. Malignant adenomyoepithelioma of the breast with mixed osteogenic, spindle cell, and carcinomatous differentiation. Am J Surg Pathol. 1998 May;22(5):631–6. PMID:9591734
**1953.** Singh K, DiazGomez B, Wang Y, et al. Invasive lobular carcinoma with extracellular mucin: not all mucinous mammary carcinomas are ductal! Int J Surg Pathol. 2019 Feb;27(1):55–8. PMID:30032676
**1954.** Singletary SE. Surgical margins in patients with early-stage breast cancer treated with breast conservation therapy. Am J Surg. 2002 Nov;184(5):383–93. PMID:12433599
**1955.** Siponen E, Hukkinen K, Heikkilä P, et al. Surgical treatment in Paget's disease of the breast. Am J Surg. 2010 Aug;200(2):241–6. PMID:20678619
**1956.** Siriaunkgul S, Tavassoli FA. Invasive micropapillary carcinoma of the breast. Mod Pathol. 1993 Nov;6(6):660–2. PMID:8302807
**1957.** Skálová A, Vanecek T, Sima R, et al. Mammary analogue secretory carcinoma of salivary glands, containing the ETV6-NTRK3 fusion gene: a hitherto undescribed salivary gland tumor entity. Am J Surg Pathol. 2010 May;34(5):599–608. PMID:20410810
**1958.** Sklair-Levy M, Sella T, Alweiss T, et al. Incidence and management of complex fibroadenomas. AJR Am J Roentgenol. 2008 Jan;190(1):214–8. PMID:18094314
**1959.** Skubitz KM. Biology and treatment of aggressive fibromatosis or desmoid tumor. Mayo Clin Proc. 2017 Jun;92(6):947–64. PMID:28578783
**1960.** Sloane JP, Amendoeira I, Apostolikas N, et al. Consistency achieved by 23 European pathologists from 12 countries in diagnosing breast disease and reporting prognostic features of carcinomas. Virchows Arch. 1999 Jan;434(1):3–10. PMID:10071228
**1961.** Sloane JP, Amendoeira I, Apostolikas N, et al. Consistency achieved by 23 European pathologists in categorizing ductal carcinoma in situ of the breast using five classifications. Hum Pathol. 1998 Oct;29(10):1056–62. PMID:9781641
**1962.** Slodkowska E, Nofech-Mozes S, Xu B, et al. Fibroepithelial lesions of the breast: a comprehensive morphological and outcome analysis of a large series. Mod Pathol. 2018 Jul;31(7):1073–84. PMID:29449684
**1964.** Smith-Warner SA, Spiegelman D, Yaun SS, et al. Alcohol and breast cancer in women: a pooled analysis of cohort studies. JAMA. 1998 Feb 18;279(7):535–40. PMID:9480365
**1965.** Sneed GM, Duncan LD. Quantifying the extent of invasive carcinoma and margin status in partial mastectomy cases having a gross lesion: Is a defined tissue processing protocol needed? Am J Clin Pathol. 2011 Nov;136(5):747–53. PMID:22031313
**1966.** Sneige N, Wang J, Baker BA, et al. Clinical, histopathologic, and biologic features of pleomorphic lobular (ductal-lobular) carcinoma in situ of the breast: a report of 24 cases. Mod Pathol. 2002 Oct;15(10):1044–50. PMID:12379750
**1967.** Sneige N, Yaziji H, Mandavilli SR, et al. Low-grade (fibromatosis-like) spindle cell carcinoma of the breast. Am J Surg Pathol. 2001 Aug;25(8):1009–16. PMID:11474284
**1968.** Soenderstrup IMH, Laenkholm AV, Jensen MB, et al. Clinical and molecular characterization of BRCA-associated breast cancer: results from the DBCG. Acta Oncol. 2018 Jan;57(1):95–101. PMID:29164974
**1969.** Sohn VY, Arthurs ZM, Kim FS, et al. Lobular neoplasia: Is surgical excision warranted? Am Surg. 2008 Feb;74(2):172–7. PMID:18306873
**1970.** Sohn VY, Causey MW, Steele SR, et al. The treatment of radial scars in the modern era–surgical excision is not required. Am Surg. 2010 May;76(5):522–5. PMID:20506884
**1971.** Soliman NA, Yussif SM. Ki-67 as a prognostic marker according to breast cancer molecular subtype. Cancer Biol Med. 2016 Dec;13(4):496–504. PMID:28154782
**1972.** Solin LJ, Gray R, Hughes LL, et al. Surgical excision without radiation for ductal carcinoma in situ of the breast: 12-year results from the ECOG-ACRIN E5194 study. J Clin Oncol. 2015 Nov 20;33(33):3938–44. PMID:26371148
**1973.** Solorzano CC, Middleton LP, Hunt KK, et al. Treatment and outcome of patients with intracystic papillary carcinoma of the breast. Am J Surg. 2002 Oct;184(4):364–8. PMID:12383904
**1974.** Sønderstrup IMH, Jensen MB, Ejlertsen B, et al. Evaluation of tumor-infiltrating lymphocytes and association with prognosis in BRCA-mutated breast cancer. Acta Oncol. 2019 Mar;58(3):363–70. PMID:30614364
**1975.** Sønderstrup IMH, Jensen MR, Ejlertsen B, et al. Subtypes in BRCA-mutated breast cancer. Hum Pathol. 2019 Feb;84:192–201. PMID:30342055
**1976.** Soo MS, Rosen EL, Baker JA, et al. Negative predictive value of sonography with mammography in patients with palpable breast lesions. AJR Am J Roentgenol. 2001 Nov;177(5):1167–70. PMID:11641195
**1977.** Soomro S, Shousha S, Taylor P, et al. c-erbB-2 expression in different histological types of invasive breast carcinoma. J Clin Pathol. 1991 Mar;44(3):211–4. PMID:1672872
**1978.** Sopik V, Sun P, Narod SA. Impact of microinvasion on breast cancer mortality in women with ductal carcinoma in situ. Breast Cancer Res Treat. 2018 Feb;167(3):787–95. PMID:29119353
**1979.** Sorrell AD, Espenschied CR, Culver JO, et al. Tumor protein p53 (TP53) testing and Li-Fraumeni syndrome: current status of clinical applications and future directions. Mol Diagn Ther. 2013 Feb;17(1):31–47. PMID:23355100
**1980.** Southey MC, Goldgar DE, Winqvist R, et al. PALB2, CHEK2 and ATM rare variants and cancer risk: data from COGS. J Med Genet. 2016 Dec;53(12):800–11. PMID:27595995
**1981.** Sparano JA, Gray RJ, Makower DF, et al. Adjuvant chemotherapy guided by a 21-gene expression assay in breast cancer. N Engl J Med. 2018 Jul 12;379(2):111–21. PMID:29860917
**1982.** Sparano JA, Gray RJ, Makower DF, et al. Prospective validation of a 21-gene expression assay in breast cancer. N Engl J Med. 2015 Nov 19;373(21):2005–14. PMID:26412349
**1983.** Speirs V, Shaaban AM. The rising incidence of male breast cancer. Breast Cancer Res Treat. 2009 May;115(2):429–30. PMID:18478326
**1984.** Spillane AJ, Thomas JM, Fisher C. Epithelioid sarcoma: the clinicopathological complexities of this rare soft tissue sarcoma. Ann Surg Oncol. 2000 Apr;7(3):218–25. PMID:10791853
**1985.** Spurdle AB, Couch FJ, Parsons MT, et al. Refined histopathological predictors of BRCA1 and BRCA2 mutation status: a large-scale analysis of breast cancer characteristics from the BCAC, CIMBA, and ENIGMA consortia. Breast Cancer Res. 2014 Dec 23;16(6):3419. PMID:25857409
**1986.** Sreekantaiah C, Karakousis CP, Leong SP, et al. Cytogenetic findings in liposarcoma correlate with histopathologic subtypes. Cancer. 1992 May 15;69(10):2484–95. PMID:1568170
**1987.** Srivastava S, Zou ZQ, Pirollo K, et al. Germ-line transmission of a mutated p53 gene in a cancer-prone family with Li-Fraumeni syndrome. Nature. 1990 Dec 20-27;348(6303):747–9. PMID:2259385
**1988.** Stacey SN, Manolescu A, Sulem P, et al. Common variants on chromosome 5p12 confer susceptibility to estrogen receptor-positive breast cancer. Nat Genet. 2008 Jun;40(6):703–6. PMID:18430407
**1989.** Stacey SN, Manolescu A, Sulem P, et al. Common variants on chromosomes 2q35 and 16q12 confer susceptibility to estrogen receptor-positive breast cancer. Nat Genet. 2007 Jul;39(7):865–9. PMID:17529974
**1990.** Stafyla V, Kotsifopoulos N, Grigoriades K, et al. Lobular carcinoma in situ of the breast within a fibroadenoma. A case report. Gynecol Oncol. 2004 Aug;94(2):572–4. PMID:15297206
**1991.** Stålhammar G, Rosin G, Fredriksson I, et al. Low concordance of biomarkers in histopathological and cytological material from breast cancer. Histopathology. 2014 Jun;64(7):971–80. PMID:24320941
**1992.** Stankovic T, Kidd AM, Sutcliffe A, et al. ATM mutations and phenotypes in ataxia-telangiectasia families in the British Isles: expression of mutant ATM and the risk of leukemia, lymphoma, and breast cancer. Am J Hum Genet. 1998 Feb;62(2):334–45. PMID:9463314
**1993.** Stephens PJ, Tarpey PS, Davies H, et al. The landscape of cancer genes and mutational processes in breast cancer. Nature. 2012 May 16;486(7403):400–4. PMID:22722201
**1994.** Stewart RL, Caron JE, Gulbahce EH, et al. HER2 immunohistochemical and fluorescence in situ hybridization discordances in invasive breast carcinoma with micropapillary features. Mod Pathol. 2017 Nov;30(11):1561–6. PMID:28752841
**1995.** Stone J, Thompson DJ, Dos Santos Silva I, et al. Novel associations between common breast cancer susceptibility variants and risk-predicting mammographic density measures. Cancer Res. 2015 Jun 15;75(12):2457–67. PMID:25862352
**1996.** Stone JP, Hartley RL, Temple-Oberle C. Breast cancer in transgender patients: a systematic review. Part 2: female to male. Eur J Surg Oncol. 2018 Oct;44(10):1463–8. PMID:30037639
**1997.** Stoppa-Lyonnet D. The biological effects and clinical implications of BRCA mutations: Where do we go from here? Eur J Hum Genet. 2016 Sep;24 Suppl 1:S3–9. PMID:27514841
**1998.** Stracker TH, Usui T, Petrini JH. Taking the time to make important decisions: the checkpoint effector kinases Chk1 and Chk2 and the DNA damage response. DNA Repair (Amst). 2009 Sep 2;8(9):1047–54. PMID:19473886
**1999.** Straver ME, Glas AM, Hannemann J, et al. The 70-gene signature as a response predictor for neoadjuvant chemotherapy in breast cancer. Breast Cancer Res Treat. 2010 Feb;119(3):551–8. PMID:19214742
**2000.** Stuebs F, Heidemann S, Caliebe A, et al. CDH1 mutation screen in a BRCA1/2-negative familial breast-/ovarian cancer cohort. Arch Gynecol Obstet. 2018 Jan;297(1):147–52. PMID:28993866
**2001.** Stutz JA, Evans AJ, Pinder S, et al. The radiological appearances of invasive cribriform carcinoma of the breast. Clin Radiol. 1994 Oct;49(10):693–5. PMID:7955831
**2002.** Su Y, Swift M. Outcomes of adjuvant radiation therapy for breast cancer in women with ataxia-telangiectasia mutations. JAMA. 2001 Nov 14;286(18):2233–4. PMID:11710885
**2003.** Subhawong AP, Subhawong TK, Khouri N, et al. Incidental minimal atypical lobular hyperplasia on core needle biopsy: correlation with findings on follow-up excision. Am J Surg Pathol. 2010 Jun;34(6):822–8. PMID:20431477
**2004.** Sullivan ME, Khan SA, Sullu Y, et al. Lobular carcinoma in situ variants in breast cores: potential for misdiagnosis, upgrade rates at surgical excision, and practical implications. Arch Pathol Lab Med. 2010 Jul;134(7):1024–8. PMID:20586632
**2005.** Sullivan SG, Hussain R, Threlfall T, et al. The incidence of cancer in people with intellectual disabilities. Cancer Causes Control. 2004 Dec;15(10):1021–5. PMID:15801486
**2006.** Sun HF, Zhao Y, Gao SP, et al. Clinicopathological characteristics and survival outcomes of male breast cancer according to race: a SEER population-based study. Oncotarget. 2017 May 26;8(41):69680–90. PMID:29050233
**2007.** Sung HJ, Maeng YI, Kim MK, et al. Breast carcinoma with choriocarcinomatous features: a case report. J Breast Cancer. 2013 Sep;16(3):349–53. PMID:24155767
**2008.** Surov A, Holzhausen HJ, Ruschke K, et al. Breast plasmacytoma. Acta Radiol. 2010 Jun;51(5):498–504. PMID:20429767
**2009.** Suryawanshi A, Middleton T, Ganda K. An unusual presentation of X-linked adrenoleukodystrophy. Endocrinol Diabetes Metab Case Rep. 2015;2015:150098. PMID:26609365
**2010.** Susnik B, Day D, Abeln E, et al. Surgical outcomes of lobular neoplasia diagnosed in core biopsy: prospective study of 316 cases. Clin Breast Cancer. 2016 Dec;16(6):507–13. PMID:27425222
**2011.** Sutton B, Davion S, Feldman M, et al. Mucocele-like lesions diagnosed on breast core biopsy: assessment of upgrade rate and need for surgical excision. Am J Clin Pathol. 2012 Dec;138(6):783–8. PMID:23161710
**2012.** Sutton T, Farinola M, Johnson N, et al. Atypical ductal hyperplasia: clinicopathologic factors are not predictive of upgrade after excisional biopsy. Am J Surg. 2019 May;217(5):848–50. PMID:30611396
**2013.** Suzuki R, Orsini N, Mignone L, et al. Alcohol intake and risk of breast cancer defined by estrogen and progesterone receptor status–a meta-analysis of epidemiological studies. Int J Cancer. 2008 Apr 15;122(8):1832–41. PMID:18067133
**2014.** Švajdler M, Baník P, Poliaková K, et al. Sebaceous carcinoma of the breast: report of four cases and review of the literature. Pol J Pathol. 2015 Jun;66(2):142–8. PMID:26247527
**2015.** Swisher EM, Lin KK, Oza AM, et al. Rucaparib in relapsed, platinum-sensitive high-grade ovarian carcinoma (ARIEL2 Part 1): an international, multicentre, open-label, phase 2 trial. Lancet Oncol. 2017 Jan;18(1):75–87. PMID:27908594
**2016.** Sy SM, Huen MS, Zhu Y, et al. PALB2 regulates recombinational repair through chromatin association and oligomerization. J Biol Chem. 2009 Jul 3;284(27):18302–10. PMID:19423707
**2017.** Symmans WF, Peintinger F, Hatzis C, et al. Measurement of residual breast cancer

burden to predict survival after neoadjuvant chemotherapy. J Clin Oncol. 2007 Oct 1;25(28):4414–22. PMID:17785706
**2018.** Syngal S, Brand RE, Church JM, et al. ACG clinical guideline: genetic testing and management of hereditary gastrointestinal cancer syndromes. Am J Gastroenterol. 2015 Feb;110(2):223–62, quiz 263. PMID:25645574
**2019.** Szabo J, Garcia D, Ciomek N, et al. Spuriously aggressive features of a lactating adenoma prompting repeated biopsies. Radiol Case Rep. 2017 Feb 24;12(2):215–8. PMID:28491154
**2020.** Szychta P, Westfal B, Maciejczyk R, et al. Intraoperative diagnosis of sentinel lymph node metastases in breast cancer treatment with one-step nucleic acid amplification assay (OSNA). Arch Med Sci. 2016 Dec 1;12(6):1239–46. PMID:27904514
**2021.** Tadros AB, Wen HY, Morrow M. Breast cancers of special histologic subtypes are biologically diverse. Ann Surg Oncol. 2018 Oct;25(11):3158–64. PMID:30094484
**2022.** Tait R, Pinder SE, Ellis IO, et al. Adenomyoepithelioma of the breast; a case report and literature review. J BUON. 2005 Jul-Sep;10(3):393–5. PMID:17357195
**2023.** Tajima S, Koda K, Ishii Y, et al. A case of matrix-producing metaplastic carcinoma of the breast exhibiting similarities to pleomorphic adenoma on fine-needle aspiration cytology. Int J Clin Exp Pathol. 2015 Nov 1;8(11):15333–7. PMID:26823890
**2024.** Talman ML, Jensen MB, Rank F. Invasive lobular breast cancer. Prognostic significance of histological malignancy grading. Acta Oncol. 2007;46(6):803–9. PMID:17653904
**2025.** Talwalkar SS, Miranda RN, Valbuena JR, et al. Lymphomas involving the breast: a study of 106 cases comparing localized and disseminated neoplasms. Am J Surg Pathol. 2008 Sep;32(9):1299–309. PMID:18636016
**2026.** Talwalkar SS, Valbuena JR, Abruzzo LV, et al. MALT1 gene rearrangements and NF-kappaB activation involving p65 and p50 are absent or rare in primary MALT lymphomas of the breast. Mod Pathol. 2006 Nov;19(11):1402–8. PMID:16917511
**2027.** Tamimi RM, Baer HJ, Marotti J, et al. Comparison of molecular phenotypes of ductal carcinoma in situ and invasive breast cancer. Breast Cancer Res. 2008;10(4):R67. PMID:18681955
**2028.** Tamura G, Monma N, Suzuki Y, et al. Adenomyoepithelioma (myoepithelioma) of the breast in a male. Hum Pathol. 1993 Jun;24(6):678–81. PMID:8389319
**2029.** Tan BY, Acs G, Apple SK, et al. Phyllodes tumours of the breast: a consensus review. Histopathology. 2016 Jan;68(1):5–21. PMID:26768026
**2030.** Tan BY, Tan PH. A diagnostic approach to fibroepithelial breast lesions. Surg Pathol Clin. 2018 Mar;11(1):17–42. PMID:29413655
**2031.** Tan EY, Tan PH, Yong WS, et al. Recurrent phyllodes tumours of the breast: pathological features and clinical implications. ANZ J Surg. 2006 Jun;76(6):476–80. PMID:16768772
**2032.** Tan H, Zhang S, Liu H, et al. Imaging findings in phyllodes tumors of the breast. Eur J Radiol. 2012 Jan;81(1):e62–9. PMID:21353414
**2033.** Tan J, Ong CK, Lim WK, et al. Genomic landscapes of breast fibroepithelial tumors. Nat Genet. 2015 Nov;47(11):1341–5. PMID:26437033
**2034.** Tan MH, Mester J, Peterson C, et al. A clinical scoring system for selection of patients for PTEN mutation testing is proposed on the basis of a prospective study of 3042 probands. Am J Hum Genet. 2011 Jan 7;88(1):42–56. PMID:21194675
**2035.** Tan MH, Mester JL, Ngeow J, et al. Lifetime cancer risks in individuals with germline PTEN mutations. Clin Cancer Res. 2012 Jan 15;18(2):400–7. PMID:22252256
**2036.** Tan PH, Ellis IO. Myoepithelial and epithelial-myoepithelial, mesenchymal and fibroepithelial breast lesions: updates from the WHO Classification of Tumours of the Breast 2012. J Clin Pathol. 2013 Jun;66(6):465–70. PMID:23533258
**2037.** Tan PH, Harada O, Thike AA, et al. Histiocytoid breast carcinoma: an enigmatic lobular entity. J Clin Pathol. 2011 Aug;64(8):654–9. PMID:21398688
**2038.** Tan PH, Jayabaskar T, Chuah KL, et al. Phyllodes tumors of the breast: the role of pathologic parameters. Am J Clin Pathol. 2005 Apr;123(4):529–40. PMID:15743740
**2039.** Tan PH, Jayabaskar T, Yip G, et al. p53 and c-kit (CD117) protein expression as prognostic indicators in breast phyllodes tumors: a tissue microarray study. Mod Pathol. 2005 Dec;18(12):1527–34. PMID:16258510
**2040.** Tan PH, Schnitt SJ, van de Vijver MJ, et al. Papillary and neuroendocrine breast lesions: the WHO stance. Histopathology. 2015 May;66(6):761–70. PMID:24845113
**2041.** Tan PH, Thike AA, Tan WJ, et al. Predicting clinical behaviour of breast phyllodes tumours: a nomogram based on histological criteria and surgical margins. J Clin Pathol. 2012 Jan;65(1):69–76. PMID:22049216
**2042.** Tan PH, Tse GM, Bay BH. Mucinous breast lesions: diagnostic challenges. J Clin Pathol. 2008 Jan;61(1):11–9. PMID:17873114
**2043.** Tan WJ, Cima I, Choudhury Y, et al. A five-gene reverse transcription-PCR assay for pre-operative classification of breast fibroepithelial lesions. Breast Cancer Res. 2016 Mar 9;18(1):31. PMID:26961242
**2044.** Tan WJ, Thike AA, Bay BH, et al. Immunohistochemical expression of homeoproteins Six1 and Pax3 in breast phyllodes tumours correlates with histological grade and clinical outcome. Histopathology. 2014 May;64(6):807–17. PMID:24438019
**2045.** Tan WJ, Thike AA, Tan SY, et al. CD117 expression in breast phyllodes tumors correlates with adverse pathologic parameters and reduced survival. Mod Pathol. 2015 Mar;28(3):352–8. PMID:25216225
**2046.** Tanaka K, Imoto S, Wada N, et al. Invasive apocrine carcinoma of the breast: clinicopathologic features of 57 patients. Breast J. 2008 Mar-Apr;14(2):164–8. PMID:18248561
**2047.** Tanaka N, Ueno T, Takama Y, et al. Fibroadenoma in adolescent females after living donor liver transplantation. Pediatr Transplant. 2017 Sep;21(6):e12947. PMID:28556594
**2048.** Tang F, Wei B, Tian Z, et al. Invasive mammary carcinoma with neuroendocrine differentiation: histological features and diagnostic challenges. Histopathology. 2011 Jul;59(1):106–15. PMID:21668471
**2049.** Tang SL, Yang JQ, Du ZG, et al. Clinicopathologic study of invasive micropapillary carcinoma of the breast. Oncotarget. 2017 Jun 27;8(26):42455–65. PMID:28418916
**2050.** Taniguchi K, Takata K, Chuang SS, et al. Frequent MYD88 L265P and CD79B mutations in primary breast diffuse large B-cell lymphoma. Am J Surg Pathol. 2016 Mar;40(3):324–34. PMID:26752547
**2051.** Tao L, Gomez SL, Keegan TH, et al. Breast cancer mortality in African-American and non-Hispanic white women by molecular subtype and stage at diagnosis: a population-based study. Cancer Epidemiol Biomarkers Prev. 2015 Jul;24(7):1039–45. PMID:25969506
**2052.** Tao L, Schwab RB, San Miguel Y, et al. Breast cancer mortality in older and younger patients in California. Cancer Epidemiol Biomarkers Prev. 2019 Feb;28(2):303–10. PMID:30333222
**2053.** Tavassoli FA. Myoepithelial lesions of the breast. Myoepitheliosis, adenomyoepithelioma, and myoepithelial carcinoma. Am J Surg Pathol. 1991 Jun;15(6):554–68. PMID:1709559
**2054.** Tavassoli FA, editor. Pathology of the breast. 2nd ed. Stamford (CT): Appleton & Lange; 1999.
**2055.** Tavassoli FA, Eusebi V. Tumors of the mammary gland. Washington, DC: American Registry of Pathology; 2009. (AFIP atlas of tumor pathology, series 4; fascicle 10).
**2056.** Tavassoli FA, Norris HJ. A comparison of the results of long-term follow-up for atypical intraductal hyperplasia and intraductal hyperplasia of the breast. Cancer. 1990 Feb 1;65(3):518–29. PMID:2297643
**2057.** Tavassoli FA, Norris HJ. Breast carcinoma with osteoclastlike giant cells. Arch Pathol Lab Med. 1986 Jul;110(7):636–9. PMID:3013119
**2058.** Tavassoli FA, Norris HJ. Mammary adenoid cystic carcinoma with sebaceous differentiation. A morphologic study of the cell types. Arch Pathol Lab Med. 1986 Nov;110(11):1045–53. PMID:3022669
**2059.** Tavassoli FA, Norris HJ. Secretory carcinoma of the breast. Cancer. 1980 May 1;45(9):2404–13. PMID:6445777
**2060.** Tavtigian SV, Oefner PJ, Babikyan D, et al. Rare, evolutionarily unlikely missense substitutions in ATM confer increased risk of breast cancer. Am J Hum Genet. 2009 Oct;85(4):427–46. PMID:19781682
**2061.** Tawasil J, Go EM, Tsang JY, et al. Associations of epithelial c-kit expression in phyllodes tumours of the breast. J Clin Pathol. 2015 Oct;68(10):808–11. PMID:26056158
**2062.** Tay TK, Chang KT, Thike AA, et al. Paediatric fibroepithelial lesions revisited: pathological insights. J Clin Pathol. 2015 Aug;68(8):633–41. PMID:25998513
**2063.** Tay TKY, Guan P, Loke BN, et al. Molecular insights into paediatric breast fibroepithelial tumours. Histopathology. 2018 Nov;73(5):809–18. PMID:29969836
**2064.** Taylor AM, Lam Z, Last JI, et al. Ataxia telangiectasia: more variation at clinical and cellular levels. Clin Genet. 2015 Mar;87(3):199–208. PMID:25040471
**2065.** Tejpar S, Nollet F, Li C, et al. Predominance of beta-catenin mutations and beta-catenin dysregulation in sporadic aggressive fibromatosis (desmoid tumor). Oncogene. 1999 Nov 11;18(47):6615–20. PMID:10597266
**2066.** Telesinghe PU, Anthony PP. Primary lymphoma of the breast. Histopathology. 1985 Mar;9(3):297–307. PMID:3922871
**2067.** Teng CY, Diego EJ. Case report of a large lactating adenoma with rapid antepartum enlargement. Int J Surg Case Rep. 2016;20:127–9. PMID:26855073
**2068.** Teo ZL, Provenzano E, Dite GS, et al. Tumour morphology predicts PALB2 germline mutation status. Br J Cancer. 2013 Jul 9;109(1):154–63. PMID:23787919
**2069.** Terada T. Ductal adenoma of the breast: immunohistochemistry of two cases. Pathol Int. 2008 Dec;58(12):801–5. PMID:19067857
**2070.** Tessier Cloutier B, Costa FD, Tazelaar HD, et al. Aberrant expression of neuroendocrine markers in angiosarcoma: a potential diagnostic pitfall. Hum Pathol. 2014 Aug;45(8):1618–24. PMID:24846674
**2071.** The Non-Hodgkin's Lymphoma Classification Project. A clinical evaluation of the International Lymphoma Study Group classification of non-Hodgkin's lymphoma. Blood. 1997 Jun 1;89(11):3909–18. PMID:9166827
**2072.** Thomas A, Link BK, Altekruse S, et al. Primary breast lymphoma in the United States: 1975-2013. J Natl Cancer Inst. 2017 Jun 1;109(6):djw294. PMID:28376147
**2073.** Thomas G, Jacobs KB, Kraft P, et al. A multistage genome-wide association study in breast cancer identifies two new risk alleles at 1p11.2 and 14q24.1 (RAD51L1). Nat Genet. 2009 May;41(5):579–84. PMID:19330030
**2074.** Thomas JS, Julian HS, Green RV, et al. Histopathology of breast carcinoma following neoadjuvant systemic therapy: a common association between letrozole therapy and central scarring. Histopathology. 2007 Aug;51(2):219–26. PMID:17650216
**2075.** Thompson AM, Clements K, Cheung S, et al. Management and 5-year outcomes in 9938 women with screen-detected ductal carcinoma in situ: the UK Sloane Project. Eur J Cancer. 2018 Sep;101:210–9. PMID:30092498
**2076.** Thompson D, Duedal S, Kirner J, et al. Cancer risks and mortality in heterozygous ATM mutation carriers. J Natl Cancer Inst. 2005 Jun 1;97(11):813–22. PMID:15928302
**2077.** Thompson D, Easton DF, Breast Cancer Linkage Consortium. Cancer incidence in BRCA1 mutation carriers. J Natl Cancer Inst. 2002 Sep 18;94(18):1358–65. PMID:12237281
**2079.** Thompson S, Kaplan SS, Poppiti RJ Jr, et al. Solitary neurofibroma of the breast. Radiol Case Rep. 2015 Dec 7;7(4):462. PMID:27330588
**2080.** Thor AD, Eng C, Devries S, et al. Invasive micropapillary carcinoma of the breast is associated with chromosome 8 abnormalities detected by comparative genomic hybridization. Hum Pathol. 2002 Jun;33(6):628–31. PMID:12152162
**2081.** Tierney RJ, Shannon-Lowe CD, Fitzsimmons L, et al. Unexpected patterns of Epstein-Barr virus transcription revealed by a high throughput PCR array for absolute quantification of viral mRNA. Virology. 2015 Jan 1;474:117–30. PMID:25463610
**2082.** Tilve A, Mallo R, Pérez A, et al. Breast hemangiomas: correlation between imaging and pathologic findings. J Clin Ultrasound. 2012 Oct;40(8):512–7. PMID:22434703
**2083.** Tischkowitz M, Xia B. PALB2/FANCN: recombining cancer and Fanconi anemia. Cancer Res. 2010 Oct 1;70(19):7353–9. PMID:20858716
**2084.** Tiulpakov A, Kalintchenko N, Semitcheva T, et al. A potential rearrangement between CYP19 and TRPM7 genes on chromosome 15q21.2 as a cause of aromatase excess syndrome. J Clin Endocrinol Metab. 2005 Jul;90(7):4184–90. PMID:15811932
**2085.** Tjalma WA, Verslegers IO, De Loecker PA, et al. Low and high grade mucoepidermoid carcinomas of the breast. Eur J Gynaecol Oncol. 2002;23(5):423–5. PMID:12440816
**2086.** To T, Wall C, Baines CJ, et al. Is carcinoma in situ a precursor lesion of invasive breast cancer? Int J Cancer. 2014 Oct 1;135(7):1646–52. PMID:24615647
**2087.** Tognon C, Garnett M, Kenward E, et al. The chimeric protein tyrosine kinase ETV6-NTRK3 requires both Ras-Erk1/2 and PI3-kinase-Akt signaling for fibroblast transformation. Cancer Res. 2001 Dec 15;61(24):8909–16. PMID:11751416
**2088.** Tognon C, Knezevich SR, Huntsman D, et al. Expression of the ETV6-NTRK3 gene fusion as a primary event in human secretory breast carcinoma. Cancer Cell. 2002 Nov;2(5):367–76. PMID:12450792
**2089.** Toi PC, Neelaiah S, Dharanipragada K, et al. Evaluation of estrogen and progesterone receptors and Her-2 expression with grading in the fine-needle aspirates of patients with breast carcinoma. J Cytol. 2018 Oct-Dec;35(4):223–8.

PMID:30498294
**2090.** Toikkanen S, Kujari H. Pure and mixed mucinous carcinomas of the breast: a clinicopathologic analysis of 61 cases with long-term follow-up. Hum Pathol. 1989 Aug;20(8):758–64. PMID:2545592
**2091.** Toikkanen S, Pylkkänen L, Joensuu H. Invasive lobular carcinoma of the breast has better short- and long-term survival than invasive ductal carcinoma. Br J Cancer. 1997;76(9):1234–40. PMID:9365176
**2092.** Toker C. Clear cells of the nipple epidermis. Cancer. 1970 Mar;25(3):601–10. PMID:4313654
**2093.** Tomlinson IP, Alam NA, Rowan AJ, et al. Germline mutations in FH predispose to dominantly inherited uterine fibroids, skin leiomyomata and papillary renal cell cancer. Nat Genet. 2002 Apr;30(4):406–10. PMID:11865300
**2094.** Torres-Mora J, Dry S, Li X, et al. Malignant melanotic schwannian tumor: a clinicopathologic, immunohistochemical, and gene expression profiling study of 40 cases, with a proposal for the reclassification of "melanotic schwannoma". Am J Surg Pathol. 2014 Jan;38(1):94–105. PMID:24145644
**2095.** Tosi AL, Ragazzi M, Asioli S, et al. Breast tumor resembling the tall cell variant of papillary thyroid carcinoma: report of 4 cases with evidence of malignant potential. Int J Surg Pathol. 2007 Jan;15(1):14–9. PMID:17172492
**2096.** Toss A, Grandi G, Cagnacci A, et al. The impact of reproductive life on breast cancer risk in women with family history or BRCA mutation. Oncotarget. 2017 Feb 7;8(6):9144–54. PMID:27880720
**2097.** Toss MS, Billingham K, Egbuniwe IU, et al. Breast tumours resembling the tall cell variant of thyroid papillary carcinoma: Are they part of the papillary carcinoma spectrum or a distinct entity? Pathobiology. 2019;86(2-3):83–91. PMID:30308500
**2098.** Toss MS, Pinder SE, Green AR, et al. Breast conservation in ductal carcinoma in situ (DCIS): What defines optimal margins? Histopathology. 2017 Apr;70(5):681–92. PMID:28000325
**2099.** Tozbikian G, Brogi E, Vallejo CE, et al. Atypical ductal hyperplasia bordering on ductal carcinoma in situ. Int J Surg Pathol. 2017 Apr;25(2):100–7. PMID:27481892
**2099A.** Tozbikian GH, Zynger DL. A combination of GATA3 and SOX10 is useful for the diagnosis of metastatic triple-negative breast cancer. Hum Pathol. 2019 Mar;85:221–7. PMID:30468800
**2100.** Tramm T, Kim JY, Tavassoli FA. Diminished number or complete loss of myoepithelial cells associated with metaplastic and neoplastic apocrine lesions of the breast. Am J Surg Pathol. 2011 Feb;35(2):202–11. PMID:21263240
**2101.** Trentham-Dietz A, Newcomb PA, Storer BE, et al. Risk factors for carcinoma in situ of the breast. Cancer Epidemiol Biomarkers Prev. 2000 Jul;9(7):697–703. PMID:10919740
**2102.** Trojani M, De Mascarel I, Coquet M, et al. [Osteoclastic type giant cell carcinoma of the breast]. Ann Pathol. 1989;9(3):189–94. French. PMID:2757703
**2103.** Trovik CS, Bauer HC, Alvegård TA, et al. Surgical margins, local recurrence and metastasis in soft tissue sarcomas: 559 surgically-treated patients from the Scandinavian Sarcoma Group Register. Eur J Cancer. 2000 Apr;36(6):710–6. PMID:10762742
**2104.** Troxell ML. Merkel cell carcinoma, melanoma, metastatic mimics of breast cancer. Semin Diagn Pathol. 2017 Sep;34(5):479–95. PMID:28645508
**2105.** Troxell ML. Reversed MUC1/EMA polarity in both mucinous and micropapillary breast carcinoma. Hum Pathol. 2014 Feb;45(2):432–4. PMID:24439232
**2106.** Troxell ML, Levine J, Beadling C, et al. High prevalence of PIK3CA/AKT pathway mutations in papillary neoplasms of the breast. Mod Pathol. 2010 Jan;23(1):27–37. PMID:19898424
**2107.** Troxell ML, Masek M, Sibley RK. Immunohistochemical staining of papillary breast lesions. Appl Immunohistochem Mol Morphol. 2007 Jun;15(2):145–53. PMID:17525625
**2108.** Tsai ML, Lillemoe TJ, Finkelstein MJ, et al. Utility of Oncotype DX risk assessment in patients with invasive lobular carcinoma. Clin Breast Cancer. 2016 Feb;16(1):45–50. PMID:26385397
**2109.** Tsang JY, Mendoza P, Lam CC, et al. Involvement of α- and β-catenins and E-cadherin in the development of mammary phyllodes tumours. Histopathology. 2012 Oct;61(4):667–74. PMID:22571452
**2110.** Tsang JY, Mendoza P, Putti TC, et al. E-cadherin expression in the epithelial components of mammary phyllodes tumors. Hum Pathol. 2012 Dec;43(12):2117–23. PMID:22820000
**2111.** Tsang JYS, Hui YK, Lee MA, et al. Association of clinicopathological features and prognosis of TERT alterations in phyllodes tumor of breast. Sci Rep. 2018 Mar 1;8(1):3881. PMID:29497099
**2112.** Tsang WY, Chan JK. Endocrine ductal carcinoma in situ (E-DCIS) of the breast: a form of low-grade DCIS with distinctive clinicopathologic and biologic characteristics. Am J Surg Pathol. 1996 Aug;20(8):921–43. PMID:8712293
**2113.** Tse GM, Law BK, Chan KF, et al. Multinucleated stromal giant cells in mammary phyllodes tumours. Pathology. 2001 May;33(2):153–6. PMID:11358046
**2114.** Tse GM, Law BK, Ma TK, et al. Hamartoma of the breast: a clinicopathological review. J Clin Pathol. 2002 Dec;55(12):951–4. PMID:12461066
**2115.** Tse GM, Ma TK, Lui PC, et al. Fine needle aspiration cytology of papillary lesions of the breast: How accurate is the diagnosis? J Clin Pathol. 2008 Aug;61(8):945–9. PMID:18552172
**2116.** Tse GM, Ma TK, Pang LM, et al. Fine needle aspiration cytologic features of mammary phyllodes tumors. Acta Cytol. 2002 Sep-Oct;46(5):855–63. PMID:12365219
**2117.** Tse GM, Tan PH. Diagnosing breast lesions by fine needle aspiration cytology or core biopsy: Which is better? Breast Cancer Res Treat. 2010 Aug;123(1):1–8. PMID:20526738
**2118.** Tseng WH, Martinez SR. Metaplastic breast cancer: To radiate or not to radiate? Ann Surg Oncol. 2011 Jan;18(1):94–103. PMID:20585866
**2119.** Tsubura A, Hatano T, Murata A, et al. Breast carcinoma in patients receiving neuroleptic therapy. Morphologic and clinicopathologic features of thirteen cases. Acta Pathol Jpn. 1992 Jul;42(7):494–9. PMID:1357916
**2120.** Turashvili G, Brogi E, Morrow M, et al. The 21-gene recurrence score in special histologic subtypes of breast cancer with favorable prognosis. Breast Cancer Res Treat. 2017 Aug;165(1):65–76. PMID:28577081
**2121.** Turnbull C, Ahmed S, Morrison J, et al. Genome-wide association study identifies five new breast cancer susceptibility loci. Nat Genet. 2010 Jun;42(6):504–7. PMID:20453838
**2122.** Tuttle R, Kane JM 3rd. Biopsy techniques for soft tissue and bowel sarcomas. J Surg Oncol. 2015 Apr;111(5):504–12. PMID:25663366
**2123.** Uchida N, Yokoo H, Kuwano H. Schwannoma of the breast: report of a case. Surg Today. 2005;35(3):238–42. PMID:15772796
**2124.** Uchida T, Ishii M, Motomiya Y. Fibroadenoma associated with gynaecomastia in an adult man. Case report. Scand J Plast Reconstr Surg Hand Surg. 1993 Dec;27(4):327–9. PMID:8159950
**2125.** Udler MS, Ahmed S, Healey CS, et al. Fine scale mapping of the breast cancer 16q12 locus. Hum Mol Genet. 2010 Jun 15;19(12):2507–15. PMID:20332101
**2126.** Ueng SH, Mezzetti T, Tavassoli FA. Papillary neoplasms of the breast: a review. Arch Pathol Lab Med. 2009 Jun;133(6):893–907. PMID:19492881
**2127.** UICC [Internet]. Geneva (Switzerland): Union for International Cancer Control; 2019. TNM Publications and Resources; updated 2019 Feb 4. Available from: https://www.uicc.org/resources/tnm/publications-resources.
**2128.** Uluoğlu O, Akyürek N, Uner A, et al. Interdigitating dendritic cell tumor with breast and cervical lymph-node involvement: a case report and review of the literature. Virchows Arch. 2005 May;446(5):546–54. PMID:15806378
**2128A.** University of Pittsburgh Department of Pathology [Internet]. Pittsburgh (PA): University of Pittsburgh Medical Center; 2018. Estimating tumor volume reduction in the breast after neoadjuvant (a.k.a. pre-operative) therapy - Magee method. Available from: https://path.upmc.edu/onlineTools/ptvr.html.
**2128B.** University of Texas MD Anderson Cancer Center [Internet]. Houston (TX): University of Texas MD Anderson Cancer Center; 2019. Residual cancer burden calculator. Available from: http://www3.mdanderson.org/app/medcalc/index.cfm?pagename=jsconvert3.
**2129.** Upadhyaya M. Neurofibromatosis type 1: diagnosis and recent advances. Expert Opin Med Diagn. 2010 Jul;4(4):307–22. PMID:23496147
**2130.** Upasham SP, VinodKiri M, Sudhamani S. One more common tumor in an uncommon location: squamous cell carcinoma on nipple areola complex. Indian J Cancer. 2014 July-September;51(3):376–7. PMID:25494146
**2131.** Ustün M, Berner A, Davidson B, et al. Fine-needle aspiration cytology of lobular carcinoma in situ. Diagn Cytopathol. 2002 Jul;27(1):22–6. PMID:12112810
**2132.** Uusitalo E, Kallionpää RA, Kurki S, et al. Breast cancer in neurofibromatosis type 1: overrepresentation of unfavourable prognostic factors. Br J Cancer. 2017 Jan 17;116(2):211–7. PMID:27931045
**2133.** Uziel T, Savitsky K, Platzer M, et al. Genomic organization of the ATM gene. Genomics. 1996 Apr 15;33(2):317–20. PMID:8660985
**2134.** Seema V, Kalyani R, Srinivasa Murthy V. Multinucleate giant cells in FNAC of benign breast lesions: its significance. J Clin Diagn Res. 2014 Dec;8(12):FC01–04. PMID:25653953
**2135.** Vainio H, Kaaks R, Bianchini F. Weight control and physical activity in cancer prevention: international evaluation of the evidence. Eur J Cancer Prev. 2002 Aug;11 Suppl 2:S94–100. PMID:12570341
**2136.** Valbuena JR, Admirand JH, Gualco G, et al. Myeloid sarcoma involving the breast. Arch Pathol Lab Med. 2005 Jan;129(1):32–8. PMID:15628906
**2137.** Valdez JM, Nichols KE, Kesserwan C. Li-Fraumeni syndrome: a paradigm for the understanding of hereditary cancer predisposition. Br J Haematol. 2017 Feb;176(4):539–52. PMID:27984644
**2138.** Valero MG, Raut CP, Lotfi P, et al. Atypical lipomatous tumor of the breast. J Clin Oncol. 2011 Nov 1;29(31):e766–8. PMID:21931026
**2139.** Validire P, Capovilla M, Asselain B, et al. Primary breast non-Hodgkin's lymphoma: a large single center study of initial characteristics, natural history, and prognostic factors. Am J Hematol. 2009 Mar;84(3):133–9. PMID:19199367
**2140.** van Broekhoven DL, Verhoef C, Grünhagen DJ, et al. Prognostic value of CTNNB1 gene mutation in primary sporadic aggressive fibromatosis. Ann Surg Oncol. 2015 May;22(5):1464–70. PMID:25341748
**2141.** van de Vijver MJ, He YD, van't Veer LJ, et al. A gene-expression signature as a predictor of survival in breast cancer. N Engl J Med. 2002 Dec 19;347(25):1999–2009. PMID:12490681
**2142.** van den Broek AJ, Schmidt MK, van 't Veer LJ, et al. Worse breast cancer prognosis of BRCA1/BRCA2 mutation carriers: What's the evidence? A systematic review with meta-analysis. PLoS One. 2015 Mar 27;10(3):e0120189. PMID:25816289
**2143.** Van den Eynden GG, Colpaert CG, Couvelard A, et al. A fibrotic focus is a prognostic factor and a surrogate marker for hypoxia and (lymph)angiogenesis in breast cancer: review of the literature and proposal on the criteria of evaluation. Histopathology. 2007 Oct;51(4):440–51. PMID:17593207
**2144.** van den Munckhof P, Christiaans I, Kenter SB, et al. Germline SMARCB1 mutation predisposes to multiple meningiomas and schwannomas with preferential location of cranial meningiomas at the falx cerebri. Neurogenetics. 2012 Feb;13(1):1–7. PMID:22038540
**2145.** van der Pol CC, Lacle MM, Witkamp AJ, et al. Prognostic models in male breast cancer. Breast Cancer Res Treat. 2016 Nov;160(2):339–46. PMID:27671991
**2145A.** van der Post RS, Bult P, Vogelaar IP, et al. HNF4A immunohistochemistry facilitates distinction between primary and metastatic breast and gastric carcinoma. Virchows Arch. 2014 Jun;464(6):673–9. PMID:24711169
**2145B.** van der Post RS, Vogelaar IP, Carneiro F, et al. Hereditary diffuse gastric cancer: updated clinical guidelines with an emphasis on germline CDH1 mutation carriers. J Med Genet. 2015 Jun;52(6):361–74. PMID:25979631
**2146.** van Deurzen CH, Bult P, de Boer M, et al. Morphometry of isolated tumor cells in breast cancer sentinel lymph nodes: metastases or displacement? Am J Surg Pathol. 2009 Jan;33(1):106–10. PMID:18852675
**2147.** van Deurzen CH, de Bruin PC, Koelemij R, et al. Isolated tumor cells in breast cancer sentinel lymph nodes: displacement or metastases? An immunohistochemical study. Hum Pathol. 2009 Jun;40(6):778–82. PMID:19200573
**2148.** van Deurzen CH, Lee AH, Gill MS, et al. Metaplastic breast carcinoma: tumour histogenesis or dedifferentiation? J Pathol. 2011 Aug;224(4):434–7. PMID:21462188
**2149.** Van Hoeven KH, Drudis T, Cranor ML, et al. Low-grade adenosquamous carcinoma of the breast. A clinocopathologic study of 32 cases with ultrastructural analysis. Am J Surg Pathol. 1993 Mar;17(3):248–58. PMID:8434705
**2150.** van Lier MG, Westerman AM, Wagner A, et al. High cancer risk and increased mortality in patients with Peutz-Jeghers syndrome. Gut. 2011 Feb;60(2):141–7. PMID:21205875
**2151.** van Maaren MC, Lagendijk M, Tilanus-Linthorst MMA, et al. Breast cancer-related deaths according to grade in ductal carcinoma

in situ: a Dutch population-based study on patients diagnosed between 1999 and 2012. Eur J Cancer. 2018 Sep;101:134–42. PMID:30059817

**2152.** van 't Veer LJ, Dai H, van de Vijver MJ, et al. Gene expression profiling predicts clinical outcome of breast cancer. Nature. 2002 Jan 31;415(6871):530–6. PMID:11823860

**2153.** Vandenbussche CJ, Khouri N, Sbaity E, et al. Borderline atypical ductal hyperplasia/low-grade ductal carcinoma in situ on breast needle core biopsy should be managed conservatively. Am J Surg Pathol. 2013 Jun;37(6):913–23. PMID:23598968

**2154.** van der Groep P, van der Wall E, van Diest PJ. Pathology of hereditary breast cancer. Cell Oncol (Dordr). 2011 Apr;34(2):71–88. PMID:21336636

**2155.** Varga Z, Kolb SA, Flury R, et al. Sebaceous carcinoma of the breast. Pathol Int. 2000 Jan;50(1):63–6. PMID:10692180

**2156.** Varga Z, Robl C, Spycher M, et al. Metaplastic lipid-rich carcinoma of the breast. Pathol Int. 1998 Nov;48(11):912–6. PMID:9832063

**2157.** Varga Z, Theurillat JP, Filonenko V, et al. Preferential nuclear and cytoplasmic NY-BR-1 protein expression in primary breast cancer and lymph node metastases. Clin Cancer Res. 2006 May 1;12(9):2745–51. PMID:16675566

**2158.** Varga Z, Zhao J, Ohlschlegel C, et al. Preferential HER-2/neu overexpression and/or amplification in aggressive histological subtypes of invasive breast cancer. Histopathology. 2004 Apr;44(4):332–8. PMID:15049898

**2159.** Vargas AC, Lakhani SR, Simpson PT. Pleomorphic lobular carcinoma of the breast: molecular pathology and clinical impact. Future Oncol. 2009 Mar;5(2):233–43. PMID:19284381

**2160.** Varley JM. Germline TP53 mutations and Li-Fraumeni syndrome. Hum Mutat. 2003 Mar;21(3):313–20. PMID:12619118

**2161.** Venable JG, Schwartz AM, Silverberg SG. Infiltrating cribriform carcinoma of the breast: a distinctive clinicopathologic entity. Hum Pathol. 1990 Mar;21(3):333–8. PMID:2312110

**2162.** Vengoechea J, Tallo C. A germline deletion of 9p21.3 presenting as familial melanoma, astrocytoma and breast cancer: clinical and genetic counselling challenges. J Med Genet. 2017 Oct;54(10):682–4. PMID:28754699

**2163.** Ventura K, Cangiarella J, Lee I, et al. Aspiration biopsy of mammary lesions with abundant extracellular mucinous material. Review of 43 cases with surgical follow-up. Am J Clin Pathol. 2003 Aug;120(2):194–202. PMID:12931549

**2164.** Vera-Badillo FE, Templeton AJ, de Gouveia P, et al. Androgen receptor expression and outcomes in early breast cancer: a systematic review and meta-analysis. J Natl Cancer Inst. 2014 Jan;106(1):djt319. PMID:24273215

**2165.** Vereide DT, Seto E, Chiu YF, et al. Epstein-Barr virus maintains lymphomas via its miRNAs. Oncogene. 2014 Mar 6;33(10):1258–64. PMID:23503461

**2166.** Vergine M, Musella A, Gulotta E, et al. Paget's disease of the male breast: case report and a point of view from actual literature. G Chir. 2018 Mar-Apr;39(2):114–7. PMID:29694313

**2167.** Verhagen MM, Last JI, Hogervorst FB, et al. Presence of ATM protein and residual kinase activity correlates with the phenotype in ataxia-telangiectasia: a genotype-phenotype study. Hum Mutat. 2012 Mar;33(3):561–71. PMID:22213089

**2168.** Vermeulen MA, Doebar SC, van Deurzen CHM, et al. Copy number profiling of oncogenes in ductal carcinoma in situ of the male breast. Endocr Relat Cancer. 2018 Mar;25(3):173–84.

PMID:29203614

**2169.** Vermeulen MA, Slaets L, Cardoso F, et al. Pathological characterisation of male breast cancer: results of the EORTC 10085/TBCRC/BIG/NABCG International Male Breast Cancer Program. Eur J Cancer. 2017 Sep;82:219–27. PMID:28292559

**2170.** Verschoor AJ, Cleton-Jansen AM, Wijers-Koster P, et al. Radiation-induced sarcomas occurring in desmoid-type fibromatosis are not always derived from the primary tumor. Am J Surg Pathol. 2015 Dec;39(12):1701–7. PMID:26414222

**2171.** Verschuur-Maes AH, de Bruin PC, van Diest PJ. Epigenetic progression of columnar cell lesions of the breast to invasive breast cancer. Breast Cancer Res Treat. 2012 Dec;136(3):705–15. PMID:23104224

**2172.** Verschuur-Maes AH, Kornegoor R, de Bruin PC, et al. Do columnar cell lesions exist in the male breast? Histopathology. 2014 May;64(6):818–25. PMID:24267518

**2173.** Verschuur-Maes AH, Moelans CB, de Bruin PC, et al. Analysis of gene copy number alterations by multiplex ligation-dependent probe amplification in columnar cell lesions of the breast. Cell Oncol (Dordr). 2014 Apr;37(2):147–54. PMID:24692099

**2174.** Viale G, Rotmensz N, Maisonneuve P, et al. Lack of prognostic significance of "classic" lobular breast carcinoma: a matched, single institution series. Breast Cancer Res Treat. 2009 Sep;117(1):211–4. PMID:18629634

**2175.** Vieira CC, Mercado CL, Cangiarella JF, et al. Microinvasive ductal carcinoma in situ: clinical presentation, imaging features, pathologic findings, and outcome. Eur J Radiol. 2010 Jan;73(1):102–7. PMID:19026501

**2176.** Vielh P, Validire P, Kheirallah S, et al. Paget's disease of the nipple without clinically and radiologically detectable breast tumor. Histochemical and immunohistochemical study of 44 cases. Pathol Res Pract. 1993 Mar;189(2):150–5. PMID:8391688

**2176A.** Vincent-Salomon A, Gruel N, Lucchesi C, et al. Identification of typical medullary breast carcinoma as a genomic sub-group of basal-like carcinomas, a heterogeneous new molecular entity. Breast Cancer Res. 2007;9(2):R24. PMID:17417968

**2177.** Vincent-Salomon A, Lucchesi C, Gruel N, et al. Integrated genomic and transcriptomic analysis of ductal carcinoma in situ of the breast. Clin Cancer Res. 2008 Apr 1;14(7):1956–65. PMID:18381933

**2178.** Vingiani A, Maisonneuve P, Dell'orto P, et al. The clinical relevance of micropapillary carcinoma of the breast: a case-control study. Histopathology. 2013 Aug;63(2):217–24. PMID:23763700

**2179.** Virk RK, Khan A. Pseudoangiomatous stromal hyperplasia: an overview. Arch Pathol Lab Med. 2010 Jul;134(7):1070–4. PMID:20586640

**2180.** Virnig BA, Tuttle TM, Shamliyan T, et al. Ductal carcinoma in situ of the breast: a systematic review of incidence, treatment, and outcomes. J Natl Cancer Inst. 2010 Feb 3;102(3):170–8. PMID:20071685

**2181.** Visscher DW, Nassar A, Degnim AC, et al. Sclerosing adenosis and risk of breast cancer. Breast Cancer Res Treat. 2014 Feb;144(1):205–12. PMID:24510013

**2181A.** Visvader JE, Stingl J. Mammary stem cells and the differentiation hierarchy: current status and perspectives. Genes Dev. 2014 Jun 1;28(11):1143–58. PMID:24888586

**2182.** Visvanathan K, Hurley P, Bantug E, et al. Use of pharmacologic interventions for breast cancer risk reduction: American Society of Clinical Oncology clinical practice guideline. J Clin Oncol. 2013 Aug 10;31(23):2942–62.

PMID:23835710

**2183.** Viswanathan K, McMillen B, Cheng E, et al. Juvenile papillomatosis (Swiss-cheese disease) of breast in an adult male with sequential diagnoses of ipsilateral intraductal, invasive, and widely metastatic carcinoma: a case report and review of the disease in males. Int J Surg Pathol. 2017 Sep;25(6):536–42. PMID:28420303

**2184.** Vladescu T, Klijanienko J, Caillaud JM, et al. Fine-needle sampling in malignant phyllodes tumors: clinicopathologic study of 22 cases seen at the Institut Curie. Diagn Cytopathol. 2004 Aug;31(2):71–6. PMID:15282716

**2185.** Vo T, Xing Y, Meric-Bernstam F, et al. Long-term outcomes in patients with mucinous, medullary, tubular, and invasive ductal carcinomas after lumpectomy. Am J Surg. 2007 Oct;194(4):527–31. PMID:17826073

**2186.** Vo TN, Meric-Bernstam F, Yi M, et al. Outcomes of breast-conservation therapy for invasive lobular carcinoma are equivalent to those for invasive ductal carcinoma. Am J Surg. 2006 Oct;192(4):552–5. PMID:16978974

**2187.** Vogel WH. Li-Fraumeni syndrome. J Adv Pract Oncol. 2017 Nov-Dec;8(7):742–6. PMID:30333936

**2188.** Vogelstein B, Lane D, Levine AJ. Surfing the p53 network. Nature. 2000 Nov 16;408(6810):307–10. PMID:11099028

**2189.** Volckmar AL, Leichsenring J, Flechtenmacher C, et al. Tubular, lactating, and ductal adenomas are devoid of MED12 exon2 mutations, and ductal adenomas show recurrent mutations in GNAS and the PI3K-AKT pathway. Genes Chromosomes Cancer. 2017 Jan;56(1):11–7. PMID:27438523

**2190.** von Minckwitz G, Untch M, Blohmer JU, et al. Definition and impact of pathologic complete response on prognosis after neoadjuvant chemotherapy in various intrinsic breast cancer subtypes. J Clin Oncol. 2012 May 20;30(15):1796–804. PMID:22508812

**2191.** Vorburger SA, Xing Y, Hunt KK, et al. Angiosarcoma of the breast. Cancer. 2005 Dec 15;104(12):2682–8. PMID:16288486

**2192.** Vos CB, Cleton-Jansen AM, Berx G, et al. E-cadherin inactivation in lobular carcinoma in situ of the breast: an early event in tumorigenesis. Br J Cancer. 1997;76(9):1131–3. PMID:9365159

**2193.** Vos S, Elias SG, van der Groep P, et al. Comprehensive proteomic profiling-derived immunohistochemistry-based prediction models for BRCA1 and BRCA2 germline mutation-related breast carcinomas. Am J Surg Pathol. 2018 Sep;42(9):1262–72. PMID:29979200

**2194.** Vos S, Moelans CB, van Diest PJ. BRCA promoter methylation in sporadic versus BRCA germline mutation-related breast cancers. Breast Cancer Res. 2017 May 31;19(1):64. PMID:28569220

**2195.** Vos S, van Diest PJ, Ausems MG, et al. Ethical considerations for modern molecular pathology. J Pathol. 2018 Dec;246(4):405–14. PMID:30125358

**2196.** Vos S, van Diest PJ, Moelans CB. A systematic review on the frequency of BRCA promoter methylation in breast and ovarian carcinomas of BRCA germline mutation carriers: mutually exclusive, or not? Crit Rev Oncol Hematol. 2018 Jul;127:29–41. PMID:29891109

**2197.** Vourtsi A, Zervoudis S, Pafiti A, et al. Male breast hemangioma–a rare entity: a case report and review of the literature. Breast J. 2006 May-Jun;12(3):260–2. PMID:16684325

**2198.** Voz ML, Aström AK, Kas K, et al. The recurrent translocation t(5;8)(p13;q12) in pleomorphic adenomas results in upregulation of PLAG1 gene expression under control

of the LIFR promoter. Oncogene. 1998 Mar;16(11):1409–16. PMID:9525740

**2199.** Vranic S, Feldman R, Gatalica Z. Apocrine carcinoma of the breast: a brief update on the molecular features and targetable biomarkers. Bosn J Basic Med Sci. 2017 Feb 21;17(1):9–11. PMID:28027454

**2200.** Vranic S, Marchiò C, Castellano I, et al. Immunohistochemical and molecular profiling of histologically defined apocrine carcinomas of the breast. Hum Pathol. 2015 Sep;46(9):1350–9. PMID:26208846

**2201.** Vranic S, Schmitt F, Sapino A, et al. Apocrine carcinoma of the breast: a comprehensive review. Histol Histopathol. 2013 Nov;28(11):1393–409. PMID:23771415

**2202.** Vranic S, Tawfik O, Palazzo J, et al. EGFR and HER-2/neu expression in invasive apocrine carcinoma of the breast. Mod Pathol. 2010 May;23(5):644–53. PMID:20208479

**2203.** Wachter DL, Wachter PW, Fasching PA, et al. Characterization of molecular subtypes of Paget disease of the breast using immunohistochemistry and in situ hybridization. Arch Pathol Lab Med. 2019 Feb;143(2):206–11. PMID:30124327

**2204.** Wagner N, Schmidt S, Yerlikaya G, et al. Superficial papillary adenomatosis of the nipple: a rare disease diagnosed by sonography and histopathologically confirmed by nipple-preserving total excision. J Ultrasound Med. 2013 Feb;32(2):373–4. PMID:23341397

**2204A.** Wahl GM, Spike BT. Cell state plasticity, stem cells, EMT, and the generation of intra-tumoral heterogeneity. NPJ Breast Cancer. 2017 Apr 19;3:14. PMID:28649654

**2205.** Wahner-Roedler DL, Sebo TJ, Gisvold JJ. Hamartomas of the breast: clinical, radiologic, and pathologic manifestations. Breast J. 2001 Mar-Apr;7(2):101–5. PMID:11328316

**2206.** Waldman FM, Hwang ES, Etzell J, et al. Genomic alterations in tubular breast carcinomas. Hum Pathol. 2001 Feb;32(2):222–6. PMID:11230710

**2207.** Walford N, ten Velden J. Histiocytoid breast carcinoma: an apocrine variant of lobular carcinoma. Histopathology. 1989 May;14(5):515–22. PMID:2472346

**2208.** Walker GV, Smith GL, Perkins GH, et al. Population-based analysis of occult primary breast cancer with axillary lymph node metastasis. Cancer. 2010 Sep 1;116(17):4000–6. PMID:20564117

**2209.** Walker L, Thompson D, Easton D, et al. A prospective study of neurofibromatosis type 1 cancer incidence in the UK. Br J Cancer. 2006 Jul 17;95(2):233–8. PMID:16786042

**2210.** Wallden B, Storhoff J, Nielsen T, et al. Development and verification of the PAM50-based Prosigna breast cancer gene signature assay. BMC Med Genomics. 2015 Aug 22;8:54. PMID:26297356

**2211.** Walsh MM, Bleiweiss IJ. Invasive micropapillary carcinoma of the breast: eighty cases of an underrecognized entity. Hum Pathol. 2001 Jun;32(6):583–9. PMID:11431712

**2212.** Walters LL, Pang JC, Zhao L, et al. Ductal carcinoma in situ with distorting sclerosis on core biopsy may be predictive of upstaging on excision. Histopathology. 2015 Mar;66(4):577–86. PMID:25231210

**2213.** Wang C, Wang X, Ma R. Diagnosis and surgical treatment of nipple adenoma. ANZ J Surg. 2015 Jun;85(6):444–7. PMID:24975720

**2214.** Wang F, Jia Y, Tong Z. Comparison of the clinical and prognostic features of primary breast sarcomas and malignant phyllodes tumor. Jpn J Clin Oncol. 2015 Feb;45(2):146–52. PMID:25387733

**2215.** Wang J, Wei B, Albarracin CT, et al. Invasive neuroendocrine carcinoma of the breast: a population-based study from the

Surveillance, Epidemiology and End Results (SEER) database. BMC Cancer. 2014 Mar 4;14:147. PMID:24589259

**2216.** Wang P, Yu XM. A primary nipple lymphoma diagnosed by a modified fine-needle aspiration method. Diagn Cytopathol. 2012 Aug;40(8):719–23. PMID:22988573

**2217.** Wang SS, Deapen D, Voutsinas J, et al. Breast implants and anaplastic large cell lymphomas among females in the California Teachers Study cohort. Br J Haematol. 2016 Aug;174(3):480–3. PMID:26456010

**2218.** Wang W, Ding J, Yang W, et al. MRI characteristics of intraductal papilloma. Acta Radiol. 2015 Mar;56(3):276–83. PMID:24696194

**2219.** Wang W, Zhu W, Du F, et al. The demographic features, clinicopathological characteristics and cancer-specific outcomes for patients with microinvasive breast cancer: a SEER database analysis. Sci Rep. 2017 Feb 6;7:42045. PMID:28165014

**2220.** Wang X, Levin AM, Smolinski SE, et al. Breast cancer and other neoplasms in women with neurofibromatosis type 1: a retrospective review of cases in the Detroit metropolitan area. Am J Med Genet A. 2012 Dec;158A(12):3061–4. PMID:22965642

**2221.** Wang Y, Dai B, Ye D. CHEK2 mutation and risk of prostate cancer: a systematic review and meta-analysis. Int J Clin Exp Med. 2015 Sep 15;8(9):15708–15. PMID:26629066

**2222.** Wapnir IL, Dignam JJ, Fisher B, et al. Long-term outcomes of invasive ipsilateral breast tumor recurrences after lumpectomy in NSABP B-17 and B-24 randomized clinical trials for DCIS. J Natl Cancer Inst. 2011 Mar 16;103(6):478–88. PMID:21398619

**2223.** Waraya M, Hayashi K, Oshida S, et al. [A case report of ipsilateral nipple skin recurrence]. Gan To Kagaku Ryoho. 2017 Nov;44(12):1595–7. Japanese. PMID:29394713

**2224.** Ward BA, McKhann CF, Ravikumar TS. Ten-year follow-up of breast carcinoma in situ in Connecticut. Arch Surg. 1992 Dec;127(12):1392–5. PMID:1365682

**2225.** Ward EM, DeSantis CE, Lin CC, et al. Cancer statistics: breast cancer in situ. CA Cancer J Clin. 2015 Nov-Dec;65(6):481–95. PMID:26431342

**2226.** Wargotz ES, Deos PH, Norris HJ. Metaplastic carcinomas of the breast. II. Spindle cell carcinoma. Hum Pathol. 1989 Aug;20(8):732–40. PMID:2473024

**2227.** Wargotz ES, Norris HJ. Metaplastic carcinomas of the breast. I. Matrix-producing carcinoma. Hum Pathol. 1989 Jul;20(7):628–35. PMID:2544506

**2228.** Wargotz ES, Norris HJ. Metaplastic carcinomas of the breast. III. Carcinosarcoma. Cancer. 1989 Oct 1;64(7):1490–9. PMID:2776108

**2229.** Wargotz ES, Norris HJ. Metaplastic carcinomas of the breast. IV. Squamous cell carcinoma of ductal origin. Cancer. 1990 Jan 15;65(2):272–6. PMID:2153044

**2230.** Wargotz ES, Norris HJ, Austin RM, et al. Fibromatosis of the breast. A clinical and pathological study of 28 cases. Am J Surg Pathol. 1987 Jan;11(1):38–45. PMID:3789257

**2231.** Wargotz ES, Weiss SW, Norris HJ. Myofibroblastoma of the breast. Sixteen cases of a distinctive benign mesenchymal tumor. Am J Surg Pathol. 1987 Jul;11(7):493–502. PMID:3037930

**2232.** Warner ET, Tamimi RM, Hughes ME, et al. Racial and ethnic differences in breast cancer survival: mediating effect of tumor characteristics and sociodemographic and treatment factors. J Clin Oncol. 2015 Jul 10;33(20):2254–61. PMID:25964252

**2233.** Warner NE. Lobular carcinoma of the breast. Cancer. 1969 Apr;23(4):840–6. PMID:5775975

**2234.** Watanabe Y, Anan K, Saimura M, et al. Upstaging to invasive ductal carcinoma after mastectomy for ductal carcinoma in situ: predictive factors and role of sentinel lymph node biopsy. Breast Cancer. 2018 Nov;25(6):663–70. PMID:29786772

**2235.** Watermann DO, Tempfer C, Hefler LA, et al. Ultrasound morphology of invasive lobular breast cancer is different compared with other types of breast cancer. Ultrasound Med Biol. 2005 Feb;31(2):167–74. PMID:15708454

**2236.** Waters EA, McNeel TS, Stevens WM, et al. Use of tamoxifen and raloxifene for breast cancer chemoprevention in 2010. Breast Cancer Res Treat. 2012 Jul;134(2):875–80. PMID:22622807

**2237.** Weaver DL, Rosenberg RD, Barlow WE, et al. Pathologic findings from the Breast Cancer Surveillance Consortium: population-based outcomes in women undergoing biopsy after screening mammography. Cancer. 2006 Feb 15;106(4):732–42. PMID:16411214

**2238.** Weaver J, Downs-Kelly E, Goldblum JR, et al. Fluorescence in situ hybridization for MDM2 gene amplification as a diagnostic tool in lipomatous neoplasms. Mod Pathol. 2008 Aug;21(8):943–9. PMID:18500263

**2239.** Weaver MG, Abdul-Karim FW, al-Kaisi N. Mucinous lesions of the breast. A pathological continuum. Pathol Res Pract. 1993 Sep;189(8):873–6. PMID:8302709

**2240.** Wechselberger G, Schoeller T, Piza-Katzer H. Juvenile fibroadenoma of the breast. Surgery. 2002 Jul;132(1):106–7. PMID:12110805

**2241.** Wei S. Papillary lesions of the breast: an update. Arch Pathol Lab Med. 2016 Jul;140(7):628–43. PMID:27362568

**2242.** Weidner N, Levine JD. Spindle-cell adenomyoepithelioma of the breast. A microscopic, ultrastructural, and immunocytochemical study. Cancer. 1988 Oct 15;62(8):1561–7. PMID:2844382

**2243.** Weidner N, Semple JP. Pleomorphic variant of invasive lobular carcinoma of the breast. Hum Pathol. 1992 Oct;23(10):1167–71. PMID:1398644

**2244.** Weigelt B, Bi R, Kumar R, et al. The landscape of somatic genetic alterations in breast cancers from ATM germline mutation carriers. J Natl Cancer Inst. 2018 Sep 1;110(9):1030–4. PMID:29506079

**2245.** Weigelt B, Eberle C, Cowell CF, et al. Metaplastic breast carcinoma: more than a special type. Nat Rev Cancer. 2014 Mar;14(3):147–8. PMID:25688406

**2246.** Weigelt B, Geyer FC, Horlings HM, et al. Mucinous and neuroendocrine breast carcinomas are transcriptionally distinct from invasive ductal carcinomas of no special type. Mod Pathol. 2009 Nov;22(11):1401–14. PMID:19633645

**2247.** Weigelt B, Geyer FC, Natrajan R, et al. The molecular underpinning of lobular histological growth pattern: a genome-wide transcriptomic analysis of invasive lobular carcinomas and grade- and molecular subtype-matched invasive ductal carcinomas of no special type. J Pathol. 2010 Jan;220(1):45–57. PMID:19877120

**2248.** Weigelt B, Geyer FC, Reis-Filho JS. Histological types of breast cancer: How special are they? Mol Oncol. 2010 Jun;4(3):192–208. PMID:20452298

**2249.** Weigelt B, Horlings HM, Kreike B, et al. Refinement of breast cancer classification by molecular characterization of histological special types. J Pathol. 2008 Oct;216(2):141–50. PMID:18720457

**2250.** Weigelt B, Kreike B, Reis-Filho JS. Metaplastic breast carcinomas are basal-like breast cancers: a genomic profiling analysis. Breast Cancer Res Treat. 2009 Sep;117(2):273–80. PMID:18815879

**2251.** Weigelt B, Ng CK, Shen R, et al. Metaplastic breast carcinomas display genomic and transcriptomic heterogeneity [corrected]. Mod Pathol. 2015 Mar;28(3):340–51. PMID:25412848

**2252.** Weischer M, Bojesen SE, Ellervik C, et al. CHEK2*1100delC genotyping for clinical assessment of breast cancer risk: meta-analyses of 26,000 patient cases and 27,000 controls. J Clin Oncol. 2008 Feb 1;26(4):542–8. PMID:18172190

**2253.** Weischer M, Nordestgaard BG, Pharoah P, et al. CHEK2*1100delC heterozygosity in women with breast cancer associated with early death, breast cancer-specific death, and increased risk of a second breast cancer. J Clin Oncol. 2012 Dec 10;30(35):4308–16. PMID:23109706

**2254.** Weisman PS, Ng CK, Brogi E, et al. Genetic alterations of triple negative breast cancer by targeted next-generation sequencing and correlation with tumor morphology. Mod Pathol. 2016 May;29(5):476–88. PMID:26939876

**2255.** Weiss HA, Brinton LA, Brogan D, et al. Epidemiology of in situ and invasive breast cancer in women aged under 45. Br J Cancer. 1996 May;73(10):1298–305. PMID:8630296

**2256.** Weiss JB, Do WS, Forte DM, et al. Is bigger better? Twenty-year institutional experience of atypical ductal hyperplasia discovered by core needle biopsy. Am J Surg. 2019 May;217(5):906–9. PMID:30771862

**2257.** Weitzel JN, Pooler PA, Mohammed R, et al. A unique case of breast carcinoma producing pancreatic-type isoamylase. Gastroenterology. 1988 Feb;94(2):519–20. PMID:2446952

**2258.** Wellcome Sanger Institute [Internet]. Hinxton (UK): Wellcome Sanger Institute, Genome Research Limited; 2018. Catalogue Of Somatic Mutations In Cancer (COSMIC); cited 2018 Oct 18. Available from: https://cancer.sanger.ac.uk/cosmic.

**2259.** Wells CA, Ferguson DJ. Ultrastructural and immunocytochemical study of a case of invasive cribriform breast carcinoma. J Clin Pathol. 1988 Jan;41(1):17–20. PMID:3343375

**2259A.** Wells CA, McGregor IL, Makunura CN, et al. Apocrine adenosis: a precursor of aggressive breast cancer? J Clin Pathol. 1995 Aug;48(8):737–42. PMID:7560201

**2260.** Wen HY, Brogi E. Lobular carcinoma in situ. Surg Pathol Clin. 2018 Mar;11(1):123–45. PMID:29413653

**2261.** Wen X, Cheng W. Nonmalignant breast papillary lesions at core-needle biopsy: a meta-analysis of underestimation and influencing factors. Ann Surg Oncol. 2013 Jan;20(1):94–101. PMID:22878621

**2262.** Wen YH, Weigelt B, Reis-Filho JS. Microglandular adenosis: a non-obligate precursor of triple-negative breast cancer? Histol Histopathol. 2013 Sep;28(9):1099–108. PMID:23584829

**2263.** Wendroth SM, Mentrikoski MJ, Wick MR. GATA3 expression in morphologic subtypes of breast carcinoma: a comparison with gross cystic disease fluid protein 15 and mammaglobin. Ann Diagn Pathol. 2015 Feb;19(1):6–9. PMID:25544392

**2264.** Werling RW, Hwang H, Yaziji H, et al. Immunohistochemical distinction of invasive from noninvasive breast lesions: a comparative study of p63 versus calponin and smooth muscle myosin heavy chain. Am J Surg Pathol. 2003 Jan;27(1):82–90. PMID:12502930

**2265.** Wesseling J, van der Valk SW, Vos HL, et al. Episialin (MUC1) overexpression inhibits integrin-mediated cell adhesion to extracellular matrix components. J Cell Biol. 1995 Apr;129(1):255–65. PMID:7698991

**2266.** Wesseling J, van der Valk SW, Hilkens J. A mechanism for inhibition of E-cadherin-mediated cell-cell adhesion by the membrane-associated mucin episialin/MUC1. Mol Biol Cell. 1996 Apr;7(4):565–77. PMID:8730100

**2267.** Weston VJ, Oldreive CE, Skowronska A, et al. The PARP inhibitor olaparib induces significant killing of ATM-deficient lymphoid tumor cells in vitro and in vivo. Blood. 2010 Nov 25;116(22):4578–87. PMID:20739657

**2268.** Westra WH, Lewis JS Jr. Update from the 4th Edition of the World Health Organization Classification of Head and Neck Tumours: Oropharynx. Head Neck Pathol. 2017 Mar;11(1):41–7. PMID:28247229

**2269.** White SR, Auguste LJ, Guo H, et al. Periductal stromal sarcoma of the breast with liposarcomatous differentiation: a case report with 10-year follow-up and literature review. Int J Surg Pathol. 2015 May;23(3):221–4. PMID:25614463

**2270.** White W, Shiu MH, Rosenblum MK, et al. Cellular schwannoma. A clinicopathologic study of 57 patients and 58 tumors. Cancer. 1990 Sep 15;66(6):1266–75. PMID:2400975

**2270A.** WHO Classification of Tumours Editorial Board. Digestive system tumours. Lyon (France): International Agency for Research on Cancer; 2019. (WHO classification of tumours series, 5th ed.; vol. 1). http://publications.iarc.fr/579.

**2271.** Williams KE, Amin A, Hill J, et al. Radiologic and pathologic features associated with upgrade of atypical ductal hyperplasia at surgical excision. Acad Radiol. 2019 Jul;26(7):893–9. PMID:30318287

**2272.** Williams LA, Pankratz N, Lane J, et al. Klinefelter syndrome in males with germ cell tumors: a report from the Children's Oncology Group. Cancer. 2018 Oct 1;124(19):3900–8. PMID:30291793

**2273.** Williams RF, Fernandez-Pineda I, Gosain A. Pediatric sarcomas. Surg Clin North Am. 2016 Oct;96(5):1107–25. PMID:27542645

**2274.** Williams SA, Ehlers RA 2nd, Hunt KK, et al. Metastases to the breast from nonbreast solid neoplasms: presentation and determinants of survival. Cancer. 2007 Aug 15;110(4):731–7. PMID:17582626

**2275.** Wilsher M, McKessar M, Mak C. Phyllodes tumour of the nipple presenting with nipple discharge. Pathology. 2014 Aug;46(5):455–7. PMID:24977745

**2276.** Wilsher MJ, Owens TW, Allcock RJ. Next generation sequencing of the nidus of early (adenosquamous proliferation rich) radial sclerosing lesions of the breast reveals evidence for a neoplastic precursor lesion. J Pathol Clin Res. 2017 Mar 20;3(2):115–22. PMID:28451460

**2277.** Wilson CH, Griffith CD, Shrimankar J, et al. Gynaecomastia, neurofibromatosis and breast cancer. Breast. 2004 Feb;13(1):77–9. PMID:14759722

**2278.** Wilson JR, Bateman AC, Hanson H, et al. A novel HER2-positive breast cancer phenotype arising from germline TP53 mutations. J Med Genet. 2010 Nov;47(11):771–4. PMID:20805372

**2279.** Wilson PC, Chagpar AB, Cicek AF, et al. Breast cancer histopathology is predictive of low-risk Oncotype DX recurrence score. Breast J. 2018 Nov;24(6):976–80. PMID:30230117

**2280.** Winchester DJ, Chang HR, Graves TA, et al. A comparative analysis of lobular and ductal carcinoma of the breast: presentation, treatment, and outcomes. J Am Coll Surg. 1998 Apr;186(4):416–22. PMID:9544955

**2281.** Winham SJ, Mehner C, Heinzen EP, et al.

NanoString-based breast cancer risk prediction for women with sclerosing adenosis. Breast Cancer Res Treat. 2017 Nov;166(2):641–50. PMID:28798985

**2282.** Wiseman C, Liao KT. Primary lymphoma of the breast. Cancer. 1972 Jun;29(6):1705–12. PMID:4555557

**2283.** Wolff AC, Hammond ME, Hicks DG, et al. Recommendations for human epidermal growth factor receptor 2 testing in breast cancer: American Society of Clinical Oncology/College of American Pathologists clinical practice guideline update. Arch Pathol Lab Med. 2014 Feb;138(2):241–56. PMID:24099077

**2284.** Wolff AC, Hammond MEH, Allison KH, et al. Human epidermal growth factor receptor 2 testing in breast cancer: American Society of Clinical Oncology/College of American Pathologists clinical practice guideline focused update. Arch Pathol Lab Med. 2018 Nov;142(11):1364–82. PMID:29846104

**2285.** Wolff AC, Hammond MEH, Allison KH, et al. Human epidermal growth factor receptor 2 testing in breast cancer: American Society of Clinical Oncology/College of American Pathologists clinical practice guideline focused update. J Clin Oncol. 2018 Jul 10;36(20):2105–22. PMID:29846122

**2286.** Wolfram D, Rabensteiner E, Grundtman C, et al. T regulatory cells and TH17 cells in peri-silicone implant capsular fibrosis. Plast Reconstr Surg. 2012 Feb;129(2):327e–37e. PMID:22286447

**2287.** Wong AY, Salisbury E, Bilous M. Recent developments in stereotactic breast biopsy methodologies: an update for the surgical pathologist. Adv Anat Pathol. 2000 Jan;7(1):26–35. PMID:10640199

**2288.** Wong LK, Kereke AR, Wright AE, et al. Microcystic adnexal carcinoma of the nipple. Wounds. 2018 Jun;30(6):E65–7. PMID:30059333

**2289.** Wong SM, Freedman RA, Sagara Y, et al. The effect of Paget disease on axillary lymph node metastases and survival in invasive ductal carcinoma. Cancer. 2015 Dec 15;121(24):4333–40. PMID:26376021

**2290.** Wong WW, Schild SE, Halyard MY, et al. Primary non-Hodgkin lymphoma of the breast: the Mayo Clinic experience. J Surg Oncol. 2002 May;80(1):19–25, discussion 26. PMID:11967901

**2291.** Wong YN, Jack RH, Mak V, et al. The epidemiology and survival of extrapulmonary small cell carcinoma in South East England, 1970-2004. BMC Cancer. 2009 Jun 29;9:209. PMID:19563623

**2292.** Woodard AH, Yu J, Dabbs DJ, et al. NY-BR-1 and PAX8 immunoreactivity in breast, gynecologic tract, and other CK7+ carcinomas: potential use for determining site of origin. Am J Clin Pathol. 2011 Sep;136(3):428–35. PMID:21846919

**2293.** Work ME, Andrulis IL, John EM, et al. Risk factors for uncommon histologic subtypes of breast cancer using centralized pathology review in the Breast Cancer Family Registry. Breast Cancer Res Treat. 2012 Aug;134(3):1209–20. PMID:22527103

**2294.** Worsham MJ, Abrams J, Raju U, et al. Breast cancer incidence in a cohort of women with benign breast disease from a multiethnic, primary health care population. Breast J. 2007 Mar-Apr;13(2):115–21. PMID:17319851

**2295.** Wrba F, Ellinger A, Reiner G, et al. Ultrastructural and immunohistochemical characteristics of lipid-rich carcinoma of the breast. Virchows Arch A Pathol Anat Histopathol. 1988;413(5):381–5. PMID:2845641

**2296.** Wright DH. Burkitt's lymphoma: a review of the pathology, immunology, and possible etiologic factors. Pathol Annu. 1971;6:337–63.

PMID:4342309

**2297.** Wu CC, Shete S, Amos CI, et al. Joint effects of germ-line p53 mutation and sex on cancer risk in Li-Fraumeni syndrome. Cancer Res. 2006 Aug 15;66(16):8287–92. PMID:16912210

**2298.** Wu Y, Zhang N, Yang Q. The prognosis of invasive micropapillary carcinoma compared with invasive ductal carcinoma in the breast: a meta-analysis. BMC Cancer. 2017 Dec 11;17(1):839. PMID:29228910

**2299.** Wynveen CA, Nehhozina T, Akram M, et al. Intracystic papillary carcinoma of the breast: an in situ or invasive tumor? Results of immunohistochemical analysis and clinical follow-up. Am J Surg Pathol. 2011 Jan;35(1):1–14. PMID:21084964

**2300.** Wyszynski A, Hong CC, Lam K, et al. An intergenic risk locus containing an enhancer deletion in 2q35 modulates breast cancer risk by deregulating IGFBP5 expression. Hum Mol Genet. 2016 Sep 1;25(17):3863–76. PMID:27402876

**2301.** Xia B, Dorsman JC, Ameziane N, et al. Fanconi anemia is associated with a defect in the BRCA2 partner PALB2. Nat Genet. 2007 Feb;39(2):159–61. PMID:17200672

**2302.** Xia B, Sheng Q, Nakanishi K, et al. Control of BRCA2 cellular and clinical functions by a nuclear partner, PALB2. Mol Cell. 2006 Jun 23;22(6):719–29. PMID:16793542

**2303.** Xie ZM, Li LS, Laquet C, et al. Germline mutations of the E-cadherin gene in families with inherited invasive lobular breast carcinoma but no diffuse gastric cancer. Cancer. 2011 Jul 15;117(14):3112–7. PMID:21271559

**2304.** Xu S, Cao X. Interleukin-17 and its expanding biological functions. Cell Mol Immunol. 2010 May;7(3):164–74. PMID:20383173

**2305.** Xu X, Bi R, Shui R, et al. Micropapillary pattern in pure mucinous carcinoma of the breast - Does it matter or not? Histopathology. 2019 Jan;74(2):248–55. PMID:30066338

**2306.** Yahara T, Yamaguchi R, Yokoyama G, et al. Adenomyoepithelioma of the breast diagnosed by a mammotome biopsy: report of a case. Surg Today. 2008;38(2):144–6. PMID:18239872

**2307.** Yamada M, Otsuki Y, Shimizu S, et al. Cytological study of 20 cases of solid-papillary carcinoma of the breast. Diagn Cytopathol. 2007 Jul;35(7):417–22. PMID:17580353

**2308.** Yamaguchi R, Horii R, Maeda I, et al. Clinicopathologic study of 53 metaplastic breast carcinomas: their elements and prognostic implications. Hum Pathol. 2010 May;41(5):679–85. PMID:20153509

**2309.** Yamaguchi R, Horii R, Maki K, et al. Carcinoma in a solitary intraductal papilloma of the breast. Pathol Int. 2009 Mar;59(3):185–7. PMID:19261097

**2310.** Yamaguchi R, Tanaka M, Kondo K, et al. Characteristic morphology of invasive micropapillary carcinoma of the breast: an immunohistochemical analysis. Jpn J Clin Oncol. 2010 Aug;40(8):781–7. PMID:20444748

**2311.** Yamamoto H, Yoshida A, Taguchi K, et al. ALK, ROS1 and NTRK3 gene rearrangements in inflammatory myofibroblastic tumours. Histopathology. 2016 Jul;69(1):72–83. PMID:26647767

**2312.** Yang M, Moriya T, Oguma M, et al. Microinvasive ductal carcinoma (T1mic) of the breast. The clinicopathological profile and immunohistochemical features of 28 cases. Pathol Int. 2003 Jul;53(7):422–8. PMID:12828606

**2313.** Yang WT, Hennessy BT, Dryden MJ, et al. Mammary angiosarcomas: imaging findings in 24 patients. Radiology. 2007 Mar;242(3):725–34. PMID:17325063

**2314.** Yang XR, Chang-Claude J, Goode EL, et al. Associations of breast cancer risk factors with tumor subtypes: a pooled analysis from the Breast Cancer Association Consortium studies. J Natl Cancer Inst. 2011 Feb 2;103(3):250–63. PMID:21191117

**2315.** Yang Y, Wang Y, He J, et al. Malignant adenomyoepithelioma combined with adenoid cystic carcinoma of the breast: a case report and literature review. Diagn Pathol. 2014 Jul 23;9:148. PMID:25056281

**2316.** Yap J, Chuba PJ, Thomas R, et al. Sarcoma as a second malignancy after treatment for breast cancer. Int J Radiat Oncol Biol Phys. 2002 Apr 1;52(5):1231–7. PMID:11955733

**2317.** Yap YS, Munusamy P, Lim C, et al. Breast cancer in women with neurofibromatosis type 1 (NF1): a comprehensive case series with molecular insights into its aggressive phenotype. Breast Cancer Res Treat. 2018 Oct;171(3):719–35. PMID:29926297

**2318.** Yaziji H, Gown AM, Sneige N. Detection of stromal invasion in breast cancer: the myoepithelial markers. Adv Anat Pathol. 2000 Mar;7(2):100–9. PMID:10721417

**2319.** Yeong J, Thike AA, Young Ng CC, et al. A genetic mutation panel for differentiating malignant phyllodes tumour from metaplastic breast carcinoma. Pathology. 2017 Dec;49(7):786–9. PMID:29066183

**2320.** Yiannakopoulou E. Etiology of familial breast cancer with undetected BRCA1 and BRCA2 mutations: clinical implications. Cell Oncol (Dordr). 2014 Feb;37(1):1–8. PMID:24306927

**2321.** Yilmaz E, Sal S, Lebe B. Differentiation of phyllodes tumors versus fibroadenomas. Acta Radiol. 2002 Jan;43(1):34–9. PMID:11972459

**2322.** Yilmaz R, Akkavak G, Ozgur E, et al. Myofibroblastoma of the breast: ultrasonography, mammography, and magnetic resonance imaging features with pathologic correlation. Ultrasound Q. 2018 Jun;34(2):99–102. PMID:29420368

**2323.** Yılmaz R, Bayramoğlu Z, Emirikçi S, et al. MR imaging features of tubular carcinoma: preliminary experience in twelve masses. Eur J Breast Health. 2018 Jan 1;14(1):39–45. PMID:29322118

**2324.** Yin M, Wang W, Drabick JJ, et al. Prognosis and treatment of non-metastatic primary and secondary breast angiosarcoma: a comparative study. BMC Cancer. 2017 Apr 27;17(1):295. PMID:28449661

**2325.** Yokouchi M, Nagano S, Kijima Y, et al. Solitary breast metastasis from myxoid liposarcoma. BMC Cancer. 2014 Jul 4;14:482. PMID:24994066

**2326.** Yoo JL, Woo OH, Kim YK, et al. Can MR imaging contribute in characterizing well-circumscribed breast carcinomas? Radiographics. 2010 Oct;30(6):1689–702. PMID:21071383

**2327.** Yoo SJ, Lee DS, Oh HS, et al. Male breast adenoid cystic carcinoma. Case Rep Oncol. 2013 Oct 12;6(3):514–9. PMID:24403896

**2328.** Yoon JY, Chitale D. Adenomyoepithelioma of the breast: a brief diagnostic review. Arch Pathol Lab Med. 2013 May;137(5):725–9. PMID:23627458

**2329.** Yoshida M, Ogawa R, Yoshida H, et al. TERT promoter mutations are frequent and show association with MED12 mutations in phyllodes tumors of the breast. Br J Cancer. 2015 Oct 20;113(8):1244–8. PMID:26355235

**2330.** Yoshida S, Nakamura N, Sasaki Y, et al. Primary breast diffuse large B-cell lymphoma shows a non-germinal center B-cell phenotype. Mod Pathol. 2005 Mar;18(3):398–405. PMID:15492762

**2331.** Young RH, Clement PB.

Adenomyoepithelioma of the breast. A report of three cases and review of the literature. Am J Clin Pathol. 1988 Mar;89(3):308–14. PMID:2831705

**2332.** Young RJ, Natukunda A, Litière S, et al. First-line anthracycline-based chemotherapy for angiosarcoma and other soft tissue sarcoma subtypes: pooled analysis of eleven European Organisation for Research and Treatment of Cancer Soft Tissue and Bone Sarcoma Group trials. Eur J Cancer. 2014 Dec;50(18):3178–86. PMID:25459395

**2333.** Yu BH, Tang SX, Xu XL, et al. Breast carcinoma in sclerosing adenosis: a clinicopathological and immunophenotypical analysis on 206 lesions. J Clin Pathol. 2018 Jun;71(6):546–53. PMID:29436376

**2334.** Yu J, Bhargava R, Dabbs DJ. Invasive lobular carcinoma with extracellular mucin production and HER-2 overexpression: a case report and further case studies. Diagn Pathol. 2010 Jun 15;5:36. PMID:20550696

**2335.** Yu JI, Choi DH, Park W, et al. Differences in prognostic factors and patterns of failure between invasive micropapillary carcinoma and invasive ductal carcinoma of the breast: matched case-control study. Breast. 2010 Jun;19(3):231–7. PMID:20304650

**2336.** Yu SN, Li J, Wong SI, et al. Atypical aspirates of the breast: a dilemma in current cytology practice. J Clin Pathol. 2017 Dec;70(12):1024–32. PMID:28554890

**2337.** Yu XF, Yang HJ, Yu Y, et al. A prognostic analysis of male breast cancer (MBC) compared with post-menopausal female breast cancer (FBC). PLoS One. 2015 Aug 27;10(8):e0136670. PMID:26313461

**2338.** Yun SU, Choi BB, Shu KS, et al. Imaging findings of invasive micropapillary carcinoma of the breast. J Breast Cancer. 2012 Mar;15(1):57–64. PMID:22493629

**2339.** Zafrani B, Aubriot MH, Mouret E, et al. High sensitivity and specificity of immunohistochemistry for the detection of hormone receptors in breast carcinoma: comparison with biochemical determination in a prospective study of 793 cases. Histopathology. 2000 Dec;37(6):536–45. PMID:11122436

**2340.** Zagars GK, Ballo MT, Pisters PW, et al. Prognostic factors for patients with localized soft-tissue sarcoma treated with conservation surgery and radiation therapy: an analysis of 1225 patients. Cancer. 2003 May 15;97(10):2530–43. PMID:12733153

**2341.** Zakaria S, Pantvaidya G, Ghosh K, et al. Paget's disease of the breast: accuracy of preoperative assessment. Breast Cancer Res Treat. 2007 Apr;102(2):137–42. PMID:17028984

**2342.** Zandrino F, Calabrese M, Faedda C, et al. Tubular carcinoma of the breast: pathological, clinical, and ultrasonographic findings. A review of the literature. Radiol Med. 2006 Sep;111(6):773–82. PMID:16896563

**2343.** Zarbo RJ, Oberman HA. Cellular adenomyoepithelioma of the breast. Am J Surg Pathol. 1983 Dec;7(8):863–70. PMID:6318584

**2344.** Zardavas D, Te Marvelde L, Milne RL, et al. Tumor PIK3CA genotype and prognosis in early-stage breast cancer: a pooled analysis of individual patient data. J Clin Oncol. 2018 Apr 1;36(10):981–90. PMID:29470143

**2345.** Zeggini E, Weedon MN, Lindgren CM, et al. Replication of genome-wide association signals in UK samples reveals risk loci for type 2 diabetes. Science. 2007 Jun 1;316(5829):1336–41. PMID:17463249

**2346.** Zekioglu O, Erhan Y, Ciris M, et al. Invasive micropapillary carcinoma of the breast: high incidence of lymph node metastasis with extranodal extension and its immunohistochemical profile compared with invasive ductal carcinoma. Histopathology. 2004 Jan;44(1):18–23. PMID:14717664

**2347.** Zhang F, Ma J, Wu J, et al. PALB2 links BRCA1 and BRCA2 in the DNA-damage response. Curr Biol. 2009 Mar 24;19(6):524–9. PMID:19268590

**2348.** Zhang G, Ataya D, L Lebda P, et al. Mucocele-like lesions diagnosed on breast core biopsy: low risk of upgrade and subsequent carcinoma. Breast J. 2018 May;24(3):314–8. PMID:29024198

**2349.** Zhang J, White NM, Schmidt HK, et al. INTEGRATE: gene fusion discovery using whole genome and transcriptome data. Genome Res. 2016 Jan;26(1):108–18. PMID:26556708

**2350.** Zhang LJ, Su Z, Liu X, et al. Peutz-Jeghers syndrome with early onset of pre-adolescent gynecomastia: a predigree case report and clinical and molecular genetic analysis. Am J Transl Res. 2017 May 15;9(5):2639–44. PMID:28560011

**2351.** Zhang N, Zhang H, Chen T, et al. Dose invasive apocrine adenocarcinoma has worse prognosis than invasive ductal carcinoma of breast: evidence from SEER database. Oncotarget. 2017 Apr 11;8(15):24579–92. PMID:28445946

**2352.** Zhang X, Chiang HC, Wang Y, et al. Attenuation of RNA polymerase II pausing mitigates BRCA1-associated R-loop accumulation and tumorigenesis. Nat Commun. 2017 Jun 26;8:15908. PMID:28649985

**2353.** Zhang Y, Kleer CG. Phyllodes tumor of the breast: histopathologic features, differential diagnosis, and molecular/genetic updates. Arch Pathol Lab Med. 2016 Jul;140(7):665–71. PMID:27362571

**2354.** Zhang Y, Lv F, Yang Y, et al. Clinicopathological features and prognosis of metaplastic breast carcinoma: experience of a major Chinese cancer center. PLoS One. 2015 Jun 26;10(6):e0131409. PMID:26115045

**2355.** Zhao C, Desouki MM, Florea A, et al. Pathologic findings of follow-up surgical excision for lobular neoplasia on breast core biopsy performed for calcification. Am J Clin Pathol. 2012 Jul;138(1):72–8. PMID:22706860

**2356.** Zhao HD, Wu T, Wang JQ, et al. Primary inflammatory myofibroblastic tumor of the breast with rapid recurrence and metastasis: a case report. Oncol Lett. 2013 Jan;5(1):97–100. PMID:23255901

**2357.** Zhao S, Ma D, Xiao Y, et al. Clinicopathologic features and prognoses of different histologic types of triple-negative breast cancer: a large population-based analysis. Eur J Surg Oncol. 2018 Apr;44(4):420–8. PMID:29429597

**2358.** Zhen DB, Rabe KG, Gallinger S, et al. BRCA1, BRCA2, PALB2, and CDKN2A mutations in familial pancreatic cancer: a PACGENE study. Genet Med. 2015 Jul;17(7):569–77. PMID:25356972

**2359.** Zheng Z, Liebers M, Zhelyazkova B, et al. Anchored multiplex PCR for targeted next-generation sequencing. Nat Med. 2014 Dec;20(12):1479–84. PMID:25384085

**2360.** Zhong E, Scognamiglio T, D'Alfonso T, et al. Breast tumor resembling the tall cell variant of papillary thyroid carcinoma: molecular characterization by next-generation sequencing and histopathological comparison with tall cell papillary carcinoma of thyroid. Int J Surg Pathol. 2018 Sep 18:1066896918800779. PMID:30227763

**2361.** Zhong F, Bi R, Yu B, et al. Carcinoma arising in microglandular adenosis of the breast: triple negative phenotype with variable morphology. Int J Clin Exp Pathol. 2014 Aug 15;7(9):6149–56. PMID:25337263

**2362.** Zhong Q, Peng HL, Zhao X, et al. Effects of BRCA1- and BRCA2-related mutations on ovarian and breast cancer survival: a meta-analysis. Clin Cancer Res. 2015 Jan 1;21(1):211–20. PMID:25348513

**2363.** Zhou M, Wang X, Jiang L, et al. The diagnostic value of one step nucleic acid amplification (OSNA) in differentiating lymph node metastasis of tumors: a systematic review and meta-analysis. Int J Surg. 2018 Aug;56:49–56. PMID:29753955

**2363A.** Zhou Z, Kinslow CJ, Hibshoosh H, et al. Clinical features, survival and prognostic factors of glycogen-rich clear cell carcinoma (GRCC) of the breast in the U.S. population. J Clin Med. 2019 Feb 14;8(2). PMID:30769905

**2364.** Zhou ZR, Wang CC, Sun XJ, et al. Prognostic factors in breast phyllodes tumors: a nomogram based on a retrospective cohort study of 404 patients. Cancer Med. 2018 Apr;7(4):1030–42. PMID:29479819

**2365.** Zhu D, Qian HS, Han HX, et al. An unusual magnetic resonance imaging of a giant cystic volume of tubular adenoma of the breast. Breast J. 2017 Mar;23(2):225–6. PMID:27868357

**2366.** Zhu J, Ni G, Wang D, et al. Lobulated adenomyoepithelioma: a case report showing immunohistochemical profiles. Int J Clin Exp Pathol. 2015 Nov 1;8(11):15407–11. PMID:26823903

**2367.** Zhu Y, Wu J, Zhang C, et al. BRCA mutations and survival in breast cancer: an updated systematic review and meta-analysis. Oncotarget. 2016 Oct 25;7(43):70113–27. PMID:27659521

**2368.** Zimmerman A, Locke FL, Emole J, et al. Recurrent systemic anaplastic lymphoma kinase-negative anaplastic large cell lymphoma presenting as a breast implant-associated lesion. Cancer Control. 2015 Jul;22(3):369–73. PMID:26351895

**2369.** Zucca-Matthes G, Urban C, Vallejo A. Anatomy of the nipple and breast ducts. Gland Surg. 2016 Feb;5(1):32–6. PMID:26855906

# Subject index

**Bold** page numbers indicate the main discussion(s) of the topic.

## Numbers and symbols

34βE12   14, 137
α1-antichymotrypsin   140
α-catenin   70, 115, 117
α-lactalbumin   33, 36, 108
α-SMA   116, 205
β-catenin   70, 72, 117, 137, 202–203, 205–208
γ-catenin   117

## A

ABO   296
acid phosphatase   106
acinar cell carcinoma   10, 139
acinic cell carcinoma   139–141, 147
actin   26, 49, 106, 212, 214, 230, 284
activation-induced cytidine deaminase   243
activin   25
ADAM29   295
ADCY3   294
adenoid cystic carcinoma (AdCC)   10, 38–39, 44, 47, 91, 120, **142–145,** 151, 160
adenomyoepithelioma (AME)   10, 38–39, **41–48,** 54, 143–144
adenosis   10, 13, 15, **22–30,** 33, 37, 44, 72, 79, 85, 93–94, 112, 120, 131–132, 140, 143, 169–170, 182–183, 276
adenosquamous   31, 47–48, 120, 135–136, 138, 180
ADH5   58, 160
adipophilin   107–109, 244
ADSSL1   297
AE1/AE3   117, 137
AHRR   295
AKAP9   296
AKT   13, 132, 226, 258, 276
AKT1   37, 39, 43, 53, 96, 115, 123
alcohol   84–85, 114, 252–253, 258
ALK   205, 209–210, 245, 247
alkaline phosphatase   106
ALS2CR12   See *FLACC1*
American Society of Clinical Oncology (ASCO)   74, 89–91, 98, 100
AMFR   297
amyloid   236
androgen   25, 84, 97, 99, 252–254, 258
angiolipoma   188, 221, 223–224
angiomatosis   188, 193–194

angiosarcoma   94, 136, 188–190, 192–194, 196–201, 224, 230
ANKRD16   296
APC   190, 207–208
APOBEC3A   298
APOBEC3B   298
apocrine adenocarcinoma   10, 131
apocrine adenoma   10, 25–27
apocrine adenosis (AAA)   25–27, 131–132
AR   26–27, 72, 96, 99, 108–109, 125, 131–133, 137, 139, 141, 147, 150, 158, 205, 251–253, 255, 258–259, 262
ARHGEF6   296
ARID1A   115, 137, 244
aromatase   100, 252–254
ARRDC3   295
ASCL1   65
ASTN2   296
ATAD5   297
ataxia–telangiectasia (AT)   277–278
ATG10   295
ATM   119, 242, 268–269, 272, **277–278,** 292–293
ATP6AP1   215–216
ATP6AP2   215–216
ATR   272
ATXN1   295
ATXN7   294
atypical ductal hyperplasia (ADH)   **10–21,** 49–50, 54, 56, 78–79, 85, 91, 120, 125, 165, 174, 254
atypical lipomatous tumour (ALT)   189, 221, 225–227
atypical lobular hyperplasia (ALH)   10, 16–17, 56, **68–70,** 74, 116
atypical vascular lesion   188–189, **195–196,** 198–199
autosomal dominant   213, 268, 270, 274–275, 279, 288, 290
autosomal recessive   277, 286
axilla   25, 35, 245

## B

B72.3   89
Bannayan–Riley–Ruvalcaba syndrome   215, 275
basal-like   7, 39, 80, 85, **95–97,** 104–105, 115, 134, 137, 258, 273

B-cell receptor (BCR)   242, 244
BCL2   89, 151–152, 161, 205, 236–237, 239, 241, 243–244, 258, 273
BCL2L11   294
BCL6   236–237, 239, 241, 243–244
BCOR   169
biphasic   39, 41, 43–45, 47, 106, 134–135, 137, 151, 165, 168, 171, 175, 203, 254
BIRC3   236
BLM   242
BMI1   207
BRAF   132, 142, 154, 173, 179, 182
BRCA1   7, 77, 83–84, 92, 96, 104, 140, 257–258, 268–274, 278, 281–282, 292–294, 297
BRCA1/2   84, 96, 257, 268–274, 278, 292–293, 297
BRCA1/2-associated hereditary breast and ovarian cancer syndrome   **270,** 274
BRCA2   77, 83–84, 91, 96, 257–259, 268–274, 278, 281, 286, 288, 292–293, 295, 297
BRCAPRO model   274, 293
Breast and Ovarian Analysis of Disease Incidence and Carrier Estimation Algorithm (BOADICEA)   274, 293
Breast Cancer Association Consortium (BCAC)   274, 292
breastfeeding   35–36, 84, 271
breast implant–associated anaplastic large cell lymphoma (ALCL)   232, 234, **245–248**
bromocriptine   36
Burkitt lymphoma (BL)   232, 234, **242–244**

## C

C/EBP   226
CA125   262
cadherin   39, 69–73, 89, 103, 115–118, 120, 129, 132, 134, 137, 151–152, 234, 268, 273, 282, 284–285
calcification   14–16, 18, 26, 28, 32, 34, 37, 70–73, 76, 83, 85, 114, 119, 121, 124–125, 128, 132, 134, 165, 169–170, 173, 180, 191, 207, 211, 229, 273
CALCOCO1   282
caldesmon   39, 219
calponin   24, 31, 34, 39, 41, 49–50, 53, 94, 112, 143, 205, 207
calretinin   154

CAM5.2 185

carcinoid 7, 155–157

carcinoma in situ 10–11, 13–16, 18–21, 23–25, 31, 34, 38, 40, 49–51, 54–64, 68–80, 85, 93, 97, 104, 107, 110–113, 116, 120–121, 125–127, 131, 134, 136–137, 140, 147, 156–158, 160–161, 164–165, 169, 174, 178, 182–185, 188, 232, 250, 254–256, 259, 265, 272–273, 276, 279–281, 284, 292

carcinoma with apocrine differentiation 131–133, 147

carcinosarcoma 47, 134

CARD11 241

Carney complex 37, 168, 211–212, 252–253

CASP8 294

catenin 70, 72, 115, 117–118, 137, 202–203, 205–208, 284

cathepsin D 29

caveolin-1 273

CBFB 72

CCDC88C 297

CCN6 137

CCND1 12, 129, 258, 296–297

CCND3 244

CD3 89, 236, 247

CD4 242, 247

CD5 236–237, 241, 244, 247

CD10 26, 39, 137, 143, 205, 236–239, 241, 243–244

CD19 241, 244

CD20 89, 236, 238–239, 241, 243–244

CD21 237, 239

CD22 241, 244

CD23 236–237, 239, 244

CD24 134

CD30 201, 241, 246–248

CD31 192, 194, 196, 198, 201, 230

CD34 89, 137, 165, 196, 198, 201–203, 205, 207, 209, 214, 228, 230

CD38 244

CD43 236, 244, 247

CD44 134

CD45 247

CD45RB 247

CD56 158, 161

CD63 216

CD68 106, 131–132, 216

CD77 244

CD79a 236, 239, 241, 244

CD79B 241

CD99 205

CD138 89, 244

CDCA7 294

CDCA7L 296

CDH1 12, 69, 71–72, 96, 114–116, 268, 282, 284–285, 292

CDH1-associated breast cancer 268, 284

CDK4 175, 225, 227

CDKAL1 295

CDKN2A 44, 46, 134, 213–214, 296

CDKN2B 213, 296

CDX2 89, 127

CDYL2 297

CEA 89, 147, 185

CEP17 90–91, 129

childhood 242, 286

CHK2, CHEK2 257, 268–269, 278, **282–283,** 292–293, 298

Chompret criteria 279–281

chromogranin 50, 64–65, 154–157, 160–161, 201

CHST9 297

cirrhosis 252–253, 257

CK5/6 14, 16, 20–21, 39, 49–50, 59, 89, 104, 108, 117, 126, 135, 137, 143, 147, 154, 253, 273

CK5/14 14, 16, 20–21, 39, 49–50, 53–55, 58–59, 79, 89, 104, 108, 110, 117, 120, 126, 135, 137, 143, 147, 154, 160, 180, 183, 253, 273

CK7 14, 58, 79, 89, 118, 127, 137, 143, 150–152, 154, 160, 179, 185, 262, 265

CK8 14, 26–27, 34, 49, 89, 120, 137, 143, 147, 180, 273

CK8/18 14, 26–27, 34, 49, 89, 120, 137, 143, 147, 180, 273

CK10 180

CK14 14, 39, 41, 47, 49–50, 53–54, 58–59, 61, 79, 89, 104, 108, 117, 137, 143, 150, 180, 253, 273

CK17 39, 89

CK18 14, 49, 58, 160, 180

CK19 34, 89, 137

CK20 89, 127, 262

c-KIT See KIT

claudin 95, 137, 214

CLCA1 282

clear cell 7, 53, 79, 104, 108, 157, 179, 190, 264

clinging carcinoma 11, 15

CMSS1 294

CNTNAP1 297

collagen IV 28, 112, 143

collagenous spherulosis 38, 44, 53, 72, 144

College of American Pathologists (CAP) 89–91

columnar cell lesion (CCL) 10–12, 15–16, 20, 68, 120

comedonecrosis 58, 72–73, 75, 77–78, 80,

111, 132, 255

comparative genomic hybridization 12, 15–16, 25, 28, 69, 71, 119, 128, 282

complex sclerosing lesion 10, 13, 22, 30–31, 135, 144

contraceptive 33, 271

core needle biopsy (CNB) 6, 17, 20–23, 31, 43, 45, 51–52, 68, 70, 74, 88, 94–95, 97, 114, 120, 122, 181, 190, 192, 200, 212, 214, 227, 254, 256, 258

Cowden syndrome (CS) 131, 166, 189, 268–269, **275–276**

CREB5 295

CREBBP 241

cribriform carcinoma 10, 51, 80, 106, 121, 144

CRTC1 150

CTCF 115

CTLA-4 101

CTNNB1 140, 190, 207–208

CUX1 296

cyclin A 273

cyclin D1 236–237, 258, 273

cyclin E 273

cytochrome P450 252

cytokeratin 14, 16, 20, 29, 39–41, 44, 47, 49–50, 54, 58–59, 61, 64–65, 79, 89, 111–112, 117–118, 120, 131–132, 137, 139–140, 143, 150, 154, 161, 180, 185, 202, 205, 207, 214, 220, 226–227, 230, 254, 273

cytokine 246

D

D2-40 39, 194, 198, 201, 230

DAB 160

DCLRE1B 294

DDIT3 225–227

desmin 137, 202, 204–205, 207, 209, 212, 214, 217, 219–220, 230

desmoplastic 51, 64, 80, 111, 119, 121, 135

diffuse large B-cell lymphoma (DLBCL) 232–233, 235–237, 240–241, 244, 265

DIRC3 294

DLX2-AS1 See DLX2-DT

DLX2-DT 294

DNAH11 296

DNAJC1 296

DNMT3A 246

DOK7 65

ductal adenoma 26, 32, **37–38,** 41, 44, 53

ductal carcinoma in situ (DCIS) 10–16, 18–21, 23, 25, 31, 34, 40, 49–51, 54–59, 61–65, 68, 70–81, 85–86, 91–94, 98, 104, 110–113, 116, 120–122, 125–127,

131–132, 134, 136–137, 140, 156–158, 160–161, 165, 174, 182–185, 250, 254–256, 273, 276, 279–281, 292

ductulolobular   116–117

DUSP22   247

**E**

E2A   See *TCF3*

EBF1   295

EBV   189, 237, 241–243

EBV-encoded small RNA (EBER)   247

E-cadherin   69–73, 89, 103, 115–118, 120, 129, 132, 134, 137, 151–152, 234, 268, 282, 284–285

EGFR (HER1)   29, 89, 104, 117, 120, 126, 134, 137, 147, 169, 173, 273

EGOT   295

ELL   297

EMA   27, 29, 34, 41, 89, 96, 99, 106, 108, 125, 128–130, 140–141, 143, 185, 198, 205, 209, 214, 219

EMBP1   294

EMID1   298

EP300   142

epithelial-myoepithelial carcinoma   10, 39, 43–44, 46–48

epithelioid   47, 94, 135–136, 188, 190, 197–198, 200–201, 205, 209, 211–212, 215, 226

ER   14, 16, 19–21, 26–27, 29, 39, 43–44, 46–47, 50–51, 53–55, 58–62, 64–65, 71–72, 77–86, 88–92, 94–100, 102, 104, 106–109, 114–115, 117–118, 120, 122–123, 125–129, 131–134, 137, 139, 141, 144–145, 147–148, 150–152, 156–158, 161, 180, 183, 185, 205, 207, 212, 214, 229–230, 251, 253–254, 256, 258–259, 262, 265, 272–274, 277–278, 281–283, 285, 288, 290–297

ERBB2 (HER2)   6, 29, 47, 51, 61–62, 64, 72, 77, 79–80, 82–86, 89–92, 94–100, 102, 104–110, 112–117, 119–122, 125–126, 129–133, 137–139, 141–142, 144, 147, 150–152, 154, 158, 161, 180, 185, 207, 256, 258–259, 273, 277, 281–283, 285, 288, 290–291

ERBB2 (HER2)-enriched   80, 91, 95, 256

ERBB3 (HER3)   89, 115–116, 140

ERBB4 (HER4)   89, 140, 169

ERG   198, 201, 229–230

ERK1/2   293

ESR1   12, 96, 258, 295

ESRRG   294

estrogen   19, 36, 74, 83–84, 168, 252–254, 257–258

ETV6   141, 146–148

EWSR1   225, 227

EXO1   294

extranodal marginal zone lymphoma of mucosa-associated lymphoid tissue (MALT lymphoma)   233, 235–239

**F**

factor VIII   229

familial adenomatous polyposis   207, 288

FANCD2   278

Fanconi   280, 286

FAT1   137

FBXW7   142

Fédération Nationale des Centres de Lutte Contre le Cancer (FNCLCC)   190

FGF   293

FGF1   273

FGF10   295

FGFR1   129, 142, 273

FGFR2   140, 142, 258, 273, 296

FGFR3   33

FH   217

FHIT   119

fibroadenoma   13–14, 18, 25–27, 32–36, 38, 40, 45, 72, 140, 146, 164–165, **167–176,** 219, 225, 229, 276, 279

fibrocystic   25–26, 45, 169, 275–276

fibromatosis   135–136, 138, 188–190, 202–203, **206–208,** 220

fibronectin   37

FILIP1L   294

FLACC1   294

flat epithelial atypia (FEA)   10–12, 15–17, 20, 85, 91, 120

FLI1   198, 201

FLJ43663   See *LINC-PINT*

FLNA   169, 173

FLT1   197

FLT4   197

fluorescence in situ hybridization (FISH)   129–130, 133, 142, 148, 196, 198–199, 203, 205, 227, 244, 281

follicular lymphoma (FL)   232–233, 235, 237–239

FOXA1   115

FOXP1   241, 294

FOXQ1   295

FTO   297

fumarate hydratase   217–218

FUS   225, 227

**G**

GAREM1   297

gastric cancer   71, 114, 262, 284–285

GATA3   79, 89, 115, 118, 125, 129, 131–132, 134, 147, 150, 154, 161, 185, 247, 255, 258, 262, 265

GATAD2A   297

GCDFP   26, 44, 89, 118, 131–132, 140, 154, 158, 185, 258, 262, 265

GCET1   241

gene expression signature   85, 99–100

genome-wide association study   84, 271, 292–293

GFAP   39, 216

GIPR   297

GLUT1   214

glycogen   7, 10, 44, 102, 104, 108

glycogen-rich carcinoma   10, 102

GNAS   37

granular cell tumour   116, 131–132, 188, 215–216

granzyme B   247

GRHL1   294

GSTP1   258

gynaecomastia   14, 168, 204, 229, 250, **252–255,** 258

**H**

haemangioma   179, 188–189, **191–192,** 195–198, 200–201

haemosiderin   27, 51, 106

hamartoma   164–167, 219, 222, 275–276

H+-ATPase   216

h-caldesmon   219–220

hCG   106, 253

HELQ   295

HER1   See *EGFR (HER1)*

HER2   See *ERBB2 (HER2)*

HER3   See *ERBB3 (HER3)*

HER4   See *ERBB4 (HER4)*

HHV8   189

hidradenoma papilliferum   54

HIF1α   273

high-grade transformation   10, 142–145

high-molecular-weight cytokeratin   14, 16, 20, 40, 44, 50, 54, 59, 61, 64–65, 89, 120, 137, 150, 154, 180, 185, 220, 226

histiocytoid   108, 116–117, 132, 285

histone   293

HIV   242

HIVEP3   294

HMB45   89, 185, 212, 216, 263

HMGA2   40, 221

HNF4G   296

HRAS   39, 43, 46

HRDetect   96

HSPA4   295

I

ID3  244
IDH2  7, 153–154
IG  242
IGF  253
IGFBP5  294
IGFR  226
IgG4  236–237
IGH  236–237, 239, 241, 243
IGHV  239
IgM  236–237, 244
IL-13  247
immune checkpoint  101, 272
immunodeficiency  232, 235, 242, 277
immunoglobulin (Ig)  236–237, 241–242
infarction  33, 35, 37, 52–53, 173
infiltrating duct carcinoma  10, 102, 250, 257
inflammatory breast carcinoma  82–83
inflammatory myofibroblastic tumour  188, 190, **209–210,** 220
INPP4B  140
intraductal carcinoma, non-infiltrating  10, 76, 250, 255
intraductal papilloma  10, 13, 32, 37–38, 44, 50, 52–56
invasive breast carcinoma of no special type (IBC-NST)  61, 89, 91–92, 94, 102–105, 107–109, 114–118, 123–124, 130, 134, 136–137
invasive micropapillary carcinoma  10, 66, 124, 128–130
IRF4  241
iron  26–27
isolated tumour cell  97–98, 130, 181
ITPR1  295

J

JAK1  246

K

KANSL1  297
KCNN4  297
KDR  197, 201
keloid  206–207
Ki-67  6, 27, 38, 61, 64, 72, 95–96, 98–100, 104, 109, 117–118, 120, 147, 154, 157–158, 194, 216, 236, 241, 243–244
KIT  143–144, 147, 173, 201, 214
KLHDC7A  294
Klinefelter syndrome (47,XXY)  252–254, 257
KMT2D  140, 169, 173, 241
KRAS  132, 137, 179, 182

L

L3MBTL3  295

lactalbumin  89
lactating adenoma  10, 32, 35–36
lactoferrin  108
laminin  112, 143, 273
LDH  244
LEF1  237
leiomyoma  168, 179, 188, **217**
leiomyosarcoma  188, 190, **219–220,** 281
LEOPARD syndrome  215
leptin  253
LGR6  294
LH  253
Li–Fraumeni syndrome (LFS)  173, 246, 268, 279–282
LIN7A  129
LINC00536  296
LINC-PINT  296
lipid-rich carcinoma  10, 102, 107–108
lipofuscin  27, 107
lipoma  167, 188–189, 205, 221–222, 275
lipopolysaccharide  246
liposarcoma  7, 172, 174–176, 188–189, **225–227,** 281
LKB1  See *STK11*
LMO2  241
LMP1  247
LMP2A  243
LMX1B  296
lobular carcinoma  7, 10, 16, 19, 24, 38, 47, 56, 68–74, 79, 83, 94, 98, 102–104, 110–111, **114–117,** 119, 124, 132, 151, 169, 185, 205, 233–234, 239, 250, 255–256, 258, 264, 272–273, 284–285, 292
lobular carcinoma in situ (LCIS)  10, 16, 19, 24, 38, 56, **68–74,** 79, 110–111, 116, 169, 250, 255–256, 272–273, 284
LOC101929626  294
LOC105369192  295
loss of heterozygosity  12, 15, 19, 25, 53, 69, 107, 115, 119, 252, 285–286
low-molecular-weight cytokeratin  14, 41, 47, 89, 137, 139–140, 143, 150, 180, 185
low-penetrance allele  84, 292–293
LRP1  282
LSP1  296
luminal A  61, 80, 95–96, 99, 110, 114–115, 118–121, 123, 128, 157, 256, 273, 282–283
luminal B  61, 65, 80, 91, 95–96, 99, 110, 115, 128–129, 256, 273, 278, 282–283
lymphatic atypical vascular lesion  188, 195
lymphoedema  98, 189, 197, 199
lymphovascular  86, 98, 104, 109, 116, 124, 130, 150, 180, 263, 273
LYPD5  297
lysozyme  106, 140

LZTR1  212

M

MALT1  236
MAML2  150
mammaglobin  89, 147, 150, 154, 258, 262, 265
MAP2K4  115, 129
MAP3K1  115, 169, 293, 295
MAPK  132, 137, 146, 290
maspin  39, 137
massively parallel sequencing  72, 207
mastectomy  68, 75, 98, 185, 189, 194–195, 197, 201, 215, 220, 272–274
MCM8  297
MDM2  7, 96, 175, 225, 227, 280
MDM4  294
MECT1  See *CRTC1*
MED12  33, 36, 165, 168–169, 173
medullary  7, 104–105, 272–274
melan-A  89, 107, 185, 212, 216, 262
melanin  107, 184, 212, 288–289
melanoma  94, 96, 106–107, 160, 179, 184–185, 216, **262–263,** 265, 270, 275–276, 279, 292
menarche  14, 33, 83–84, 168, 271
menopause  14, 32–33, 58, 60, 63, 71, 77, 83–84, 99, 119, 126, 165, 169, 184, 204, 229, 251, 257, 271, 279
merlin (NF2)  211–212
MET  33
metachronous  168
metaplasia  15, 25–27, 30, 37, 41, 44, 49–50, 53, 131–132, 134, 169–170, 174, 182, 205, 207, 221, 254
metaplastic carcinoma  10, 31, 39, 41, 47–48, 91, 134–138, 160, 173, 175, 189, 203, 207, 220, 226–227, 258, 272, 290
metastasis  7, 39, 45, 48, 62, 65–66, 82, 94, 97–98, 100, 106–107, 112, 114, 117–118, 124–125, 127–128, 130, 137, 141, 145, 148, 150, 152–154, 157, 159, 173, 176, 190, 194, 199, 201, 208, 210, 216, 220, 226–227, 258–259, 262–265, 273
methylation  12, 77, 115, 123, 258, 271, 292
MIB1  117, 273
microcalcification  11, 13, 16–19, 22–23, 25, 40, 52, 57, 71–72, 75, 77–78, 121, 123, 131, 192, 204, 215, 256, 258, 262
microenvironment  6–7, 77, 92, 116, 247
microglandular adenosis  10, **28–29,** 85, 93–94, 140, 143
microinvasive carcinoma  79, **110–113**
micrometastasis  97, 113
micropapillary  10, 14, 16, 19, 50, 55, 57–58,

61, 66, 77–79, 124–125, **128–130,** 132, 182, 255, 258

microRNA   143, 242, 244, 258

microsatellite instability   123

milk fat globule   89

MIR640   297

MITF   185, 216

mitotic count   6, 47, 64, 87–88, 92, 115–118, 144, 150, 157–158, 176, 205, 259

MKL1   See *MRTFA*

MLL2   See *KMT2D*

MNF116   137

MRPS30   295

MRTFA   298

MSA   39

mTOR, MTOR   13, 140, 213, 258

MUC2   123

MUC4   147

mucinous carcinoma (MC)   105, **123–125,** 130, 155, 157

mucinous cystadenocarcinoma   7, 10, **126–127**

MUCL1   282

mucoepidermoid carcinoma (MEC)   149–150

multigene breast cancer susceptibility   268

MUTYH   271

MYB   44, 142–144

MYC   129, 131, 196–199, 201, 241–244, 296

MYD88   241

myeloid sarcoma   233–234

myeloperoxidase   233

MYH9   203

myofibroblast   39, 49, 202, 204, 228–230

myofibroblastoma   188–189, **203–205,** 207, 220–221, 229

myosin   143

# N

National Surgical Adjuvant Breast and Bowel Project (NSABP)   81, 99

NBN   292

NBPF10   129

NBS1   See *NBN*

NEB   140

neoadjuvant   85–86, 88, 92–93, 95–96, 98, 100–101, 118, 133, 201

neuroendocrine   7, 10, 50, 59, 63–65, 79–80, 104–105, 123–124, 144, 155–161, 263

neuroendocrine carcinoma (NEC)   7, 105, 123, 144, 155–161

neuroendocrine tumour (NET)   7, 105, 155–157, 161, 263

neurofibroma   188, 213–214, 291

neurofibromatosis type 1 (NF1)   43, 46, 137, 169, 173, 213–215, 229, 254, 268,

290–291

neurofibromin (NF1)   137, 169, 173, 213–214, 268, 290–291

next-generation sequencing   33, 36–37, 96, 148, 223, 244, 280–281, 287

NF1   137, 169, 173, 213–214, 268, 290–291

NF2   211–212

NF-κB   236, 241

NFIB   142–143

NFIX   297

NFP   216

nipple   6, 13, 25, 32, 35, 37, 43, 52, 54, 60, 63, 75–76, 78, 82, 86, 107, 111, 135, 146, 149, 172–173, 178–185, 188, 202, 206, 211, 213, 215, 217, 219, 250, 253, 255, 257–258

nipple adenoma   13, 54, 179–180, 182–183

NKX2-1   154

NKX3-1   258

NOBOX   296

nodular fasciitis   188, 202–203

Noonan syndrome   215

NOTCH1   142

Nottingham grade   51, 62, 65–66, **86–87,** 103, 105, 120, 122, 129, 147, 156–157

NRAS   132, 137

NREP   295

NRIP1   298

NSE   106, 161, 216

NTN4   297

NTRK1   148

NTRK2   148

NTRK3   141, 146–148, 209

NY-BR-1   262, 265

# O

oncocytic   7, 10, 102, 104, 107–108, 131–132

oncocytic carcinoma   10, 102, 107–108, 132

osseous   41, 134, 136–137, 174, 205

osteoclast-like giant cell   106, 122, 129, 137

OTUD7B   294

ovarian cancer   270–272, 274, 277, 292

overdiagnosis   36, 49, 51, 93, 112–113

# P

p16   173, 214

p21(ras)   213

p40   34, 39, 49

p53   38, 104, 117, 120, 165, 185, 225, 262, 268, 273, 278, 280, 282

p63   14, 24, 31, 34, 39–41, 49–50, 53–54, 57–59, 89, 94, 111–112, 117, 120, 134–135, 137, 143, 150, 154, 160, 175, 180–181, 207, 220, 273

p75   39

p120   117, 129

p120-catenin   70, 72, 115, 117–118

Paget disease   75–76, 78, 107, 111, 178–179, **182–185,** 250, 255–256

PALB2   257, 268–269, 286–287, 292–293

PALB2-associated cancer   286

papillary carcinoma

encapsulated papillary carcinoma   10, 50, 54–55, 57–62, 66–67, 126, 256

invasive papillary carcinoma   49–50, 61, 66

papillary carcinoma   7, 10, 49–51, 53–67, 105, 126, 146, 153, 155, 157, 256, 258

papillary ductal carcinoma in situ (DCIS)   49–51, 54–59, 61, 64, 78

solid papillary carcinoma   7, 10, 49–50, 54, 56–59, 61, 63–67, 105, 153, 155, 157

solid papillary carcinoma in situ   10, 56, 58–59, 63–64

paraneoplastic syndrome   173

PARP1   278

PAS   26, 108, 146

PAX5   239, 241, 244

PAX8   89, 262

PAX9   297

P-cadherin   39, 120, 273

PD1   101, 247

PDE4D   295

PDGF   293

PDGFRB   209

PDL1   101, 247

perforin   247

periductal stromal tumour   164–165, 172, **175–176**

Peutz–Jeghers syndrome (PJS)   252–253, 268, **288–289**

PEX14   294

PGP9.5   161

PHLDA3   294

phyllodes tumour   7, 94, 137, 164–165, 169–170, **172–176,** 189, 202–203, 207, 220, 225–227, 229, 279, 281

PI3K   13, 96, 137, 146, 154, 226, 244, 258, 276, 278

PIDD1   296

PIK3CA   7, 37, 39, 43, 46, 53, 60, 65, 72, 85, 96, 115, 123, 129, 132, 134, 137, 140, 154, 157, 169, 173, 179, 182, 255, 258

PIK3R1   137

PIK3R3   294

PIM1   241

PKD2   223

PLA2G6   298

PLAG1 40

plasmacytoma 234

PLCG1 197, 201

pleomorphic adenoma (PA) 10, **39–42,** 44, 137

podoplanin 196, 198

poly (ADP-ribose) polymerase (PARP) 96, 269, 272, 274, 278, 287

polygenic component of breast cancer susceptibility 268, 292

polygenic risk score (PRS) 293

polymorphous adenocarcinoma (PmA) 10, 151–152

population-based screening 11, 77, 97, 269

PR 27, 29, 44, 50–51, 61–62, 64, 77, 80–81, 84, 86, 88–90, 94–98, 100, 102, 104, 106–109, 114, 117–118, 120, 122, 125–127, 129, 132–133, 137, 139, 141, 144–145, 147–148, 150–152, 158, 161, 185, 205, 207, 229–230, 251, 253, 256, 258–259, 273, 277–278, 281–283, 288, 291

PRC1 297

PRDM1 241

predictive 75, 81, 95, 98, 100–101, 109, 137, 190, 208, 227, 251, 274, 286

pregnancy 32–33, 35–37, 165, 168–169, 193, 233, 242, 244, 271

PRKAR1A 212

PRKD2 223

progesterone 36, 84, 229, 253

progestogen 83

prolactin 26, 36, 242, 253

Proteus syndrome 275

Prussian blue 26

PSA 258

pseudoangiomatous stromal hyperplasia (PASH) 188, 202–204, **228–230,** 254

PSMA 258

PTEN 72, 96, 115, 131–132, 134, 137, 167, 173, 268–269, 275–276, 292

PTPRB 197

puberty 12, 25, 165, 242, 244, 252, 254

Q

quality assurance 88, 90

R

RAB3C 295

RAD17 278

RAD51 269, 271–272, 286

RAD51B 297

RAD51C 268

RAD51D 268–269

radial scar 10, 13, 22, **30–31,** 37, 72, 94, 120, 135

radiation 35, 74, 93, 96, 98, 161, 188–189, 194–201, 208, 258, 277, 281

RALY 298

RANBP9 295

RARA 169, 173

RAS 142, 146, 213, 268, 290

RB1 96, 137, 160, 169, 173, 205, 226, 272

receptor tyrosine kinase (RTK) 197, 209

RECQ 280

RET 65, 154, 209

retroareolar 40, 43, 52, 57–58, 142, 149, 211, 251–252, 255, 257

rhabdomyosarcoma 189, 262–263, 279, 281

RHOA 244

RIN3 297

RNF115 294

ROS1 209–210

RUNX1 115

S

S100 29, 39, 89, 106, 108, 131–132, 140, 143, 147, 185, 202, 205, 209, 212–216, 230, 262

salivary gland–like 89, 94, 140, 150

SBEM See *MUCL1*

schwannoma 188–189, 205, **211–212,** 214, 220

schwannomatosis 211–212

sclerosing adenosis 10, 13, **22–25,** 30, 37, 72, 79, 94, 112, 120, 169–170, 182–183

screening 11, 14–15, 18–19, 43, 71, 75–77, 83, 97, 110, 119, 142, 173, 211, 213, 225, 238, 240, 269, 273, 276, 284, 287, 291

SDH 275

sebaceous 7, 10, 44, 53, 102, 104, 108–109, 143–144

sebaceous carcinoma 7, 10, 102, 104, 108–109

secretory carcinoma 10, 108, 140–141, **146–148**

SEER Program 108, 113, 125, 133, 201, 233, 239–240, 274

sentinel lymph node biopsy 75, 113

SETBP1 297

SETD2 169, 173

SF3B1 142

SH2D1A 242

signet-ring cell 64, 69–70, 72, 79, 95, 116–117, 124, 147, 265, 285

single nucleotide polymorphism (SNP) 71, 292, 294–298

SLC4A7 294

SMA 24, 28, 34, 39–41, 47, 49, 117, 137, 196, 198, 202, 207, 209–210, 217, 219–220

SMARCA4 244

SMARCA5 142

SMARCB1 212

SMC1 278

SMM 23, 31, 50

SMMHC 24, 31, 39–40, 49, 53–54, 76, 94, 120, 137

smoking 84–85, 159, 258

SNAI1 134

SNAI2 134

sonography 35, 37, 114, 123, 128, 173, 193, 229

SOX10 147, 185, 209, 212–214, 262, 265

SOX11 236

spindle cell carcinoma 47, 106, 136–137, 189, 202

squamous cell carcinoma 47, 94, 134–136, 179, 185, 263, 292

STAT3 246–247

STAT6 205

Stewart–Treves syndrome 189, 197

STK11 252, 268, 288, 292

synaptophysin 50, 64, 105, 154–159, 161, 201

syringoma 178–181

syringomatous tumour (SyT) 179–181, 183

T

TAB2 295

tall cell carcinoma with reversed polarity (TCCRP) 7, 10, 49, 54, 147, **153–154**

tamoxifen 21, 75, 99–100

TBX3 115, 297

TCF3 244

TCF7L2 296

TdT 244

TEK 197

terminal duct lobular unit (TDLU) 11, 13, 15–16, 18, 22, 25, 32–33, 68–75, 168, 229, 272

TERT 137, 169, 173, 176, 295

testosterone 252

TET2 295

TFAP2A 295

TFE3 216

TGFBR2 294

thrombosis 192

thyroglobulin 154

TIA1 247

TIE1 197

TNFAIP3 241

Toker cell 179, 184–185

TOX3 297

TP53 46, 72, 85, 96, 115, 129, 132, 134, 137, 140, 143, 160, 169, 173, 190, 226–227, 244, 246, 255, 258, 268, 272–273,

278–281, 292
TP63  247
TR  241
transcriptome  72, 82, 95–96, 119, 121, 123,
    137, 157
TRB  247
TRD  247
TRG  247
TRIM46  294
triple-negative  62, 72, 84–85, 91–92,
    **95–97,** 100–101, 104–105, 108, 110, 129,
    132–134, 137–141, 143–145, 147–148,
    150, 154, 258, 262, 265, 269, 272–274
TRK  147–148
TTF1  89, 159, 161, 262–263, 265
tubular adenoma  10, 26, **32–34,** 36, 44, 279
tubular carcinoma (TC)  10, 15–16, 51, 64,
    87, 94, **119–122,** 143–144, 180, 279
tubulolobular  116, 118, 285
tumour-infiltrating lymphocyte (TIL)  6–7, 77,
    86, 92–93, 100–101, 103–105, 109, 115,
    272, 278
TWIST  134
tyrosine kinase  146, 197, 209

U

ultrasonography  25, 32, 40, 52–53, 63, 76,
    83, 98, 114, 119, 124, 134, 153, 165–166,
    172, 180, 182, 200, 204, 211, 213, 221,
    223, 225, 245, 262, 276
underdiagnosis  113
USP6  203
usual ductal hyperplasia (UDH)  10–15,
    19–20, 30, 40, 49–50, 53–55, 65, 72, 79,
    165, 169, 171, 174, 182–183

V

vascular malformation  191
VEGFR  197, 201
VEGFR3  See *FLT4*
VGLL3  294
vimentin  134, 147, 205, 273

W

WDR43  294
whole-exome sequencing  69, 137, 148, 269
WISP3  See *CCN6*
WNT  137, 173, 206–208, 293
WT1  39, 89, 125

X

XRCC6  298

Z

ZBTB38  295
ZC3H11A  294
ZFPM2  296
ZMIZ1  296
ZNF365  296

# The World Health Organization Classification of Tumours

## Soft tissue and bone
Fletcher CDM, Bridge JA, Hogendoorn PCW, et al., editors. WHO classification of tumours of soft tissue and bone. Lyon (France): International Agency for Research on Cancer; 2013. (WHO classification of tumours series, 4th ed.; vol. 5). https://publications.iarc.fr/15.

## Female reproductive organs
Kurman RJ, Carcangiu ML, Herrington CS, et al., editors. WHO classification of tumours of female reproductive organs. Lyon (France): International Agency for Research on Cancer; 2014. (WHO classification of tumours series, 4th ed.; vol. 6). https://publications.iarc.fr/16.

## Lung, pleura, thymus and heart
Travis WD, Brambilla E, Burke AP, et al., editors. WHO classification of tumours of the lung, pleura, thymus and heart. Lyon (France): International Agency for Research on Cancer; 2015. (WHO classification of tumours series, 4th ed.; vol. 7). https://publications.iarc.fr/17.

## Urinary system and male genital organs
Moch H, Humphrey PA, Ulbright TM, et al., editors. WHO classification of tumours of the urinary system and male genital organs. Lyon (France): International Agency for Research on Cancer; 2016. (WHO classification of tumours series, 4th ed.; vol. 8). https://publications.iarc.fr/540.

## Central nervous system
Louis DN, Ohgaki H, Wiestler OD, et al., editors. WHO classification of tumours of the central nervous system. Lyon (France): International Agency for Research on Cancer; 2016. (WHO classification of tumours series, 4th rev. ed.; vol. 1). https://publications.iarc.fr/543.

## Head and neck
El-Naggar AK, Chan JKC, Grandis JR, et al., editors. WHO classification of head and neck tumours. Lyon (France): International Agency for Research on Cancer; 2017. (WHO classification of tumours series, 4th ed.; vol. 9). https://publications.iarc.fr/548.

## Endocrine organs
Lloyd RV, Osamura RY, Klöppel G, et al., editors. WHO classification of tumours of endocrine organs. Lyon (France): International Agency for Research on Cancer; 2017. (WHO classification of tumours series, 4th ed.; vol. 10). https://publications.iarc.fr/554.

## Haematopoietic and lymphoid tissues
Swerdlow SH, Campo E, Harris NL, et al., editors. WHO classification of tumours of haematopoietic and lymphoid tissues. Lyon (France): International Agency for Research on Cancer; 2017. (WHO classification of tumours series, 4th rev. ed.; vol. 2). https://publications.iarc.fr/556.

## Skin
Elder DE, Massi D, Scolyer RA, et al., editors. WHO classification of skin tumours. Lyon (France): International Agency for Research on Cancer; 2018. (WHO classification of tumours series, 4th ed.; vol. 11). https://publications.iarc.fr/560.

## Eye
Grossniklaus HE, Eberhart CG, Kivelä TT, editors. WHO classification of tumours of the eye. Lyon (France): International Agency for Research on Cancer; 2018. (WHO classification of tumours series, 4th ed.; vol. 12). https://publications.iarc.fr/561.

## Digestive system
WHO Classification of Tumours Editorial Board. Digestive system tumours. Lyon (France): International Agency for Research on Cancer; 2019. (WHO classification of tumours series, 5th ed.; vol. 1). https://publications.iarc.fr/579.

## Breast
WHO Classification of Tumours Editorial Board. Breast tumours. Lyon (France): International Agency for Research on Cancer; 2019. (WHO classification of tumours series, 5th ed.; vol. 2). https://publications.iarc.fr/581.